To our families, friends, teachers, and students

Walsh and Hoyt's
Clinical
Neuro-Ophthalmology:
THE ESSENTIALS
SECOND EDITION

Walsh and Hoyt's
Clinical
Neuro-Ophthalmology:
THE ESSENTIALS

SECOND EDITION

EDITORS

Neil R. Miller, MD
Professor of Ophthalmology, Neurology,
   and Neurosurgery
Frank B. Walsh Professor of Neuro-Ophthalmology
Director, Neuro-Ophthalmology and Orbit Units
Wilmer Eye Institute
Johns Hopkins Hospital
Baltimore, Maryland

Nancy J. Newman, MD
LeoDelle Jolley Professor of Ophthalmology
Professor of Ophthalmology and Neurology
Instructor in Neurological Surgery
Director, Neuro-Ophthalmology Unit
Emory University School of Medicine
Atlanta, Georgia
Lecturer in Ophthalmology
Harvard Medical School
Boston, Massachusetts

Valérie Biousse, MD
Cyrus H. Stoner Professor of Ophthalmology
Associate Professor of Ophthalmology
   and Neurology
Emory University School of Medicine
Atlanta, Georgia

John B. Kerrison, MD
Charleston Neuroscience Institute
Division of Retina and Neuro-Ophthalmology
Charleston, South Carolina

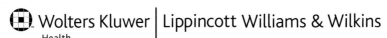

Wolters Kluwer | Lippincott Williams & Wilkins
Health

Philadelphia · Baltimore · New York · London
Buenos Aires · Hong Kong · Sydney · Tokyo

Acquisitions Editor: Jonathan W. Pine, Jr.
Developmental Editor: Anne E. Jacobs
Project Manager: Jennifer Harper
Senior Manufacturing Manager: Benjamin Rivera
Associate Director of Marketing: Adam Glazer
Associate Marketing Manager: Lisa Parry
Design Coordinator: Steve Druding
Production Services: Aptara, Inc.

Library of Congress Cataloging-in-Publication Data

Walsh and Hoyt's clinical neuro-ophthalmology : the essentials / [edited by]
Neil R. Miller . . . [et al.].—2nd ed.
   p. ; cm.
Includes index.
Rev. ed. of: The essentials: Walsh and Hoyt's clinical neuro-ophthalmology, 5th edition. 1999.
Condensed clinical information found in the 1st volume of: Walsh and Hoyt's clinical
neuro-ophthalmology, 6th ed.
   ISBN-13: 978-0-7817-6379-0
   ISBN-10: 0-7817-6379-7
   1. Neuroophthalmology.   I. Walsh, Frank Burton.   II. Hoyt, William Fletcher.
III. Miller, Neil R.   IV. Essentials.   V. Title: Clinical neuro-ophthalmology.
   [DNLM: 1. Eye Diseases.   2. Neurologic Manifestations.   WW 140 W2235 2008]
   RE725.E86 2008
   617.7′—dc22

                                                                                    2007031529

Care has been taken to confirm the accuracy of the information presented and to describe generally accepted practices. However, the authors, editors, and publisher are not responsible for errors or omissions or for any consequences from application of the information in this book and make no warranty, expressed or implied, with respect to the currency, completeness, or accuracy of the contents of the publication. Application of this information in a particular situation remains the professional responsibility of the practitioner; the clinical treatments described and recommended may not be considered absolute and universal recommendations.

The authors, editors, and publisher have exerted every effort to ensure that drug selection and dosage set forth in this text are in accordance with current recommendations and practice at the time of publication. However, in view of ongoing research, changes in government regulations, and the constant flow of information relating to drug therapy and drug reactions, the reader is urged to check the package insert for each drug for any change in indications and dosage and for added warnings and precautions. This is particularly important when the recommended agent is a new or infrequently employed drug.

Some drugs and medical devices presented in this publication have Food and Drug Administration (FDA) clearance for limited use in restricted research settings. It is the responsibility of health care providers to ascertain the FDA status of each drug or device planned for use in their clinical practice.

The publishers have made every effort to trace copyright holders for borrowed material. If they have inadvertently overlooked any, they will be pleased to make the necessary arrangements at the first opportunity.

To purchase additional copies of this book, call our customer service department at (800) 638-3030 or fax orders to 1-301-223-2400. Lippincott Williams & Wilkins customer service representatives are available from 8:30 am to 6:00 pm, EST, Monday through Friday, for telephone access. Visit Lippincott Williams & Wilkins on the Internet: http://www.lww.com.

10 9 8 7 6 5 4 3 2 1

After the 5th edition of *Walsh and Hoyt's Clinical Neuro-Ophthalmology* was published in 1998, we recognized that not every practitioner required such an in-depth exposure to neuro-ophthalmology, especially as regards the detailed referencing. Indeed, we believed there was a need to distill the material found primarily in the first volume of the 5th edition down to the basics of neuro-ophthalmic disease, to "just the essentials." Two of us (NRM, NJN) therefore put together the first edition of *Walsh and Hoyt's Clinical Neuro-Ophthalmology: The Essentials*, which consisted of a single text, divided into five sections: the afferent visual system, the pupil, the efferent (ocular motor) system, the eyelid, and non-organic disorders. The various portions of the five volumes of the 5th edition pertinent to a particular chapter in *The Essentials* were referenced at the end of each chapter.

The 6th edition of Walsh and Hoyt's Clinical Neuro-Ophthalmology was published in 2005. Although it is a svelte 3500 pages (down from 6000 pages in the 5th edition), it nevertheless continues to provide more information than many physicians and students want or need for their practice or learning. Accordingly, we have provided this second edition of "*The Essentials*." As in the last edition, this edition contains what we believe to be the most important aspects of the diagnosis and management of neuro-ophthalmologic disorders. Once again, there are five main sections containing a total of 23 chapters adapted from those written by contributors to the 6th edition. To help readers peruse the chapters for content, there is a summary of major and minor headings at the beginning of each chapter. Also, as in the first edition of this text, there are no references in the chapters; however, the reference to those portions of the 6th edition from which the chapter has been adapted can be found on the first chapter page to assist the reader who wishes to obtain more information (including references) from that edition.

We sincerely hope that those who use this second edition of *Walsh and Hoyt's Clinical Neuro-Ophthalmology: The Essentials* find it convenient and useful.

Neil R. Miller, MD
Nancy J. Newman, MD
Valérie Biousse, MD
John B. Kerrison, MD

ACKNOWLEDGMENTS

We wish to thank the Wolters Kluwer/Lippincott Williams & Wilkins team for making this second edition happen. In particular, Jonathan W. Pine, Jr., our Senior Executive Editor, and Anne E. Jacobs, our Senior Managing Editor, fought for us every step of the way and dedicated themselves to seeing it through to completion. We also wish to thank Adam Glazer, our Associate Marketing Director, Jennifer Harper, our Project Manager, and Stephen Druding, our Design Coordinator. Without them, this book would most certainly have not seen the light of day. Finally, we thank all the contributors to the 6th edition of Walsh and Hoyt's Clinical Neuro-Ophthalmology, particularly those whose chapters have been adapted for this book.

Madhu R. Agarwal, MD
Assistant Professor of Ophthalmology
Division of Neuro-Ophthalmology and Orbital
   Surgery
Loma Linda University Medical Center
Loma Linda, California
Clinical Instructor of Ophthalmology
Doheny Eye Institute
University of Southern California Keck School
   of Medicine
Los Angeles, California

Anthony C. Arnold, MD
Professor and Chief
Neuro-Ophthalmology Division
Jules Stein Eye Institute
Department of Ophthalmology
University of California-Los Angeles
Los Angeles, California

Laura J. Balcer, MD, MSCE
Associate Professor of Neurology and
   Ophthalmology
University of Pennsylvania
Neuro-Ophthalmologist
Hospital of the University of Pennsylvania
Scheie Eye Institute
Philadelphia, Pennsylvania

Jason J. S. Barton, MD, PhD, FRCP(C)
Associate Professor of Neurology
Harvard Medical School
Adjunct Professor of Bioengineering
Boston University
Director of Neuro-Ophthalmology
Beth Israel Deaconess Medical Center
Boston, Massachusetts

Ghassan K. Bejjani, MD
Clinical Assistant Professor of Neurosurgery
University of Pittsburgh School of Medicine
Pittsburgh, Pennsylvania

Valérie Biousse, MD
Cyrus H. Stoner Professor of Ophthalmology
Associate Professor of Ophthalmology and
   Neurology
Emory University School of Medicine
Atlanta, Georgia

Mark S. Borchert, MD
Associate Professor of Ophthalmology and
   Neurology
University of Southern California Keck School
   of Medicine
Division Head
Department of Ophthalmology
Childrens Hospital of Los Angeles
Los Angeles, California

Michael C. Brodsky, MD
Professor of Ophthalmology and Pediatrics
University of Arkansas for Medical Sciences
Chief of Pediatric Ophthalmology
Arkansas Childrens Hospital
Little Rock, Arkansas

Preston C. Calvert, MD
Assistant Professor of Neurology
Johns Hopkins University School of Medicine
Baltimore, Maryland
Attending Physician in Neurology
Fairfax Hospital
Fairfax, Virginia

Kimberley P. Cockerham, MD
Associate Professor of Ophthalmology
University of California-San Francisco
San Francisco, California

Kathleen B. Digre, MD
Professor of Neurology and Ophthalmology
Moran Eye Center
University of Utah
Departments of Neurology and Ophthalmology
University of Utah Hospital
Salt Lake City, Utah

Deborah I. Friedman, MD
Associate Professor of Ophthalmology and
   Neurology
University of Rochester
Rochester, New York

Steven L. Galetta, MD
Van Meter Professor of Neurology
Professor of Neurology and Ophthalmology
University of Pennsylvania Medical Center
Chief, Division of Neuro-Ophthalmology
Philadelphia, Pennsylvania

Robert A. Goldberg, MD
Professor of Ophthalmology
Chief, Orbital and Ophthalmic Plastic
    Surgeon Division
Jules Stein Eye Institute
University of California-Los Angeles
Los Angeles, California

Steven R. Hamilton, MD
Clinical Associate Professor of Ophthalmology
    and Neurology
University of Washington
Neuro-Ophthalmic Consultants Northwest
Seattle, Washington

Thomas R. Hedges III, MD
Professor of Ophthalmology and Neurology
Tufts University
Director of Neuro-Ophthalmology
Tufts New England Medical Center
Boston, Massachusetts

Paul N. Hoffman, MD, PhD
Research Associate of Ophthalmology and Neurology
Wilmer Ophthalmological Institute
The Johns Hopkins School of Medicine
Baltimore, Maryland

Chris A. Johnson, PhD
Director of Diagnostic Research in Ophthalmology
Devers Eye Institute
Legacy Health Systems
Portland, Oregon

Barrett Katz, MD, MBA
Clinical Professor of Ophthalmology
The Weill Medical College of Cornell University
New York-Presbyterian Hospital
New York, New York
Chief Medical Officer
Fovea Pharmaceuticals, SA
Paris, France

Aki Kawasaki, MD, MER
Mantre d'Enseignement et de Recherche
    of Ophthalmology
University of Lausanne
Medécin Associée in Neuro-Ophthalmology
Hopital Ophtalmique Jules Gonin
Lausanne, Switzerland

John S. Kennerdell, MD
Professor of Ophthalmology
Drexel University College of Medicine
Philadelphia, Pennsylvania
Chairman of Ophthalmology
Allegheny General Hospital
Pittsburgh, Pennsylvania

John B. Kerrison, MD
Charleston Neuroscience Institute
Division of Retina and Neuro-Ophthalmology
Charleston, South Carolina

R. John Leigh, MD
Blair-Daroff Professor of Neurology
Case Western Reserve University
Staff Neurologist
Louis Stokes Veterans Affairs Medical Center
Cleveland, Ohio

Leonard A. Levin, MD, PhD
Associate Professor of Ophthalmology and Visual
    Sciences, Neurology, and Neurological Surgery
University of Wisconsin
Madison, Wisconsin

Joseph C. Maroon, MD
Professor of Neurosurgery
Heindl Scholar
Tristate Neurosurgical Associates
University of Pittsburgh Medical Center
Pittsburgh, Pennsylvania

Neil R. Miller, MD
Professor of Ophthalmology, Neurology, and
    Neurosurgery
Frank B. Walsh Professor of Neuro-Ophthalmology
Director, Neuro-Ophthalmology and Orbit
    Units
Wilmer Eye Institute
Johns Hopkins Hospital
Baltimore, Maryland

Nancy J. Newman, MD
LeoDelle Jolley Professor of Ophthalmology
Professor of Ophthalmology and Neurology
Instructor in Neurological Surgery
Director, Neuro-Ophthalmology Unit
Emory University School of Medicine
Atlanta, Georgia
Lecturer in Ophthalmology
Harvard Medical School
Boston, Massachusetts

David E. Newman-Toker, MD
Assistant Professor of Neurology and
    Ophthalmology
The Johns Hopkins University School of
    Medicine
Active Staff in Neurology
Johns Hopkins Hospital
Baltimore, Maryland

Paul H. Phillips, MD
Associate Professor of Ophthalmology
University of Arkansas for Medical Sciences
Department of Ophthalmology
Arkansas Childrens Hospital
Little Rock, Arkansas

Valerie Purvin, MD
Clinical Professor of Ophthalmology and Neurology
Indiana University Medical Center
Chief, Neuro-Ophthalmology Service
Midwest Eye Institute
Methodist Hospital
Indianapolis, Indiana

Michael X. Repka, MD
Professor of Ophthalmology and Pediatrics
The Johns Hopkins School of Medicine
Department of Ophthalmology
The Johns Hopkins Hospital
Baltimore, Maryland

Joseph F. Rizzo III, MD
Associate Professor of Ophthalmology
The Massachusetts Eye and Ear Infirmary
Harvard Medical School
Director, Center for Innovative Visual Rehabilitation
Boston Veterans Administration Hospital
Boston, Massachusetts

Matthew Rizzo, MD
Professor of Neurology, Engineering,
    and Public Policy
Director, Division of Neuroergonomics
Carver College of Medicine
University of Iowa
Iowa City, Iowa

Janet C. Rucker, MD
Assistant Professor of Neurology
Case Western Reserve University
Staff Neurologist
University Hospitals
Cleveland, Ohio

Alfredo A. Sadun, MD, PhD
Thornton Chair
Professor of Ophthalmology and Neurological
    Surgery
Doheny Eye Institute
University of Southern California Keck School
    of Medicine
Los Angeles, California

Jane C. Sargent, MD
Professor of Clinical Neurology and Clinical
    Surgery
University of Massachusetts Medical School
Department of Neurology
University of Massachusetts Memorial Medical
    Center
Worcester, Massachusetts

Barry Skarf, MD, PhD
Adjunct Associate Professor of Ophthalmology
University of Toronto
Toronto, Ontario, Canada
Director of Neuro-ophthalmology service
Henry Ford Hospital
Detroit, Michigan

Craig H. Smith, MD
Clinical Professor of Neurology, Medicine,
    and Ophthalmology
University of Washington
President, MS Hub Medical Group
Seattle, Washington

Kenneth David Steinsapir, MD
Assistant Clinical Professor of Ophthalmology
Jules Stein Eye Institute
David Geffen School of Medicine at the University of
    California-Los Angeles
Los Angeles, California

Nicholas J. Volpe, MD
Adele Niessen Associate Professor of Ophthalmology
    and Neurology
University of Pennsylvania School of Medicine
Vice Chairman, Residency Program Director
Scheie Eye Institute
Philadelphia, Pennsylvania

Michael Wall, MD
Professor of Neurology and Ophthalmology
University of Iowa College of Medicine
Veterans Administration Hospital
Iowa City, Iowa

David S. Zee, MD
Professor of Neurology and Ophthalmology
The Johns Hopkins University School of
    Medicine
Baltimore, Maryland

CONTENTS

SECTION I

THE AFFERENT VISUAL SYSTEM

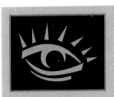

CHAPTER 1

Examination of the Visual Sensory System *

Despite continuous advances in neurodiagnostic imaging and other new techniques, the examination of the afferent visual sensory system is still the core of the neuro-ophthalmologic examination. This chapter describes the most common subjective and objective testing parameters used in the afferent visual system examination. In addition, it discusses recent developments in perimetry, clinical psychophysics, and electrophysiology.

Evaluation of the afferent system begins with a thorough medical history, followed by an ophthalmologic examination (refraction, slit lamp examination, funduscopy, assessment of pupillary function, etc.), evaluation of selected psychophysical visual functions (acuity, stereoacuity, color vision, visual fields, contrast sensitivity, etc.) and relevant ancillary test procedures. After the examiner has performed these functions, providing a diagnosis, or at least a differential diagnosis, for the

etiology of an afferent visual system deficit should be possible.

HISTORY

An examination of patients experiencing dysfunction of the afferent visual system begins with a careful history about the details of the visual loss. A thorough history is one of the most important parts of the examination, because it determines the initial strategy for differential diagnostic evaluation. It is essential to establish if the visual loss is monocular or binocular; if its location is central, peripheral, altitudinal, or hemianopic, and if the onset of the loss is gradual, sudden, or intermittent.

It is also important to ask about photopsias (visual phenomena such as flashing black squares, flashes of lights, or showers of sparks) distortions in vision (metamorphopsia or micropsia), and positive scotomas. A positive scotoma is one that is seen by the patient, like the purple spot that is often seen after a flash bulb goes off, whereas a negative scotoma refers to a nonseeing area of the visual field. Metamorphopsia, micropsia, and positive scotomas often occur in patients with maculopathies, whereas photopsias may be

---

*Adapted from: Wall M, Johnson CA. Principles and techniques of the examination of the visual sensory system. In: Miller NR, Newman NJ, Biousse V, Kerrison JB, eds. *Walsh & Hoyt's Clinical Neuro-Ophthalmology.* 6th ed. Vol. I. Philadelphia: Lippincott Williams & Wilkins; 2005:83–149.

present in patients with retinal disease, optic nerve dysfunction, or cerebral dysfunction from migraine and other disorders.

CLINICAL OFFICE EXAMINATION

Clinical evaluation of the afferent visual system for each eye incorporates the items in Table 1.1, which can be performed in the office. The first goal for the neuro-ophthalmology examination is to determine if the visual loss is caused by a disorder anterior to the retina (ocular media), in the retina, in the optic nerve, in the optic chiasm, in the retrochiasmal pathways, or is nonorganic (i.e., hysteria or malingering). The second goal is to establish a differential and working diagnosis. By examining various parameters of afferent visual

Table 1.1. *Components of the Clinical Neuro-Ophthalmologic Examination*

I. REFRACTION
    Retinoscopy
    Keratometry
    Manifest refraction
    Cycloplegic refraction
II. VISUAL FUNCTION
    Visual acuity (distance and near)
    Stereoacuity
    Color vision, color comparison
    Brightness comparison
    Photostress test
    Pulfrich phenomenon
    Visual fields
    Confrontation fields
    Amsler grid
    Tangent screen
    Manual kinetic perimetry (Goldmann Perimeter)
    Automated static perimetry
III. PUPILS
    Size
    Direct and consensual response
    Accommodation response
    Afferent pupillary defect
IV. CRANIAL NERVES I, III, IV, V, VI, VII, VIII
V. EXOPHTHALMOMETRY
VI. EXTERNAL AND ANTERIOR SEGMENT
    External examination
    Slit lamp examination
    Applanation tonometry
VII. FUNDUS
    Optic nerve head and nerve fiber layer
    Macula and retinal vessels
    Peripheral retina

function, the examiner can frequently make a determination as to the anatomic site of the afferent system abnormality and the most probable cause or causes.

REFRACTION AND VISUAL ACUITY

A thorough refraction is an essential part of all clinical neuro-ophthalmologic examinations. Identification of a previously undetermined refractive error, corneal pathology, or a subtle lens problem can prevent initiation of an expensive and time-consuming evaluation. It is essential to have the best refraction possible when measuring visual acuity to distinguish whether visual acuity loss is caused by optical factors or damage to neural elements in the visual system. Refractive problems cannot only cause loss of visual acuity but may also produce symptoms such as monocular diplopia. A cycloplegic refraction is important, not only to obtain the correct refraction, but also to observe the red reflex through the retinoscope as a means of identifying corneal irregularities and lens opacities that may not be as apparent with a slit lamp examination. Visual acuity measurements obtained with the patient viewing through a pinhole can also help identify problems with the optics of the eye. In many instances, it is useful to dilate the patient in conjunction with the use of a pinhole to maximize the likelihood of finding a clear pinhole region around an opacity. Improvement of visual acuity with the use of a pinhole indicates that the cause of the visual loss is optical in nature. The Potential Acuity Meter (PAM), which utilizes the pinhole principle, can be helpful. Keratoconus and surface irregularities of the cornea can be diagnosed by improvement in visual acuity with the use of a hard contact lens. A Placido's disk, keratometry readings, or corneal topography maps can also help to identify corneal surface irregularities and associated problems.

Subtle central vision loss can often be identified by the use of low contrast visual acuity charts or contrast sensitivity measurements. In addition, low luminance visual acuity can be compared with similar measures made under standard lighting conditions. For example, placing a 2.0 log unit neutral density filter before the eye (i.e., producing a 100-fold reduction in the luminance of the visual acuity chart) causes a normal eye to be reduced from 20/20 to 20/40 visual acuity (a factor of 2 or 0.3 logMAR). Patients with optic nerve conduction abnormalities, such as optic neuritis or multiple sclerosis with optic atrophy, have a disproportionately greater reduction in visual acuity (e.g., from 20/30 down to 20/200) when the neutral density filter is placed before the affected eye. Other anomalies such as amblyopia do not demonstrate this disproportionate drop in visual acuity with the neutral density filter.

Measuring visual acuity in children requires skill, patience, and an enthusiastic attitude. By creating a friendly, relaxed environment for the child in which vision testing is presented as a game, the chances of success will be greater. A system of positive rewards, ranging from a verbal "Hooray!" or "That's Terrific!" to the use of mechanical animal toys and projected cartoons, is essential. A video demonstration of many techniques for evaluating children and infants is available from the American Academy of Ophthalmology.

During any neuro-ophthalmologic examination, it is essential to measure not only distance visual acuity but also near visual acuity. In some instances (e.g., an in-hospital consultation on a patient who is unable to come to the examination room), near visual acuity is the only measurement that is possible. Near visual acuity measurements can be performed with any of the standard near acuity cards, which are held at 13 to 14 inches from the eyes with the patient wearing an appropriate near refractive correction. In patients with normal visual function, there is little or no difference between distance and near visual acuity. A discrepancy between near and distance visual acuity suggests several possible etiologies. Patients with cataracts often perform better on near acuity than distance acuity. Young patients with head trauma may complain of reading problems from loss of accommodation, resulting in poorer near acuity than distance acuity. Patients with nonorganic loss of vision may not understand the relationship between near and distance acuity and may provide inconsistent responses with the two measurements. One must be careful, however, to ensure that optical factors (e.g., cataract, accommodation loss) are not responsible for the differences.

STEREOACUITY

Stereoacuity requires good visual acuity in both eyes and normal cortical development. As such, stereoacuity can be helpful in establishing if a patient has visual loss from congenital amblyopia or monofixation syndrome, as well as verifying the extent of any monocular visual acuity loss. Using the Titmus Stereo Tester, stereoacuity in normal observers with good binocular function and visual acuity should be 40 seconds of arc or better when both eyes have 20/20 visual acuity. If plus lenses are placed before one eye, stereoacuity is reduced to 60 seconds of arc when the eye is blurred to 20/40 and 100 seconds of arc when the eye is blurred to 20/100. Although this correlation does not hold for all clinical conditions, it provides a useful reference for cross-checking mild losses of monocular visual acuity, especially when nonorganic visual loss is suspected (see Chapter 23).

COLOR VISION AND BRIGHTNESS COMPARISON

Color vision testing, using pseudoisochromatic plates, the Farnsworth 100 Hue and D-15 tests, or the Lanthony 15 Desaturated D-15 panel can be helpful in detecting subtle signs of optic neuropathy or macular disease. **Acquired** color vision loss usually does not respect color vision axes. On the other hand, **congenital** loss respects these axes, with red/green deficits occurring in approximately 8% of the male population and in 0.4% of females. Congenital blue/yellow deficits are much less common, occurring in 0.005% of the population. Nevertheless, both types of congenital color vision deficits need to be distinguished from acquired color vision loss. A comparison of color vision between the two eyes can be helpful, because both the type and severity of congenital color vision deficits are the same for each eye, a situation that is often not true for acquired color vision loss. In addition, congenital color vision deficits are stable over time and are almost always red/green deficits.

A comparison of the saturation of colors, between eyes and across the vertical midline, can sometimes identify subtle optic nerve dysfunction or chiasmal lesions. The same is true for brightness comparisons between the two eyes and across the vertical midline. Although such tests can be used to corroborate other evidence of optic neuropathy, subjective brightness differences between the two eyes as an isolated finding with an otherwise normal examination is often of no significance.

VISUAL FIELD EXAMINATION

Examination of the visual field is one of the fundamental portions of the afferent system evaluation. A variety of visual field test procedures can be employed, including confrontation fields, the Amsler grid, the tangent (Bjerrum) screen, manual kinetic testing using a Goldmann perimeter, and automated static perimetry. When evaluating a patient with an afferent system deficit, it is important to keep in mind the advantages and disadvantages of the various procedures.

Confrontation visual fields should be part of every afferent system examination. Although testing by confrontation may lack the sophistication of modern techniques, it is the most flexible form of visual field testing, can be performed almost anywhere, and may be the only form of visual field testing that is possible. In skilled hands, confrontation testing can provide information equivalent to that obtained with more extensive forms of visual field testing, although only one third of optic nerve-related defects are detected by this method.

The **Amsler grid** can be useful in identifying patients with retinal pathology. Amsler grid testing is performed at 30 cm, where each 5-mm square subtends 1 degree of visual angle (total extent is 20 degrees in diameter, or 10 degrees in radius). The patient is shown the Amsler grid with and is told to look at the center spot and report if there is absence or distortion of

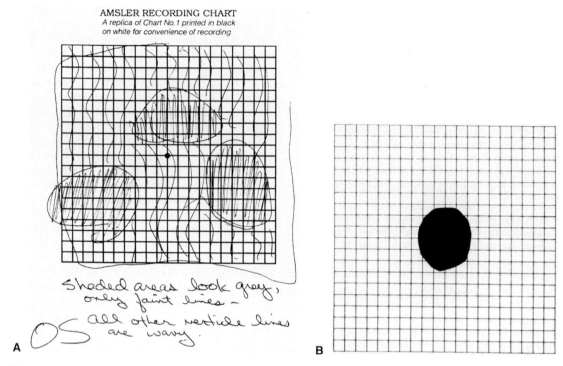

Figure 1.1. Amsler grid defects. **A:** Metamorphopsia and paracentral scotomas in a patient with a maculopathy. **B:** A small central scotoma in a patient with optic neuritis.

the central fixation spot, if any portions of the Amsler grid are missing, and if any of the lines are wavy or bent (metamorphopsia). This type of image distortion is usually indicative of macular disease (Fig. 1.1A), whereas inability to see the central fixation point may indicate a central scotoma (Fig. 1.1B).

Tangent screen testing permits evaluation of the central 30-degree radius of the visual field. A 1-meter tangent screen can be placed on the wall of an examining room for easy use. It can provide more detailed, quantitative visual field information than that afforded by confrontation field testing. In the hands of a skilled perimetrist, the tangent screen examination may provide information that is equal to or better than that obtained with automated perimetric test procedures.

Sophisticated, quantitative evaluations can be achieved with **kinetic perimetry** on the Goldmann perimeter, which provides flexibility through close interaction between the patient and the perimetrist to obtain the most accurate responses from the patient. In children, the elderly, or patients with dementia, this may be the only form of quantitative visual field test that can be performed. The Goldmann perimeter also makes it possible to evaluate efficiently the far peripheral visual field beyond a radius of 30 degrees. In some instances, this information can be useful in determining the extent of visual field loss and in establishing a differential diagnosis. The major disadvantages of this form of perimetry include the lack of standards and normative values and the high dependence on the skills of the perimetrist.

Automated perimetry is the most popular form of visual field testing. The major advantages of automated perimetry include standardized test procedures, age-related normal population values, and statistical analysis procedures for evaluating the data. Its major disadvantages include long testing times, high variability in areas of visual loss, inflexibility, and learning and fatigue effects.

PHOTO STRESS TEST

The differentiation between unilateral retinal disease and retrobulbar optic neuropathy may be aided using the **photo stress recovery test.** This test is based on the principle that visual pigments bleach when exposed to an intense light source, resulting in a transient state of sensitivity loss and reduced central visual acuity. Recovery of retinal sensitivity is dependent upon regeneration of visual pigments, which is determined by the anatomic and physiologic apposition of the photoreceptors and retinal pigment epithelium. It is independent of neural mechanisms. Diseases that produce visual loss by damaging the photoreceptors or the adjacent retinal pigment epithelium cause a lag in regeneration of pigment, resulting in a delay in visual recovery following light stress.

The photo stress test is performed by determining best-corrected visual acuity, shielding one eye, and then asking the patient to look directly at a bright focal light held 2 to 3 cm from the eye for about 10 seconds. The time needed to return to within one line of best-corrected visual acuity level is called the photo stress recovery time (PSRT). The PSRT in normal eyes averages 27 seconds with a standard deviation of 11 seconds. Ninety-nine percent of normal eyes have a PSRT of 50 seconds or less. In eyes with macular disease, PSRT is likely to be significantly prolonged, even when the retina appears to be relatively normal, whereas the PSRT is relatively normal in eyes with optic neuropathies. The photo stress test is especially useful in the differential diagnosis of subtle macular disease from subtle optic neuropathies.

PULFRICH PHENOMENON

When a small target oscillating in a frontal plane is viewed binocularly with one eye covered with a filter to reduce light intensity, the target appears to move in an elliptic path, rather than a to-and-fro path—the **Pulfrich phenomenon.** When the filter is placed over the right eye, the rotation appears counterclockwise; if it is placed over the left eye, the rotation appears clockwise. The explanation for this stereo phenomenon is that the covered eye is more weakly stimulated than the uncovered eye, resulting in a delay in the transmission of visual signals to the striate cortex. This disparity in latency between eyes results in a difference in the apparent position of the target in the two eyes, thereby producing a retinal disparity cue underlying the stereoscopic effect.

Because optic nerve damage results in delayed transmission of impulses to the occipital cortex, patients with unilateral or markedly asymmetric optic neuropathy sometimes observe the Pulfrich phenomenon under natural viewing conditions without a filter in front of one eye. This can present difficulties for the patient driving an automobile, mobility over uneven terrain, or with recreational activities such as tennis and baseball. The Pulfrich phenomenon has a similar clinical implication as a relative afferent pupillary defect.

PUPILLARY EXAMINATION

Examination of the pupils is an essential part of the afferent system evaluation. Pupil size for each eye should be noted, as should the magnitude and latency of the direct and consensual responses to light and near stimulation. The presence of a relative afferent pupil defect

(RAPD) is the hallmark of a unilateral afferent sensory abnormality or bilateral asymmetric visual loss. The etiology is usually an optic neuropathy, but other abnormalities such as a central retinal artery occlusion, retinal detachment, or a large macular scar may be responsible (see Chapter 2). In the case of a retrobulbar optic neuropathy with a relatively normal-appearing fundus examination, **the RAPD may be the only objective sign of anterior visual pathway dysfunction.** Cataracts, refractive errors, and nonorganic visual loss do not cause a RAPD. A patient with a dense strabismic or anisometropic amblyopia (visual acuity of 20/200 or worse) may demonstrate a small RAPD. The RAPD can be quantified by placing graded neutral density filters over the normal or lesser affected eye until the RAPD can no longer be appreciated.

CRANIAL NERVES, EXOPHTHALMOMETRY, EXTERNAL EXAMINATION, AND ANTERIOR SEGMENT EXAMINATION

Cranial nerves I, III, IV, V, VI, VII, and VIII should be tested as part of the afferent visual system examination, because lesions in the orbit, cavernous sinus, suprasellar cistern, and brainstem may directly or indirectly produce afferent system dysfunction. Exophthalmometry is essential for someone who may have an orbital mass or thyroid orbitopathy causing visual loss. External examination of the eye and anterior segment evaluation may suggest various causes of afferent visual loss, such as a carotid-cavernous sinus fistula or thyroid eye disease. A slit lamp examination will establish whether or not corneal or anterior segment problems are the cause of the visual loss. It may also demonstrate iris abnormalities, such as transillumination defects characteristic of albinism or Lisch nodules seen in neurofibromatosis type 1. Applanation tonometry should also be performed. This test not only will establish the intraocular pressure (IOP) but also will detect a significant asymmetry of IOP between the two eyes, such as occurs in patients with unilateral severe carotid artery stenosis or carotid-cavernous sinus fistula.

FUNDUS EXAMINATION

A fundus examination is essential for evaluating the macula, retina, nerve fiber layer, and optic nerve. This can be performed by several methods, including direct ophthalmoscopy and indirect ophthalmoscopy with a 20-diopter handheld lens. Examination of the macula with a 78- or 90-diopter handheld lens or a corneal contact lens viewed through a slit lamp may identify the cause of visual loss as being from retinal dysfunction rather than neuro-ophthalmologic disease.

Performing a fundus examination on infants and young children can be a challenge. It is best to leave the room after performing the afferent system and motility evaluations, allowing a nurse or technician to administer dilating drops to preserve your rapport with the child. In the case of infants, it is best to ask the parents to withhold a feeding bottle until you return to the room. Most infants will readily accept a bottle at this point and will be cooperative during a cycloplegic refraction and dilated fundus examination. The soporific effect of the cycloplegic drops may also cause them to fall asleep.

After completing the cycloplegic refraction, the physician should perform a dilated fundus examination using both a handheld direct ophthalmoscope and a 20-diopter lens in conjunction with an indirect ophthalmoscope, using a low level of illumination for both assessments. A lid speculum is not necessary for most pediatric neuro-ophthalmologic examinations, because the macula and optic disc are the primary areas of interest. If a child becomes uncooperative, it may be necessary for the parents to hold the child in a "lock-down" position (one parent holding the arms outstretched over the ears with the other parent holding the feet) to complete the examination. This is a stressful and difficult situation for all concerned, and all rapport with the child is gone when this occurs. If it is not possible to perform an adequate dilated examination of the infant or child, it may be necessary to conduct an evaluation with light sedation.

OTHER PROCEDURES

Other tests beyond a conventional office examination may be needed to establish the site of the pathology in the afferent visual system. Fluorescein angiography and indocyanine green angiography (ICG) may be necessary to identify retinal pathology. An electroretinogram (ERG), focal or maculoscope ERG, pattern ERG (PERG), dark adaptation, visual-evoked potential (VEP), multifocal ERG, multifocal VEP, or a combination of these tests may be needed to establish the locus of the afferent system disorder. Finally, neuroimaging with magnetic resonance imaging or computed tomographic scanning may be needed to establish the anatomic site of the afferent system abnormality.

PSYCHOPHYSICAL TESTS

Light represents a very small portion of the electromagnetic spectrum (wavelengths between 400 and 700 nm), is emitted by natural and artificial sources, and is reflected by objects in the environment, thereby serving as the stimulus for vision. Light entering the eye is first refracted by the tear film, cornea, and lens to form an inverted image on the retina. Photoreceptors convert this light energy into electric signals that are subsequently processed by neural elements in the retina, optic nerve, and higher visual centers of the brain. The relationship between the physical properties of light and perceptual and behavioral responses is known as **visual psychophysics,** which serves as the foundation for the clinical assessment of visual function.

Because subpopulations of neural elements have distinct response characteristics to particular visual attributes (see Chapters 2 and 12), it is possible to design psychophysical tests that isolate (or at least are dominated by) the activity of specific visual mechanisms. These psychophysical tests can thus serve as probes to evaluate different neural populations throughout the visual pathways. Early detection of eye disease, differential diagnosis of various ocular and neurologic disorders, and monitoring the efficacy of therapeutic regimens are just a few of the purposes that psychophysical tests can subserve in a clinical setting. This section provides a brief overview of some of the more common psychophysical test procedures that can be used in the clinical evaluation of patients.

VISUAL ACUITY

The most common measurement of visual function in a clinical setting is visual acuity. It is the primary method of assessing the integrity of the optics of the eye and the neural mechanisms subserving the fovea. Visual acuity is used to monitor central visual function in patients, is an essential part of clinical refraction procedures, and is important to the patient for reading, face recognition, and other tasks involving fine visual detail. Visual acuity is specified in terms of the visual angle subtended by the finest spatial detail that can be identified by the observer. The physical size of an object and its distance from the observer determines its visual angle.

There are three basic types of visual acuity measurements: detection acuity, resolution acuity, and identification acuity. Detection acuity is the smallest stimulus object or pattern of elements (the minimum angle of detection) that can be distinguished from a uniform field and it is primarily limited by stimulus contrast. The optics of the eye are the main factors limiting detection acuity for normal human foveal vision, producing an attenuation of contrast for small stimuli imaged on the retina. Resolution acuity is the smallest spatial detail that can be discriminated to permit one stimulus pattern to be distinguished from another (e.g., distinguishing horizontal from vertical stripes), and it is usually measured by grating patterns of alternating light and dark lines of varying widths. Resolution acuity also is limited by contrast.

Identification acuity, the measure used for clinical purposes, is the smallest spatial detail that can be

Table 1.2. *Visual Acuity Notation Systems*

Distance (Feet)	Snellen	Distance (Meters)	Metric	Mar (Minutes)	LogMAR	Cycles/Degree
10	20/10	3.0	6/3	0.50	−0.3	60.0
12	20/12	3.6	6/3.8	0.60	−0.2	50.0
16	20/16	4.8	6/4.8	0.80	−0.1	38.0
20	20/20	6.0	6/6	1.00	0.0	30.0
25	20/25	7.5	6/7.5	1.25	0.1	24.0
30	20/30	9.0	6/9	1.50	0.2	20.0
40	20/40	12.0	6/12	2.00	0.3	15.0
50	20/50	15.0	6/15	2.50	0.4	12.0
60	20/60	18.0	6/18	3.00	0.5	10.0
80	20/80	24.0	6/24	4.00	0.6	7.5
100	20/100	60.0	6/60	5.00	0.7	6.0
200	20/200	120.0	6/120	10.00	1.0	3.0
400	20/400	240.0	6/240	20.00	1.3	1.5

MAR = Minimum angle of resolution.

resolved in order to recognize objects (e.g., letters of the alphabet). It is specified in terms of the Minimum Angle of Resolution (MAR), logMAR, or values such as Snellen notation or metric equivalents based on MAR. Table 1.2 presents a comparison of the various methods of designating visual acuity. For clinical visual acuity charts, the MAR is the angle subtended by the thickness or stroke of a letter, with the overall height and width of the letter typically being five times larger than the thickness. Figure 1.2 presents an example of a typical eye chart used for clinical evaluation of visual acuity. This design is essentially the same as that introduced by Snellen in 1862, and the most common form of reporting visual acuity is still in terms of "Snellen notation," consisting of a fraction in which the numerator is the testing distance (20 feet or 6 meters) and the denominator is the distance at which a "normal" observer is able to read the letter. By definition, a visual acuity of 20/20 (6/6) refers to a MAR of one minute of arc letter thickness. The standard of 20/20 for "normal" vision was developed more than 100 years ago, and with today's high contrast eye charts and better light sources, most normal persons under the age of 50 can be corrected to better than 20/20.

Another type of visual acuity chart is known by various names, including the Early Treatment for Diabetic Retinopathy Study (ETDRS) chart, the Bailey-Lovie chart, and the logMAR chart (Fig. 1.3). This chart has several advantages over the standard Snellen chart. First, the letters used are equally detectable for normal observers. Second, each line has an equal number of letters. Third, the spacing between letters is proportional to the letter size. Fourth, the change in visual acuity from one line to another is in equal logarithmic steps. Fifth, better specification of visual acuity with either Snellen notation, MAR or logMAR values can be achieved. Finally, new methods of scoring responses can be implemented that produce greater sensitivity and reliability.

The measurement of visual acuity in special populations (e.g., young children and physically challenged persons) is not always possible with a standard letter chart. Testing of central visual function of infants begins with an assessment of how well the infant fixes and follows the examiner's face, a small toy, or other objects of interest. For older children, the "Tumbling E Cube" can be used for visual acuity testing. This cube is a white block with black E letters of different sizes on each of its sides. By rotating the cube, an individual E can be presented in four different orientations to test the patient's ability to distinguish the direction of the E. The cube can be placed at various distances from the patient, and different-sized E targets can be evaluated to make a determination of visual acuity. The Tumbling E Cube thus relies on a child's ability to orient the hand according to the direction of the E. For older children the "E game" can be performed using a projected "E" acuity chart. The "HOTV" test involves matching each test letter to one of four letters (H, O, T, or V) printed on a card held by the child. Some visual acuity tests use pictures or symbols. These may be more reliable than the HOTV test. The most popular of the picture visual acuity tests are the Allen Cards. Projector slides with the familiar cake, bird, telephone, and other pictures are also available. Other devices like the B-VAT vision tester can generate many random sequences of characters and figures to avoid memorization by the child.

"Preferential-looking" techniques, oculomotor responses such as optokinetic nystagmus, and electrophysiologic measures such as the VEP can also be

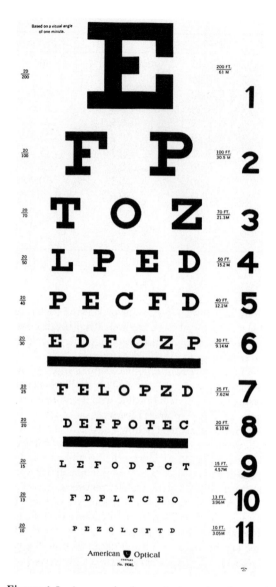

Figure 1.2. An example of a standard eye chart for visual acuity testing.

the examiner to ensure that the nontested eye is properly occluded to avoid peeking. The examiner must work quickly, may need to use more than one procedure to establish visual acuity capabilities, and should continually provide positive feedback to the child to maintain cooperation.

In patients suspected of having nonorganic visual loss, several additional methods of assessing visual acuity may be useful (see Chapter 23). The Tumbling E cube can be used as a cross-check of the eye chart visual acuity determination (e.g., a patient that can see the 20/200 E on the eye chart at 20 feet should be able to see an E that is five times smaller at a distance of 4 feet, because they subtend the same visual angle). By moving the cube from one distance to another, the consistency of visual acuity responses can be ascertained. If this is done quickly, it is extremely difficult for a patient with nonorganic visual loss to maintain consistent responses (i.e., select appropriate target sizes for different distances to maintain a constant visual angle). Often the patient will pick the same physical target size, irrespective of the distance at which it is presented.

A helpful device that can be used to test patients with suspected nonorganic monocular visual acuity loss is a cross-Polaroid projection chart (the American Optical Vectograph Project-O-Chart slide). This consists of a projector eye chart that is combined with polarizing material. The left or right half of the eye chart is projected through horizontally polarized material, and the other half is projected through vertically polarized material. The patient views the chart wearing a pair of glasses with polarized material that has different orientations over the two eyes (e.g., horizontal left eye polarization, vertical right eye polarization). Thus, one eye sees only the left half of the eye chart, and the other eye sees only the right half. The chart is viewed by the patient with both the "good" eye and the "bad" eye open. Patients with nonorganic visual loss in one eye will often read all of the eye chart, even though the "good" eye can only see half of the chart. Another portion of the American Optical Vectograph slide has randomly arranged visual acuity letters (ranging from 20/20 to 20/40) that can be seen with the left eye only, the right eye only, or with both eyes. This is especially useful in patients with nonorganic monocular visual acuity loss.

In normal observers, visual acuity is highest for the foveal region and decreases rapidly with increasing visual field eccentricity. In many instances, central visual field loss and reduced visual acuity appear to be closely related. However, visual acuity can also be reduced when there is generalized depression of the central visual field and no scotoma is apparent. There are also several conditions for which the visual field

used to estimate visual acuity. In addition, a number of eye charts and behavior test procedures can be used to assess visual acuity in nonverbal or physically challenged patients. These tests utilize patterned stimuli and caricatures of faces (e.g., Mr. Happy Face) or common objects with "critical detail" (e.g., Cheerios) that can be used to obtain an indication of the individual's level of visual acuity.

Visual acuity measurements in children present special problems, in part because the child wants to do well and please the examiner. It is therefore important for

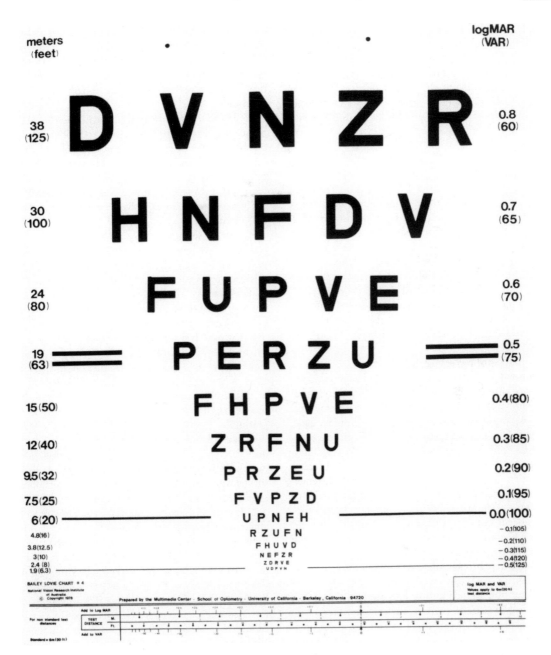

Figure 1.3. An example of the Bailey-Lovie LogMAR visual acuity chart.

may be at or near normal sensitivity, but visual acuity may be dramatically reduced. These conditions include refractive errors, corneal surface irregularities, cataract, retinal edema or serous detachment, and amblyopia.

CONTRAST SENSITIVITY

Visual acuity defines the smallest spatial detail that can be resolved for high-contrast stimuli, but it does not specify the responses of the visual system to objects of different sizes and contrasts. Measurement of the spatial contrast sensitivity function (CSF) is necessary to obtain this information. The CSF is most commonly determined by measuring contrast thresholds for sinusoidal gratings, an alternating pattern of light and dark bars with luminance that varies sinusoidally in a direction perpendicular to orientation of the grating. The size of the grating is specified according to spatial frequency, which is the number of cycles (pairs of light and dark bars) of the grating pattern per degree of visual angle. Typically, between 3 and 10 spatial frequencies from 0.5 to 30 cycles per degree are measured for the CSF. Contrast is defined by the luminance of the peaks (L_{max}) and troughs (L_{min}) of the sinusoidal grating, according to the equation:

$$\text{Contrast} = \frac{L_{max} - L_{min}}{L_{max} + L_{min}}$$

Contrast can vary from a minimum of 0 for a uniform field ($L_{max} = L_{min}$) to a maximum of 1 ($L_{min} = 0$). A contrast threshold is the minimum amount of contrast needed to detect the presence of the grating, and contrast sensitivity is the reciprocal of the contrast threshold (sensitivity = 1/threshold). The CSF describes the behavior of the visual system at **threshold** contrast levels, which is not completely representative of the visual system's characteristics for processing suprathreshold contrast information.

A number of factors influence the measurement of the normal CSF, including background adaptation luminance, stimulus size, visual field eccentricity, pupil size, temporal characteristics, stimulus orientation, and various optical factors such as defocus, dioptric blur, diffusive blur, and astigmatism. The CSF can be used to evaluate optical properties of the human eye, including refractive error and defocus, corneal disease, cataract, refractive surgery, intraocular lenses, retinal degenerations, glaucoma, and the normal aging properties of the optics of the eye. Contrast sensitivity deficits sometimes occur in patients with normal visual acuity and optical conditions that produce subtle changes in the quality of their vision.

From a neuro-ophthalmologic standpoint, measurement of the CSF can reveal subtle deficits in patients with optic neuritis and multiple sclerosis, but also in patients with a variety of other optic neuropathies and cerebral abnormalities, amblyopia, and other conditions such as Alzheimer's disease and Parkinson's disease.

In general, the CSF is clinically useful for detecting early or subtle visual loss (especially when visual acuity is normal), making comparisons between the two eyes, or for monitoring the progression or improvement of visual function. One of the shortcomings of the CSF, however, is that sensitivity losses have little specificity for differential diagnostic purposes. The main patterns of contrast sensitivity loss are (a) generalized contrast sensitivity loss at all spatial frequencies; (b) greater high spatial frequency contrast sensitivity loss; (c) greater low spatial frequency contrast sensitiv-

ity loss; and (d) a "notch" produced by contrast sensitivity loss for a particular group of spatial frequencies (Fig. 1.4). Generalized and high-frequency contrast sensitivity deficits are by far the most common patterns of loss across a wide variety of pathologic ocular conditions.

The CSF may be helpful in predicting the performance for various daily tasks, such as the identification of distant objects, reading highway signs and books, recognizing faces, and mobility. Thus, the CSF is not only useful for revealing subtle visual deficits associated with ocular disorders but is also helpful in identifying problems that a patient is likely to encounter during daily activities.

Contrast sensitivity may be measured with wall charts in a manner similar to the way in which visual acuity is typically measured. One of these methods uses the Vistech chart (Fig. 1.5). This chart has a series of five rows (A to E), each with a different spatial frequency. Each row consists of a group of nine circular targets containing a sinusoidal grating that is either vertical, tilted to the left, or tilted to the right. From the left side of the chart to the right, there is a successive reduction in the contrast of the grating. Patients are positioned 10 feet from the chart and are asked to read each row from left to right by indicating the orientation of the grating.

A second method of testing contrast sensitivity utilizes the typical letter charts for testing visual acuity, but there is a low contrast between the letters and the background. Although normal observers show a small reduction in visual acuity for low contrast targets (about two lines), patients with early or subtle abnormalities sometimes demonstrate quite profound reductions in visual acuity for low contrast targets compared with high contrast letters. Thus, this approach to contrast sensitivity testing can reveal mild disturbances of visual sensory function not detectable by standard visual acuity testing. The advantage of a low contrast acuity chart is that it uses a test procedure that is highly familiar to most patients and clinicians.

A third method of testing contrast sensitivity is the Pelli-Robson chart (Fig. 1.6), consisting of letters of a fixed size that vary in contrast. Each line consists of six letters, with the three left-most and three right-most letters having the same amount of contrast. The patient reads the chart in a manner similar to a standard visual acuity chart, and the minimum contrast at which the letters can be detected is recorded. This method of testing contrast sensitivity is highly reproducible and is capable of detecting disturbances in visual function that are not evident with standard visual acuity testing.

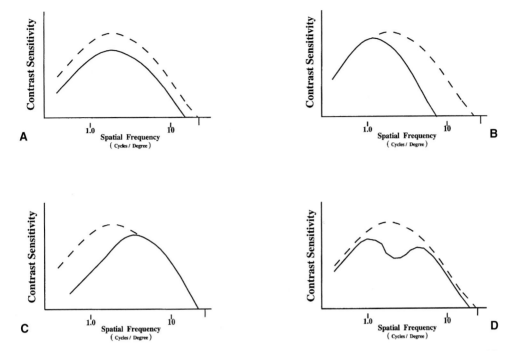

Figure 1.4. Examples of the various types of contrast sensitivity loss. **A:** Generalized depression. **B:** High spatial frequency loss. **C:** Low spatial frequency loss. **D:** Middle spatial frequency loss.

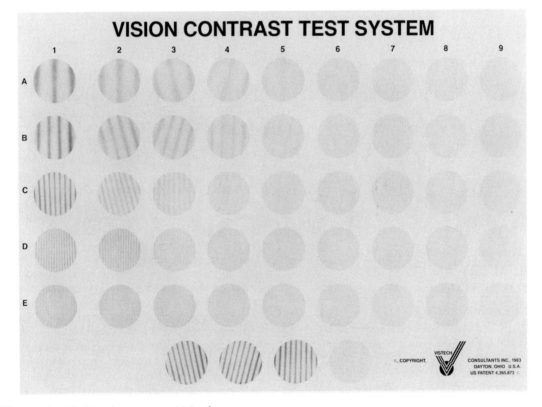

Figure 1.5. The Vistech contrast sensitivity chart.

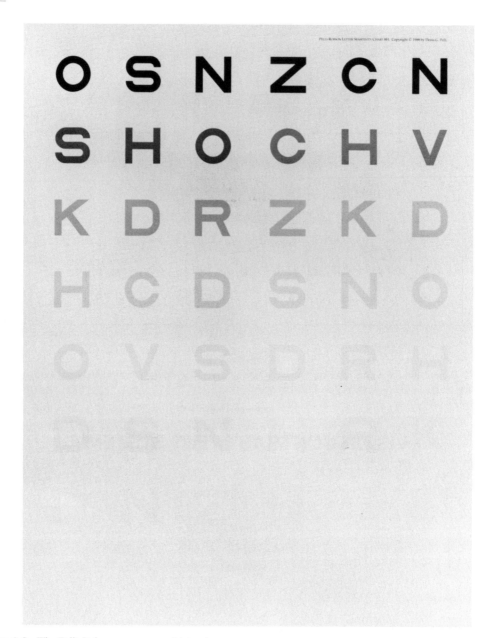

Figure 1.6. The Pelli-Robson contrast sensitivity chart.

PERIMETRY AND VISUAL FIELD TESTING

GENERAL PRINCIPLES

Perimetry and visual field testing have been clinical diagnostic test procedures for more than 150 years. Although instrumentation and testing strategies have changed dramatically over this time, the basic principle underlying conventional perimetry has remained the same. Detection sensitivity is determined for a number of locations throughout the visual field using a small target presented against a uniform background. The loss of sensitivity at various visual field locations serves as a noninvasive marker for identifying pathology or dysfunction of the visual pathways. The ability of perimetry to provide helpful clinical information has been responsible for its long-term use as a diagnostic procedure. Because perimetry can provide information about both the likely anatomic locus and disease process or processes for afferent system abnormalities, it remains a vital part of the neuro-ophthalmologic evaluation.

Perimetry and visual field testing fulfill several important diagnostic functions:

1. **Early detection of abnormalities.** Because many ocular and neurologic disorders are initially expressed as sensitivity loss in the peripheral visual field, perimetry is an important factor in identifying early signs of afferent system dysfunction. Perimetry is typically the only clinical procedure that evaluates the status of the afferent visual pathways for locations outside the macular region.
2. **Differential diagnosis.** The spatial pattern of visual field deficits and comparison of patterns of visual field loss between the two eyes also provide valuable differential diagnostic information. Not only can this information be helpful in defining the location of damage along the visual pathways, it can also assist in identifying the specific type of disease that has caused the damage.
3. **Monitoring progression and remission.** The ability to monitor a patient's visual field over time is important for verifying a working diagnosis, establishing whether a condition is stable or progressive, and evaluating the effectiveness of therapeutic interventions.
4. **Revealing hidden visual loss.** Perhaps the most important role subserved by perimetry is the ability to find afferent visual pathway loss that may not be apparent to the patient. Changes in foveal visual function are typically symptomatic. Peripheral vision loss, on the other hand, can often go unnoticed, especially if it is gradual and monocular. Paradoxically, even though a patient may be unaware of peripheral visual field loss, it can significantly affect the performance of daily activities such as driving, orientation, and mobility.

Some form of visual field testing should be performed on all patients, particularly those at greater risk of having visual field loss: (a) patients over the age of 60; (b) individuals with high myopia, elevated intraocular pressure, diabetes, vascular disease, systemic disease, family history of glaucoma or other eye disease, or other risk factors for development of ocular or neurologic disorders; (c) individuals with visual symptoms or complaints, but minimal findings on their eye examination; and (d) individuals with significant problems involving orientation and mobility, balance, driving, night vision and related activities. It is not feasible or necessary to perform a long quantitative visual field examination on all patients. However, a confrontation visual field or brief tangent screen evaluation should be performed as part of a standard neuroophthalmologic examination. When more sensitive measurements of the visual field are needed, automated static perimetry or manual kinetic perimetry can be performed.

Manual perimetry with the Goldmann perimeter has many advantages. Because the perimetric stimulus presentation is done by a human, subjects can be cajoled into performing. When the perimetrist senses subject fatigue, a rest break is given. Unlike the fixed, 6-degree spaced grid of conventional automated perimetry, Goldmann perimetry allows for custom test point locations along with improvisation of strategies based on coexisting findings. Specific exploration strategies can be used for individual concerns. This allows for much more accurate mapping of defect shape and can be invaluable for the topographic localization of visual field defects. However, manual perimetry is less sensitive than conventional automated perimetry and it may be more time-consuming. Its most severe limitation, though, is that many perimetrists are not adequately trained. This may be worse than no perimetry at all.

Automated perimetry has had a dramatic impact on improving the quality of care for patients with ocular disorders. Automatic calibration of instruments, standardized test procedures, high sensitivity and specificity, reliability checks ("catch trials"), and quantitative statistical analysis procedures are some of the many advantages of this method of perimetry. However, there are also disadvantages of automated perimetry, including prolonged test time, increased cognitive demands, fatigue, and lack of flexibility for evaluating difficult patient populations. We believe that there is no single method of visual field testing that is best for all circumstances and all patients. Automated perimetry is but one of many tools that the clinician can use to evaluate peripheral visual function, and the various forms of visual field testing should be regarded as **complementary** techniques, the utility and appropriateness of which are determined by the clinical circumstances and the question that is being addressed. There is no single method of data representation, analysis procedure, visual field index, or other method of evaluating visual field data that provides all of the essential clinical information. It is important to consider all of the information available, including reliability characteristics and the subjective clinical interpretation of the visual field. In addition, it should be kept in mind that although the test may be automated, the patient is not. It is unreasonable to begin an automated visual field test, leave a patient alone in a dark room, and expect the patient to remain alert, energetic, attentive, interested, and to maintain proper alignment and fixation throughout the test procedure. Some patients require periodic rest breaks, encouragement, and personal contact to perform visual field examinations in a reliable manner. It is also important to insure that proper test conditions, refractive characteristics, and other factors have been properly established before initiating the examination.

Psychophysical Basis for Perimetry and Visual Field Testing

The primary psychophysical concept underlying perimetry and visual field testing is the increment or differential light threshold. The increment threshold (Weberian contrast) is the minimum amount of light that must be added to a stimulus (gdL) to make it just detectable from the background (L). At very low background luminances, the amount of light needed to detect a stimulus is constant. At higher background luminances, the increment threshold increases in direct proportion to the background luminance. For example, a doubling of the background luminance requires a doubling of the stimulus luminance for detection. This relationship, which holds over a large range of background luminance levels, is known as Weber's law. The standard background luminance used by most perimetric devices is 31.5 apostilbs (asb), or 10 cd/m².

Increment threshold determinations are usually made at a number of visual field locations during quantitative perimetry. For a normal visual field, the increment threshold varies as a function of visual field location. Visual field results are usually represented in terms of sensitivity, the reciprocal of threshold (sensitivity = 1/threshold). At the 31.5 asb background luminance, the fovea has the highest sensitivity and is able to detect both the dimmest and the smallest targets. Sensitivity drops rapidly between the fovea and 3 degrees decreases gradually out to 30 degrees, and then drops off more rapidly again beyond 50 degrees (Fig. 1.7). The characteristic three-dimensional representation of the visual field sensitivity profile is often called the "hill of vision" or an "island of vision in a sea of blindness." In addition to eccentricity-dependent changes in the slope of the visual field profile, the temporal visual field (to the right of the foveal peak) extends farther than the nasal visual field, and the inferior visual field extends farther than the superior visual field. The location of the blind spot, approximately 15 degrees temporal to the foveal peak, is indicated in most representations by a darkened vertically oval area.

Visual field sensitivity can be affected by many different stimulus attributes, including background luminance, stimulus size, stimulus duration, chromaticity, and other factors. Of these parameters, stimulus size is the most important for clinical perimetry. Next to stimulus luminance, it is the most common method of adjusting the detectability of perimetric stimuli. Not only does a change in stimulus size affect the overall sensitivity to light, but the slope of the sensitivity profile is also changed. Small targets produce steeper sensitivity profiles, and larger targets result in a flatter sensitivity profile, especially for the central 30 to

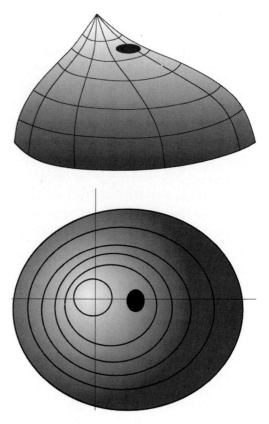

Figure 1.7. Three-dimensional representation of the normal visual field represented as a hill of vision. Sensitivity is plotted as a function of visual field eccentricity.

40 degrees eccentricity. Response variability is also reduced as stimulus size is increased.

Certain patient characteristics that are not associated with ocular or neurologic pathology can also influence the increment or differential light threshold. Blur and refractive error, media opacities such as cataract, ptosis, and pupil size can affect visual field sensitivity characteristics. In addition, procedural circumstances related to trial lens rim obstructions, fixation instability, response errors, and other artifacts of testing can produce the appearance of visual field loss or can obscure visual field deficits that are actually present.

Cognition, attention, and other higher-order functions in patients undergoing visual field testing can influence visual field sensitivity, as well as attention, practice, and learning. Fatigue effects can reduce visual field sensitivity, particularly after the test procedure has taken more than 5 to 7 minutes of testing. Patients with visual field loss typically demonstrate greater fatigue effects than those with normal perimetric function, and this may be especially true for some conditions such as optic neuritis.

Techniques for Perimetry and Visual Field Testing

Perimetry and visual field test procedures may be categorized in several different ways: (a) the amount of information obtained by the test (i.e., screening versus quantitative); (b) the type of stimulus used to perform the test (kinetic, static, or suprathreshold static); and (c) the manner in which the test is administered (manually vs. computer-driven). There are both advantages and disadvantages for each method. Automated perimetry, for example, provides greater standardization, calibration, and statistical analysis of results than manual visual field testing, but it is less efficient, less flexible, and too demanding for some patients. Kinetic perimetry, when performed appropriately, is a more efficient method of performing an evaluation of the full visual field than static perimetry and the technique can yield exquisite information about defect shape, but the technique varies from one test to another. Quantitative procedures provide a better ability to detect subtle anomalies and monitor changes over time, but they are more time-consuming than screening procedures and may cause fatigue in some patients.

Confrontation Visual Fields   Confrontation visual fields are usually performed with the patient seated in the examination chair and the examiner seated facing the patient at a distance of 2 to 3 feet. One of the patient's eyes is occluded using the palm of the patient's hand, an occluder paddle, or a patch, and the patient is asked to fixate with the uncovered eye on the examiner's nose or opposite eye. A variety of stimuli can be employed for confrontation visual fields (Fig. 1.8). The basic intent is to use a small, localized target whose presence or absence in the visual field can be readily determined by the patient. A confrontation visual field should include an examination of each of the four visual field quadrants, including the superior and inferior hemifields along the horizontal midline, the nasal and temporal hemifields along the vertical midline, and the central and peripheral visual field. Most examiners test patients using double simultaneous finger counting to survey the visual field for any dense quadrantic defect. Finger counting is followed by a test of the central visual field to evaluate for the presence of relative visual field defects. One such test is to use two red objects and compare perception of the two eyes or parts of the visual field. Unfortunately, for optic nerve-related visual field defects, finger confrontation identifies only about 10% of defects while bedside color techniques yield defects in about one-third of patients with abnormalities on formal perimetry. Color confrontation

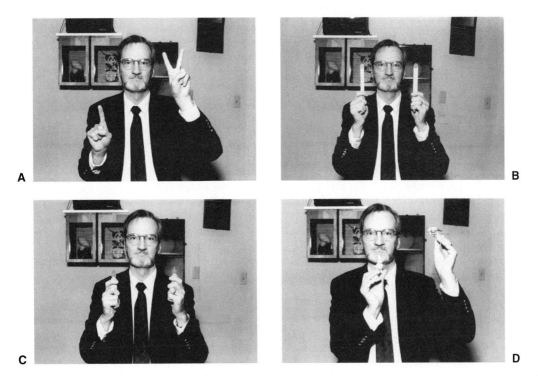

Figure 1.8.   Common objects used for confrontation visual field testing. **A:** Hands and fingers. **B:** Tongue depressors with colored dots. **C:** Medicine bottle caps. **D:** Small toys.

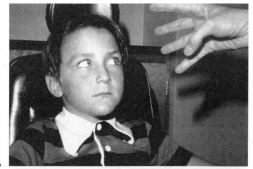

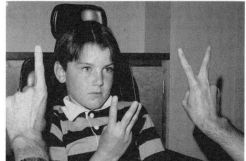

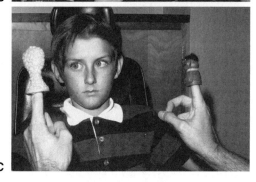

Figure 1.9. Examples of confrontation visual field testing in children. **A:** Startle response. **B:** Finger counting. **C:** Finger puppets.

techniques fare better with chiasmal defects, detecting about three quarters of patients. Even by combining several confrontation visual field tests, only about half of the perimetrically identified defects are found. Therefore, formal perimetry is usually necessary when the patient has visual loss not explained by a general ophthalmologic examination.

Confrontation visual field techniques for infants and children can be quite challenging (Fig. 1.9). For infants and young children, a visually mediated startle response can be used to detect hemianopic defects and other substantial defects in the peripheral field. A child who sees a startle stimulus will look in that direction. For older children, finger mimicking or a "Simon says" game can be used to evaluate the peripheral visual field. The child mimics the examiner by holding up the same number of fingers he or she observes. "Finger puppet

perimetry" can be performed, with one puppet used to direct central fixation and the other puppet used as a peripheral stimulus for saccadic eye movements.

In many instances, simultaneous comparison of color saturation or brightness of stimuli between hemifields or between the two eyes is useful in distinguishing subtle anomalies. When the stimuli are presented in a double simultaneous fashion to the right and left of fixation, it is possible to detect homonymous defects. Subtle deficits across the vertical midline can be detected by asking the patient to indicate which of the two test objects is clearer or brighter. In addition, double simultaneous presentation can be used to detect the phenomenon of visual extinction—the lack of awareness of an object in a seeing area of the visual field when other seeing areas of the visual field are stimulated simultaneously.

The obvious advantages of confrontation visual field testing include its simplicity, flexibility, speed of administration, and ability to be performed in any setting, including at the bedside. The disadvantages of confrontation visual field testing include the lack of standardization, the qualitative nature of the results, and the limited ability to detect subtle deficits and monitor progression or remission of visual loss. Because it is quick and easy to perform, confrontation visual field should be performed on all patients, regardless of their visual complaints.

Amsler Grid   Amsler grids are a series of charts, specifically designed to qualitatively analyze the disturbances of visual function which accompany the beginning and evolution of maculopathies. The charts are a series of lined and patterned grids that test the central visual field within 10 degrees of fixation when the plates are held at one third of a meter from the eyes. Each square of the grid subtends 1 degree of visual angle, making the ability to define the location of small defects rather easy. The patient is asked to fixate a central spot on the grid, using one eye at a time, and is asked if he or she can see the spot. If not, the patient's finger can be placed on the center to help fixation. The patient is then asked to point out any regions in which the lines are missing, blurred, distorted, bent, or irregular.

This technique is well known to ophthalmologists who routinely examine patients with known or suspected macular disease, because Amsler grids can be used to identify and plot small scotomas and other visual field defects that occur with macular scars, mild macular degeneration, central serous chorioretinopathy, and related disorders. It is perhaps less well recognized that small central or paracentral scotomas that occur with optic nerve disease can also be identified with these plates. The Amsler grid (Fig. 1.1) is particularly useful for identifying small central scotomas and other subtle central visual disturbances that are difficult to detect with more sophisticated automated and manual perimeters. The Amsler grid is very quick and easy to administer. Its main disadvantages are related to the qualitative, subjective nature of the information derived from the test.

Tangent (Bjerrum) Screen The central visual field can be studied in detail using a tangent or Bjerrum screen. The screen is made of black felt or other black matte material and can be mounted on the wall or hung from the ceiling. The screen has several concentric circles and radial lines imprinted on it to provide a reference for the examiner. A dark wand with circular targets of various sizes and colors mounted on the end is used to examine the central visual field, usually within 30 degrees of fixation. In its most common application, testing is performed at a distance of 1 meter, and a light source is employed to provide a relatively uniform illumination of 7 foot-candles on the screen. Targets are specified in terms of their diameter, their color, and the testing distance in millimeters. For example, a 1-mm-diameter white target used with the patient located 1 meter from the tangent screen would be designated as 1/1000W, and a 5-mm red target used with the patient located 2 meters from the screen would be designated as 5/2000R.

A kinetic technique is usually performed to test the visual field during a tangent screen examination. The patient fixates a central target, and a stimulus is slowly moved from the periphery towards the center of the screen along a particular meridian until the patient reports detection of the stimulus. By repeating this procedure along different meridians, a contour of equal sensitivity—an **isopter**—can be plotted. The use of several different target sizes generates several different isopters and creates a map of visual field sensitivity. Scotomas, areas of low sensitivity or nonseeing areas surrounded by normal visual field regions, are also plotted. A well-performed kinetic tangent screen examination can detect subtle defects and provide quantitative information for the central visual field that is comparable to that obtained by more sophisticated automated procedures.

Suprathreshold static visual field screening can also be accomplished with the tangent screen. Using targets that are white on one side and black on the other, the wand can be rotated to present and then extinguish the stimulus at key locations throughout the visual field. The target size employed is typically one that can be readily detected by persons with normal visual fields. In this manner, it is possible to quickly determine whether or not visual field abnormalities are present.

The main advantages of the tangent screen are its flexibility (i.e., variable distance from the patient, different colored objects, single versus multiple stimuli used simultaneously), speed, and ease of use. Varying the distance of the patient from the screen can be helpful in differentiating organic from nonorganic constriction of the visual field (Fig. 1.10). The main disadvantages are the strong dependence of results on the skill and technique of the perimetrist, the lack of standardization, difficulty in monitoring the patient's fixation while performing the visual field examination, and the need to establish age-related population norms.

Goldmann Manual Projection Perimeter The Goldmann perimeter is a white hemispheric bowl of uniform luminance (31.5 asb) onto which a small bright stimulus is projected. It is generally used to perform kinetic perimetry, although static and suprathreshold static perimetry can also be tested with this perimeter. Unlike the Amsler grid and tangent screen, the Goldmann perimeter can be used to evaluate the entire visual field. With one eye occluded, the patient fixates a small target in the center of the bowl, and the perimetrist monitors eye position by means of a telescope. A particular stimulus size and luminance is projected onto the bowl, the target is moved from the far periphery toward fixation at a constant rate of speed, typically 4 to 5 degrees per second, and the patient is instructed to press a response button when he or she first detects the stimulus. The location of target detection is noted on a chart, and the process is repeated for different meridians around the visual field. Isopters and scotomas are plotted in a manner similar to that described for the tangent screen examination, except that both the target size and luminance can be adjusted to vary stimulus detectability. This process produces a two-dimensional representation of the hill of vision that is basically a topographical contour map of the eye's sensitivity to light (Fig. 1.11). Kinetic testing (at least 1 or 2 isopters) on the Goldmann perimeter can be performed in cooperative children as young as 5 or 6 years of age.

Static Perimetry Static perimetry uses a stationary target, the luminance of which is adjusted to vary its visibility. Although it can be performed manually using either the Goldmann or Tübingen perimeters, it is most often performed with an automated perimeter such as the Humphrey Field Analyzer or the Octopus perimeter. Measurements of the increment threshold are obtained at a variety of visual field locations that are usually arranged in a grid pattern or along meridians. A bracketing or staircase procedure may be used to measure threshold sensitivity, although new techniques such as SITA and ZEST use Bayesian forecasting methods.

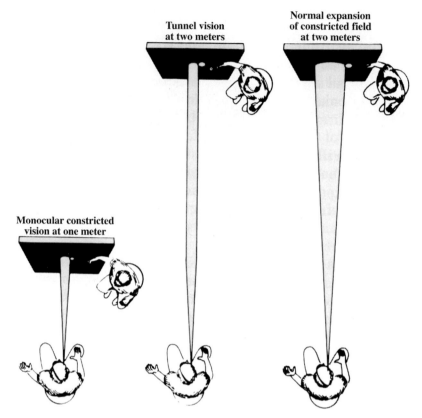

Figure 1.10. A demonstration of physiologically invalid tunnel vision ("tubular vision") associated with nonorganic visual field loss, and the normal cone-shaped expansion of the normal visual field as testing distance is increased. (Reprinted from: Beck RW, Smith CH. The neuro-ophthalmologic examination. *Neurol Clin.* 1983;1:807–830, with permission.)

Introduction of the SITA algorithm has resulted in a 50% reduction in test time. Thresholds are 1 to 2 db higher than with the use of the full staircase (full threshold) method. The shortening of test time is likely the result of a combination of less patient fatigue and interruption of the staircase procedure before threshold is reached. The algorithm has been so successful in cutting down test time that full threshold testing has largely been replaced.

The presentation of visual field sensitivity for grid patterns is typically a gray scale representation (Fig. 1.11B), rather than the three-dimensional "hill of vision" that is produced during kinetic perimetry. Areas of high sensitivity near the peak of the hill of vision are denoted by lighter shading and areas of low sensitivity by dark shading. Determinations along meridians are usually represented by a sensitivity profile plot (Fig. 1.11A).

Both static and kinetic perimetry are quantitative procedures that require a considerable amount of testing time. **Suprathreshold static perimetry** is a procedure that is faster than quantitative techniques and is typically used for screening purposes. There are a num-

ber of variations in test procedures, strategies, and theoretical bases for suprathreshold static perimetry. The basic technique, however, is that stimuli that can be easily detected by persons with normal peripheral vision are presented at specific locations throughout the visual field. These locations are selected to evaluate areas that are frequently affected by various ocular or neurologic disorders that damage the visual pathways (e.g., glaucoma, chiasmal tumors). Locations at which the target is seen are denoted by one symbol and locations where the target is not seen are denoted by another (Fig. 1.12).

Interpretation of Visual Field Information

A large amount of visual field information is derived from perimetric testing, especially from automated perimetry. Test conditions and stimulus parameters used, indicators of patient reliability and cooperation, physiologic factors (pupil size, refractive state, visual acuity, etc.), summary statistics and visual field indices, and other items are presented in conjunction with sensitivity values for various locations in the patient's visual field. Visual field sensitivity can also be represented

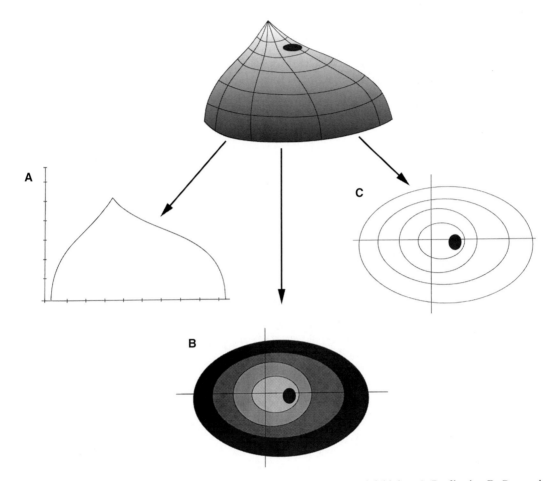

Figure 1.11. A comparison of the various graphic methods of representing visual field data. **A:** Profile plot. **B:** Gray-scale plot. **C:** Isopter/scotoma plot.

in many different forms (numerical values, deviations from normal, gray scale representations, probability plots, etc.). The following discussion presents a brief overview of the various types of information provided on the final printed outputs. Because of its current popularity and widespread use, this discussion and most of the examples are derived from automated static perimetry. However, some examples of kinetic testing using the Goldmann perimeter are presented for certain clinical cases, especially for situations in which kinetic testing provides more information about visual field status.

Graphic Representation of Visual Field Data   In most instances, the numeric representation of visual field information, whether by means of summary values such as visual field indices or by sensitivity values for individual visual field locations, is difficult to interpret. A graphic representation of visual field data makes it easier to evaluate, particularly for detecting

specific patterns of visual field loss or for assessing progression or other visual field changes over time. There are three primary methods of graphically representing visual field data: isopter/scotoma plots, profile plots, and gray scale plots (Fig. 1.11).

Ancillary Information   Several important pieces of information that should be checked on each visual field examination are the position of the eyelids, the refractive correction used for testing, pupil size, and visual acuity. Ptosis can produce a superior visual field defect that may be minimal or significant (Fig. 1.13A). High refractive corrections (>6-diopter spherical equivalent) can sometimes produce trial lens rim artifacts (Fig. 1.13B. When a patient's spherical equivalent correction for perimetric testing exceeds 6 diopters, it is advisable to use a soft contact lens correction that is appropriate for the testing distance to avoid lens rim artifacts. Proper near refractive corrections that are appropriate for the near testing distance of the perimeter

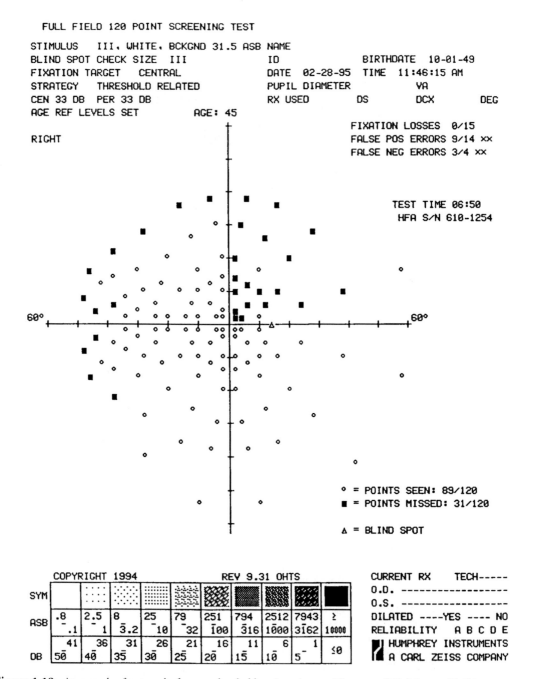

```
FULL FIELD 120 POINT SCREENING TEST

STIMULUS    III. WHITE, BCKGND 31.5 ASB NAME
BLIND SPOT CHECK SIZE   III                ID                        BIRTHDATE  10-01-49
FIXATION TARGET    CENTRAL                 DATE  02-28-95  TIME  11:46:15 AM
STRATEGY    THRESHOLD RELATED              PUPIL DIAMETER            VA
CEN 33 DB   PER 33 DB                      RX USED        DS         DCX         DEG
AGE REF LEVELS SET          AGE: 45
```

FIXATION LOSSES 0/15
FALSE POS ERRORS 9/14 xx
FALSE NEG ERRORS 3/4 xx

RIGHT

TEST TIME 06:50
HFA S/N 610-1254

60°   60°

o = POINTS SEEN: 89/120
■ = POINTS MISSED: 31/120

△ = BLIND SPOT

SYM									
ASB	.8 -.1	2.5 -1	8 -3.2	25 -10	79 -32	251 -100	794 -316	2512 -1000	7943 -3162	≥ 10000
DB	41 -50	36 -40	31 -35	26 -30	21 -25	16 -20	11 -15	6 -10	1 -5	≤0

COPYRIGHT 1994   REV 9.31 OHTS

CURRENT RX   TECH-----
O.D. ------------------
O.S. ------------------
DILATED ----YES ---- NO
RELIABILITY   A B C D E
HUMPHREY INSTRUMENTS
A CARL ZEISS COMPANY

Figure 1.12. An example of test results for suprathreshold static perimetry. (Courtesy of CA Johnson, Ph.D.)

bowl and the patient's age must be used to minimize the likelihood of refraction scotomas and sensitivity reductions from blur (Fig. 1.13C). Small pupils (<2 mm diameter) can produce spurious test results, especially in older persons who may have early lenticular changes. If pupil size is small, the patient should be dilated to 3 mm or greater (Fig. 1.13D). Finally, the patient's visual acuity can also provide useful informa-

tion when assessing generalized visual field sensitivity loss and the potential sources responsible for the loss.

Reliability Indices   The quality of information obtained from perimetry and visual field testing depends on a patient's cooperation, willingness, and ability to respond in a reliable fashion and maintain a consistent

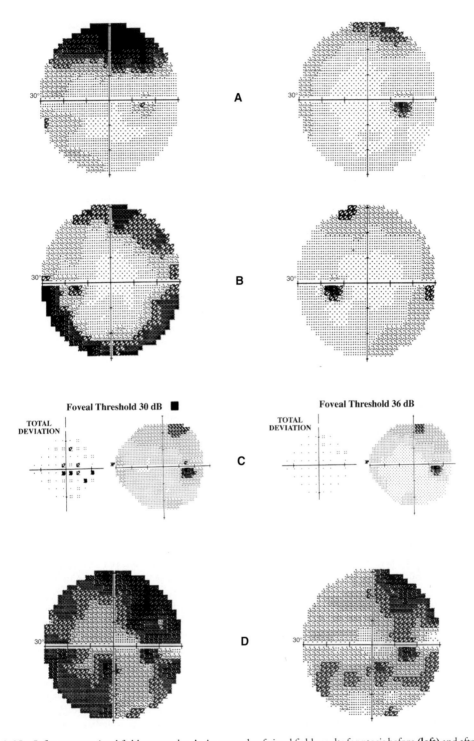

Figure 1.13. Influences on visual field test results. **A:** An example of visual field results for ptosis before **(left)** and after **(right)** taping up the upper lid and brow. **B:** Example of trial lens rim artifact **(left)** and its disappearance **(right)** after realigning the patient. **C:** Refractive error introduced by improper lens correction **(left)** and results after proper lens was employed **(right)**. **D:** Visual field results obtained in the same eye with a 1-mm **(left)** and a 3-mm **(right)** pupil diameter.

response criterion. It is important to have an assessment of patient reliability and consistency in order to properly evaluate the significance of visual field information. With manual perimetry, it is possible to monitor the patient's fixation behavior directly by means of a telescopic viewer. False-positive errors (responses when no stimulus is presented) and false-negative errors (failure to respond to a stimulus presented in a region previously determined to be able to detect equal or less detectable targets) can be monitored throughout the test procedure.

Automated test procedures not only have the capability of monitoring false-positive errors, false-negative errors, and fixation behavior in the same manner as described previously, but also can obtain an assessment of response fluctuation by retesting a sample of visual field locations. Also, indirect indicators of fixation accuracy (e.g., whether or not a patient responds to a target presented to the physiologic blind spot) can be monitored. An additional advantage of automated test procedures is that these **reliability indices** (false positives, false negatives, fixation losses, short-term fluctuations) can be immediately compared with those of age-adjusted normal control subjects, thereby providing an indication as to whether or not the patient's reliability parameters are within normal population characteristics.

Some of the reliability indices for automated perimetry are not always accurate indicators of a patient's true performance. For example, false-negative rates are correlated with visual field deficits, that is, there is an increase in false-negative responses with increased field loss. Thus, high false-negative rates may be more indicative of disease severity than of unreliable patient responses. Excessive fixation losses can be caused by factors such as mislocalization of the blind spot during the initial phases of testing, misalignment or head tilt of the patient midway through testing, or inattention on the part of the technician administering the visual field examination. Also, one should be careful not to consider reliability indices as a replacement for technician interaction and monitoring of patients. Some patients are uncomfortable when left alone in a darkened room during automated perimetry testing. In addition, misalignment of the patient, drowsiness, and related factors can occur during testing and go undetected if the patient is not adequately monitored. It is important to remember that it is the test procedure that is automated, not the patient.

Although reliability indices are helpful in determining if the visual field is accurate, they are not sufficient to eliminate the possibility that a visual field defect is nonorganic in nature. It has been shown that both patients and otherwise normal subjects can "fool" the automated perimeter, producing a variety of abnormal fields despite maintaining reliability indices that are within normal limits.

Visual Field Indices A distinct advantage afforded by automated perimeters is the ability to provide summary statistics, usually called **visual field indices.** The Mean Deviation (MD) on the Humphrey Field Analyzer and the Mean Defect (MD) on the Octopus perimeters refer to the average deviation of sensitivity at each test location from age-adjusted normal population values. They provide an indication of the degree of generalized or widespread loss in the visual field. The Pattern Standard Deviation (PSD) on the Humphrey Field Analyzer and the Loss Variance (LV) on the Octopus perimeter present a summary measure of the average deviation of individual visual field sensitivity values from the normal slope after correcting for any overall sensitivity differences. They represent the degree of irregularity of visual field sensitivity about the normal slope and therefore indicate the amount of localized visual field loss, because scotomas produce significant departures from the normal slope of the visual field. Corrected Pattern Standard Deviation (CPSD) and Corrected Loss Variance (CLV) take into account the patient's short-term fluctuation (STF) during testing. STF is derived by testing a sample of ten locations twice to determine the average deviation of repeated measures. This correction minimizes the influence of patient variability on the local deviation measures. Note that CPSD and STF are not evaluated by the SITA test algorithm.

Probability Plots Another advantage of automated static perimetry is that a patient's test results are compared with age-adjusted normal population values. Thus, it is possible to determine the amount of deviation from normal population sensitivity values on a point by point basis for all visual field locations tested. A useful means of expressing this information is by means of **probability plots.** The Humphrey Field Analyzer has two methods of presenting this type of information. One is called the "Total Deviation Plot" and the other is called the "Pattern Deviation Plot." For the Total Deviation Plot, each visual field location has one of a group of different symbols indicating whether the sensitivity is within normal limits, or is below the 5%, 2%, 1%, or 0.5% of normal limits, respectively. In other words, visual field locations or indices that have a probability corresponding to $p < 1\%$ mean that this value is observed $<1\%$ of the time in a normal population of the same age. This provides an immediate graphic representation of the locations that are abnormal

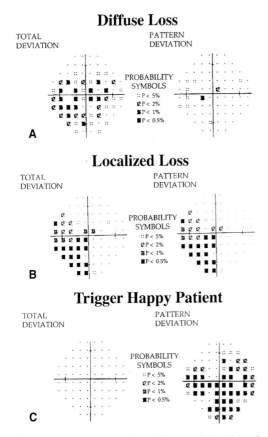

Figure 1.14. Patient results as they are depicted on the total deviation and pattern deviation probability plots for the Humphrey Field Analyzer. **A:** Diffuse loss. **B:** Localized loss. **C:** "Trigger happy" patient.

and the degree to which they vary from normal levels.

The Pattern Deviation Plot is similar to the Total Deviation Plot, except that the determinations are performed after the average or overall sensitivity loss has been subtracted, thereby revealing specific locations with **localized** deviations from normal sensitivity values. The value of these representations is twofold. First, they provide an immediate indication of the locations with sensitivity loss. Second, the comparison of the Total and Pattern Deviation Plots provides a clear indication of the degree to which the loss is diffuse or localized. If the loss is predominantly diffuse, the abnormal locations will appear on the Total Deviation Plot, but all or most of these locations will be within normal limits on the Pattern Deviation Plot (Fig. 1.14A). If the deficit is predominantly localized, the Total and Pattern Deviation Plots will look almost identical (Fig. 1.14B). The degree of similarity between the Total and Pattern Deviation Plots thus gives an in-

dication of the proportion of loss that is diffuse and localized. In a few instances, the Total Deviation Plot may appear to be normal, but the Pattern Deviation Plot reveals a number of abnormal locations (Fig. 1.14C). This occurs when the patient's measured sensitivity is significantly better than normal, and it is most often caused by a patient who presses the response button too often ("trigger happy").

Progression of Visual Field Loss   The determination of whether a patient's visual field improves, worsens, or remains stable over time is the most difficult aspect of visual field interpretation. Although there are several quantitative analysis procedures available for evaluating visual field progression, none of them enjoys complete acceptance by the clinical ophthalmic community. Nevertheless, the use of quantitative statistical analysis procedures may be helpful in monitoring a patient's visual field status.

There are several important factors to consider when evaluating a patient's visual field status over time. First, it is necessary to examine the test conditions that were present for each visual field examination. If different test strategies, target sizes or other test conditions are different from one examination to another, it is difficult to compare the results, because the type of test procedure and the stimulus size (and characteristics) can significantly alter the appearance of the visual field (Figs. 1.15 and 1.16). Second, it is important to determine if there are any differences in patient conditions from one visual field to another. If there are meaningful differences in pupil size, refractive corrections, visual acuity, time of day, or other factors (e.g., upper lid taped on one occasion and not on another occasion), this can have a dramatic effect on the visual field results obtained on different visits (Fig. 1.13). Third, unless the visual field changes are dramatic, it is important to base judgments of visual field progression or stability on the basis of the entire series of visual fields that are available. It is not possible to distinguish subtle visual field changes from long-term variation on the basis of two visual fields (e.g., comparing the current visual field to the previous visual field). In particular, patients with moderate to advanced visual field loss can sometimes exhibit considerable variations from one visual field to another. Also, factors such as fatigue and experience can produce significant differences in visual field characteristics. If it is suspected that a change in visual field loss has occurred, it is best to repeat the examination on a separate visit to confirm the suspected change. Depending on which part of the sequence and which eye is examined, any two successive visual fields can reflect apparent improvement, progression, or stability of the visual field.

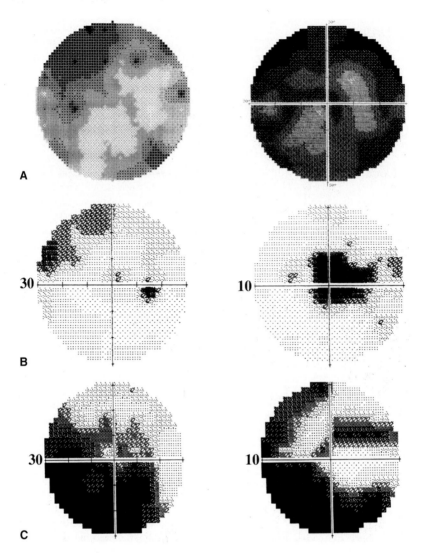

Figure 1.15. Examples of different fields obtained when patients with a field defect are tested with different strategies on an automated perimeter or with different perimeters. **A:** A patient with an optic neuropathy who was tested on two different automated perimeters. Note marked difference in results. **B:** A macular scotoma using a central 30-degree test **(left)** and central 10-degree test **(right)**. Note appearance of scotoma when 10-degree test is performed. **C:** Advanced glaucoma using a central 30-degree test **(left)** and a central 10-degree test **(right)**.

Five-Step Approach to Visual Field Interpretation
One of the common errors that occurs in visual field interpretation is the lack of attention to details and specific patterns of visual field loss before obtaining a global evaluation of the visual field. To avoid this tendency, we suggest a simple five-step approach to visual field interpretation:

1. Determine if the visual field is normal or abnormal for each eye separately. Automated perimetry results provide assistance with this task, because they show both point-by-point and summary comparisons of the patient's test results with age-matched

normal population values. If both eyes are normal, both in terms of statistical comparison and clinical assessment, then further evaluation is not necessary. However, subtle visual field loss can sometimes be present despite visual field indices that are within normal limits. Perhaps the most common of these occurrences are the subtle vertical steps in the superior visual field that may reflect an early bitemporal chiasmal lesion.

2. If one or both visual fields are abnormal, examine the ancillary information to determine if proper test conditions were employed, the appropriate near correction was used, and the pupil size was

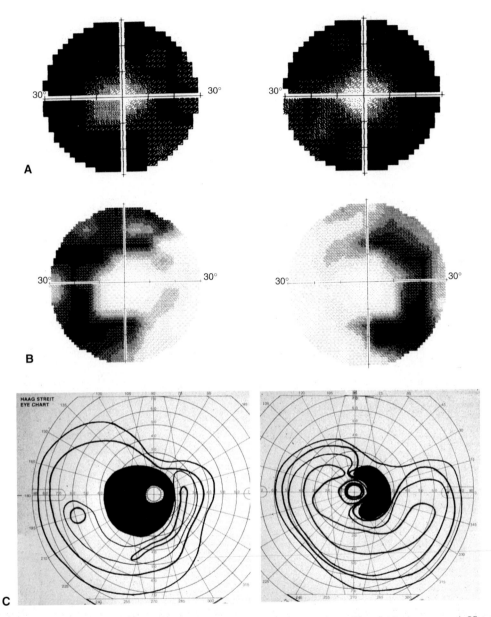

Figure 1.16. Appearance of visual fields obtained by different techniques in a patient with retinitis pigmentosa. **A:** Visual field defects with static perimetry using a Humphrey 30-2 test with a size III target for the left and right eyes shows diffuse reduction in sensitivity in each eye with a small area of central sparing. **B:** Results using a Size V target for the central 30 degrees. Note expansion of the clear central area. **C:** Results obtained by full field kinetic perimetry using a Goldmann perimeter. Note that with static perimetry the true extent of the field defects cannot be appreciated. With kinetic perimetry, the scotomatous nature of the defects can be appreciated.

sufficiently large. Also, check for patterns of visual field loss that are indicative of a trial lens rim artifact, a droopy upper eyelid, or other nonpathologic conditions that may account for the visual field loss. Fatigue, drowsiness, and related conditions can also produce apparent visual field loss. It is crucial that the person who performs the perimetric test-

ing, especially with automated perimetric tests, be attentive to these factors. A surprising number of visual field deficits can be attributed to nonpathologic influences.

3. Determine if the visual field is abnormal in both eyes or in only one eye. If the visual field is abnormal in only one eye, the defect is almost always caused by

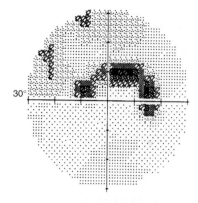

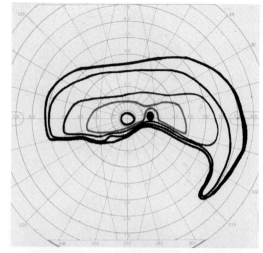

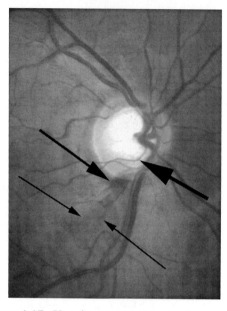

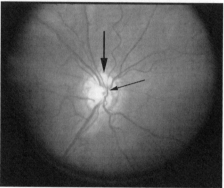

Figure 1.17. Humphrey visual field **(top)** and corresponding fundus photo **(bottom)** from a patient with low tension glaucoma in the right eye. Note moderate cupping (*large arrow*), small peripapillary nerve fiber layer hemorrhage (*medium arrow*), and wedge-shaped nerve fiber layer defect (*small arrows*) that corresponds to the superior arcuate field defect detected by perimetry.

Figure 1.18. Unilateral visual field defect in a patient with segmental hypoplasia of the right optic nerve. Visual acuity was 20/20 in the eye. **Top:** Kinetic perimetry using a Goldmann perimeter shows marked inferior altitudinal defect that does not obey the horizontal midline. Note preservation of the central field to small isopters. **Bottom:** Fundus photograph shows absence of the upper part of the disc substance. The thin arrow indicates the location of the optic disc, and the thick arrow indicates the scleral crescent.

a disorder anterior to the optic chiasm (Figs. 1.17 and 1.18). If the visual field of both eyes is abnormal, it means that the deficit is at or posterior to the optic chiasm (Figs. 1.19 and 1.20) **or** that the patient has bilateral intraocular or optic nerve disease (Figs. 1.21 and 1.22).

4. Determine the general location of the visual field loss for each eye independently. Specifically, determine if the visual field loss is in the superior or inferior hemifield, the nasal or temporal hemifield, or the central portion of the field. This is especially important for the nasal and temporal hemifield assessment. If the loss is extensive, determine where the greatest amount of visual field loss is present. If the visual field loss is bitemporal and respects the vertical midline, then a chiasmal locus should be strongly suspected, especially if the deficit is in the superior temporal quadrant in each eye (Fig. 1.19). If the visual field loss is nasal in one eye and temporal in the other eye (i.e., homonymous), then a retrochiasmal location should be suspected (Fig. 1.20). Binasal defects or a nasal deficit in only one eye should generate a suspicion of glaucoma, various nonglaucomatous optic neuropathies, or certain types of retinal disorders (Figs. 1.21 and 1.22). A central deficit in one or both eyes may indicate a macular

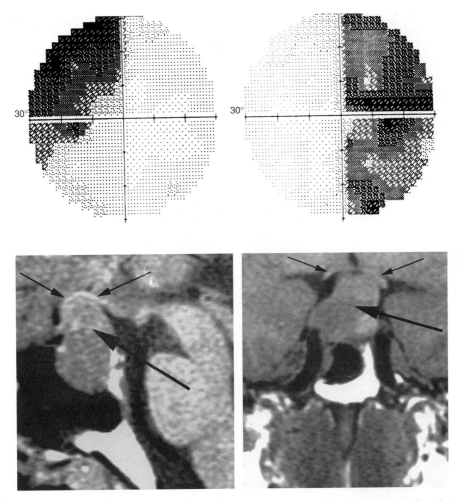

Figure 1.19. Bilateral visual field defect in a patient with a tumor in the region of the optic chiasm. **Top:** Static perimetry reveals a bilateral temporal hemianopia that is worse in the right eye (right side of illustration). **Bottom:** Sagittal **(left)** and coronal **(right)** T1-weighted magnetic resonance images show a large mass in the sella turcica with suprasellar extension (*large arrows*). The mass compresses and elevates the optic chiasm (*small arrows*).

disorder (especially if the visual field defect does not connect to the blind spot) or an optic neuropathy (Figs. 1.23 and 1.24). With this simple step, a global view of visual field properties is generated, and a hierarchy of potential locations of damage along the visual pathway and probable disease entities is hypothesized.

5. Look at the specific shapes, patterns, and features of the visual field loss (Figs. 1.17 to 1.25 and Table 1.3). Does the defect respect either the horizontal or vertical meridians? What is the shape of the deficit (arcuate, oval, circular, pie-shaped, irregular)? Does the deficit "point" to the blind spot or to fixation? If there is visual field loss in both eyes, is it congruous (symmetric in the two eyes) or incongruous (more extensive visual field loss in one eye than in the other)? Do the edges of the defect have a steep or a gradual sloping profile? These and other specific features of the visual field should provide confirmatory information for the location of the damage determined by Step 4 or allow one to differentiate among several possible alternative locations. However, it should not be used as the initial basis for generating a hypothesis about location of damage. Attention to specific features of the visual field before getting a global view of the visual field from Step 4 may lead to misinterpretation of visual field information.

The approach to visual field interpretation outlined above is not intended to cover all possible scenarios but is rather meant as a guide to identify most kinds

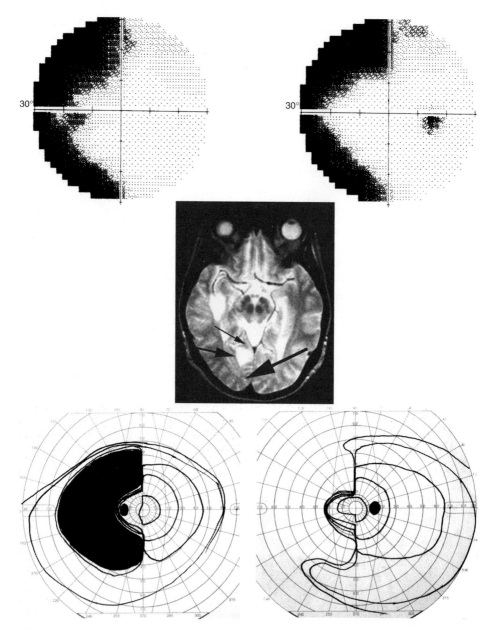

Figure 1.20. Bilateral visual field defects in a patient with an occipital lobe infarct. **Top:** Static perimetry using a Humphrey visual field analyzer shows a left homonymous field defect with macular sparing. **Middle:** T2-weighted axial magnetic resonance image shows a hyperintense region consistent with an infarct (*medium arrow*) in the right occipital lobe. Note the normal appearance of the posterior aspect of the right occipital lobe (*large arrow*), which corresponds to the macular sparing. In addition, the deep portion of the calcarine fissure (*thin arrow*), which has only monocular representation and is responsible for the temporal crescent, also appears normal. **Bottom:** Kinetic perimetry confirms a left homonymous hemianopia with macular sparing and sparing of the temporal crescent of the visual field of the left eye.

of visual field deficits and to avoid many of the common pitfalls. Once the pattern and degree of visual field loss has been established, a differential diagnosis needs to be determined. If there is doubt about the validity of visual field results, the test should be repeated when the patient is well-rested. Pathologic visual field changes usually are replicable, whereas nonpathologic visual field changes typically are not. If there is concern about fatigue affecting visual field results, a shorter test procedure should be employed.

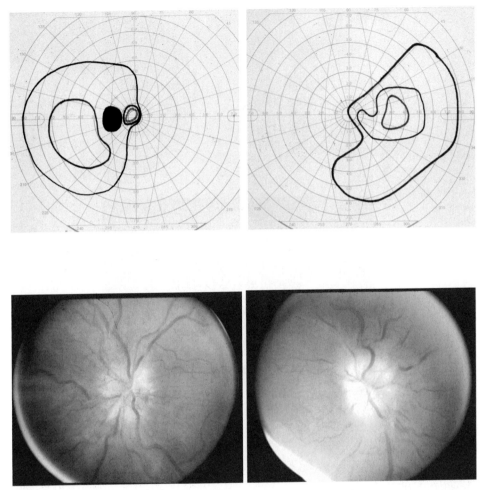

Figure 1.21. Bilateral visual field defects in a patient with pseudotumor cerebri. **Top:** Kinetic perimetry demonstrates complete loss of the nasal visual field of both eyes with involvement of the temporal fields as well. **Bottom:** Fundus photographs show bilateral chronic papilledema with early atrophy.

New Perimetry Tests

In order to improve sensitivity of visual field testing, several test procedures have been modified for use in perimetry. Although the tests vary widely in terms of the visual functions that they measure, they have a common objective: by creating a unique stimulus display, these tests attempt to isolate (or strongly bias) threshold responses to be mediated by a specific subpopulation of neural mechanisms, instead of the wide range of neural mechanisms stimulated by conventional perimetry.

These test procedures have several theoretical advantages. First, because these tests are designed to target specific visual mechanisms, their response properties bear a strong linkage to the underlying physiology and anatomy of the visual pathways. Second, if certain diseases cause selectively greater amounts of damage to some visual mechanisms than others, these new test procedures may be able to detect early losses or changes in visual function that may not otherwise be noticed with conventional perimetry. Finally, because these test procedures are designed to isolate specific subpopulations of neural mechanisms, they eliminate much of the redundancy and overlap that is normally present in the visual pathways. By reducing this redundancy, it becomes easier to detect early, subtle losses or changes in visual function, even if these losses are not selective.

Perimetry tests that appear to have the greatest potential for clinical utility in neuro-ophthalmologic diagnosis include Short Wavelength Automated Perimetry [SWAP], High-Pass Resolution Perimetry (HRP), Flicker Perimetry, Motion and Displacement Perimetry, and Frequency Doubling Perimetry.

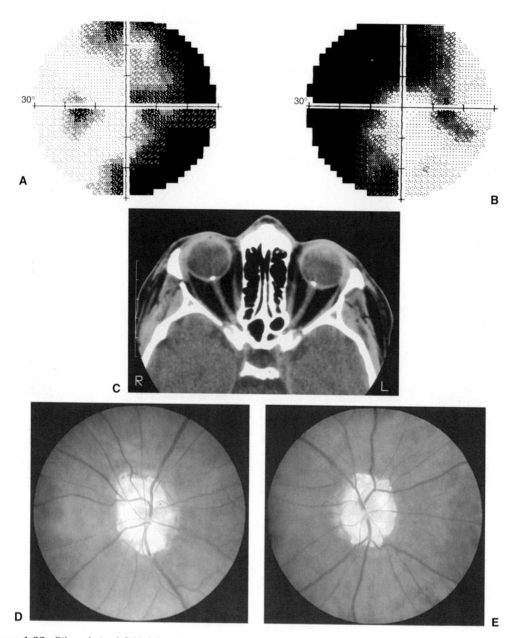

Figure 1.22. Bilateral visual field defects in a patient with bilateral optic disc drusen. **A and B:** Static perimetry reveals significant nasal field loss in both eyes. **C:** Axial computed tomographic scan set at bone window density shows calcified drusen. **D and E:** Fundus photographs show extensive optic disc drusen. Note absence of visible nerve fiber layer and constriction of retinal arteries.

COLOR VISION

NORMAL COLOR VISION MECHANISMS

There are two different theories concerning the mechanisms underlying normal color vision. The trichromatic theory of color vision is that there are three different receptors that are maximally sensitive to wavelengths in different regions of the visual spectrum, with sensitivity peaks at short (blue), middle (green), and long (red) wavelengths, respectively. Although maximally sensitive to a specific part of the spectrum, each of these receptor types is proposed to have some degree of sensitivity to wavelengths throughout most of the visual spectrum. An efficient means of uniquely

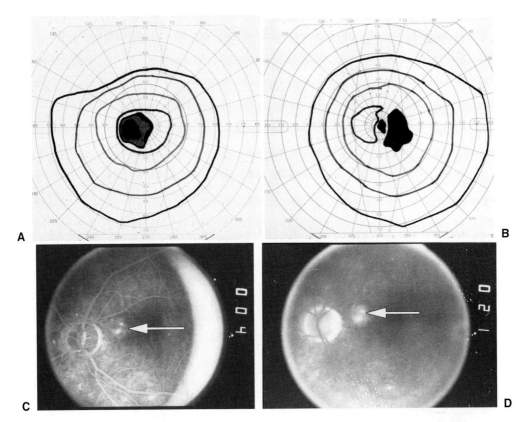

Figure 1.23. Bilateral visual field defects in a patient with bilateral central serous chorioretinopathy. **A and B:** Kinetic perimetry reveals bilateral central defects with normal peripheral fields. **C and D:** Early (**C**) and late (**D**) phases of fluorescein angiography show leakage of dye consistent with central serous chorioretinopathy in the posterior pole of the left eye (*arrows*).

signaling thousands of different colors should therefore be achieved by examining the ratio of excitation of the three receptors.

An alternate view of color vision, the opponent-process theory, is that there are two chromatic mechanisms (red-green and blue-yellow) and one achromatic mechanism (black-white) that pair sensations in an opposing or antagonistic manner. The opponent-process theory is proposed as a means of accounting for six distinct color sensations (blue, green, yellow, red, black, and white).

Abundant psychophysical and physiologic evidence supports both theories. Initially, visual stimuli are processed by three types of cone photoreceptors, one with peak sensitivity in the short-wavelength region (approximately 440 nm), one with peak sensitivity in

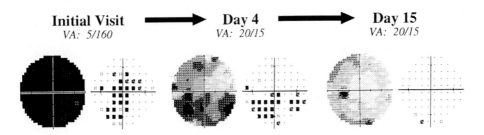

Figure 1.24. Improvement in a visual field defect as detected by static perimetry in a patient with optic neuritis over a 15-day period. (Reprinted from: Keltner JL, Johnson CA, Spurr JO, et al. Visual field profile of optic neuritis: one-year follow-up in the Optic Neuritis Treatment Trial. *Arch Ophthalmol.* 1994;112:946–953, with permission.)

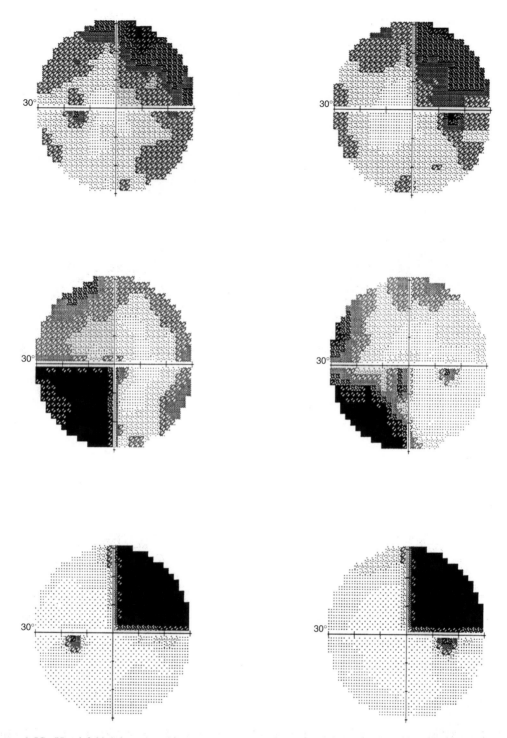

Figure 1.25. Visual field defects caused by postgeniculate lesions in the temporal **(top)**, parietal **(middle)**, and occipital **(bottom)** lobes as defined by static perimetry. **Top:** Right incomplete incongruous homonymous hemianopia, denser above, from the left temporal lobe lesion. **Middle:** Left incomplete incongruous homonymous hemianopia, denser below, from the lesion of the right parietal lobe. **Bottom:** Right congruous superior quadrantanopia from the lesion of the inferior aspect of the left occipital lobe.

Table 1.3. *Differential Diagnosis of Visual Field Deficits*

I. GENERAL DEPRESSION
  A. Cataract (diffuse depression from cataracts may improve with dilation)
  B. Corneal Disease (shows no improvement with dilation)
  C. Other Media Opacities
  D. Some Optic Neuropathies
II. ENLARGED BLIND SPOT
  A. Optic Nerve Disease
    1. Papilledema and Big Blind Spot syndrome
    2. Drusen of the optic nerve head
    3. Congenital optic nerve lesion (coloboma, staphyloma)
    4. Optic neuritis
  B. Retinal Disease
    1. Multiple evanescent white dot syndrome (MEWDS)
    2. Acute zonal occult outer retinopathy (AZOOR)
  C. High Myopia
III. ARCUATE, ALTITUDINAL, NASAL STEP, NASAL DEPRESSION
  A. Optic Nerve Disease
    1. Glaucoma
    2. Papilledema
    3. Drusen of the optic nerve head
    4. Other optic neuropathies (AION, optic neuritis, etc)
  B. Branch Artery Occlusion
IV. CROSSES THE VERTICAL AND HORIZONTAL MERIDIANS
  A. Retinal Disease
    1. Ring scotomas, peripheral depression, "scalloped" field loss
  B. Optic Neuropathy
    1. Generalized depression, sparing of central vision

  C. Fatigue, Poor Testing Ability
    1. Fatigue in conjunction with visual pathology
  D. Malingering
    1. Peripheral depression, square visual fields, spiraling or crossed isopters, inconsistent patterns of loss
V. CENTRAL OR CENTROCECAL DEFECTS
  A. Maculopathy (visual acuity often more affected than visual field)
  B. Optic Neuropathies of All Types
VI. BITEMPORAL DEFECTS
  A. Superior Bitemporal Defects (pituitary adenoma)
  B. Inferior Bitemporal Defects (craniopharyrngioma, hypothalamic tumor)
VII. HOMONYMOUS HEMIANOPIA
  A. Complete Homonymous Hemianopia
    1. Retrochiasmal defect with no further localizing value
  B. Tongue- or Keyhole-Shaped Homonymous Defect, or Remaining Visual Field
    1. Lateral geniculate lesion
  C. Incongruous Homonymous Hemianopia (anterior optic tract, radiations)
    1. Optic tract
    2. Temporal lobe ("pie in the sky" defect)
    3. Parietal lobe ("pie on the floor" defect)
  D. Highly Congruous Homonymous Hemianopia
    1. Occipital lobe lesion
      a. "Cookie cutter" punched-out lesion
      b. Macular sparing
      c. Temporal crescent
      d. Static-kinetic dissociation

the middle-wavelength region (approximately 530 to 540 nm), and one with peak sensitivity in the long-wavelength region (approximately 560 to 580 nm), in accordance with the trichromatic theory. The output from the three cone photoreceptors is then transmitted to neurons in the inner retina that process information according to two opponent chromatic mechanisms (yellow-blue and red-green) and one achromatic mechanism, in accordance with the opponent-process theory. Although there is additional spatial and temporal processing of this information at different levels of the visual pathways, this opponent coding of chromatic information is carried through to the higher visual centers. The processing of color

information is conducted by parvocellular mechanisms (see Chapter 13).

CLINICAL TESTS OF COLOR VISION

A wide variety of color vision tests are available to the clinician. Because most of them were designed to evaluate congenital red-green color vision deficiencies, many do not permit adequate testing of blue-yellow deficits or optimum characterization of acquired color vision losses. As with any test of visual function, it is important that the testing conditions be standardized and performed in the proper manner. A particularly important factor for all clinical color vision test procedures is the use of proper lighting, both in terms of having an adequate amount of light for the test and having a light source with the proper spectral distribution.

Pseudoisochromatic Plates   Pseudoisochromatic plates are the most common color vision tests employed in clinical practice. A number of pseudoisochromatic plate tests are available, although the Ishihara and Hardy-Rand-Rittler are the most commonly used versions. Each of these tests consists of a series of plates that contain colored dots of varying size and brightness. The tests are designed so that persons with normal color vision see numbers, shapes, or letters as a consequence of grouping certain colored dots together to form a figure against the background of other dots. Depending on how the particular test is designed, persons with color deficiencies are either unable to see the figure because the figure dots are confused with the background dots, or they see a figure different from that seen by persons with normal color vision because figure dots and background dots are grouped together in an abnormal pattern. The variation in size and brightness of the dots is used to ensure that recognition of figures is made on the basis of color discrimination and not other cues. Other variations of pseudoisochromatic plates include winding paths of colored dots that the patient can trace. These are useful in young children, illiterates, and some neurologically ill patients who are unable to identify letters, numbers, or shapes.

The main advantage of color vision tests using pseudoisochromatic plates is that they are quick and easy to perform and are therefore an excellent screening procedure for distinguishing normal color vision from any type of color vision abnormality. The disadvantages of pseudoisochromatic plate tests are that they have rather limited ability to classify acquired color vision deficits and to determine their severity, and that they have little or no ability (depending on the particular test) to test for either congenital or acquired blue-yellow color vision deficits.

Farnsworth Panel D-15 Test

The Farnsworth Panel D-15 test is a color arrangement test consisting of 15 color caps that form a color circle covering the visual spectrum. A reference cap is permanently fixed in the arrangement tray; the other 15 caps are placed in a scrambled order in front of the patient. The patient's task is to select the cap that is closest in hue to the reference cap and place it next to the reference cap in the tray. The patient is then asked to continue to place the caps in the tray, one at a time, so that they are arranged in an orderly transition of hue. Patients with moderate to severe protan, deutan, or tritan color vision deficits will confuse colors across the color circle, so that the arrangement contains misplaced caps. On the back of each cap is a number to assist in scoring the test. On the D-15 scoring chart, the caps along the color circle are connected in a dot-to-dot fashion in the order represented in the tray, and the specific arrangement indicates the type of color deficiency. The Panel D-15 test does not indicate the degree of color deficiency, other than to separate color normals and mild anomalous trichromats from those with moderate to severe color vision deficiencies.

Farnsworth-Munsell 100 Hues Test

The Farnsworth-Munsell 100 Hues test permits both classification of the type of color vision deficiency and its severity. Despite its name, it consists of **85** colored caps that are arranged in roughly equal small steps around the color circle. The caps are divided into four boxes, and arrangements of caps are performed one box at a time. In each box, there are two reference caps, one at each end, that are permanently attached to the box. The other caps are taken out of the box, scrambled, and placed before the patient. The patient is then asked to arrange the caps so that there is an orderly transition in hue from one reference cap to another. As with the panel D-15 test, the Farnsworth-Munsell 100 Hues test is designed so that certain caps across the color circle will be confused by persons with both congenital and acquired color deficiencies. The caps are numbered on the back, and scoring is determined by the arrangement of the caps in the box. Depending on the type of color deficiency, specific caps across the color circle will be confused, resulting in greater arrangement errors in those locations. In this manner, the type of color vision deficit can be classified (Fig. 1.26). In addition, the severity of the color deficiency can be quantified by determining an overall error score for arrangement errors.

GENERAL PRINCIPLES OF COLOR TESTING

From a clinical diagnostic standpoint, it is important to distinguish if a color vision deficiency is congenital or acquired. Congenital color vision deficits are usually easy to classify using standard clinical color vision tests because color discrimination is usually impaired for a specific region of the visual spectrum, and the deficits are long-standing, stable, symmetric in the two eyes, and unassociated with other visual symptoms or complaints. In patients with acquired color vision loss, however, color discrimination may be impaired throughout the visual spectrum or along a specific axis, and the deficits may be mild or severe, of sudden onset, asymmetric, and often associated with other visual symptoms or complaints. In acquired color vision deficiencies, tritan (blue) and blue-yellow deficiencies are most commonly associated with diseases affecting the photoreceptors and the outer plexiform layer, whereas red-green deficiencies are most commonly associated with diseases affecting the optic nerve and posterior visual pathways.

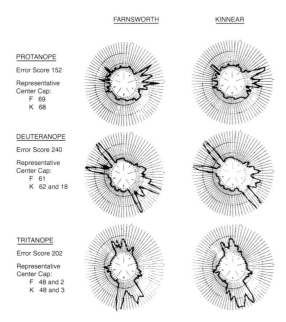

FARNSWORTH   KINNEAR

PROTANOPE
Error Score 152
Representative
Center Cap:
  F 69
  K 68

DEUTERANOPE
Error Score 240
Representative
Center Cap:
  F 61
  K 62 and 18

TRITANOPE
Error Score 202
Representative
Center Cap:
  F 48 and 2
  K 48 and 3

Figure 1.26. Examples of tritan (blue), protan (red), and deutan (green) color vision deficiencies as determined by the Farnsworth-Munsell 100 Hues Test. **Left:** The figures depict the results scored according to the method originally described by Farnsworth. **Right:** The figures depict a modified scoring system. (Reprinted from: Kinnear PR. Proposals for scoring and assessing the 100-hue test. *Vision Res.* 1970;10:423–433, with permission.)

Some notable exceptions include glaucoma, dominant hereditary optic atrophy, and chronic papilledema, which demonstrate blue-yellow deficits, and Stargardt's and Best's disease, which produce red-green deficits. Optic neuritis produces a mixture of red-green and blue-yellow deficits, although one axis is usually more affected than the other.

Color comparison tests, although only qualitative in nature, can provide valuable information concerning subtle visual anomalies. Using pages from the pseudoisochromatic plates, colored bottle caps, or other brightly colored objects, comparisons of color appearance can be very effective in detecting subtle differences between the two eyes. The brightness or saturation of the colored objects may be less in one eye, making the object's color appear dim or washed out. Similarly, comparisons within the same eye across the vertical and horizontal midline or between central vision and the mid-periphery can detect subtle differences in color appearance that are indicative of damage to the visual pathways.

ELECTROPHYSIOLOGIC TESTS

Frequently, the physician is confronted with a patient who has unexplained loss of vision and an apparently normal fundus examination. Because electrophysiologic testing often provides diagnostic clues as to the etiology of the unexplained visual loss, it should be part of the neuro-ophthalmologic examination in selected patients. Electrophysiology provides an objective method for evaluating the function of the visual system from the retina to the visual cortex. Several electrodiagnostic methods can be used to evaluate the status of individual components of the afferent visual pathways (Table 1.4).

ELECTRORETINOGRAM (ERG)
Components of the Electroretinogram

The alteration in the electric potential that occurs when light falls on the retina determines the **ERG.** There are three main components of the ERG: (a) an early cornea-negative "a-wave," (b) a cornea-positive "b-wave," and (c) a slower, usually cornea-positive "c-wave." The photoreceptors are responsible for the generation of the leading edge of the a-wave. The cellular origin of the b-wave is a combination of cells in the Müller and bipolar cell layers. The retinal pigment epithelium must be present to generate the c-wave, but the photoreceptors also contribute to this part of the ERG.

Table 1.4. *Isolation of Components of the Afferent Visual Pathways Using Electrophysiology*

Anatomical Structure	Technique
Retinal pigment epithelium	Electro-oculogram (EOG) Electro-retinogram (Flash ERG) c-wave
Photoreceptors	
Rods	Rod-flash ERG (scotopic) a-wave
Cones	Cone-flash ERG (photopic) a-wave 30 Hz Flicker ERG
Middle retinal layers	Scotopic Threshold Response (STR) Flash ERG b-wave Oscillatory Potentials Pattern ERG (P50)
Ganglion cell layer	Pattern ERG (N95)
Macula or other local region	Focal ERG 30 Hz Flicker ERG
Optic tract, radiations and cortex	VEP

Reprinted from: Weisinger HS, Vingrys AJ, Sinclair AJ, et al. Electrodiagnostic methods in vision. I. Clinical application and measurement. *Clin Exp Optom.* 1996;79:50–61, with permission.

The rod and cone components of the ERG may be separated on the basis of their respective spectral sensitivities by altering the retinal state of adaptation or by using different flicker rates for the stimulus. Although the rods are more sensitive than the cones across most of the visible spectrum, this difference decreases with increasing wavelength so that it is possible to isolate a cone response if the stimulus wavelength is >680 nm. The rod contribution to the ERG can be separated by recording from a dark-adapted subject and stimulating with a short-wavelength or long-wavelength light that has been scotopically matched for their luminances.

ERGs are often described as having photopic (light-adapted) and scotopic (dark-adapted) responses (Fig. 1.27). ERG waveforms obtained from relatively intense white stimuli usually represent contributions from both the rod and cone systems (mixed response), whereas scotopic ERGs to relatively dim blue light can be generated by the rods alone. Photopic ERGs obtained on an adapting background represent responses from the cone system. The wavelength, intensity, and temporal properties of the stimulus, as well as the state of retinal adaptation are all important in separating rod and cone system contributions. International standards for ERG testing should be followed.

By stimulating the eye in the presence of a background light sufficient to eliminate the rod response, it is possible to obtain a reasonably isolated cone response. The cone and rod ERG responses have temporal aspects that are dependent on stimulus intensity and state of retinal adaptation. Dim, short-wavelength light elicits slow, small responses from the rod system, and more intense light stimuli result in faster and larger responses. Flickering stimuli presented at 25 to 30 flashes per second (25 to 30 Hz) isolate cone responses. The ERG elicited with a white stimulus of high luminance after 30 minutes of dark adaptation has both rod and cone components. The major contributor to both the increased amplitude and implicit time is the rod component. However, an isolated rod response can be evoked by a low-intensity short-wavelength (blue) stimulus.

In normal persons, low-amplitude, rapid oscillations are superimposed on the ascending limb of the b-wave. These are called the oscillatory potentials (OPs). Bandpass filtering over 70 to 300 Hz will extract these oscillations from the underlying a- and b-waves, and they can then be quantified by giving their summed and rectified amplitudes. OPs are thought to reflect activity in the inner retinal layers. They are of clinical importance because they are often absent in patients with diabetic retinopathy and other diseases that are associated with ischemia of the inner retina.

The ERG is described by the temporal characteristics and amplitudes of the recorded waveform

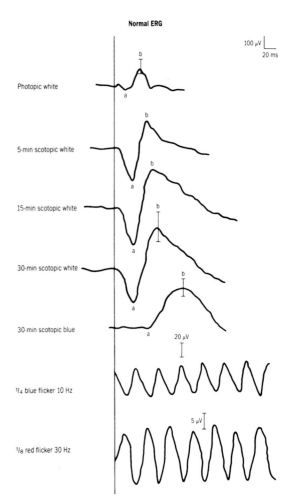

Normal ERG

Figure 1.27. Normal electroretinographic response under photopic and scotopic conditions. Cone responses are generally isolated using photopic adaptation conditions and 30 Hz flicker. Rod responses are isolated after 30 minutes of dark adaptation with a low luminance short-wavelength stimulus either as a single flash or with 10 Hz flicker. A dark-adapted scotopic white flash measures a combined rod-cone response. (Reprinted from: Fishman GA, Sokol S. *Electrophysiologic Testing in Disorders of the Retina, Optic Nerve, and Visual Pathway.* San Francisco: American Academy of Ophthalmology; 1990, with permission.)

(Fig. 1.28). The temporal aspects of the waveform can be described by the latency and implicit times. Latency refers to the time between stimulus onset and response onset, whereas implicit time refers to the time needed for the response to reach maximum amplitude. Waveform amplitudes are measured from the baseline (which is usual for the a-wave) or as a peak-to-peak comparison (which is usual for the b-wave). The b/a wave ratio can be used as an index of inner to outer retinal function.

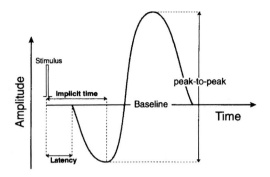

Figure 1.28. Amplitude, latency, and implicit time measurements for the standard single-flash electroretinogram. (Reprinted from: Weisinger HS, Vingrys AJ, Sinclair AJ, et al. Electrodiagnostic methods in vision. I. Clinical application and measurement. *Clin Exp Optom.* 1996;79:50–61, with permission.)

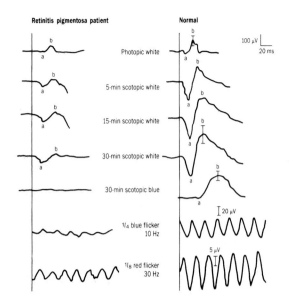

Testing Conditions and Interpretation

One of the major advances in ERG technology was the development of low-impedence, user-friendly electrodes. The Burian-Allen electrode contains a silver annulus implanted into a plastic (hard) contact lens that is placed on a topically anesthetized cornea. The contact lens is insulated and kept separate from a lid speculum that is used to keep the eyelids open during testing. The speculum is impregnated with silver granules. It thus serves as an inactive electrode, permitting a difference potential to be measured. This is called a bipolar electrode.

The ERG can be affected by a number of additional factors. The implicit time of the waveform does not mature until 4 to 6 months of age, and the amplitude may be reduced until 1 year of age. The ERG may be greater in women than in men and may be reduced in myopes with more than 6 diopters of refractive error. There may be as much as a 13% reduction in ERG amplitude in the morning, which corresponds to the time of the maximum photoreceptor disk shedding. Systemic drugs and anesthetics may also alter the ERG.

An ERG can provide important information about a number of retinal disorders that may simulate neuroophthalmologic problems. These include congenital stationary night blindness, congenital achromatopsia, retinitis pigmentosa (rod-cone dystrophy), retinitis pigmentosa sine pigmenta, cone-rod dystrophy, cone dystrophy, cancer-associated retinopathy (CAR), melanoma-associated retinopathy (MAR), and toxic retinopathies (Figs. 1.29 and 1.30).

The ERG is often helpful in establishing a diagnosis in children with nystagmus or unexplained visual loss. ERGs can be performed on infants without sedation if the infant is sleepy and is given a bottle.

Figure 1.29. An example of electroretinogram (ERG) recordings from a patient with autosomal-dominant retinitis pigmentosa **(left)** compared with normal ERG responses **(right)**. (Reprinted from: Fishman GA, Sokol S. *Electrophysiologic Testing in Disorders of the Retina, Optic Nerve, and Visual Pathway.* San Francisco: American Academy of Ophthalmology; 1990, with permission.)

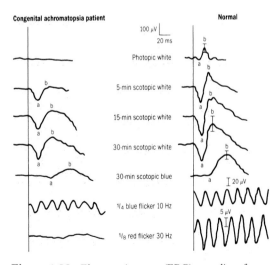

Figure 1.30. Electroretinogram (ERG) recordings from a patient with congenital achromatopsia **(left)** compared with normal ERG responses **(right)**. (Reprinted from: Fishman GA, Sokol S. *Electrophysiologic Testing in Disorders of the Retina, Optic Nerve, and Visual Pathway.* San Francisco: American Academy of Ophthalmology; 1990, with permission.)

In addition, conjunctival electrodes made of thin microfibers (Dawson-Trick-Litzkow electrodes) can be used in children of almost any age. Depending on the procedures employed, however, different laboratories may obtain widely differing results for infants and young children. Thus, it is important that each laboratory establish normal ERG standards for infants and young children in order to properly interpret the results. When analyzing ERG results for an infant, caution must be exercised. The ERG b-wave amplitude only becomes equivalent to that of adults at 5 to 6 months of age, and some authors believe that b-wave amplitudes do not reach adult levels until 1 year of age.

Pattern Electroretinogram

The **pattern electroretinogram** (PERG) is produced by a phase-reversing patterned stimulus that maintains a constant overall mean luminance. The stimulus may be an alternating pattern of light and dark regions, such as a checkerboard or bar grating generated on a television monitor. When the pattern reverses (light regions become dark and vice versa) once or twice per second, an isolated response is obtained; when faster reversal rates are used (>9 Hz), a steady-state signal is generated.

The isolated PERG has three major components that are reliably used to define it. The first is a negative lobe found at about 30 msec (called N1 or N30). This is followed by a positive lobe at about 50 msec (called P1 or P50) and a second negative lobe at about 95 msec (called N2 or N95). In normal eyes, the P1 occurs between 48 and 55 msec, and the N2 occurs between 87 and 100 msec. Normal persons have exquisite symmetry in the waveforms between the two eyes, and amplitude ratios are typically 0.8 to 0.9 in each eye. It is believed that the N2 reflects ganglion cell activity, whereas the P1 reflects outer retinal function. The PERG is abnormal in a variety of retinal and optic nerve disorders.

Focal and Multifocal Electroretinogram (Topographical ERG)

The human ERG recorded at the cornea in response to a full-field stimulus is a mass response generated by cells across the entire retina. Loss of half the retinal photoreceptors across the retina is associated with about a 50% reduction in ERG amplitude. Because the total cone population in the human retina is approximately 7 million, and the number of cones in the macula is at most 440,000, the macula contains only about 7% of the total retinal cone population. The full-field ERG system is thus unable to detect abnormalities confined to the fovea, or macula, because these structures contribute only about 7% to the total signal. Moreover, recording a foveal or macular ERG using conventional full-field equipment is prevented by the scattered light produced by a focal light stimulus that evokes a response from many receptors outside of the tested area. In addition, the macula contains as many rods as cones, and the macular rod response may obscure the contribution from the macular cones.

Focal ERGs that measure macular function can be exceptionally helpful in a neuro-ophthalmologic practice. In our experience, patients with visual loss are frequently referred to the neuro-ophthalmologist by a retinal specialist or general ophthalmologist who can find no abnormalities of the macula or fovea on funduscopic examination or fluorescein angiography. The visual field frequently shows only a mild to modest reduction in foveal threshold or depression in the central field. Because of this, the referring ophthalmologist may suspect that the visual loss is caused by an optic neuropathy or that the patient has nonorganic visual loss. In these cases, a focal ERG using a hand-held device (sometimes called a "maculoscope") that generates a repetitive, small, focused beam of light can be used to distinguish subtle macular dysfunction from optic neuropathies and nonorganic visual loss.

A technique is now available for simultaneously recording ERG signals from a large number of retinal locations (up to 256) (Fig. 1.31). This **topographical ERG** is able to detect localized abnormalities in a variety of retinal diseases, including age-related macular degeneration, macular holes, retinitis pigmentosa, branch retinal artery occlusion, and is especially useful for evaluation of patients with apparently normal clinical retinal examinations.

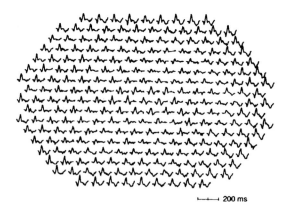

Figure 1.31. Example of a topographic electroretinogram obtained at 255 locations throughout the central 30 degrees of the visual field. (Reprinted from: Sutter EE, Tran D. The field topography of ERG components in man. I. The photopic luminance response. *Vision Res.* 1992;32:433–446, with permission.)

ELECTRO-OCULOGRAM

The human eye acts as a dipole, with the cornea positive with respect to the retina. If two electrodes are placed near the inner and outer canthi respectively, movement of the eye will produce a change in the potential measured between the two electrodes, with the electrode closest to the cornea being more positive. A recording of this potential change produced by movement of the eye is called the electro-oculogram. The EOG consists of two different potentials, one that is sensitive to light, and the other that is insensitive to light.

Under typical recording conditions, the EOG is measured under conditions of dark adaptation after prior exposure to a pre-adapting illumination. The patient is asked to make saccades every second between two stimuli (usually LEDs) spaced approximately 30 degrees apart that are alternately illuminated. These saccadic eye movements produce the change in potential that comprises the EOG signal, with the average of several saccades being taken as the potential at that time. The light-insensitive potential (also called the standing potential) decreases slightly over a period of 8 or 9 minutes, at which time the lowest potential recorded in the dark-adapted state can be measured (the dark trough). Following reexposure to light, the potential gradually increases and reaches its peak in another 10 to 15 minutes (the light peak). The amplitude of the light peak is approximately twice that of the dark trough (light rise of the EOG) in normal persons. Because the standing potential can vary considerably, in part related to the placement of the electrodes, the EOG is most appropriately represented as a ratio of the light peak to the dark trough. This ratio is called the **Arden ratio** and is typically >1.8 in normal persons.

Clinical studies suggest that the retinal pigment epithelium is probably responsible for generating the EOG. The light-sensitive, large, slow, cornea-positive component must depend upon the activity of the photoreceptors and on cells in the inner nuclear layers of the retina, because it is induced by light and can be eliminated by central retinal artery occlusion. Based on studies of the action spectrum of the EOG in both dark-adapted and light-adapted states, as well as the observation that human subjects without rod function may have a large, light-rise response, this response is thought to represent both rod and cone activity. The light-insensitive potential of the EOG provides a way to measure the function of the pigment epithelium without having to stimulate the photoreceptors.

The EOG has limited usefulness in the diagnosis of visual dysfunction. When the EOG is abnormal, the ERG is also usually abnormal. There are four exceptions, however, in which patients may have a normal or nearly normal ERG with an abnormal EOG light-rise to dark-trough ratio. The conditions are (a) butterfly-shaped pigment dystrophy of the fovea, (b) Stargardt's disease (fundus flavimaculatus), (c) advanced drusen, and (d) vitelliform dystrophy or Best's disease. From a neuro-ophthalmologic standpoint, the EOG is more important for the recording and analysis of ocular motility than in diagnosing causes of visual loss.

VISUAL-EVOKED POTENTIAL

If the spontaneous occipital electroencephalogram (EEG) is recorded while brief flashes of light are presented to an eye, changes result in the occipital potential. These changes are called the **visual-evoked potential** (VEP), visual-evoked response (VER), or the visual-evoked cortical potential (VECP). The VEP is thus a gross electric potential of the visual cortex in response to visual stimulation. The VEP is limited mainly to the occipital region of the brain, with an amplitude between 1 and 20 microvolts. The VEP depends on the integrity of the entire visual pathway, although it remains to be determined if its components can truly be separated into anatomic correlates.

Methodology and Interpretation

The VEP is measured by placing scalp electrodes over the occipital region (O_z) of both hemispheres, with reference electrodes attached to the ear (Fig. 1.32). The patient then views the display, typically a xenon-arc photostimulator for flash VEPs and a television screen display with patterned stimuli for pattern VEPs. Recordings of the VEP may be made from either hemisphere with one or both eyes fixating. Typically, 100 to 150 stimulus presentations are generated, and time-locked signal averaging procedures are used to extract the VEP waveform from the spontaneous EEG activity. The amplitude and latency of the waveform are then measured. A flash stimulus is generally used only when no response is produced using a pattern stimulus. Thus, infants and patients with extremely poor acuity, dense media opacities, or poor fixation are most commonly tested with flash VEP.

In most patients, however, a pattern stimulus is preferred for obtaining the VEP, because of the greater clinical utility and more reliable waveform generated with this stimulus. A repetitive pattern of light and dark areas (checkerboards, bar gratings) are phase-reversed every 1 or 2 seconds (Fig. 1.33 top). The pattern VEP is primarily generated from the central 5 degrees of the visual field. Indeed, when the central 3 degrees are occluded (Fig. 1.33 **middle**), there is a dramatic reduction in the amplitude of the pattern VEP, and the waveform almost completely disappears when the central 9 degrees are occluded (Fig. 1.33 **bottom**). These findings are consistent with the anatomic correlates that the central 10 degrees of the visual field is represented by at least 50% to 60% of the posterior striate

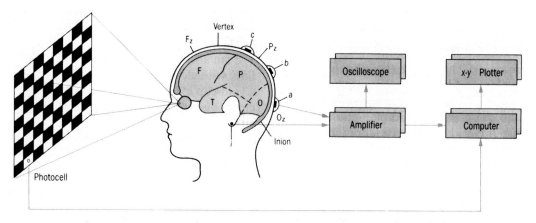

Figure 1.32. Method for generating and recording the visual-evoked potential. (Reprinted from: Fishman GA, Sokol S. *Electrophysiologic Testing in Disorders of the Retina, Optic Nerve, and Visual Pathway.* San Francisco: American Academy of Ophthalmology; 1990, with permission.)

cortex and that the central 30 degrees are represented by about 80% of the cortex (see Chapter 12).

The amplitude of the pattern VEP is affected by a number of different factors. The size of the stimulus pattern can affect the amplitude of the VEP signal,

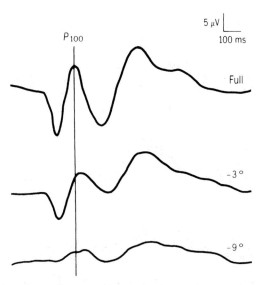

Figure 1.33. Visual-evoked potential waveforms. **Top:** From stimulation of the central 30 degrees visual field. **Middle:** With the central 3 degrees occluded. **Bottom:** With the central 9 degrees occluded. Note that the majority of the waveform is subserved by the central 9 degrees of the visual field. This is consistent with observations that the central 10 degrees of the visual field are represented by at least 50% to 60% of the posterior striate cortex. (Reprinted from: Fishman GA, Sokol S. *Electrophysiologic Testing in Disorders of the Retina, Optic Nerve, and Visual Pathway.* San Francisco: American Academy of Ophthalmology; 1990, with permission.)

as can the rate of alternation of the pattern. At low rates of alternation (1 to 2 reversals per second), the waveform typically contains two negative (N1, N2) and two positive (P1, P2) potentials. This is called the "transient" pattern VEP and is the most commonly used procedure for routine clinical purposes. As the rate of alternation is increased (>6 reversals per second), the response is not able to fully recover between presentations, and only the initial portions of the waveform are observed, similar to the waveforms obtained for ERG with rapidly flickering stimuli. This is called the "steady-state" VEP. The latencies of the first major positive and negative components of the VEP become increasingly delayed with increasing age in adults. Latency of the response is indirectly related to stimulus intensity, but amplitude tends to reach maximum at only moderate stimulus intensities and varies with electrode placement, scalp thickness, etc. Infants and young children have quite variable waveforms and prolonged latencies. The VEP also varies with stimulus size and frequency, attention, mental activity, pupil size, fatigue, state of dark adaptation, color of the stimulus, background illumination, and even the emotional content of the stimulus. All of these factors emphasize the importance of using standardized and optimized test conditions (including the best refractive correction) for clinical VEP testing, as well as establishing age-related normative standards for the procedures employed for each laboratory.

Analysis of the VEP waveform is rather complex. For transient pattern VEPs, the amplitude and latency of the N1, P1, and N2 components are typically measured (Fig. 1.33). For steady-state VEPs, the amplitude and phase of the waveform are measured. The latencies of the pattern VEP are quite consistent both within and among observers, although the amplitudes vary considerably from one person to another. Therefore, the most useful clinical features of the VEP are the latency of its major components and a comparison of the symmetry of the amplitudes between eyes and between hemispheres in the same person.

A more recent development is the use of evoked potentials to map visual field function, the **multifocal VEP.** Electrical responses to pattern reversal stimuli presented pseudo-randomly to the central visual field can be extracted from occipital scalp recordings. This test's clinical usefulness in patients with optic nerve, cerebral and nonorganic visual loss is under investigation.

FOR FURTHER INFORMATION

See *Walsh & Hoyt's Clinical Neuro-Ophthalmology*, 6th edition, Volume 1, Chapter 2, pages 83–149.

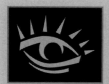

CHAPTER **2**

Anatomy and Physiology of the Retina and Optic Nerve: Distinguishing Retinal from Optic Nerve Disease *

Knowing the anatomy and physiology of the retina and optic nerve is crucial in understanding the similarities and differences in findings in patients with retinal versus optic nerve disease.

ANATOMY AND PHYSIOLOGY OF THE RETINA

The retina is a unique part of the nervous system because it can be visualized, allowing the clinician to observe directly the effects of a wide range of diseases such as an infarction in evolution, deposition of metabolic storage products, or slowing of axoplasmic flow. The retina is also a favorite tissue for study by neuroscientists because it is thin and can be easily dissected from the eye, because its cells are segregated into layers, and because there is at least a fundamental appreciation of its anatomic and physiologic organization.

---

*Adapted from: Rizzo JF III. Embryology, anatomy, and physiology of the afferent visual pathway. In: Miller NR, Newman NJ, Biousse V, Kerrison JB, eds. *Walsh & Hoyt's Clinical Neuro-Ophthalmology.* 6th ed. Vol. I. Philadelphia: Lippincott Williams & Wilkins; 2005:3–82; Sadun AA, Argarwal MR. Topical diagnosis of acquired optic nerve disorders. In: Miller NR, Newman NJ, Biousse V, Kerrison JB, eds. *Walsh & Hoyt's Clinical Neuro-Ophthalmology.* 6th ed. Vol. I. Philadelphia: Lippincott Williams & Wilkins; 2005:197–236.

The cellular structure of the retina is enormously complex. In humans, it contains over 100 million neurons, among which are about 30 different cell types that use at least ten different neurotransmitters. Most architectural schemas underrepresent the intricacy of the retina because the degree to which information is shared among various cells depends on a variety of factors, including the region of the retina being illuminated, the characteristics of the light stimulus, and the state of adaptation of the retina to light. Given this complexity, one might imagine that a large number of symptoms would result from dysfunction of these many cell types. On the contrary, most clinically recognized diseases of the retina are caused by dysfunction of either photoreceptors or retinal ganglion cells.

The human retina covers an area approximately 2,500 mm^2 and extends from the ora serrata to the optic disc (Fig. 2.1). The retina contains six classes of neurons (photoreceptors, horizontal cells, bipolar cells, amacrine cells, interplexiform cells, and ganglion cells) and two types of glial cells (astrocytes and Müller cells) that are arranged into three parallel layers, except in the perifoveal zone, where the retina thins to a single layer (Table 2.1; Figs. 2.2 and 2.3). The human retina is roughly 120 μm thick over most of its area, with a maximum thickness of 230 μm in the macula and a minimum thickness of 100 μm in the foveal pit.

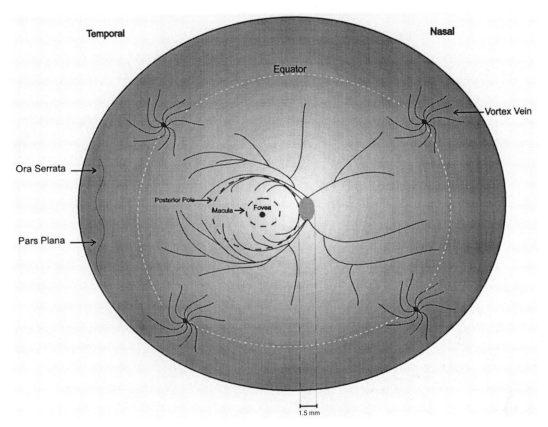

Figure 2.1. Gross anatomy of the retina. Schematic diagram of overall structure of the retina as viewed by funduscopic examination. The width of the optic nerve is indicated at the bottom of the figure.

CELL TYPES AND LAYERS OF THE RETINA

The **retinal pigment epithelium** (RPE) is a monolayer of cells derived from the outer wall of the optic vesicle that is intimately associated with the outer

Table 2.1. *Cellular Organization of the Retina*

Cell Layer	Neuronal and Glial Nuclei
Outer nuclear layer	Photoreceptors
Inner nuclear layer	Horizontal cells
	Bipolar cells
	Interplexiform cells
	Amacrine cells
	Müller cells
Ganglion cell layer	Ganglion cells
	Displaced amacrine cells
	Astrocytes

Reprinted from: Miller NR, Newman NJ. *The Essentials.* 1st ed. Philadelphia: Lippincott Williams and Wilkins; 1999, with permission.

segments of the photoreceptors (Fig. 2.4). The RPE is responsible for several essential functions; most significantly, it (a) is integrally involved in the phototransduction cascade through regeneration of chromophore; (b) provides trophic support for photoreceptors; (c) is a transport barrier between the choriocapillaris and the sensory retina; (d) participates in ocular immune responses; (e) binds reactive oxygen species; and (f) absorbs excess radiation with their melanin granules.

The visual cycle begins when the outer segment of a photoreceptor absorbs a photon, causing isomerization of 11-*cis*-retinol, the dark-adapted form of rhodopsin, to all-*trans*-retinol. This reaction initiates the phototransduction cascade that ultimately influences propagation of nerve impulses through the retina (Fig. 2.5). The 11-*cis*-retinol must be continuously regenerated to maintain the ability of the photoreceptors to respond to light, and this regeneration is performed by the RPE. Patients in whom regeneration of photopigment is abnormally slow have a prolonged recovery of central vision following exposure of the retina to bright light. This phenomenon, which is present in patients with various macular dystrophies, age-related macular

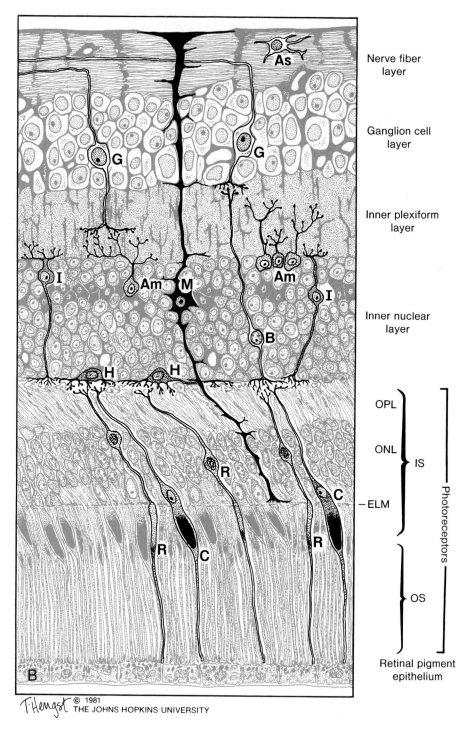

Nerve fiber layer

Ganglion cell layer

Inner plexiform layer

Inner nuclear layer

OPL

ONL

IS

ELM

OS

Photoreceptors

Retinal pigment epithelium

© 1981
THE JOHNS HOPKINS UNIVERSITY

Figure 2.2. Cellular components of the fully developed primate retina, showing cellular relationships and major synaptic interactions. *OPL,* outer plexiform layer; *ONL,* outer nuclear layer; *ELM,* external limiting membrane; *OS,* outer segment; *As,* astrocyte; *G,* ganglion cell; *Am,* amacrine cell; *I,* interplexiform cell; *H,* horizontal cell; *B,* bipolar cell; *C,* cone; *R,* rod; *M,* Müller cell. The photoreceptor nuclei lie in the ONL, and a large stretch of the photoreceptors consists of their outer segments, which lie proximal (i.e., nearer to the retinal pigment epithelium) to their nuclei. The outer segments contain chromophore, which captures the energy from incoming light and initiates the ionic exchange that hyperpolarizes the photoreceptors. The inner segments of photoreceptors (not labeled) are the segments between the outer segments and the nucleus that contain a high concentration of mitochondria and endoplasmic reticulum.

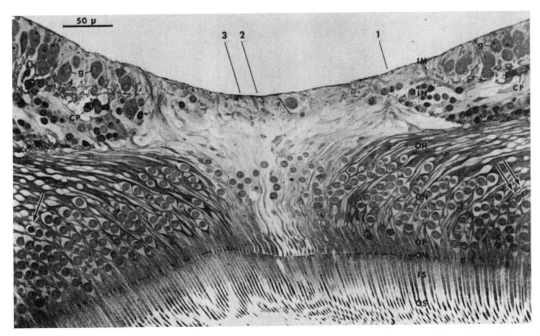

Figure 2.3. Section through center of fovea. Nuclei of rod receptor cells are indicated by arrows. Remaining receptor cells are foveal cone cells. *OS,* outer nuclear layer; *OF,* outer cone fiber; *OH,* outer fiber layer of Henle; *IN,* inner nuclear layer; *g,* ganglion cell; *CP,* capillary; *IM,* internal limiting membrane; *IS,* inner segment; *OM,* outer limiting membrane; *ON,* outer nuclear layer. (Reduced from ×400.) (Reprinted from: Yamada E. Some structural features of the fovea centralis in the human retina. *Arch Ophthalmol.* 1969;82:151–159, with permission.)

degeneration, and central serous chorioretinopathy, can be detected clinically by performing a photostress test (see Chapter 1).

The second primary function of the RPE—membrane renewal—is just as important as RPE's role in phototransduction. Outer segments of rods and cones are shed on a daily basis. The outer segment of a human rod is entirely replaced over a period of 10 days and, although the timing of cone shedding is more variable, the involvement of the RPE in this process of shedding and renewal is integral. Disruption of the interaction between the RPE and the photoreceptors can lead to retinal degeneration, as occurs in hydroxychloroquine toxicity.

The **photoreceptor cells** of the retina are the sensory transducers for the visual system. They convert electromagnetic energy (i.e., light) into a neural signal. The photoreceptors contain visual pigments that, by absorbing photons of light, initiate the phototransduction process. These pigments have evolved to absorb within the range of electromagnetic wavelengths that pass through the cornea and lens, generally between 400 and 700 nm. The two types of photoreceptors are the **rods** and the **cones.**

Photoreceptors have inner and outer segments, both of which are located outside the boundary of the outer limiting membrane (Fig. 2.6). The inner segment

contains the **ellipsoid,** a structure that is richly endowed with mitochondria. The ellipsoid is responsible for the high level of oxidative metabolism that occurs in photoreceptors. The **myoid** is the region between the ellipsoid and the nucleus of the photoreceptor. This region contains numerous cellular organelles. The outer segment is connected to the inner segment by a cilium, which contains nine pairs of microtubules arranged in a pattern that is characteristic of nonmotile cilia.

Rods contain rhodopsin, a molecule that is composed of the apoprotein, opsin, and 11-*cis*-retinol. Rhodopsin is present in very high concentrations within the membranes of the outer segment discs, which are oriented vertically to maximize capture of incident photons. Activation of the phototransduction cascade causes an intracellular decline in cyclic guanidine monophosphate (GMP) concentration within the rod outer segment, followed by closure of the cyclic GMP-gated cation channel and cessation of inflow of extracellular cations that normally generates the dark current. The rod becomes hyperpolarized upon exposure to light, which decreases the amount of neurotransmitter released at the synaptic terminal.

Vitamin A is used in the process of phototransduction and regeneration of photopigment. Vitamin A must be replenished from the circulation, and failure to do so can result in retinopathy. Because rods are

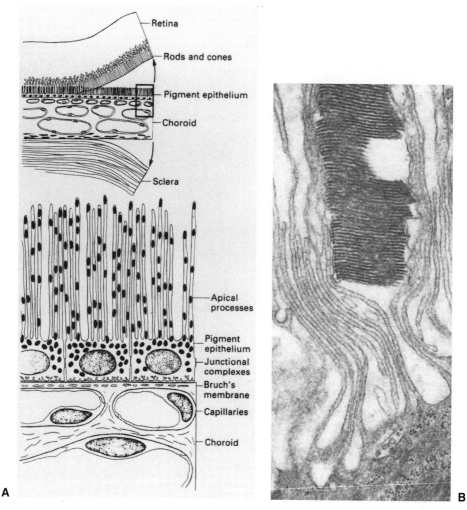

Figure 2.4. The bullfrog retina and retinal pigment epithelium (RPE). **A:** The relation between the RPE and neural retina **(top left).** Detailed drawing of the RPE and choroid **(bottom left).** The basic features of the mammalian RPE, including a convoluted basal membrane (adjacent to Bruch's membrane), junctions between cells, and apical processes, are similar to those illustrated here. (Reprinted from: Hughes BA, Steinberg RH. Voltage-dependent currents in isolated cells of the frog retinal pigment epithelium. *J Physiol.* 1990;428:273–297, with permission.) **B:** Electron micrograph showing longitudinal section of retinal pigment epithelial cell projections enveloping photoreceptor outer segments. (Reprinted from: Anderson DH, Fisher SK. The relationship of primate fovea cones to the pigment epithelium. *J Ultrastruct Res.* 1979;67:23–32, with permission.)

predominately affected in retinopathy caused by deficiency of vitamin A, **nyctalopia** (night blindness) is usually the initial manifestation of this disorder. Hypovitaminosis A is a highly significant problem in developing countries but also occurs in persons who live in developed countries but who have malabsorption syndromes or liver disease, or who adhere to restrictive diets.

Cones also contain 11-*cis*-retinol but have different apoproteins than rods. The variation of the opsin moieties produces three different spectral response curves corresponding to the blue, green, and red cones, which

are more appropriately called short (S-), medium (M-), and long (L-) wavelength cones to emphasize that their responsiveness is not limited to a single color but rather is spread across a portion of the visible spectrum. Congenital color blindness almost always results from defects in either the red or green photopigment gene, both of which are located on the X chromosome.

Humans have a cone:rod ratio of approximately 1:20, with each retina containing 140 million rods and 7 million cones. About 50% of the cones are located within the central 30 degrees of the visual field, an area

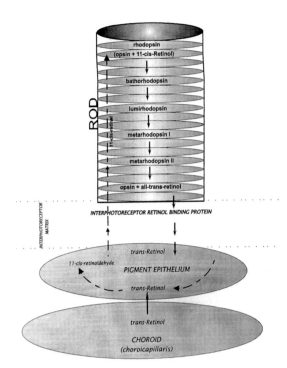

Figure 2.5. Phototransduction cascade. Schematic drawing of junction of rod, retinal pigment epithelium, and choroid to show the interrelationship among those structures required to regenerate photopigment. *trans*-Retinol is carried by the blood to the choriocapillaris where it can then enter the retinal pigment epithelium and contribute to the cycle.

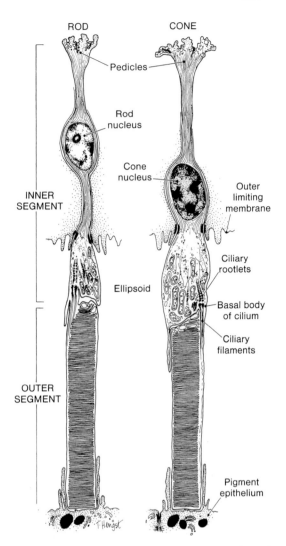

Figure 2.6. Ultrastructure of photoreceptors. Schematic drawing of photoreceptor cells showing the relationship of the inner and outer segments. The ellipsoid is located at the apex of the inner segment. (Reprinted from: Hogan MJ, Alvarado JA, Weddell JC. *Histology of the Human Eye: An Atlas and Textbook.* Philadelphia: WB Saunders; 1971, with permission.)

that roughly corresponds to the size of the macula. Rods are absent in the fovea and are in highest density in an elliptical ring, the center of which is the optic nerve head. There is an age-related decline in the number of rods in the human retina, with an annual loss of about 0.2% to 0.4%.

The density of foveal cones poses a problem in regard to their forward connections because their synaptic terminals (called cone pedicles) and the ganglion cells to which they connect have larger diameters than the cone inner segments themselves. Thus, each foveal ganglion cell soma is displaced away from the site of the cone that initiates its visual response. This realignment is accomplished by the nerve fiber layer of Henle, an elongation of cones and rods between their nuclei and synaptic terminals.

The **"midget"** system refers to the anatomic pattern of cone outflow within the most central retina, although there is no specific boundary beyond which the midget pathway cannot be found. The midget system provides the most direct communication of spatial detail from the outer to inner retina. In this system, output from one cone passes to one ON-center

and one OFF-center bipolar cell with each bipolar cell connecting in turn to a single ON- **or** OFF-center ganglion cell. Thus, the divergence of signal from a foveal cone to a ganglion cell is 1:2. In the peripheral retina, by comparison, there is marked convergence of information from outer to inner retina, with perhaps up to 1,500 rods influencing the function of one ganglion cell.

The **outer plexiform layer** (OPL) is the zone of synaptic connection between cells whose nuclei are

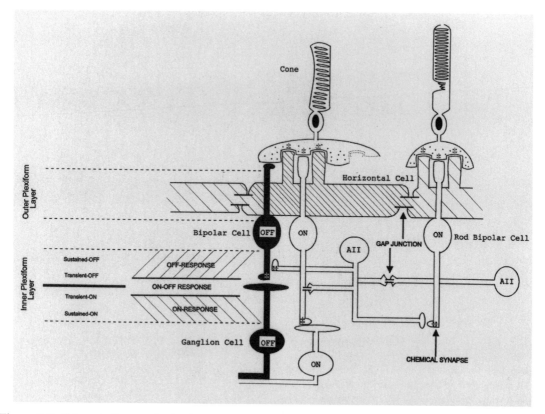

Figure 2.7. Schematic diagram of rod and cone through pathways to the retinal ganglion cells. Both cone pedicles and rod spherules have flat and invaginating surfaces upon which bipolar and horizontal cells make contact within the outer plexiform layer. AII amacrine cells and bipolar cells contact one another within the inner plexiform layer, which is subdivided into zones that contain synapses of either ON-center or OFF-center cells. Sites of chemical (i.e., ribbon) synapses and gap junctions between cells are labeled or indicated by symbols (=, gap junction; :|:, chemical synapse). *AII,* AII amacrine cell.

in the outer and inner nuclear layers. Cone pedicles and rod spherules, the synaptic specializations of cones and rods, respectively, have several invaginations into which processes of horizontal and bipolar cells extend, creating "triads" of one bipolar cell and two horizontal cells (Fig. 2.7).

The retina contains two types of **horizontal cells.** The HII cell, the smaller of the two types, makes dendritic contact with cones and axon contact with rods, whereas both ends of the HII cell synapse only with cones. Horizontal cells seem to provide the anatomic substrate for the center-surround response characteristics observed in the physiologic recordings made from ganglion cells and some other inner retinal neurons. Specifically, the response of a ganglion cell to light that falls within the center of its receptive field is opposite to that which occurs to light that falls in the surround (i.e., the portion of the receptive field beyond the center) (Fig. 2.8). The antagonistic center-surround organization emphasizes contrast within the visual scene, which enhances spatial resolution.

Bipolar cells receive input from photoreceptors and provide output to both amacrine cells and ganglion cells. Some bipolar cells receive input from rods, others from cones. Rod bipolar cells are the target of an apparent paraneoplastic immune attack in some patients with cutaneous malignant melanoma, so-called melanoma-associated retinopathy. The physiologic consequence of destruction of these cells is loss of the scotopic b-wave of the electroretinogram (ERG).

The major excitatory neurotransmitter in the retina is glutamate, and this substance has a profound effect at the level of the bipolar cells. There are two physiologic types of bipolar cells: hyperpolarizing (OFF-center cells) and depolarizing (ON-center cells). These bipolar cells respond differently to changes in the ambient glutamate concentration within the outer plexiform layer. Release of glutamate by photoreceptors initiates two opposing but parallel signals to the inner retina (Fig 2.9).

Amacrine cells are so-named because they lack axons. Their cell bodies are located primarily in the inner

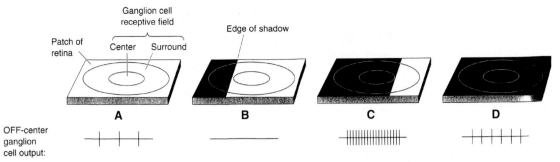

OFF-center
ganglion
cell output:

Figure 2.8. Center-surround organization of retinal ganglion cell receptive fields, and the resultant output of a ganglion cell in response to a light-dark border falling within its receptive field. Depicted is an OFF center ganglion cell, which responds most vigorously when a dark spot precisely fills its receptive field center. The responsiveness of the cell is diminished by darkness that covers its surround. The output in **(A)** is the resting, basal level of spontaneous action potentials, which are a characteristic feature of all retinal ganglion cells. In **(B)**, the output is decreased because the darkness falls only across the inhibitory surround. In **(C)**, the responsiveness is greatly enhanced because darkness fills the excitatory center of this OFF cell. In **(D)**, the cellular output is above the basal level of activity because the receptive field center is filled by darkness, despite the fact that the entire surround is also covered by darkness. (Reprinted from: Bear MF, Connors BW, Paradiso MA. *Neuroscience. Exploring the Brain.* 2nd ed. Baltimore: Lippincott Williams & Wilkins; 2001:306, with permission.)

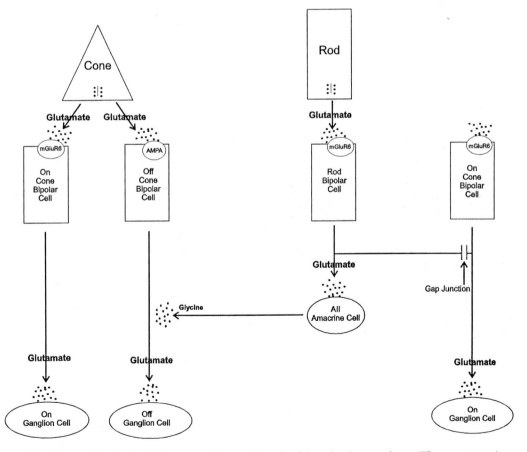

Figure 2.9. Schematic illustration of neurotransmitters used by cells of the rod and cone pathways. The neurotransmitters are released within the outer and inner plexiform layers. The mGluR6 and AMPA receptors of the bipolar cells are also depicted. The former uses a G protein to control the intracellular concentration of cGMP that, in turn, regulates the Na^+-Ca^{2+}-cGMP-gated ion channel.

nuclear layer of the retina. Some amacrine cells are interneurons between bipolar and ganglion cells. Others connect to fellow amacrine cells, forming a lateral pathway within the inner plexiform layer similar to that formed by horizontal cells in the outer plexiform layer (Fig. 2.2). There are numerous subtypes of amacrine cells.

The cell bodies of the **interplexiform cells** reside in the inner plexiform layer. These cells are postsynaptic to amacrine and bipolar cells in the inner plexiform layer and presynaptic to horizontal and bipolar cells in the outer plexiform layer. This cell thus appears to be unique in that it apparently conveys information from the inner to the outer plexiform layer, against the standard direction of neural transmission within the retina.

The retina contains several types of glial cells that have various functions. The most important are Müller cells and astrocytes. Müller cell somas are located in the inner nuclear layer, but processes from these cells extend throughout the entire retina (Fig. 2.2). The apical processes of **Müller cells** form the outer limiting membrane by making junctional complexes with one another and with photoreceptors. On the vitread side, apposed Müller cell end-feet form the inner limiting membrane. Lateral extensions from Müller cells contact neurons within cellular layers, synapses within plexiform layers, axons within the nerve fiber layer, and blood vessels.

Despite all their connections, Müller cells are not in the direct pathway of neural signal transfer. However, they exert substantial influence over signal transmission by (a) maintaining the local extracellular environment needed for proper neuronal function, particularly with respect to the extracellular concentration of potassium; (b) adjusting concentrations of extracellular neurotransmitters; and (c) possibly buffering pH levels.

Astrocytes are found only on the vitread side of the retina, within the nerve fiber and ganglion cell layers. Two morphologic types of astrocytes develop from stem cells in the optic nerve. Each cell type preferentially contacts either nerve fiber bundles or blood vessels. Oligodendrocytes are not present in the primate retina, which is consistent with the absence of myelin in these retinas. However, the observation of myelinated nerve fibers in the retinas of about 0.5% of normal persons suggests that such a migration can occur during, and even after, development (see Chapter 3).

The **inner plexiform layer** (IPL), which is much thicker than the outer plexiform layer, is the zone of synaptic connection of bipolar and amacrine cells to ganglion cells. The IPL can be divided into sublaminae a and b. Sublamina a is the more proximal layer. It is nearer the inner nuclear layer and is the zone in which bipolar, amacrine, and ganglion cells of the OFF-center pathway synapse. Sublamina b is the more distal layer. It is nearer the ganglion cell layer and is the site of synaptic connections for the ON-center cell pathway (Fig. 2.7).

The **retinal ganglion cell layer** is, in fact, composed not only of retinal ganglion cells but also of "displaced" amacrine cells, astrocytes, endothelial cells, and pericytes. The human retina contains about 1.2 million retinal ganglion cells, although there is a very wide interindividual variability. It has been calculated that 69% of the ganglion cells in the human retina subserve the central 30 degrees of the visual field and are located adjacent to the fovea. The distribution of retinal ganglion cells with respect to the Goldmann visual field map is shown in Figure 2.10.

Dendrites of ganglion cells branch in well-defined strata within the IPL, and the specific region of stratification varies with the particular cell type. ON-center and OFF-center ganglion cells have dendrites that terminate in sublamina b or a of the IPL, respectively (Fig. 2.7). Retinal ganglion cell axons terminate in either the magnocellular or parvocellular layers of the lateral geniculate nucleus (LGN), and this also depends on the cell type. In the primate retina, there may be as many as 10 or more subpopulations of ganglion cells.

Retinal ganglion cells can be subdivided into two main types based on cell size. About 80% of the cells are small cells that are called "beta" or "P" cells, for **parvocellular** cells. These cells, as their name implies, synapse in the parvocellular layers of the LGN. From 5% to 10% of primate retinal ganglion cells are large cells that are called "alpha" or "M" cells, for **magnocellular** cells. The axons of these cells synapse in the magnocellular layers of the LGN. Together, the P and M ganglion cells comprise 85% to 90% of all primate retinal ganglion cells. The ganglion cells that remain are present in small numbers, are less studied, and may have functions other than for visual perception, such as the pupillary light reflex and the retinohypothalamic pathway, the latter of which is believed to be an integral part of the pathway that regulates circadian functions.

From a clinical standpoint, the P- and M-cells have great significance. The P-cells are color-opponent (i.e., the center of the receptive field is maximally responsive to either red or green light, whereas the inverse is true for the surround), have small receptive fields, and have low sensitivity to contrast in the visual scene. Color-opponency is generated by connections at both the OPL and IPL. The receptive field center of P ganglion cells near the fovea approximately equals the diameter of a single cone. These cells have linear response characteristics, meaning that their firing rate is proportional to the degree to which the center of the

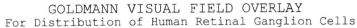

GOLDMANN VISUAL FIELD OVERLAY
For Distribution of Human Retinal Ganglion Cells

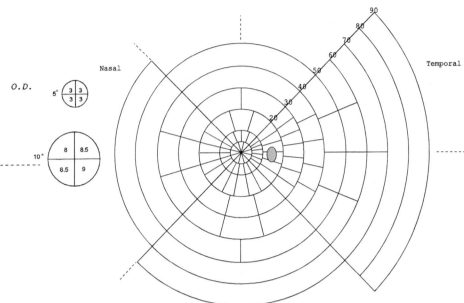

Figure 2.10. Visual field overlay for the distribution of the human retinal ganglion cells for perimetry using a Goldmann perimeter. Each sector of the map equals 1% of the total number of cells. An inset **(left)** has been provided to assist in counting of boxes when a field defect involves the central region. The blind spot is included for orientation only and should not influence the counting of boxes when field defects involve the peripapillary region. The hatched lines extending from the meridia in the nasal quadrants are a reminder that a relatively small number of ganglion cells (<1%) are present beyond the superior, inferior, and nasal borders of the map. (Map constructed by Drs. Joseph F. Rizzo and Anthony C. Castelbuono, using original data from Curcio CA, Allen KA. Topography of ganglion cells in human retina. *J Comp Neurol.* 1990;300:5–25.)

receptive field is stimulated or inhibited. Cells with this response property are also called "X" cells. Given these characteristics, the P-cells are probably the major neural input to the optic nerve for visual functions such as central (i.e., Snellen) acuity, color vision, and fine stereopsis.

The M-cells are spectrally "broad-band." Because of the combined input to these ganglion cells from all three cone types, their peak responsiveness at a given intensity of light is not determined by the wavelength. M-cells have much larger receptive fields and are more responsive to luminance contrast than P-cells. The majority of M-cells have nonlinear responses to light. These cells typically show spikes of activity in response to changes in the visual scene rather than showing activity that is proportional to the intensity of light and that matches the duration of light stimulation, which is the case with P-cells. M-cells with this physiologic profile are also called "Y" cells to distinguish their responses from the X-like response profile of P-cells. Lesions of the magnocellular pathway in monkeys impair high-temporal-frequency flicker and motion perception.

Most retinal ganglion cells have several physiologic properties in common. First, their receptive fields have a concentric and antagonistic center-surround organization. This property is probably derived at least in part from the effect of the lateral inhibition of horizontal, and possibly amacrine, cells. Second, most ganglion cells respond either in an on or off manner to change in the luminance contrast or spectral distribution of light within their receptive field centers (Fig. 2.8). This property is reflected in the location of dendritic ramification within the IPL. ON-center bipolar and ganglion cells ramify in sublamina b of the IPL, whereas OFF-center bipolar and ganglion cells ramify in sublamina a (Fig. 2.7). Third, the responses to light of most ganglion cells are either sustained or transient, depending on the pattern of interconnections with amacrine cells within the IPL (Fig. 2.11). Fourth, ganglion cells with sustained responses also show linearity of spatial summation; that is, the magnitude of their response is proportional to the degree of illumination within the center of the receptive field. In contrast, transiently responding ganglion cells briefly increase or decrease their firing

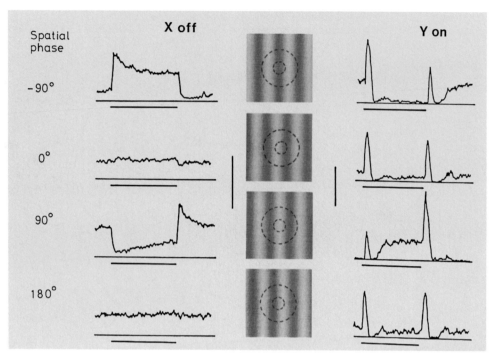

Figure 2.11. Firing-rate records from a cat retinal OFF-center X-cell **(left)** and an ON-center Y-cell **(right)** responding to the appearance and disappearance of a sine-wave grating in different positions. The pictures in the middle show the positions of the stimulus pattern in relation to the receptive field during the period in which the pattern was present (1.1 second of every 2.2 second as marked by the bar under each record). When the pattern disappeared, the stimulus screen remained at the same mean luminance. Note that the Y-cell generates a transient excitatory response at both the appearance and disappearance of the stimulus pattern, regardless of its position. The vertical scale bar corresponds to a firing rate of 100 impulses/sec. (Reprinted from: Enroth-Cugell C, Robson JG. Functional characteristics and diversity of cat retinal ganglion cells. *Invest Ophthalmol Visual Sci.* 1984;25:250–267, with permission.)

rates in response to a change in illumination. Lastly, retinal ganglion cells maintain a continuous spontaneous discharge. This activity requires considerable energy but presumably has the advantage of allowing the cell to reflect more precisely the degree of illumination by either increasing or decreasing its firing rate.

It should be emphasized that the two largest classes of retinal ganglion cells (the P- and M-cells) do not alter their mean firing rate in response to a change in the overall level of light striking the retina. Rather, they respond to differences in **contrast** between the center and surround of its receptive field. Hence, it is likely that neither cell type drives the pupillomotor responses to light.

The **axon** of a retinal ganglion cell is relatively long, and the body of the ganglion cell is the sole site for production of the components needed to maintain the health of the axon. The axon is a dynamic structure that requires nearly constant repair of its membranes, a process that is partly achieved by transport of proteins, enzymes, and other subcellular components (including

mitochondria) to, and detritus from, sites up to the synapse.

Axon transport is bidirectional and simultaneous, with velocities that can be broadly divided into fast (i.e., hundreds of mm/day) and slow (<10 mm/day). Slow anterograde transport, which largely carries components that remain within the cell such as cytoskeletal proteins, constitutes the bulk (about 85%) of all movement within the axon. At least five different classes of proteins are transported at different velocities within retinal ganglion cells, and these relationships vary during development. Fast anterograde transport is used to carry neurotransmitter-containing vesicles. Retrograde transport, which is less well understood, proceeds at roughly half the maximum velocity of anterograde transport. It returns to the cell body substances that have been taken into the cell at its terminal synapse. Axon transport, whether anterograde or retrograde, is highly energy dependent, and the adenosine triphosphate (ATP) needed to sustain it is supplied by mitochondria that are distributed along the entire length of the axon.

The final common defect in pathologic swelling of the optic disc from almost any etiology is disruption of anterograde axonal transport of the retinal ganglion cells at the lamina cribrosa (see Chapter 4). The degree to which fast versus slow transport is disrupted probably varies according to the etiology.

Axons of retinal ganglion cells synapse in the LGN, mesencephalon, pretectum, or one of several nuclei in the hypothalamus. The specific site of termination of the axon is related to the anatomy of the ganglion cell body. Generally, P- and M-cell axons synapse in the parvocellular and magnocellular layers, respectively. ON-center and OFF-center ganglion cells appear to remain functionally separated at the level of the LGN, although both channels converge at the visual cortex.

The **nerve fiber layer** (NFL) of the retina is composed of axons of ganglion cells, astrocytes, components of Müller cells, and a very small number of efferent fibers to the retina, the functions of which are unknown. The NFL is thinnest in the peripheral retina and thickest adjacent to the superior and inferior margins of the optic disc, where it measures about 200 μm in humans. The temporal and nasal NFL adjacent to the optic disc is about one-tenth as thick.

The gross organization of the NFL is characterized by three main features. The first is the papillomacular bundle, which contains nerve fibers originating from ganglion cells in the foveal area. Papillomacular fibers from ganglion cells on the nasal side of the fovea project directly to the optic disc, whereas those from ganglion cells on the temporal side of the fovea arch around the nasal fibers en route to the optic nerve (Fig. 2.12). The relatively early formation of the central retina relative to the peripheral retina gives rise to the second feature: the arching of axons from midperipheral and peripheral ganglion cells temporal to the fovea around the previously formed papillomacular bundle. A watershed line called the temporal raphe is present on the temporal side of the fovea, and this horizontal demarcation separates axons in the superior temporal retina from those in the inferior temporal retina. The raphe creates not only an anatomic separation but also a physiologic separation between the superior and inferior regions of the temporal retina. The third anatomic feature of the NFL is the radial distribution of nerve fibers that enter the nasal aspect of the optic disc.

The temporal-nasal demarcation of the retina (and, thus, the visual field) is a vertical line that passes through the **fovea,** not the optic disc. Fibers from ganglion cells located nasal to the fovea cross to the opposite side within the optic chiasm, whereas fibers from ganglion cells located temporal to the fovea remain uncrossed, passing through the chiasm into the ipsilateral optic tract. This vertical meridian, although

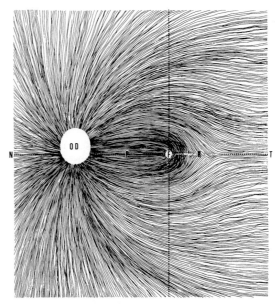

Figure 2.12. Drawing of the retinal nerve axons as they extend from the ganglion cells to the disc. The axons arising from ganglion cells in the nasal macula project directly toward the optic disc *(OD)* and comprise part of the papillomacular bundle *(P)*. Axons from ganglion cells of the temporal macula have a slight arching pattern around the nasal macular axons. They form the remainder of the papillomacular bundle. Axons from nonmacular ganglion cells that are nasal to the fovea *(F)* have a straight or gently curved course to the optic disc, whereas axons from ganglion cells temporal to the fovea must arch around the papillomacular bundle and enter the disc at its superior and inferior poles. Note that the superior and inferior portions of the temporal retina are delineated by an anatomic landmark, the temporal raphe *(R)*. The dotted lines delineate the nasal *(N)*, temporal *(T)*, superior, and inferior portions of the retina. Note that the temporal and nasal parts of the retina are defined by a vertical line through the fovea, not the optic disc. (Redrawn from: Hogan MJ, Alvarado JA, Weddell JE. *Histology of the Human Eye. An Atlas and Textbook.* Philadelphia: WB Saunders; 1971.)

reasonably precise from a clinical standpoint, is inexact at a cellular level. There is a small area of nasotemporal overlap on either side of the vertical meridian in which some axons from ganglion cells temporal to the fovea cross within the chiasm, and some axons from ganglion cells nasal to the fovea remain uncrossed. However, the mere presence of an overlap may have no significant visual consequences. A ganglion cell that is located on one side of the fovea does not necessarily receive input from a photoreceptor that is located on the same side. The much larger width of the cone pedicle compared with the foveal cone soma creates a packing problem that is only partly resolved by lateral displacement of cone pedicles and via the nerve fiber layer of Henle. This lateral shift could theoretically connect photoreceptors on one side of the vertical meridian to seemingly displaced ganglion cells on the opposite side. Such an anatomic relationship would have no adverse visual consequences, because it is the position of the photoreceptor and not the ganglion cell body that provides spatial cues to the brain.

There is, in addition to the specific arrangement of fibers in the NFL described above, an orderly arrangement of the fibers in the third dimension—that is, with respect to their vertical orientation as viewed in cross-section. The nerve fibers are generally stratified such that axons from ganglion cells in the peripheral retina occupy a position adjacent to the ganglion cell layer, whereas axons from ganglion cells located more centrally lie more superficially in the NFL, adjacent to the vitreoretinal interface. To achieve this arrangement, fibers from increasingly central ganglion cells must cross fibers from more peripheral ganglion cells. This arrangement is maintained until the fibers are near the optic disc, at which point there is significant intermingling of more central axons with those that originated peripherally. Nevertheless, near the disc margin, most of the axons with a long course (i.e., from peripheral ganglion cells) are located deep within the NFL, whereas axons with a short course (i.e., from central ganglion cells) are located superficially. This arrangement results in the longest axons being positioned in the periphery of the anterior optic disc and axons from more central ganglion cells being located more centrally in the anterior optic disc.

Table 2.2 provides a list of known neurotransmitters for the major classes of retinal cells, and Figure 2.9 shows some of the neurotransmitters used by the intraretinal cone and rod through pathways.

RETINAL BLOOD VESSELS

The human retina receives its essential nutrients—oxygen and glucose—from both the retinal and the choroidal circulations. The border between these circulations is near the outer plexiform layer. The choroidal circulation supplies the photoreceptors; the retinal arteries supply the inner retina, although the latter do not enter a small area composed of the fovea and a varying degree of perifoveal retina. This avascular area is called the **foveal avascular zone.** There is considerable inter-individual variation in the size of the foveal avascular zone. In addition, the degree to which the inner retina is vascularized appears to correlate with the degree of oxidative metabolic demand, rather than with the thickness of the retina.

The retinal vasculature is organized into specific laminae. Generally, four planes of capillaries can be recognized. The two more vitread layers bracket the inner nuclear layer, whereas the two other layers are located more superficially. Superficial retinal capillaries in humans can probably nourish ganglion cell bodies up to 45 μm away.

Retinal blood vessels are barrier vessels, analogous to the blood-brain barrier elsewhere within the central nervous system. These vessels are impermeable to particles larger than 2 nm. Astrocytes and pericytes almost certainly play a role in maintaining this nonspecific low permeability for capillaries within the nerve fiber layer, whereas Müller cells probably play a similar role within deeper retina. The blood-retinal barrier is maintained not only by physical factors, such as the cells surrounding the retinal capillaries described above, but also by chemical factors. Specifically, autoregulation of retinal (and choroidal) blood vessels may be at least partially controlled chemically by hormonal products of the local vascular endothelium. These substances include vasodilators, such as nitric oxide and prostaglandins, and vasoconstrictors, particularly endothelin and the products of the renin-angiotensin system that are produced and released via angiotensin-converting enzyme, which is located on the endothelial cell membrane. Additionally, adenosine and α_1-adrenergic receptors in retinal blood vessels have been shown to mediate vasodilation and vasoconstriction, respectively.

Table 2.2. *Retinal Neurons and Some of Their Associated Neurotransmitters*

Cell Type	Neurotransmitter		
Photoreceptors	Glutamate		
Horizontal cells	GABA		
Bipolar cells:			
ON-center (depolarizing)	Glutamate		
OFF-center (hyperpolarizing)	Glutamate		
Interplexiform cells	Dopamine	GABA	
Amacrine cells	Acetylcholine	GABA	Dopamine
	Glycine	Peptides	

Reprinted from: Miller NR, Newman NJ. *The Essentials.* 1st ed. Philadelphia: Lippincott Williams and Wilkins; 1999, with permission.

ROD AND CONE THROUGH PATHWAYS: FUNCTIONAL CONSIDERATIONS

The complex anatomic and physiologic features of the retina combine to produce a well-defined reaction when the retina is stimulated with light. Light causes the photoreceptors to hyperpolarize, decreasing the release of glutamate from both rod and cone synaptic terminals. Horizontal cells then become hyperpolarized, suppressing the light response of the photoreceptors. Rod and cone outputs then diverge. Rod signals are transmitted to the rod bipolar cells via a sign-inverting signal. Thus, bipolar cells depolarize in response to light. The signal is then carried via the axons of the rod bipolar cells to sublamina b of the IPL, where there is a sign-conserving synapse on amacrine cells. (Rod bipolar cells do not make direct contact with ganglion cells.) The amacrine cells make gap junctions with cone-depolarizing bipolar cells, the axon terminals of which also ramify in sublamina b of the IPL, where the terminal of the amacrine cells contact ON-center ganglion cells via a conventional synapse. The amacrine cells also make conventional synapses on cone-hyperpolarizing bipolar cells through sign-reversing glycinergic synapses, and these bipolar cells terminate in sublamina a of the IPL and then make contact with OFF-center ganglion cells.

Cone output in the central retina uses the midget system of interconnections in which one foveal cone contacts two bipolar cells, each of which then contacts a single ganglion cell. A sign-conserving synapse is made on a cone-hyperpolarizing (OFF-center) bipolar cell, and a sign-conserving synapse is made with a cone-depolarizing (ON-center) bipolar cell. The two bipolar cells then terminate in the proximal (sublamina a) and distal (sublamina b) laminae of the IPL, respectively, wherein they make contact with an OFF-center (sublamina a) or an ON-center (sublamina b) ganglion cell. From this location, visual information is passed to the brain via the optic nerve. Visual information (i.e., spatial detail, color, contrast) is presented in parallel fashion to the brain, with major physiologic cell types in the retina, generally maintaining anatomic segregation at the LGN.

ANATOMY AND PHYSIOLOGY OF THE OPTIC NERVE

The **optic nerve** is not really a nerve, as are the peripheral nerves. It is a part of the central nervous system. As such, it is a tract, and its axons are myelinated by oligodendrocytes, not Schwann cells. The optic nerve carries about 1.2 million axons whose cell bodies are the retinal ganglion cells and which synapse in one or more of at least eight primary visual nuclei.

Common nomenclature considers only the anterior portion of this retinofugal fiber projection to be the

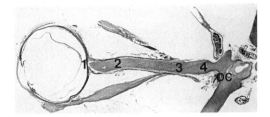

Figure 2.13. Histologic section showing the four topographic sections of the normal optic nerve. 1: intraocular. 2: intraorbital. 3: intracanalicular. 4: intracranial. *OC:* optic chiasm. (Reprinted from: Hogan MJ, Zimmerman LE. *Ophthalmic Pathology. An Atlas and Textbook.* Philadelphia: WB Saunders; 1962, with permission.)

optic nerve. The optic chiasm is the site of a partial decussation of these fibers, and the optic tract is the posterior continuation of the same fiber tract to its termination in the LGN.

The optic nerve is about 50 mm long (Fig. 2.13), although there is some individual variation in length, especially with regard to its posterior half. It may be described as having four parts: (i) the intraocular portion (the optic nerve head); (ii) the intraorbital portion; (iii) the intraosseous portion within the optic canal; and (iv) the intracranial portion. The intraocular optic nerve can be further divided into three anatomically distinct zones: the retinal or prelaminar portion (anterior), the choroidal or laminar portion (middle), and the scleral or retrolaminar portion (posterior). These zones have very different microanatomic arrangements.

OPTIC NERVE HEAD (INTRAOCULAR OPTIC NERVE)

Axons of the retinal ganglion cells form bundles that constitute the nerve fiber layer, which converges like spokes of a wheel at the optic nerve head. The optic nerve head is about 1 mm long (anterior–posterior); its diameter is 1.5 mm horizontally by 1.8 mm vertically at the level of the retina and a little wider in the retrolaminar space. It is a major zone of transition, because nerve fibers pass from an area of high tissue pressure within the eye to a zone of low pressure that correlates with the intracranial pressure. At the same time, the nerve fibers leave an area in which their blood supply is from the central retinal artery alone to zones supplied by other branches of the ophthalmic artery. In addition, the axons become myelinated immediately at the posterior end of the optic nerve head.

The optic nerve head is composed of four types of cells: ganglion cell axons, astrocytes, capillary-associated cells, and fibroblasts. It also includes an oval grouping of 200 to 300 holes that perforate the choroid and sclera, forming a specialized structure called the **lamina cribrosa,** through which all retinal axons pass to exit the eye.

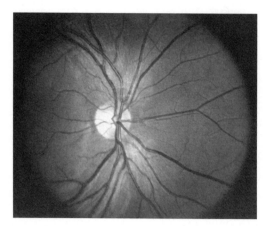

Figure 2.14. Appearance of the "disc at risk." Note that the optic disc is smaller than normal and has no central cup.

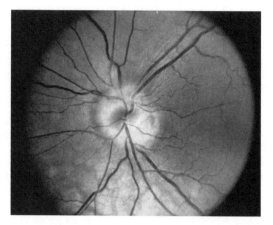

Figure 2.16. Appearance of a tilted optic disc. The elevated superior portion of the disc simulates optic disc swelling. Note inferior conus.

The anterior surface of the optic nerve head is the clinically visible **optic disc.** The appearance of the disc depends on two important features: the size of the scleral canal and the angle of exit of the canal from the eye. The size of the canal varies somewhat among individuals; however, the volume of tissue passing through the hole appears to be more constant. The scleral canal may be thought of as a hole in the sclera. The larger the scleral canal, the more leftover space is present in the center of the disc, leading to a larger physiologic cup size. The converse is also apt to be true. A small or absent physiologic cup often reflects a small scleral canal and a crowded optic nerve head (Fig. 2.14).

When the optic nerve head exits the sclera at less than a 90-degree angle, the RPE frequently ends be-

fore the edge of the canal proper, exposing a crescent-shaped halo of choroid and sclera (Fig. 2.15). In addition, with an oblique angle of exit at one side of the disc, nerve fibers must make a >90-degree turn, giving a rolled edge to this rim of the disc that may simulate true swelling (Fig. 2.16). At the opposite side of such a disc, fibers are exiting at less than a 90-degree angle, and the disc rim appears shallowly sloped.

The retinal NFL turns 90 degrees posteriorly as it enters the optic nerve head. The axons then run in bundles surrounded by glial columns as they pass through the perforations of the lamina cribrosa. The fenestrated connective tissue and glia form a tight seal that helps keep the relatively high intraocular pressure from "leaking" into the retrolaminar tissues.

Within the optic nerve head, there are two types of blood vessels: capillary-sized vessels that directly supply the cells and the central retinal vessels (the central retinal artery and one or more central retinal veins) that pass through the nerve head. The ophthalmic artery originates from the ophthalmic segment of the internal carotid artery just as that vessel emerges from the distal dural ring of the cavernous sinus (Fig. 2.17). It then turns anteriorly and passes through the optic canal along with the optic nerve but separated from it by a covering of dura. Within the orbit, the ophthalmic artery gives rise to several branches, one of which is the central retinal artery, which pierces the optic nerve sheath 10 to 12 mm behind the globe and runs anteriorly in the central aspect of the optic nerve to emerge in the center of the optic disc. This artery does not contribute directly to the circulation of the optic nerve head. Instead, the blood supply to the optic nerve head derives from the circle of Zinn-Haller which forms a ring about it. The circle of Zinn-Haller receives three major sources of blood. Much of its blood derives from

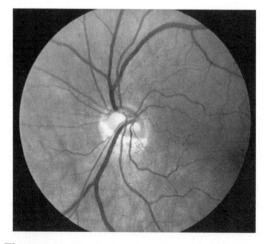

Figure 2.15. Appearance of a tilted optic disc. Note inferior conus.

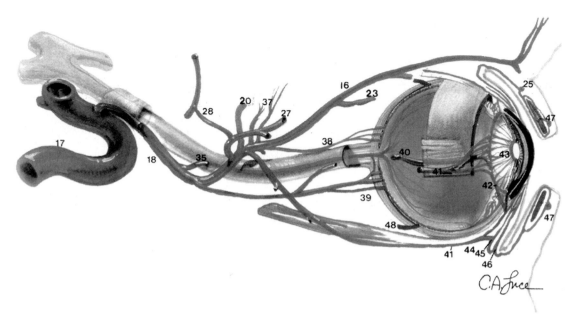

Figure 2.17. The internal carotid artery blood supply to the orbit and eye, with emphasis on the ophthalmic artery and its major branches. Key for arteries: frontal branch *(16)*; internal carotid *(17)*; ophthalmic *(18)*; posterior ethmoidal branch of the ophthalmic *(20)*; superior peripheral arcade *(25)*; lacrimal *(27)*; recurrent meningeal *(28)*; central retinal *(35)*; muscular branches for the superior rectus, superior oblique, and levator palpebrae muscles *(37)*; medial posterior ciliary *(38)*; short ciliary *(39)*; long ciliary *(40)*; anterior ciliary *(41)*; greater circle of the iris *(42)*; lesser circle of the iris *(43)*; episcleral *(44)*; subconjunctival *(45)*; conjunctival *(46)*; marginal arcade *(47)*; medial palpebral *(49)*; vortex vein *(48)*. (Reprinted from: BM Zide, GW Jelks. *Surgical Anatomy of the Orbit*. New York: Raven Press; 1985, with permission.)

the choroidal feeder vessels. A second source consists of about four short posterior arteries that feed into the circle directly. The third source of blood to this perineural arteriolar anastomosis is a small contribution from the pial arterial network. Feeding this capillary plexus are subdivisions of the ophthalmic artery via the third- and fourth-order branches of the posterior ciliary arteries, which enter the lateral aspect of the nerve head and vessels of the pial plexus and retrobulbar optic nerve posteriorly (Fig. 2.18).

The venous drainage of the optic nerve head is primarily via the central retinal venous system. Under certain conditions, however, such as chronic compression of the intraorbital optic nerve or after central retinal vein occlusion, preexisting connections between superficial disc veins and choroidal veins—opticociliary veins—may enlarge and shunt venous blood from the retina to the choroid and then, via the vortex veins, to the superior and inferior ophthalmic veins.

ORBITAL OPTIC NERVE

The orbital portion of the optic nerve is 25 mm in length and thus exceeds the anterior–posterior distance from the back of the eye to the optic foramen by about 8 mm (Fig. 2.19). The redundancy of the sinuous optic

nerve permits it to move freely during eye movements. There is also an allowance of up to 9 mm of proptosis before the optic nerve acts as a tether and distorts the globe or is stretched to the point of dysfunction.

The optic nerve increases in diameter from 3 mm just posterior to the globe to about 4.5 mm at the orbital apex. Throughout its orbital course, the nerve is surrounded by dura, arachnoid, and pia mater (Figs. 2.19 and 2.20). The dura is the outermost sheath, a dense collagenous tunic that is continuous anteriorly with the sclera. At the apex of the orbit, the dura fuses with the periosteum and with the annulus of Zinn. The arachnoid lies under the dura and is more cellular, less vascular, and less collagenous. Delicate arachnoidal trabeculae connect this membrane with the dura and underlying pia (Fig. 2.21). The pia is the most vascular of the sheaths covering the optic nerve. It invests the capillaries as they enter the substance of the nerve. The subarachnoid space is continuous with the intracranial subarachnoid space and thus contains CSF.

The cellular organization of the myelinated orbital portion of the optic nerve is similar to that of the intraocular optic nerve head, although the retrobulbar

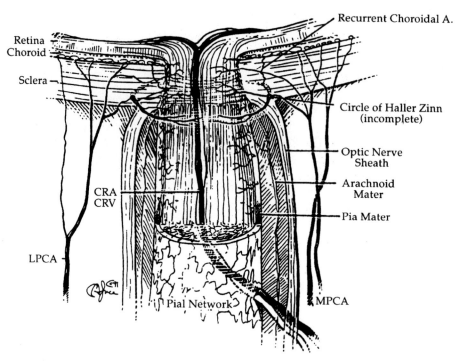

Retina
Choroid
Sclera
CRA
CRV
LPCA

Recurrent Choroidal A.

Circle of Haller Zinn
(incomplete)

Optic Nerve
Sheath

Arachnoid
Mater

Pia Mater

Pial Network

MPCA

Figure 2.18. The blood supply to the proximal optic nerve and choroid arises from the branches of the medial *(MPCA)* and lateral *(LPCA)* posterior ciliary arteries, the incomplete circle of Zinn-Haller, the pial network, and recurrent choroidal arteries. The posterior ciliary arteries send branches to the circle of Zinn-Haller and the pial network. The central retinal artery *(CRA)* provides minute branches to the optic nerve capillaries as it passes anteriorly to supply the retina. The central retinal vein *(CRV)* parallels the course of the CRA. (Reprinted from: Kupersmith MJ. *Neurovascular Neuro-Ophthalmology.* New York, Springer-Verlag; 1993, with permission.)

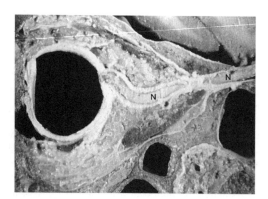

Figure 2.19. Sagittal section through a normal orbit showing the optic nerve (*N*). Note that the length of the nerve within the orbit appears to exceed the distance from the posterior aspect of the globe to the apex of the orbit. Also note that the intraorbital and intracanalicular portions of the nerve are covered by leptomeninges, the dural sheath of which is continuous with the periorbita lining the inner surface of the orbital walls and the dura lining the base of the skull. (Reprinted from: Unsöld R, DeGroot J, Newton TH. Images of the optic nerve: anatomic-CT correlation. *Am J Roentgenol.* 1980;135:767–773, with permission.)

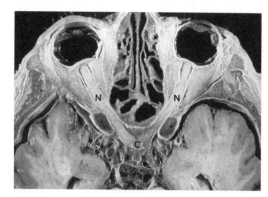

Figure 2.20. Axial section of normal optic nerves (*N*), showing relationships to other orbital and intracranial structures. Note that the intraorbital and intracanalicular portions of the nerve are covered by a dural sheath that is continuous with the periorbita lining the inner surface of the orbital walls and the dura lining the base of the skull. Optic chiasm (*C*). (Reprinted from: Unsöld R, DeGroot J, Newton TH. Images of the optic nerve: anatomic-CT correlation. *Am J Roentgenol.* 1980;135:767–773, with permission.)

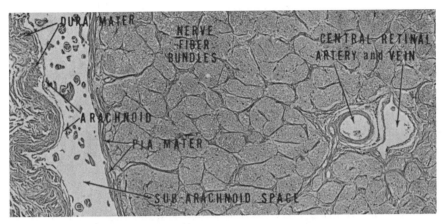

Figure 2.21. Cross-section of human optic nerve, showing relationships of the vaginal sheaths. The nerve fibers are divided into bundles by connective tissue septa that are continuous with both the connective tissue of the pia mater and the adventitia of the central retinal vessels.

nerve is twice as wide because of the addition of myelin. Bundles of nerve fibers are surrounded by connective tissue septa containing small arterioles, venules, and capillaries, forming a meshwork much like that in the lamina cribrosa. Astrocytes are here joined by oligo-dendrocytes, the specialized glial cells that provide membranes for myelination. All of the visual axons are myelinated from their exit from the eye to their synapse in the LGN. The axons from the largest reti-nal ganglion cells are surrounded by the thickest myelin sheaths, thus providing them with faster nerve conduc-tion velocities.

With the exception of the central retinal artery, there are few vessels larger than capillaries within the orbital portion of the optic nerve. The arterial input derives chiefly from the surrounding pial plexus. As the optic nerve leaves the eye, it is surrounded by about four posterior ciliary arteries that are branches of the ophthalmic artery. Within the midportion of the orbit, the ophthalmic artery initially runs inferolateral to the optic nerve until it crosses under (or occasionally over) it to proceed medially. At the optic foramen, the oph-thalmic artery lies below and lateral to the nerve. The inferior division of the oculomotor nerve, the nasocil-iary artery, the abducens nerve, and the ciliary ganglion are all located lateral to the optic nerve in the poste-rior orbit (Figs. 2.17, 2.22, and 2.23). At the apex of the orbit, the optic nerve is surrounded by the four rectus muscles that originate from the fibrous circle of Zinn.

INTRACANALICULAR (INTRAOSSEOUS) OPTIC NERVE

The optic nerve enters the optic canal through its an-terior opening in the apex of the orbital roof about 5 cm posterior and 1.5 cm inferior to the supraor-

bital margin. This anterior opening is called the **optic foramen.**

The optic canal itself is formed by the union of the two roots of the lesser wings of the sphenoid bonE. The proximal (orbital) opening of the optic canal is usually elliptical in shape, with the vertical diameter be-ing consistently greater than the horizontal. The distal (intracranial) opening is always elliptical, but its widest diameter is in the horizontal plane.

The thickness of the bony optic canal wall varies from medial (thinnest in mid-canal) to lateral (thickest in mid-canal) but also from anterior to pos-terior. The thin medial wall separates the optic nerve from the sphenoid and posterior ethmoid sinuses. The canal is about 10 mm in length, with the lateral wall be-ing shorter (9 mm) than the medial wall (about 14 mm). Inferolaterally, the optic canal is separated from the superior orbital fissure by a bony ridge that joins the lesser wing of the sphenoid to the body of the sphenoid bone—the **optic strut.**

The relationship between the paranasal sinuses and the optic canal is extremely important, particularly be-cause in about 4% of patients, the nerves have areas covered only by the nerve sheaths and sinus mucosa but without any bone separating the intracanalicular portion of the optic nerve from the adjacent paranasal sinus. The paranasal sinuses may occasionally become ballooned out without erosion of bone. This condition, called "pneumosinus dilatans," may result in the optic canals appearing as tunnels surrounded by sphenoid and posterior ethmoid air cells. Pneumosinus dilatans in this region is usually associated with an adjacent op-tic nerve sheath meningioma.

The intraorbital optic nerve moves freely as the eye moves; however, the intracanalicular optic nerve is tightly fixed within the optic canal. The dura is

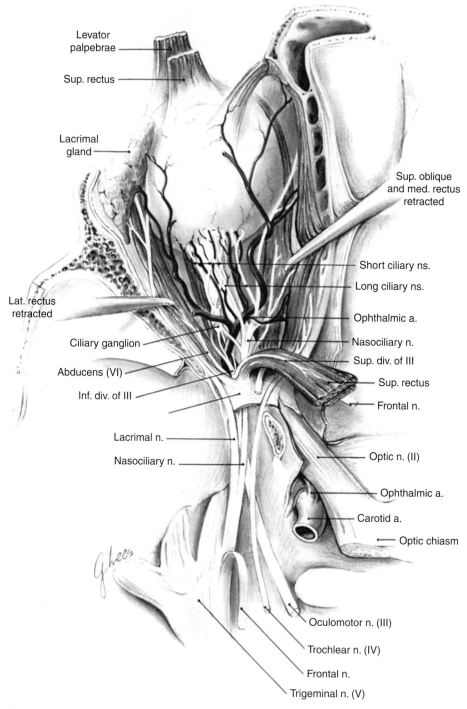

Levator palpebrae

Sup. rectus

Lacrimal gland

Sup. oblique and med. rectus retracted

Short ciliary ns.

Long ciliary ns.

Lat. rectus retracted

Ophthalmic a.

Ciliary ganglion

Nasociliary n.

Abducens (VI)

Sup. div. of III

Inf. div. of III

Sup. rectus

Frontal n.

Lacrimal n.

Optic n. (II)

Nasociliary n.

Ophthalmic a.

Carotid a.

Optic chiasm

Oculomotor n. (III)

Trochlear n. (IV)

Frontal n.

Trigeminal n. (V)

Figure 2.22. View of the intraorbital optic nerve from above showing relationships of the nerve to the ocular motor nerves and the posterior ciliary vessels. (Redrawn from: Wolff E. *Anatomy of the Eye and Orbit.* 6th ed. Philadelphia: WB Saunders; 1968.)

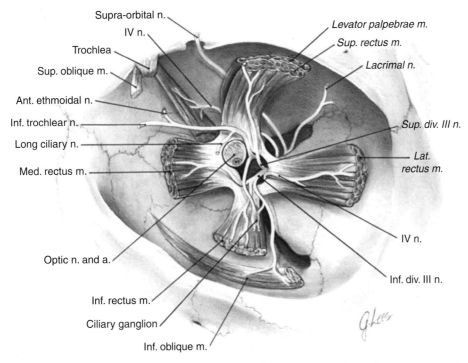

Figure 2.23. View of the posterior orbit showing the relationship of the optic nerve to the ocular motor nerves and extraocular muscles. (Redrawn from: Wolff E. *Anatomy of the Eye and Orbit.* 6th ed. Philadelphia: WB Saunders; 1968.)

adherent to the bone of the canal on one side and the optic nerve on the other (Fig. 2.24). Thus, small lesions arising within the optic canal or at either of its openings may compress and significantly damage the optic nerve while they are still quite small and difficult to visualize, even with thin-section computed tomography (CT) scanning and MRI.

INTRACRANIAL OPTIC NERVE

The intracranial portion of each optic nerve exits past a firm fold of dura that covers it superiorly and to some extent on both sides. The distance between the optic nerves as they exit from the optic canal averages 13 mm. The two nerves then extend posteriorly, superiorly, and medially to join at the optic chiasm.

The length of the intracranial segment of the normal optic nerve varies considerably. It is usually about 10 mm long, but it may be as short as 3 mm or as long as 16 mm. This portion of the nerve is about 4.5 to 5 mm in average diameter, but it is flattened and thus is wider in the horizontal plane than in the vertical plane (Fig. 2.25). When the intracranial optic nerve is shorter than about 12 mm, the optic chiasm is positioned anteriorly, or "prefixed," and sits directly over the sella turcica. When the intracranial optic nerve is long (over 18 mm), the chiasm is positioned posteriorly to the dorsum sellae, or "postfixed" (Fig. 2.26). The variation in

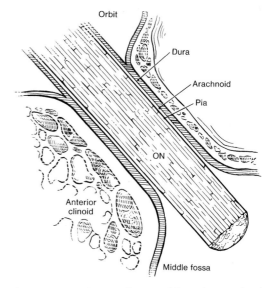

Figure 2.24. Schematic drawing of the optic nerve sheaths showing their relationship to the optic nerve (*ON*) and to the surrounding sphenoid bone. The dura is tightly adherent to the bone within the optic canal. Within the orbit it divides into two layers, one of which remains as the outer sheath of the optic nerve, and the other becomes the orbital periosteum (periorbita). Intracranially, the dura leaves the optic nerve to become the periosteum of the sphenoid bone.

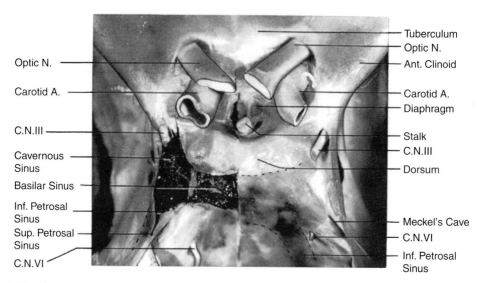

Figure 2.25. The intracranial portions of the optic nerves viewed from above and posteriorly. The optic nerves are seen almost in their entirety. Note that they have an oval or elliptical shape, with the widest diameter in the horizontal plane. (Reprinted from: Renn WH, Rhoton AL Jr. Microsurgical anatomy of the sellar region. *J Neurosurg.* 1975;43:288–298, with permission.)

the length of the optic nerve is extremely important with respect to the visual deficits caused by tumors in the suprasellar region (see Chapter 12).

The gyrus recti of the frontal lobes of the brain are above the optic nerves. On the ventral surface of each frontal lobe, the olfactory tract is separated from the optic nerve by the anterior cerebral and anterior communicating arteries. On the lateral side of the optic nerve, the internal carotid artery sometimes forms an immediate relationship as it emerges from the cavernous sinus. Because the intracranial optic nerve is in the region where the internal carotid artery bifurcates into the anterior cerebral and middle cerebral arteries, these vessels are often immediately adjacent to the optic nerve, as is the proximal portion of the posterior communicating artery (Fig. 2.27).

The internal carotid artery supplies the optic nerve via the ophthalmic artery, which enters the optic canal inferior and lateral to the optic nerve (Figs. 2.25 and 2.27). It is separated from the nerve, however, by a dural sheath that covers it throughout the length of the canal. The anatomic relationship of the optic nerve and the

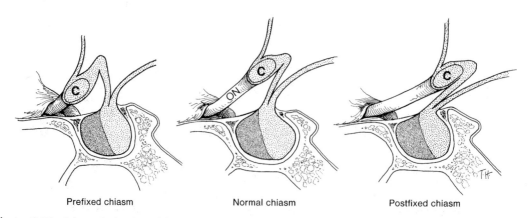

Prefixed chiasm   Normal chiasm   Postfixed chiasm

Figure 2.26. Schematic drawing of three sagittal sections of the optic chiasm and sellar region. **Left:** The position of a pre-fixed chiasm above the tuberculum sellae. *Center:* The position of a normal chiasm above the diaphragma sellae. **Right:** The position of a postfixed chiasm above the dorsum sellae. (Redrawn from: Rhoton AL Jr, Harris FS, Renn WH. Microsurgical anatomy of the sellar region and cavernous sinus. In: Glaser JS, ed. *Neuro-Ophthalmology Symposium of the University of Miami and the Bascom Palmer Eye Institute.* St. Louis: CV Mosby; 1977:75–105.)

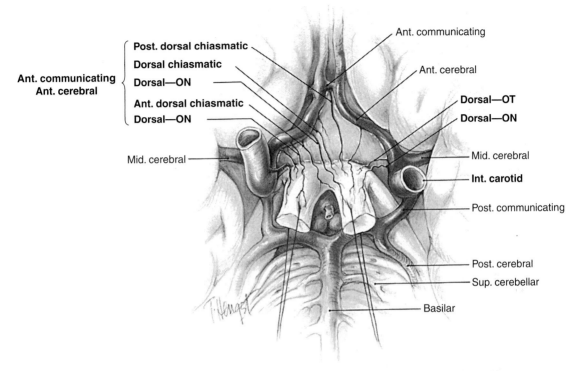

Figure 2.27. Blood supply to the dorsal aspect of the optic chiasm and intracranial optic nerves. ON, optic nerve; OT, optic tract. (Reprinted from: Wollschlaeger P, Wollschlaeger G, Ide C, et al. Arterial blood supply of the human optic chiasm and surrounding structures. *Ann Ophthalmol.* 1971;3:862–869, with permission.)

internal carotid artery and its branches account for the visual deficits that occur in some cases of dolichoectasia or aneurysms of the internal carotid, ophthalmic, and anterior cerebral arteries. Inferomedially, the sphenoid sinus has an important relationship to the optic nerve.

OPTIC NERVE PHYSIOLOGY

As noted above, there are at least two classes of retinal ganglion cells in humans. About 80% to 90% of these cells are of small to moderate size, are concentrated in the macula, have small-caliber axons, and project to the parvocellular layers of the dorsal LGN (the P-cell system). P-cells have color-opponent physiology and are thought to subserve high-contrast, high-spatial frequency resolution. In contrast, large cells with large, fast-conducting axons comprise about 10% to 20% of the retinal ganglion cell population. These M-cells project to the magnocellular layers of the LGN and are primarily involved with noncolor information of high-temporal and low-spatial frequency. Conduction velocities in optic nerve fibers are much faster than those in the unmyelinated but similar caliber fibers in the retina, ranging from 1.3 to 20 meters per second.

TOPOGRAPHIC ANATOMY OF THE OPTIC NERVE

Fibers from peripheral ganglion cells occupy a more peripheral position in the optic disc, whereas fibers from ganglion cells located closer to the optic disc occupy a more central position. The arrangement of fibers in the optic disc and distal optic nerve corresponds generally to the topographic distribution of fibers in the retina. Fibers from the superior portion of the retina are located in the superior part of the optic nerve head; fibers from the inferior retina are located inferiorly in this region; and nasal and temporal fibers are on their respective sides. The papillomacular bundle is a sector-shaped structure that occupies about one-third of the temporal optic disc, adjacent to the central vessels. This bundle of fibers gradually moves centrally in the more distal (posterior) portions of the orbital optic nerve. The gradual movement of the macular fibers to the center of the orbital optic nerve allows the uncrossed upper and lower retinal fibers to come together (Fig. 2.28). Dorsal (superior) and ventral (inferior) macular fibers retain their relative positions throughout the nerve, whereas crossed macular fibers lie nasal to the uncrossed fibers. Indeed, all the retinal fibers retain their relative positions throughout

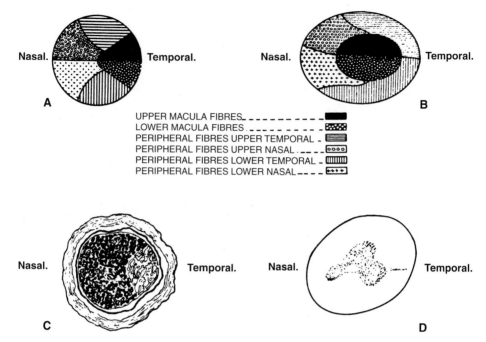

Figure 2.28. Fiber arrangement in the optic nerve. **A:** In the distal portion of the optic nerve. **B:** In the proximal portion of the optic nerve. **C:** A transverse section of the optic nerve in its distal portion in a case of atrophy of the papillomacular bundle. **D:** Secondary degeneration in the proximal portion of the optic nerve after a macular lesion. (Reprinted from: Duke-Elder S. *Textbook of Ophthalmology.* Vol 1. St. Louis: CV Mosby; 1932, with permission.)

the visual pathways; that is, upper fibers remain upper and lower remain lower, except in the optic tract and at the LGN, where there is a rotation of 90 degrees that becomes straightened out in the optic radiations (see Chapter 12).

Within the intracranial portion of the optic nerve, the axons lose their retinotopic order to some extent because some axons decussate within the optic chiasm and some do not. The macular fibers do not have a precise localization in the posterior nerve and the gradual inclination inward of the macular fibers in the most posterior portions of the nerve allows for regrouping of the peripheral visual fibers.

Most of the visual axons, whether crossed or uncrossed, pass directly through the chiasm into the ipsilateral (uncrossed) or contralateral (crossed) optic tract. However, as they enter the chiasm, some ventral crossed fibers, primarily from the inferonasal retina of the contralateral eye and serving the superotemporal portion of the contralateral visual field, were historically believed to loop anteriorly 1 to 2 mm into the terminal portion of the opposite optic nerve before turning posteriorly to continue through the chiasm and into the optic tract. This loop is called **Wilbrand's knee.** There is some evidence that Wilbrand's knee is not a true anatomic structure but is, in fact, an ar-

tifact that develops in both humans and nonhuman primates with longstanding unilateral optic atrophy. However, Wilbrand's knee clearly exists from a clinical standpoint. Patients with a monocular optic neuropathy caused by a lesion that has damaged the distal optic nerve at its junction with the optic chiasm not infrequently have an asymptomatic superior temporal defect in the visual field of the contralateral eye (see Chapter 12).

TOPOGRAPHIC DIAGNOSIS OF RETINAL LESIONS

Retinal diseases may be divided into two main groups: (i) those affecting the detecting apparatus—the receptor cells and their synapses; and (ii) those affecting the conducting apparatus—the ganglion cell and nerve fiber layers. In many cases, the diagnosis is obvious from the appearance of the affected region of the retina. In other cases, however, it is possible to diagnose retinal dysfunction only from other aspects of the clinical examination. Indeed, patients with "unexplained visual loss" may, in fact, have a disorder of the retina that may not be obvious during a clinical examination. Features that help distinguish retinal disease from optic nerve disease are noted in Table 2.3.

Table 2.3. *Distinguishing Optic Neuropathies and Maculopathies*

Features	Optic Nerve	Macula
Presenting deficit	Central dark cloud	Distortions
Pain (rarely)	Sometimes with eye movement	Rarely
Refractive error	Unchanged	Sometimes hyperopia
Visual acuity	Variable	Markedly impaired
Afferent pupillary defect	Present	Absent
Color vision	Very reduced	Slightly reduced
Brightness sense	Very reduced	Variable
Amsler grid	Scotoma	Metamorphopsia

DISTINGUISHING RETINAL DISEASE FROM AN OPTIC NEUROPATHY BY CLINICAL EXAMINATION

Central **visual acuity** may or may not be affected by disease that damages the retina. Disorders that cause dysfunction only of extramacular retina typically are unassociated with a reduction in central acuity, whereas macular disorders and disorders that damage the entire retina invariably reduce central vision. Most disorders that affect the macula are detected by a careful funduscopic examination, particularly when the macula is examined with a slit lamp biomicroscope using a corneal contact lens, a 78- or 90-diopter hand-held lens, or a Hruby lens. Nevertheless, some disorders, such as central serous chorioretinopathy, cystoid macular edema, and epiretinal membrane formation (surface wrinkling retinopathy, cellophane maculopathy) can easily be overlooked (Fig. 2.29).

In other diseases that affect the macula, such as macular cone dystrophy, there are often no changes that can be observed in the macula, even though the patient has decreased central vision and a visual field defect. In such cases, the diagnosis of retinal disease may be suspected if there is associated metamorphopsia (an irregularity or distortion in the appearance of viewed objects), photophobia, nyctalopia (night blindness), or hemeralopia (the inability to see as distinctly in a bright light as in a dim one). These symptoms occur much more often in patients with ocular disease than in patients with neurologic disease. Photophobia should be obvious during the examination. Metamorphopsia is usually caused by a distortion of the normal alignment of the photoreceptors. When there is increased separation among cones (and among rods to a lesser extent because of the central position of the lesion), there is an apparent decrease in the size of objects (micropsia). The foveal cones are already so close to each other that it is unlikely that an apparent increase in the size of objects (macropsia) can occur from further crowding together of these cells. Evidence of metamorphopsia may be detected in patients with and without the complaint of distortion of objects by using an Amsler grid. The results of a photostress test usually are abnormal in such patients, as are the results of fluorescein angiography or focal electroretinography (Fig. 2.30) (see Chapter 1).

Color vision is often but not always abnormal in patients with retinal disease. For instance, patients with central serous chorioretinopathy and epiretinal membrane formation rarely have any significant dyschromatopsia, whereas patients with macular cone or cone-rod dystrophies usually do; such patients may even develop difficulties with color vision as the initial sign of the disease. In such cases, the correct diagnosis is not made until other studies such as electroretinography are performed. Retinal disorders are more likely to produce either generalized loss of color vision or a blue-yellow dyschromatopsia, but there are sufficient exceptions that make the pattern of color vision loss an unreliable diagnostic criterion.

A **relative afferent pupillary defect** can only be detected clinically in patients with unilateral or asymmetric retinal disease if the retinal disease is severe, affects most of the retina or the entire macula, and is obvious during a funduscopic examination (Fig. 2.31). If a relative afferent pupillary defect is observed in a patient with decreased visual acuity associated with some macular drusen, central serous chorioretinopathy, cystoid macular edema, an epiretinal membrane, or a normal-appearing fundus, a lesion affecting the optic nerve should be suspected.

DISTINGUISHING RETINAL DISEASE FROM AN OPTIC NEUROPATHY BY VISUAL FIELD

When the photoreceptors are affected, the defect in the visual field corresponds to the retinal defect in position, shape, extent, and intensity. When the ganglion cell or nerve fiber layer is damaged, however, the field defect does not conform to the size and shape of the lesion but rather to the field represented by the ganglion cells whose fibers are damaged. Thus, a small lesion situated

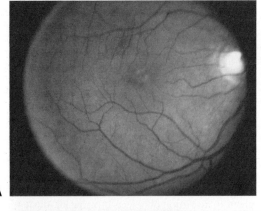

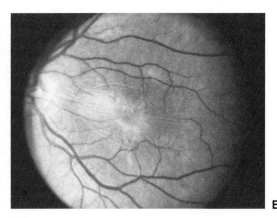

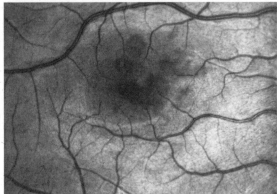

Figure 2.29. Subtle macular lesions causing visual loss. **A:** Pigment changes in the right macula of a patient with "unexplained" central visual loss. **B:** Epiretinal membrane in the left macula of a patient complaining of blurred vision in the eye. **C:** Changes in the right macula of a patient who complained of decreased central vision in the eye after blunt ocular trauma. It was initially suspected that he had a traumatic optic neuropathy or was malingering.

close to the optic disc that damages only photoreceptors usually causes a small scotoma, whereas a lesion of the same size that damages the ganglion cells and nerve fibers in the same area may result in an extensive defect in the visual field (Fig. 2.32). Conversely, a small lesion in the periphery that damages only a few fibers transmitting impulses from widely separated ganglion cells may produce such a small field defect that it may be difficult or even impossible to detect.

Diseases that cause photoreceptor damage usually produce a greater loss of the visual field when it is tested with blue stimuli than when it is tested with red stimuli. This observation is useful because the situation is reversed in disorders that damage the conducting apparatus of the retina. In lesions of the ganglion cells, retinal nerve fiber layer, and optic nerve, there usually is a more pronounced loss of the visual field for red than for blue.

If a lesion superotemporal or inferotemporal to the optic disc damages peripheral visual fibers, the field defect is arcuate in shape because the fibers from peripheral ganglion cells arch around the papillomacular bundle (Fig. 2.12). The field defect is, of course, situated nasal to the blind spot. If the lesion is nasal to

the optic disc, it damages a nasal bundle. The resultant field defect is temporal and fan-shaped, because fibers from ganglion cells located nasal to the optic disc take a direct path to the disc.

An arcuate defect in the visual field may indicate a defect in the nerve fiber layer. When such a retinal lesion is present, it usually can be identified by ophthalmoscopic examination. Because of the anatomy of the temporal raphe that separates fibers from ganglion cells located above the horizontal midline from those from ganglion cells below the horizontal midline, there is often a sharp dividing line between the area of the scotoma and the functioning upper or lower field. This is particularly evident in large arcuate scotomas, so much so that visual fields performed on tangent screen or by automated static perimetry may suggest complete loss of the superior or inferior hemifield unless the entire field is tested.

Any visual field defect that can be produced by an inner retinal lesion can also be produced by a lesion of the optic nerve. Damage to the papillomacular area of the retina results in a central scotoma that connects to the physiologic blind spot; this is a **cecocentral scotoma** (Fig. 2.33). An **arcuate visual field defect**

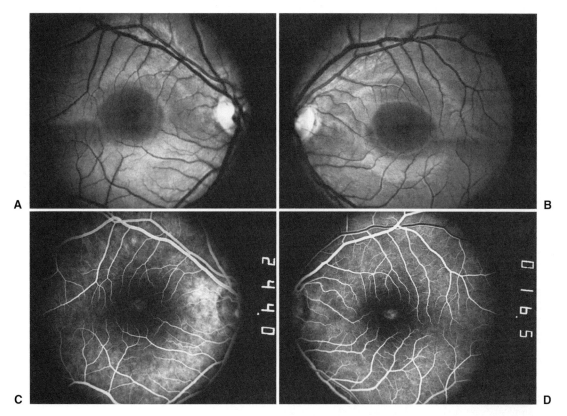

Figure 2.30. Macular lesions in a 13-year-old girl with unexplained loss of vision in both eyes. Visual acuity was 20/80 OU. **A and B:** The maculae appear fairly normal. **C and D:** However, fluorescein angiography reveals impressive pigment epithelial changes in the macula, consistent with the decreased vision. The patient was diagnosed as having a macular dystrophy of unknown cause.

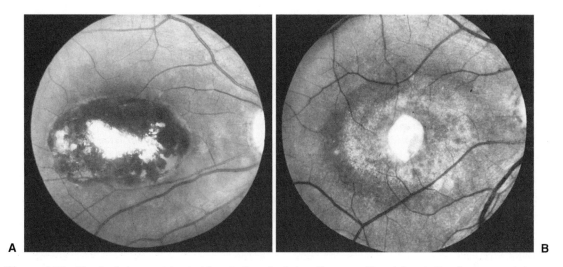

Figure 2.31. Macular lesions associated with an ipsilateral relative afferent pupillary defect. **A:** Scar from congenital toxoplasmosis. **B:** Scar from presumed ocular histoplasmosis. Note that both lesions are quite obvious and would not be overlooked during an ophthalmoscopic examination, even if the pupils were not dilated.

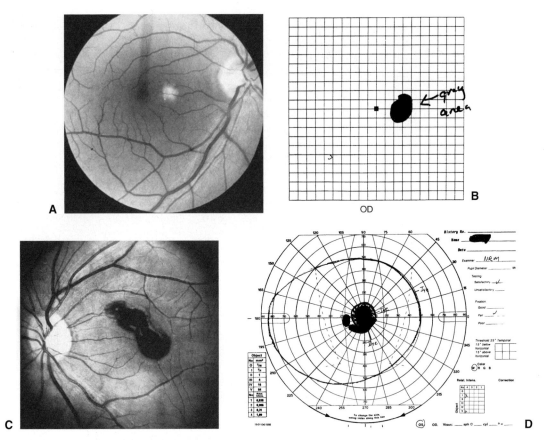

Figure 2.32. Variation in visual fields caused by posterior pole lesions. **A and B:** Small chorioretinal scar adjacent to right fovea. Because this lesion is located in the deep retina at the level of the photoreceptors and retinal pigment epithelium, it produces only a small central scotoma. **C and D:** Hemorrhage in the left macula in another patient. This lesion has produced a large central scotoma associated with an inferior arcuate defect because of its superficial location in the retina.

usually results from damage to retinal nerve fibers or ganglion cells in the superior or inferior arcuate nerve fiber bundles. In such cases, there is a central field defect that is not circular but instead is limited above or below by the horizontal meridian (Fig. 2.34). This visual field defect may occur in patients with occlusion of the blood supply of the superior or inferior portion of the macula or in patients with glaucoma. In both settings, the scotoma is associated with normal visual acuity, since it does not completely affect the macula. Virtually any lesion, whether ischemic, inflammatory, infiltrative, or compressive, can cause an arcuate field defect and may be located in either the retina or the optic nerve.

Annular or ring scotomas occur in a variety of conditions, most notably in patients with various pigmentary retinopathies. Ring scotomas may also occur in patients with open angle glaucoma, but in such cases, the ring is actually caused by the coalescence of up-

per and lower arcuate scotomas originating from the physiologic blind spot and extending across the vertical midline into the nasal visual field. Similar defects may be seen in various optic neuropathies, particularly those caused by ischemia, compression, and inflammation.

A ring scotoma can be detected in most types of pigmentary retinopathy (e.g., retinitis pigmentosa) if the visual field is carefully examined. In some cases, however, the peripheral field is so contracted and central vision so reduced that the ring scotoma may not be detected. A ring scotoma may also persist after incomplete resolution of a preexisting central scotoma in patients with retinal or optic nerve disease.

In general, a unilateral temporal or nasal hemianopia that respects the vertical midline is either nonorganic or caused by dysfunction of the optic nerve (see Chapter 4). Nevertheless, a unilateral hemianopia

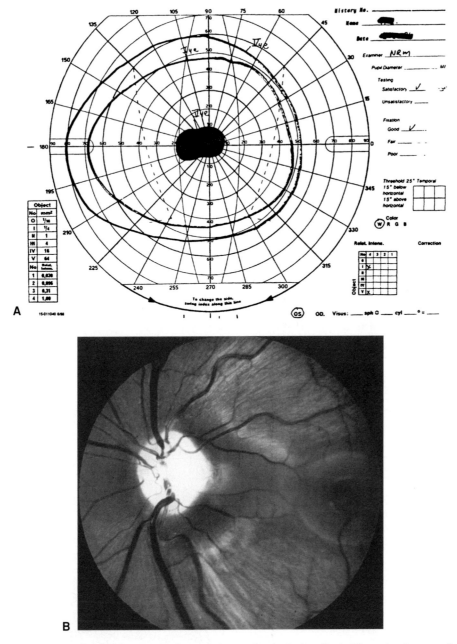

Figure 2.33. Cecocentral scotoma caused by a lesion in the papillomacular bundle. **A:** The patient has a small cecocentral scotoma in the visual field of the left eye. **B:** There is a serous detachment of the retina in the papillomacular bundle of the left eye, associated with a temporal optic pit.

very rarely can be caused by sectoral retinitis pigmentosa.

The **blind spot** also plays a role in the interpretation of the visual field. It represents the negative scotoma that is the projection of the optic disc. The optic disc is located nasal to the fovea, and its center is slightly above it. Thus, the blind spot is tempo-

ral to the point of fixation, and its center is slightly below it.

The blind spot becomes enlarged from peripapillary retinal dysfunction. This dysfunction can occur because the peripapillary retina is diseased, as occurs in patients with the so-called "big blind spot syndrome" and related disorders such as acute zonal occult outer

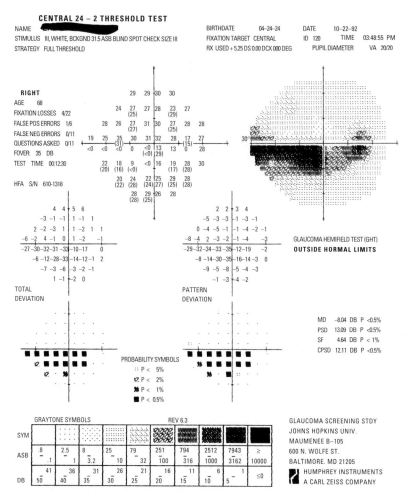

Figure 2.34. "Central" scotoma in the right eye of a patient with open-angle glaucoma. Although the visual field defect is central in location, it is actually an arcuate/altitudinal scotoma that is located adjacent but just inferior to the horizontal midline. The visual acuity in this eye is 20/20.

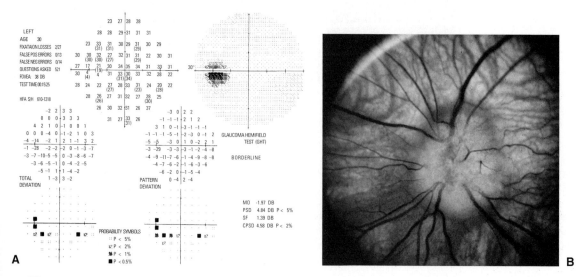

Figure 2.35. Enlargement of the blind spot in a 30-year-old obese woman with headaches. **B:** Appearance of left optic disc, showing chronic swelling. An evaluation revealed increased intracranial pressure.

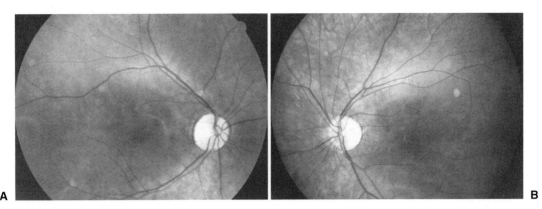

Figure 2.36. Optic atrophy in retinal dystrophy. **A and B:** The right and left optic discs, respectively, of a 20-year-old woman with visual acuity of 20/50 OU, abnormal color vision, and nonspecific visual field defects. Both optic discs show diffuse pallor, and the retinal arteries are somewhat narrowed. The patient was found to have a retinal cone dystrophy. (Reprinted from: Newman NJ, Slavin M, Newman SA. Optic disc pallor: a false localizing sign. *Surv Ophthalmol.* 1993;37:273–282, with permission.).

retinopathy (AZOOR) and the multiple evanescent white dot syndrome (MEWDS), or because expansion of the optic disc tissue encroaches on the peripapillary retina, as occurs in optic disc swelling and in pseudopapilledema (Fig. 2.35).

APPEARANCE OF THE OPTIC DISC IN RETINAL DISEASE

The optic nerve is composed primarily of axons whose cell bodies are the ganglion cells of the retina. Thus,

any retinal disorder that directly or indirectly damages the ganglion cells or their axons in the retinal nerve fiber layer will eventually produce optic atrophy. Indeed, damage to the ganglion cell body or the NFL is tantamount to damage to the optic nerve; that is, there will be visual loss, a relative afferent pupillary defect if the damage is unilateral or asymmetric, and ultimately optic atrophy. Because the central retinal arterial and venous circulations subserve the inner layers of the retina (including the ganglion cell and nerve

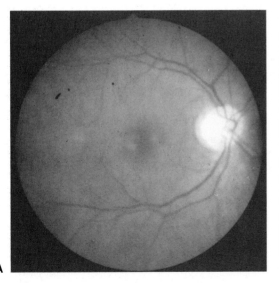
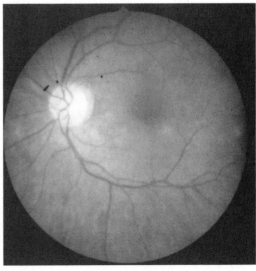

Figure 2.37. Optic atrophy in vitamin A deficiency. The patient was a woman who developed bilateral visual loss and cecocentral scotomas several years after a jejunoileal bypass for morbid obesity. An electroretinogram revealed evidence of a retinopathy affecting the photoreceptors, and laboratory studies revealed a reduced concentration of vitamin A in the patient's serum. The patient's visual function improved after vitamin A therapy. Both the right (**A**) and left (**B**) optic discs are pale. (Courtesy of Dr. Eric Eggenberger.)

fiber layers), retinal vascular occlusive events will result in inner retinal damage, visual loss, and eventual optic atrophy. Acute vascular events involving the retina—including central and branch retinal artery occlusions, ophthalmic artery occlusions, and central retinal vein occlusions—have a dramatic and distinct funduscopic appearance, permitting immediate correct diagnosis. However, over time, the retinal findings resolve, and the optic disc becomes pale. In such cases, subsequent narrowing and sheathing of the retinal arteries or the presence of a visible embolus within the retinal circulation may provide clues as to the etiology of the original event.

Loss of the NFL and optic atrophy are not uncommon in patients with various photoreceptor dystrophies and degenerations, particularly those affecting the cones (Fig. 2.36). Clues that suggest retinal cone dysfunction include profound dyschromatopsia, photophobia and hemeralopia, retinal arterial attenuation, and, eventually, changes in the appearance of the maculae, often resembling a bull's-eye (bull's-eye maculopathy). Bilateral secondary optic atrophy can be seen in patients with cone dystrophies, rod/cone dystrophies, paraneoplastic retinopathies, and the retinopathy of vitamin A deficiency (Fig. 2.37).

FOR FURTHER INFORMATION

See *Walsh & Hoyt's Clinical Neuro-Ophthalmology*, 6th edition, Volume 1, Chapter 1, pages 3–35; Chapter 4, pages 197–208.

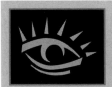

C H A P T E R 3

Congenital Anomalies of the Optic Disc *

Ophthalmologists and neurologists are frequently asked to evaluate patients with anomalous optic discs. A comprehensive evaluation requires an understanding of the ophthalmoscopic features, associated neuro-ophthalmologic findings, pathogenesis, and appropriate ancillary studies for each anomaly. Increased recognition of the ocular and systemic associations related to each anomaly has advanced our understanding of its pathogenesis. For example, different forms of excavated optic disc anomalies that were previously lumped together as colobomatous defects are now subclassified. This has enhanced our ability to predict the likelihood of associated central nervous system (CNS) anomalies based solely on the appearance of the optic disc. Additionally, the widespread clinical application of computed tomographic (CT) scans and magnetic resonance imaging (MRI) has enabled us to more accurately identify associated CNS anomalies and predict the likelihood of subsequent neurodevelopmental and endocrinologic problems.

Certain general principles are particularly useful in the evaluation and management of patients with anomalous optic discs.

1. Children with bilateral optic disc anomalies generally present in infancy with poor vision and nystagmus; those with unilateral optic disc anomalies generally present during their preschool years with sensory esotropia, or exotropia.
2. CNS malformations are common in patients with malformed optic discs. Small discs are associated with a variety of malformations of the cerebral hemispheres, pituitary infundibulum, and midline intracranial structures (septum pellucidum, corpus callosum). Large optic discs of the morning glory configuration are associated with the transsphenoidal form of basal encephalocele, whereas colobomatous optic discs may be associated with systemic anomalies and a variety of syndromes.
3. Any structural ocular abnormality that reduces visual acuity in infancy may lead to superimposed amblyopia. A trial of occlusion therapy may be warranted in young children with unilateral optic disc anomalies and decreased vision.
4. Anomalous optic discs (particularly excavated optic disc anomalies and pseudopapilledema with or without optic disc drusen) may produce episodes of transient visual loss.

*Adapted from: Brodsky MC. Congenital anomalies of the optic disc. In: Miller NR, Newman NJ, Biousse V, Kerrison JB, eds. *Walsh & Hoyt's Clinical Neuro-Ophthalmology*. 6th ed. Vol. I. Philadelphia: Lippincott Williams & Wilkins; 2005, 151–195.

OPTIC NERVE HYPOPLASIA

Optic nerve hypoplasia is the most common optic disc anomaly encountered in ophthalmologic practice.

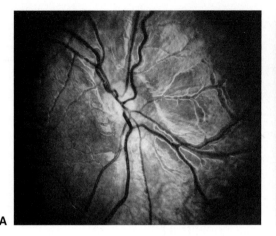
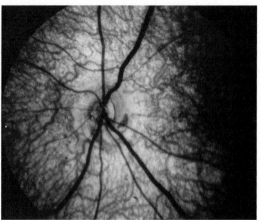

A   B

Figure 3.1. Optic nerve hypoplasia. **A:** The disc is small and pale but the retinal vessels are of normal size. **B:** The disc is small and surrounded by a rim of variably pigmented tissue.

CLINICAL FEATURES

Ophthalmoscopically, the hypoplastic disc appears as an abnormally small optic nerve head (Fig. 3.1). It may appear gray or pale and is often surrounded by a yellowish mottled peripapillary halo, bordered by a ring of increased or decreased pigmentation ("double-ring" sign), which facilitates recognition of the anomaly. Optic nerve hypoplasia is often associated with tortuosity of the retinal veins.

Optic nerve hypoplasia is characterized histopathologically by a subnormal number of optic nerve axons with normal mesodermal elements and glial supporting tissue. The double-ring sign correlates to a normal junction between the sclera and lamina cribrosa, which corresponds to the outer ring, and the termination of an abnormal extension of retina and pigment epithelium over the lamina cribrosa, which corresponds to the inner ring.

Visual acuity in optic nerve hypoplasia ranges from 20/20 to no light perception, and affected eyes show localized visual field defects, often combined with generalized constriction. Because visual acuity is determined primarily by the integrity of the papillomacular nerve fiber bundle, it does not necessarily correlate with the overall size of the disc. The strong association of astigmatism with optic nerve hypoplasia warrants careful attention to correction of refractive errors. In addition, unilateral optic nerve hypoplasia has been implicated in the pathogenesis of amblyopia.

Except when amblyopia develops in one eye, visual acuity usually remains stable throughout life.

Calculation of the disc-to-macula/disc diameter ratio reveals that in 95% of normals, the ratio is >2.94, in contrast to an average of 2.62 for patients with optic nerve hypoplasia. Calculation of this ratio has the important advantage of eliminating the magnification effect of high refractive errors (myopic refractive errors can make a hypoplastic disc appear normal in size, whereas hyperopic refractive errors can make a normal disc appear abnormally small). However, it is often difficult to distinguish between the normal and the hypoplastic disc; indeed, large optic discs can be axonally deficient, and small optic discs do not preclude normal visual function. Other variables must also be considered, including the size of the central cup, the percentage of the nerve occupied by axons (as opposed to glial tissue and blood vessels), and the cross-sectional area and density of axons. Furthermore, segmental forms of optic nerve hypoplasia (see below) may affect only one sector of the disc and thus not produce a diffuse diminution in the size of the disc. As such, it would seem prudent to reserve the diagnosis of optic nerve hypoplasia for patients with small optic discs who have reduced vision or visual field loss with corresponding nerve fiber bundle defects.

Electroretinography is normal in the majority of patients with optic nerve hypoplasia. However, some have decreased amplitudes, suggesting coexistent retinal dysgenesis. Visual-evoked responses (VER) vary from normal to extinguished. Some patients with poor vision have normal flash VEP latencies, which probably result from the normal transmission speed of residual axons.

ASSOCIATED ENDOCRINOLOGIC DEFICIENCIES

Optic nerve hypoplasia is frequently associated with other CNS anomalies. Septo-optic dysplasia (de Morsier syndrome) refers to the constellation of small anterior visual pathways, absence of the septum pellucidum, and thinning or agenesis of the corpus callosum. Growth hormone deficiency is the most common endocrinologic deficiency associated with optic nerve hypoplasia, but hypothyroidism, hypocortisolism, diabetes insipidus, and hyperprolactinemia may also occur. Children with an intact septum pellucidum and optic nerve hypoplasia may still have endocrinologic deficiency. Anterior pituitary hormone deficiencies may evolve over time in some patients; thus, longitudinal reevaluation and periodic monitoring of anterior pituitary hormone function are indicated in children with posterior pituitary ectopia. Estimates of the prevalence of pituitary hormone deficiency in children with septo-optic dysplasia are as high as 62%, but these clinical reports are strongly skewed toward cases with endocrinologic manifestations, and the true prevalence is probably closer to 15%.

Children with septo-optic dysplasia and corticotropin deficiency are at risk for sudden death during febrile illness. This is explained by an impaired ability to increase corticotropin secretion to maintain blood pressure and blood sugar in response to the physical stress of infection. These children may have coexistent diabetes insipidus that contributes to dehydration during illness and hastens the development of shock. Some also have hypothalamic thermoregulatory disturbances signaled by episodes of hypothermia during well periods and high fevers during illnesses, which may predispose to life-threatening hyperthermia. Because corticotropin deficiency represents the preeminent threat

to life in children with septo-optic dysplasia, a complete anterior pituitary hormone evaluation, including provocative serum cortisol testing and assessment for diabetes insipidus, should be performed in children who have clinical symptoms (history of hypoglycemia, dehydration, or hypothermia) or neuroimaging signs (absent pituitary infundibulum with or without posterior pituitary ectopia) of pituitary hormone deficiency.

ASSOCIATED CENTRAL NERVOUS SYSTEM MALFORMATIONS

MRI is the optimal noninvasive neuroimaging modality for delineating associated CNS malformations in patients with optic nerve hypoplasia. In optic nerve hypoplasia, coronal and sagittal T1-weighted MRI consistently demonstrate thinning and attenuation of hypoplastic prechiasmatic intracranial optic nerves (Fig. 3.2). Coronal T1-weighted MRI in bilateral optic nerve hypoplasia shows diffuse thinning of the optic chiasm (Fig. 3.2) in patients with bilateral optic nerve hypoplasia, and focal thinning or absence of the side of the chiasm corresponding to the hypoplastic nerve in unilateral optic nerve hypoplasia. When MRI shows a decrease in intracranial optic nerve size accompanied by other features of septo-optic dysplasia, a presumptive diagnosis of optic nerve hypoplasia can be made.

In approximately 45% of cases with optic nerve hypoplasia, MRI demonstrates other structural abnormalities involving the cerebral hemispheres and the

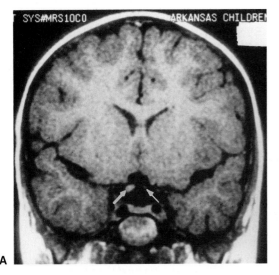
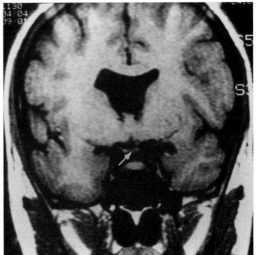

Figure 3.2. Magnetic resonance imaging in optic nerve hypoplasia. **A:** Left optic nerve hypoplasia. *Thick arrow* denotes normal right optic nerve. *Thin arrow* denotes hypoplastic intracranial prechiasmatic optic nerve. **B:** Bilateral optic nerve hypoplasia. *Arrow* denotes hypoplastic chiasm. (Reprinted from: Brodsky MC, Glasier CM, Pollock SC, et al. Optic nerve hypoplasia: identification by magnetic resonance imaging. *Arch Ophthalmol.* 1990;108:562–567, with permission.)

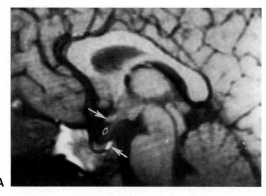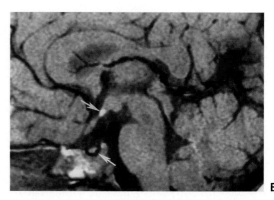

A   **B**

Figure 3.3. Posterior pituitary ectopia. **A:** MR image demonstrating the normal hyperintense signal of the posterior pituitary gland (*lower arrow*), normal pituitary infundibulum (*open arrow*), optic chiasm (*upper arrow*). **B:** MR image demonstrating posterior pituitary ectopia that appears as an abnormal focal area of increased signal intensity at the tuber cinereum (*upper arrow*). Note absence of the pituitary infundibulum and absence of the normal posterior pituitary bright spot (*lower arrow*). (Reprinted from: Brodsky MC, Glasier CM, Pollock SC, et al. Optic nerve hypoplasia: identification by magnetic resonance imaging. *Arch Ophthalmol.* 1990;108:562–567, with permission.)

pituitary infundibulum, such as hemispheric migration anomalies (schizencephaly, cortical heterotopia, polymicrogyria), intrauterine or perinatal hemispheric injury (periventricular leukomalacia, encephalomalacia, or porencephaly), midline fusion of the cerebral hemispheres (holoprosencephaly) and cerebellar hemispheres, and other intracranial anomalies including anencephaly, hydranencephaly, and transsphenoidal encephalocele.

Evidence of perinatal injury to the pituitary infundibulum (seen on MR imaging as posterior pituitary ectopia) is found in approximately 15% of patients with optic nerve hypoplasia. Normally, the posterior pituitary gland appears bright on T1-weighted images (Fig. 3.3), probably because of the phospholipid membrane component of its hormone-containing vesicles. In posterior pituitary ectopia, MRI demonstrates absence of the normal posterior pituitary bright spot, absence or attenuation of the pituitary infundibulum, and an ectopic posterior pituitary bright spot where the upper infundibulum is normally located (Fig. 3.3). It is unknown whether posterior pituitary ectopia results from defective neuronal migration during embryogenesis, or from a perinatal injury to the hypophyseal-portal system, which causes necrosis of the infundibulum.

In a child with optic nerve hypoplasia, posterior pituitary ectopia is almost pathognomonic of anterior pituitary hormone deficiency with normal posterior pituitary function, whereas absence of a normal or ectopic posterior pituitary bright spot predicts coexistent antidiuretic hormone deficiency (i.e., diabetes insipidus). Cerebral hemispheric abnormalities are highly predictive of neurodevelopmental deficits.

Absence of the septum pellucidum alone does not portend neurodevelopmental deficits or pituitary hormone deficiency. Thinning or agenesis of the corpus callosum is predictive of neurodevelopmental problems only because of its frequent association with cerebral hemispheric abnormalities. The finding of unilateral optic nerve hypoplasia does not preclude coexistent intracranial malformations. MRI thus provides critical prognostic information regarding the likelihood of neurodevelopmental deficits and pituitary hormone deficiency in the infant or young child with **unilateral** or **bilateral** optic nerve hypoplasia.

SYSTEMIC AND TERATOGENIC ASSOCIATIONS

Numerous environmental factors that are detrimental to the fetus are sporadically associated with optic nerve hypoplasia. These include maternal insulin-dependent diabetes mellitus, fetal alcohol syndrome, maternal ingestion of quinine, anticonvulsants, illicit drugs, and fetal or neonatal infection with cytomegalovirus or hepatitis B virus. Optic nerve hypoplasia occurs with increased frequency in firstborn children of young mothers. The majority of cases are sporadic, although a handful of familial cases have been reported in siblings. The growing list of systemic and ocular disorders associated with optic nerve hypoplasia includes frontonasal dysplasia, aniridia, fetal alcohol syndrome, Dandy-Walker syndrome, Kallmann syndrome, Delleman syndrome, Duane syndrome, Klippel-Trenaunay-Weber syndrome, Goldenhar syndrome, linear nevus-sebaceous syndrome, Meckel syndrome, hemifacial atrophy, blepharophimosis,

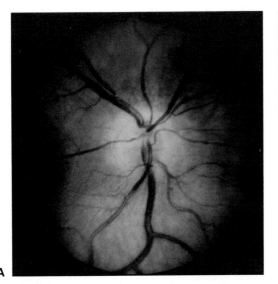
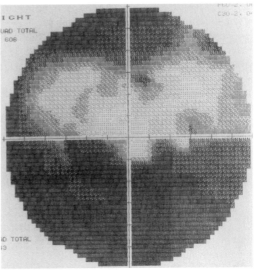

Figure 3.4. Superior segmental optic hypoplasia in a child whose mother had adult-onset diabetes mellitus. **A:** Right optic disc demonstrating an abnormal superior entrance of the central retinal artery, relative pallor of the superior disc, and a superior peripapillary halo. The superior nerve fiber layer is absent, while the inferior nerve fiber layer is clearly seen. **B:** Humphrey visual field in superior segmental hypoplasia showing a nonaltitudinal inferior visual field defect with milder superior depression. (Reprinted from: Brodsky MC, Schroeder GT, Ford R. Superior segmental optic hypoplasia in identical twins. *J Clin Neuroophthalmol.* 1993;13:152–154, with permission.)

osteogenesis imperfecta, chondrodysplasia punctata, Aicardi syndrome, Apert syndrome, Potter syndrome, chromosome 13q-syndrome, trisomy 18, neonatal isoimmune thrombocytopenia, and bilateral microphthalmos.

SEGMENTAL OPTIC NERVE HYPOPLASIA

Some forms of optic nerve hypoplasia are segmental. An isolated superior segmental optic hypoplasia with an inferior visual field defect occurs in children of insulin-dependent diabetic mothers (Fig. 3.4).

Congenital lesions of the retina, optic nerve, chiasm, tract, or retrogeniculate pathways are associated with segmental hypoplasia of the corresponding portions of each optic nerve. The term *homonymous hemioptic hypoplasia* describes the asymmetric form of segmental optic nerve hypoplasia seen in patients with unilateral congenital hemispheric lesions affecting the postchiasmal afferent visual pathways. In this setting, the nasal and temporal aspects of the optic disc contralateral to the hemispheric lesion show segmental hypoplasia and loss of the corresponding nerve fiber layers. This anomaly may be accompanied by a central band of horizontal pallor across the disc. The ipsilateral optic disc may range from normal in size to frankly hypoplastic. Homonymous hemioptic hypoplasia in

retrogeniculate lesions results from transsynaptic degeneration of the optic tract.

PATHOGENESIS

The term *optic nerve hypoplasia* implies that the nerve is deficient in axons because of a primary failure of these axons to develop. A deficiency of axon guidance molecules (such as netrin-1) at the optic disc can lead to optic nerve hypoplasia. In addition to defects in optic nerve formation, the lack of netrin-1 function during development also results in abnormalities in other parts of the CNS, such as agenesis of the corpus callosum, and cell migration and axonal guidance defects in the hypothalamus. The timing of coexistent CNS injuries would suggest that some cases of optic nerve hypoplasia result from intrauterine destruction of a normally developed structure (i.e., an encephaloclastic event), whereas others represent a primary failure of axons to develop. In human fetuses, there is a peak of 3.7 million axons at 16 to 17 weeks of gestation, with a subsequent decline to 1.1 million axons by the 31st gestational week. This massive degeneration of supernumerary axons, termed *apoptosis*, occurs as part of the normal development of the visual pathways and may serve to establish the correct topography of the visual pathways. Toxins or associated CNS malformations could augment the usual processes by which superfluous axons are eliminated from the developing visual pathways. Prenatal hemispheric injuries or malformations that injure the optic radiations can lead to retrograde transsynaptic degeneration and segmental hypoplasia of both optic nerves.

Reported cases of optic nerve hypoplasia in siblings are sufficiently rare that parents of a child with optic nerve hypoplasia can reasonably be assured that subsequent siblings are at little or no additional risk. Homozygous mutations in the *Hesx1* gene have been identified in two siblings with optic nerve hypoplasia, absence of the corpus callosum, and hypoplasia of the pituitary gland. Additional mutations in *Hesx1* have been observed in children with sporadic pituitary disease and septo-optic dysplasia. Optic nerve hypoplasia may accompany other ocular malformations in patients with mutations in the PAX6 gene.

EXCAVATED OPTIC DISC ANOMALIES

Excavated optic disc anomalies include optic disc coloboma, morning glory disc anomaly, peripapillary staphyloma, megalopapilla, optic pit, and the "vacant optic disc" associated with papillorenal syndrome. In the morning glory disc anomaly and peripapillary staphyloma, an excavation of the posterior globe surrounds and incorporates the optic disc, whereas in the other conditions, the excavation is contained within the optic disc. The terms *morning glory disc, optic disc coloboma,* and *peripapillary staphyloma* are often transposed in the literature, causing tremendous confusion regarding their diagnostic criteria, associated systemic findings, and pathogenesis. It is important to emphasize that optic disc colobomas, morning glory optic discs, and peripapillary staphylomas are distinct anomalies, each with its own specific embryologic origin, and not simply clinical variants along a broad phenotypic spectrum.

MORNING GLORY DISC ANOMALY

The morning glory disc anomaly is a congenital, funnel-shaped excavation of the posterior fundus that incorporates the optic disc, resembling the morning glory flower. Ophthalmoscopically, the disc is markedly enlarged, orange or pink in color, and may appear to be recessed or elevated centrally within the confines of a funnel-shaped peripapillary excavation (Fig. 3.5). A wide annulus of chorioretinal pigmentary disturbance surrounds the disc within the excavation. A white tuft of glial tissue overlies the central portion of the disc. The blood vessels appear increased in number and often arise from the periphery of the disc. They often curve abruptly as they emanate from the disc and run an abnormally straight

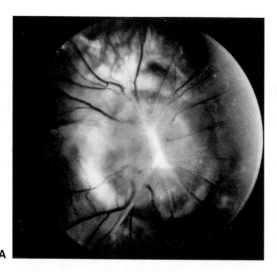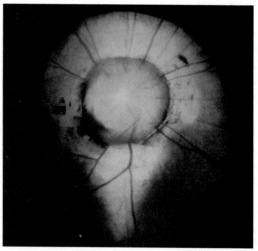

Figure 3.5. Morning glory disc anomaly. **A:** The optic disc shows the classic features of the morning glory syndrome: An enlarged, funnel-shaped, excavated and distorted optic disc that is surrounded by an elevated annulus of chorioretinal pigmentary disturbance. **B:** In another case of morning glory syndrome, a large optic disc is surrounded by an annular zone of pigmentary disturbance and a V-shaped zone of infrapapillary depigmentation. The retinal vessels appear increased in number, appear to emerge from the disc periphery, and have an abnormally straight radial configuration. A tuft of white glial overlies the center of both optic discs.

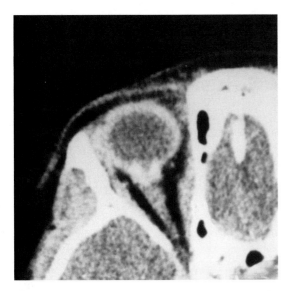

Figure 3.6. CT scan of morning glory disc anomaly. Note calcified funnel-shaped enlargement of the distal optic nerve at its junction with the globe. (Reprinted from: Brodsky MC. Congenital optic disk anomalies. *Surv Ophthalmol.* 1994;39:89–112, with permission.)

course over the peripapillary retina. It is often difficult to distinguish arterioles from venules. Close inspection may reveal the presence of peripapillary or arteriovenous communications that can be confirmed by fluorescein angiography. The macula may be incorporated into the excavation. Neuroimaging shows a funnel-shaped enlargement of the distal optic nerve at its junction with the globe (Fig. 3.6). Additional findings may include diffuse thickening with increased or decreased radiodensity of the orbital optic nerve, cavum vergae, and, most notably, transsphenoidal encephalocele.

The morning glory disc anomaly usually occurs as a unilateral condition, but bilateral cases have been reported. Visual acuity usually ranges from 20/200 to finger counting, but cases with 20/20 vision as well as no light perception have been reported. Unlike optic disc colobomas, which have no racial or gender predilection, morning glory discs are more common in females and rare in African Americans. The morning glory disc anomaly is usually not part of a multisystem genetic disorder. However, morning glory disc anomaly has been described with ipsilateral orofacial hemangioma, suggesting an association with the PHACE syndrome (**p**osterior fossa malformations, large facial **h**emangiomas, **a**rterial anomalies, **c**ardiac anomalies and aortic coarctation, and **e**ye anomalies), which occurs only in girls. This is supported by findings of ipsilateral intracranial vascular dysgenesis in

such patients. Atypical morning glory disc anomalies have also rarely been reported in patients with neurofibromatosis 2.

The association of morning glory disc anomaly with the transsphenoidal form of basal encephalocele is well established. The finding of V- or tongue-shaped infrapapillary depigmentation adjacent to a morning glory disc anomaly or other optic disc malformation (Fig. 3.7) is highly associated with transsphenoidal encephalocele. Transsphenoidal encephalocele is a rare midline congenital malformation in which a meningeal pouch, often containing the chiasm and adjacent hypothalamus, protrudes inferiorly through a large, round defect in the sphenoid bone. Patients with this occult basal meningocele have a wide head, flat nose, mild hypertelorism, a midline notch in the upper lip, and sometimes a midline cleft in the soft palate (Fig. 3.8). The meningocele protrudes into the nasopharynx, where it may obstruct the airway. Symptoms of transsphenoidal encephalocele in infancy include rhinorrhea, nasal obstruction, mouth-breathing, or snoring. These symptoms may be overlooked unless the associated morning glory disc anomaly or the characteristic facial configuration is recognized. A transsphenoidal encephalocele may appear clinically as a pulsatile posterior nasal mass or as a "nasal polyp" high in the nose, and surgical biopsy or excision of the lesion can have severe and even lethal consequences. Associated brain malformations include agenesis of the corpus callosum and posterior dilatation of the lateral ventricles. Absence of the chiasm is seen in approximately one third of patients at surgery or autopsy. Most of the affected children have no overt intellectual or neurologic deficits, but hypopituitarism is common. Morning glory disc anomaly has been associated with hypoplasia of the ipsilateral intracranial vasculature, such ipsilateral intracranial vascular dysgenesis (hypoplasia of the carotid arteries and major cerebral arteries with or without Moyamoya syndrome) (Fig 3.8B). These reports underscore the need for MR angiography in the neurodiagnostic evaluation of patients with morning glory disc anomaly.

Patients with a morning glory disc anomaly may experience both transient visual loss and permanent visual loss later in life. Serous retinal detachments occur in 26% to 38% of eyes with morning glory optic discs. These detachments typically originate in the peripapillary area and extend through the posterior pole, occasionally progressing to total detachments. In other cases with acquired visual loss, there is nonattachment and radial folding of the retina within the excavated zone.

Several authors have documented contractile movements in a morning glory optic disc, which may be related to fluctuations in subretinal fluid volume.

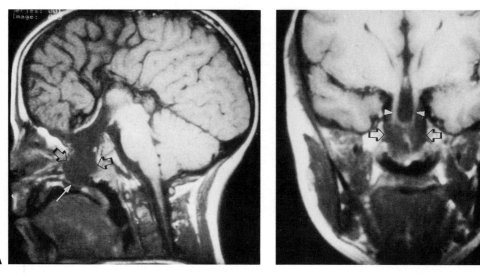

Figure 3.7. MR imaging in transsphenoidal encephalocele. **A:** Sagittal MR image shows an encephalocele (delimited by *open arrows*) extending down through the sphenoid bone into the nasopharynx with impression on the hard palate (*white arrow*). **B:** Coronal MR image shows the third ventricle and hypothalamus (*white arrowheads*) extending inferiorly into the encephalocele (delimited inferiorly by *open arrow*). (Reprinted from: Brodsky MC. Congenital optic disk anomalies. *Surv Ophthalmol.* 1994;39:89–112, with permission. Courtesy of A. James Barkovich, M.D.)

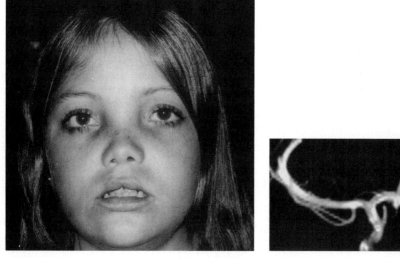

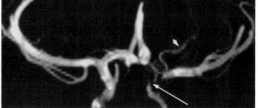

Figure 3.8. A: Photograph of a child with transsphenoidal encephalocele. Note hypertelorism, depressed nasal bridge, and subtle midline upper lip defect. **B:** MR angiography in a different patient with a morning glory disc anomaly. Note decrease in caliber of the left internal carotid artery with focal narrowing of the distal portion (*long arrow*), and narrowing of the bifurcation into middle and anterior cerebral arteries. The increased size of the lenticulostriate arteries (*short arrow*) produce a moyamoya appearance. (**A:** Reprinted from: Brodsky MC, Hoyt WF, Hoyt CS, et al. Atypical retinochoroidal coloboma in patients with dysplastic optic discs and transsphenoidal encephalocele. *Arch Ophthalmol.* 1995;113:624–628, with permission. **B:** Reprinted from: Wisotsky BJ, Magat-Gordon CB, Puklin JE. Vitreopapillary traction as a cause of elevated optic nerve head. *Am J Ophthalmol.* 1998;126:137–139, with permission.)

Subretinal neovascularization may occasionally develop within the circumferential zone of pigmentary disturbance adjacent to a morning glory disc.

The embryologic defect leading to the morning glory disc anomaly is debated. Some authors have suggested that the morning glory disc anomaly results from defective closure of the embryonic fissure and is but one phenotypic form of a colobomatous (i.e., embryonic fissure-related) defect. Others interpret the clinical findings of a central glial tuft, vascular anomalies, and a scleral defect, together with the histologic findings of adipose tissue and smooth muscle within the peripapillary sclera in presumed cases of the morning glory disc to signify a primary mesenchymal abnormality.

OPTIC DISC COLOBOMA

The term *coloboma*, of Greek derivation, means curtailed or mutilated. It is used only with reference to the eye. Colobomas of the optic disc result from incomplete or abnormal coaptation of the proximal end of the embryonic fissure.

Optic disc coloboma is characterized by a sharply delimited, glistening white, bowl-shaped excavation that occupies an enlarged optic disc (Fig. 3.9). The excavation is decentered inferiorly, reflecting the position of the embryonic fissure relative to the primitive epithelial papilla. The inferior neuroretinal rim is thin or absent, whereas the superior neuroretinal rim is relatively spared. Rarely, the entire disc appears excavated; however, the colobomatous nature of the defect can still be appreciated ophthalmoscopically because

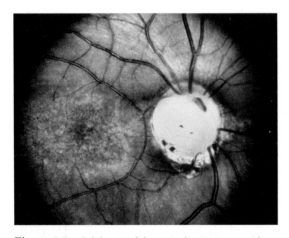

Figure 3.9. Coloboma of the optic disc in an eye with an old serous macular detachment. The disc is enlarged. A deep white excavation occupies most of the disc but spares its superior aspect. Note absence of inferior retinal nerve fiber layer and pigment epithelial disturbance in the macula. The patient had a large superior, altitudinal visual field defect.

the excavation is deeper inferiorly. The defect may extend further inferiorly to include the adjacent choroid and retina, in which case microphthalmia is frequently present. Iris and ciliary colobomas often coexist. Axial CT shows a craterlike excavation of the posterior globe at its junction with the optic nerve. Colobomatous malformations of the optic disc produce an inferior segmental hypoplasia of the optic nerve, with a C-shaped or quarter-moon-shaped neuroretinal rim confined to the superior aspect of the optic disc (Fig. 3.9).

Colobomas constitute the most common segmental form of optic nerve hypoplasia encountered in clinical practice. Coronal T1-weighted MRI confirms that the intracranial portion of the optic nerve is reduced in size. The nosological overlap between colobomatous derangement of the optic nerve and segmental hypoplasia reflects the early timing of colobomatous dysembryogenesis which results in primary failure of inferior retinal ganglion cells to develop.

Visual acuity, which depends primarily upon the integrity of the papillomacular bundle, may be mildly to severely decreased, and is difficult to predict from the appearance of the disc. Unlike the morning glory disc anomaly, which is usually unilateral, optic disc colobomas occur unilaterally or bilaterally with approximately equal frequency. As with uveal colobomas, isolated optic disc colobomas may be sporadic or inherited.

Ocular colobomas may be accompanied by other systemic anomalies, in genetic disorders such as the CHARGE association, Walker-Warburg syndrome, Goltz focal dermal hypoplasia, Aicardi syndrome, Goldenhar sequence, and linear sebaceous nevus syndrome. Optic disc coloboma has been linked to a mutation of the PAX6 gene.

Optic disc coloboma may be accompanied by other ocular malformations, including orbital cysts that communicate with atypical dark excavations of the disc that may be colobomatous in nature, retinal venous malformations, and macular hole.

Histopathologic examination in optic disc coloboma typically demonstrates intrascleral smooth muscle strands oriented concentrically around the distal optic nerve. Presumably, this pathologic finding accounts for the contractility of the optic disc seen in rare cases of optic disc coloboma. Heterotopic adipose tissue is also present within and adjacent to some optic disc colobomas. Eyes with an isolated optic disc coloboma can develop a serous macular detachment (Fig. 3.9) (in contrast to the rhegmatogenous retinal detachments that complicate retinochoroidal colobomas).

Unfortunately, many uncategorizable dysplastic optic discs (see later) are indiscriminately labeled as optic disc colobomas. This practice complicates the nosology of coloboma-associated genetic disorders. It is, therefore, crucial that the diagnosis of optic disc

Table 3.1. *Ophthalmoscopic Findings that Distinguish the Morning Glory Disc Anomaly from Optic Disc Coloboma*

Morning Glory Disc	Optic Disc Coloboma
Optic disc lies within the excavation	Excavation lies within the optic disc
Symmetrical defect (disc lies *centrally* within the excavation)	Asymmetrical defect (excavation lies *inferiorly* within the disc)
Central glial tuft	No central glial tuft
Severe peripapillary pigmentary disturbance	Minimal peripapillary pigmentary disturbance
Anomalous retinal vasculature	Normal retinal vasculature

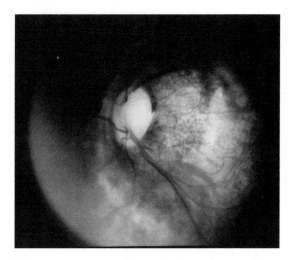

Figure 3.10. Peripapillary staphyloma. The optic disc is situated within a bowl-shaped excavation.

coloboma be reserved for discs that show an inferiorly decentered, white-colored excavation, with minimal peripapillary pigmentary changes. For example, the purported association between optic disc coloboma and basal encephalocele is deeply entrenched in the literature; however, a critical review reveals only two photographically documented cases. The ophthalmoscopic features of optic disc coloboma are most consistent with a primary structural dysgenesis of the proximal embryonic fissure, as opposed to an anomalous dilation confined to the distal optic stalk in the morning glory disc anomaly (Table 3.1). The profound differences in associated ocular and systemic findings between the two anomalies (Table 3.2) lend further credence to this hypothesis. Anomalous optic discs with overlapping features of the morning glory disc anomaly and optic disc coloboma are occasionally seen. These "hybrid" anomalies could easily represent instances of early embryonic injury affecting both the proximal

embryonic fissure and the distal optic stalk. However, the concept of "an optic disc coloboma with a morning glory configuration" should be abandoned.

PERIPAPILLARY STAPHYLOMA

Peripapillary staphyloma is an extremely rare, usually unilateral anomaly, in which a deep fundus excavation surrounds the optic disc (Fig. 3.10). In this condition, the disc is seen at the bottom of the excavated defect and may appear normal or show temporal pallor. The walls and margin of the defect may show atrophic changes in the retinal pigment epithelium (RPE) and choroid. Unlike the morning glory disc anomaly, there is no central glial tuft overlying the disc, and the retinal vascular pattern remains normal, apart from reflecting the essential contour of the lesion (Table 3.3). Several cases of contractile peripapillary staphyloma have been documented.

Table 3.2. *Associated Ocular and Systemic Findings that Distinguish the Morning Glory Disc from Isolated Optic Disc Coloboma*

Morning Glory Disc	Optic Disc Coloboma
More common in females; rare in blacks	No sex or racial predilection
Rarely familial	Often familial
Rarely bilateral	Often bilateral
No iris, ciliary, or retinal colobomas	Iris, ciliary, and retinal colobomas common
Rarely associated with multisystem genetic disorders	Often associated with multisystem genetic disorders
Basal encephalocele common	Basal encephalocele rare

Table 3.3. *Ophthalmoscopic Findings that Distinguish Peripapillary Staphyloma from the Morning Glory Disc Anomaly*

Peripapillary Staphyloma	Morning Glory Disc
Deep, cup-shaped excavation	Less depth, funnel-shaped excavation
Relatively normal, well-defined optic disc	Grossly anomalous, poorly defined optic disc
Absence of glial and vascular anomalies	Central glial bouquet, anomalous vascular pattern

Visual acuity is usually markedly reduced in eyes with a peripapillary staphyloma, but cases with nearly normal acuity have also been reported. Affected eyes are usually emmetropic or slightly myopic, and eyes with decreased vision frequently have centrocecal scotomas. Although peripapillary staphyloma is clinically and embryologically distinct from morning glory optic disc, these conditions are frequently transposed in the literature.

Although peripapillary staphyloma is usually isolated, it has been reported in association with transsphenoidal encephalocele, PHACE syndrome, linear nevus sebaceous syndrome, and 18q- (de Grouchy) syndrome.

The fairly normal appearance of the optic disc and retinal vessels in eyes with a peripapillary staphyloma suggests that the development of these structures is complete before the staphylomatous process begins. The clinical features of peripapillary staphyloma are most consistent with diminished peripapillary structural support, perhaps resulting from incomplete differentiation of sclera from posterior neural crest cells in the fifth month of gestation.

MEGALOPAPILLA

Megalopapilla is a generic term that connotes an abnormally large, excavated optic disc that lacks the numerous anomalous features of the morning glory disc anomaly, the inferior displacement of a coloboma, or the striking cilioretinal circulation of the papillorenal syndrome (see below). Megalopapilla comprises two phenotypic variants. The first is a common variant in which an abnormally large optic disc (>2.1 mm in diameter) retains an otherwise normal configuration. This form of megalopapilla is usually bilateral and is often associated with a large cup-to-disc ratio, which almost invariably raises the diagnostic consideration of normal-tension glaucoma (Fig. 3.11). However, the optic cup is usually round or horizontally oval with no vertical notching or encroachment, so that the quotient of horizontal to vertical cup-to-disc ratio remains normal, in contradistinction to the decreased quotient that characterizes glaucomatous optic atrophy. Because the axons are spread over a larger surface area, the neuroretinal rim may also appear pale, mimicking optic atrophy. Less commonly, the normal optic cup is replaced by a grossly anomalous noninferior excavation that obliterates the adjacent neuroretinal rim (Fig. 3.11). The inclusion of this rare variant under the rubric of megalopapilla serves the nosologically useful function of distinguishing it from a colobomatous defect with the latter's attendant systemic implications. Cilioretinal arteries are common in eyes with megalopapilla.

Visual acuity is usually normal with megalopapilla, but it may be mildly decreased. The visual field is also usually normal, except for an enlarged blind spot. Colobomatous discs are distinguished from megalopapilla by their predominant excavation of the inferior optic disc. Aside from glaucoma and optic disc coloboma, the differential diagnosis of megalopapilla includes orbital optic glioma, which in children can cause progressive enlargement of a previously normal-sized optic disc.

Pathogenetically, most cases of megalopapilla may simply represent a statistical variant of normal.

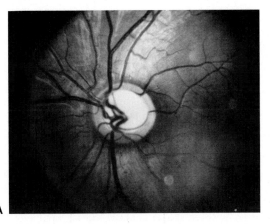 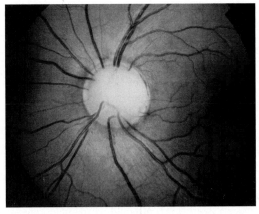

A   B

Figure 3.11. Megalopapilla. **A:** A common variant of megalopapilla in which an abnormally large optic disc contains a large central cup. Unlike glaucomatous optic atrophy, the cup is horizontally oval with an intact neuroretinal rim, and there is no nasalization of vessels at the point of origin. **B:** An uncommon variant of megalopapilla in which an anomalous superior excavation obliterates much of the temporal neuroretinal rim. (Reprinted from: Brodsky MC. Congenital optic disk anomalies. *Surv Ophthalmol.* 1994;39:89–112, with permission.)

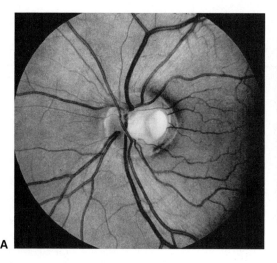
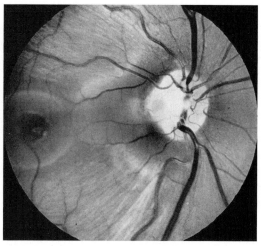

A   **B**

Figure 3.12. Optic pit. **A:** Oval white excavation occupies the temporal portion of the disc. **B:** Grayish temporal optic disc with adjacent retinoschisis cavity (*large arrows*), serous macular detachment (*small arrows*) and outer layer hole (*open arrow*).

However, it is likely that megalopapilla occasionally results from altered migration of optic axons early in embryogenesis, as evidenced by reports of megalopapilla in patients with anterior encephaloceles. Nevertheless, the rarity of an association between megalopapilla and CNS abnormalities suggests that neuroimaging is unwarranted in a patient with megalopapilla, unless midline facial anomalies (e.g., hypertelorism, cleft palate, cleft lip, depressed nasal bridge) coexist.

OPTIC PIT

An optic pit is a round or oval, gray, white, or yellowish depression in the optic disc (Fig. 3.12). The estimated frequency of optic pits is approximately 1 in 11,000. Numerous reports of familial optic pits suggest an autosomal-dominant mode of transmission.

Optic pits commonly affect the temporal portion of the optic disc but may be situated in any sector. Such temporally located pits are often accompanied by adjacent peripapillary pigment epithelial changes. One or two cilioretinal arteries emerge from the bottom or the margin of the pit in more than 50% of cases. Although optic pits are typically unilateral, bilateral pits are seen in 15% of cases. In unilateral cases, the affected disc is slightly larger than the normal disc. Visual acuity is typically normal unless there is fluid within or beneath the macula (see below). Although visual field defects are variable and often correlate poorly with the location of the pit, the most common defect appears to be a paracentral arcuate scotoma connected to an enlarged blind spot. Optic pits do not portend additional CNS malformations, although rare exceptions exist.

Serous macular elevations develop in 25% to 75% of eyes with optic pits (Fig. 3.12). Optic pit-associated maculopathy generally becomes symptomatic in the third and fourth decades of life. Vitreous traction on the margins of the pit and tractional changes in the roof of the pit may be the inciting events that ultimately lead to late-onset macular detachment. The risk of optic pit-associated macular detachment is greater in eyes with large optic pits and in eyes with temporally located pits. Spontaneous reattachment occurs in approximately 25% of cases. Laser photocoagulation to block the flow of fluid from the pit to the macula is usually unsuccessful, perhaps because of the inability of laser photocoagulation to seal a retinoschisis cavity. Vitrectomy with internal gas tamponade and laser photocoagulation can results in long-term improvement in acuity.

Histologically, optic pits consist of herniations of dysplastic retina into a collagen-lined pocket extending posteriorly, often into the subarachnoid space, through a defect in the lamina cribrosa. The source of intraretinal fluid in eyes with optic pits is controversial and include vitreous cavity via the pit, the subarachnoid space, blood vessels at the base of the pit, and the orbital space surrounding the dura.

Although the pathogenesis of optic pits remains controversial, most authors view optic pits as the mildest variant in the spectrum of optic disc colobomas; however, this is unlikely. Indeed, optic pits are usually unilateral, sporadic, and unassociated with systemic anomalies, whereas colobomas are bilateral as often as unilateral, commonly autosomal dominant, and may be associated with a variety of multisystem disorders. In addition, it is rare for optic pits to coexist

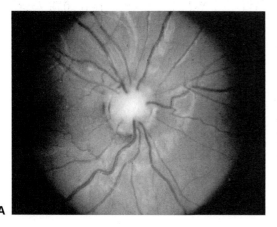
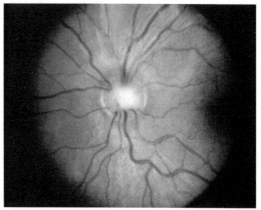

A   B

Figure 3.13. Papillorenal syndrome. Both optic discs show a central excavation with multiple cilioretinal arteries in place of the normal central retinal circulation. This 9-year-old girl with chronic renal failure had 20/20 acuity in each eye. Renal biopsy showed interstitial fibrosis. (Photographs courtesy of Erika M. Levin, M.D.)

with iris or retinochoroidal colobomas, and optic pits usually occur in locations unrelated to the embryonic fissure.

PAPILLORENAL SYNDROME (THE "UNCOLOBOMA")

The papillorenal syndrome (previously known as renal-coloboma syndrome) is characterized by a distinct optic disc malformation that bears no relationship to coloboma. In this syndrome, the excavated optic disc is normal in size, and may be surrounded by variable pigmentary disturbance. Unlike in colobomatous defects, the excavation is centrally positioned. The defining feature is the presence of multiple cilioretinal vessels which emanate from the periphery of the disc, and variable attenuation or atrophy of the central retinal vessels (Fig. 3.13). Color Doppler imaging has confirmed the absence of central retinal circulation in patients with papillorenal syndrome.

Visual acuity is usually normal but may occasionally be severely diminished secondary to choroidal and retinal hypoplasia and, in some cases, to later-onset serous retinal detachments. Peripheral visual field defects corresponding to areas of retinal hypoplasia are often present. The central optic disc excavation and peripheral field defects can simulate coloboma as well as normal tension glaucoma.

Families have been reported with an autosomal dominant mode of transmission. In some patients, mutations have been found in the developmental gene PAX2. This malformation is attributed to a primary deficiency in angiogenesis involved in vascular development. In these patients, there is a failure of the hyaloid system to convert to normal central retinal vessels.

CONGENITAL TILTED DISC SYNDROME

The tilted disc syndrome is a nonhereditary, usually bilateral condition in which the superotemporal optic disc is elevated and the inferonasal disc is posteriorly displaced, resulting in an oval-appearing optic disc, with its long axis obliquely oriented (Fig. 3.14). This configuration is accompanied by *situs inversus* of the retinal vessels, congenital inferonasal conus, thinning of the inferonasal RPE and choroid, and bitemporal hemianopia that do not respect the vertical midline. Histopathologically, the optic nerve enters at an extremely oblique angle, the superior or superotemporal portion of the disc is elevated, and there is posterior ectasia of the inferior or inferonasal fundus and optic disc. The cause of the tilted disc syndrome is unknown, but the inferonasal or inferior location of the excavation suggests a pathogenetic relationship to retinochoroidal coloboma.

Affected patients often have myopic astigmatism, with the plus-axis oriented parallel to the ectasia. The ocular imagery resulting from a tilted retina creates a type of curvature of field that may subjectively simulate astigmatic blur. The congenital tilted disc syndrome is bilateral in about 80% of cases. Familiarity with the tilted disc syndrome is crucial for the ophthalmologist, since affected patients may present with bitemporal hemianopia, suggesting a chiasmal syndrome. The bitemporal hemianopia in patients with tilted discs, however, is typically incomplete and confined primarily to the superior quadrants. It is, in fact, a refractive scotoma, secondary to regional myopia localized to the inferonasal retina (Fig. 3.15). Unlike the visual field loss that results from damage to the optic chiasm, the field defects seen in the tilted disc syndrome

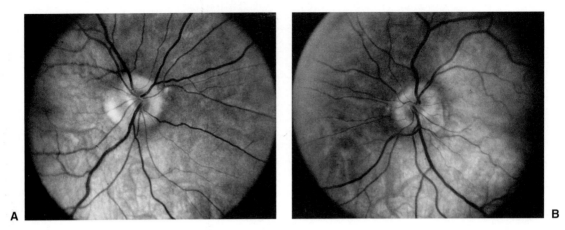

Figure 3.14. Congenital tilted disc syndrome. Both optic discs are oval with relative elevation of the superior-temporal portion compared to the inferior-nasal portion. This elevation is often mistaken for true disc swelling. Note situs inversus of the vessels and inferior retinochoroidal hypopigmentation.

fail to respect the vertical meridian on both kinetic and static perimetry. Furthermore, the superotemporal depression on Goldmann perimetry is selectively detected with mid-sized isopters, whereas the large and small isopters give fairly normal results because the ectasia that occurs in such cases is confined to the midperipheral fundus. Despite the regional retinal ectasia, recent topography studies have suggested that an irregular corneal curvature underlies the associated astigmatism. Repeat perimetry with a spectacle lens in place to correct myopic astigmatism may reduce or eliminate the superotemporal defect, confirming its refractive nature. In some cases, retinal sensitivity may be decreased in the area of the ectasia, and the defect thus persists to some degree despite appropriate refractive correction. Other quadrants also show mildly decreased sensitivities on threshold perimetry and suggested that the tilted disc syndrome may actually include some degree of diffuse retinal or optic nerve hypoplasia. In some cases, elevation of the superior-temporal portion of the disc mimics optic disc swelling.

It should be emphasized that a true bitemporal hemianopia may occur in patients with the tilted disc syndrome who also harbor a congenital suprasellar

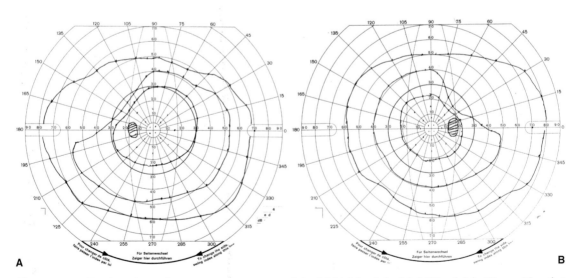

Figure 3.15. Kinetic perimetry demonstrates a supertemporal visual field defect in both left (**A**) and right (**B**) eyes. Note that the defect is confined to the midperipheral isopter that does not respect the horizontal meridian.

tumor. As with optic nerve hypoplasia, these two seemingly disparate lesions may reflect the disruptive effect of a suprasellar lesion on the migration of optic axons during embryogenesis. This sinister association mandates neuroimaging in any patient with a tilted disc syndrome whose bitemporal hemianopia either respects the vertical meridian or fails to preferentially involve the midperipheral isopter on kinetic perimetry. The tilted disc syndrome has also been documented in patients with craniofacial anomalies, including Crouzon's disease and Apert's disease.

Tilted discs without retinal ectasia occur in patients with transsphenoidal encephalocele, congenital tumors of the anterior visual pathways, X-linked congenital stationary night blindness, Ehlers-Danlos syndrome (type III), and familial dextrocardia.

OPTIC DISC DYSPLASIA

Optic disc dysplasia is a term that connotes a markedly deformed optic disc that fails to conform to any recognizable diagnostic category (Fig. 3.16). The distinction between a nonspecifically "anomalous" disc and a "dysplastic" disc is somewhat arbitrary and based primarily upon the severity of the lesion.

Dysplastic optic discs in patients with transsphenoidal encephalocele tend to be associated with a discrete infrapapillary zone of V-or tongue-shaped retinochoroidal depigmentation. This finding should prompt neuroimaging. These juxtapapillary defects differ from typical retinochoroidal colobomas, which widen inferiorly and are not associated with basal encephalocele. Unlike the typical retinochoroidal

coloboma, this distinct juxtapapillary defect is associated with minimal scleral excavation and no visible disruption in the integrity of the overlying retina.

CONGENITAL OPTIC DISC PIGMENTATION

Congenital optic disc pigmentation is a condition in which melanin deposition anterior to or within the lamina cribrosa imparts a slate-gray appearance to the entire optic disc. True congenital optic disc pigmentation is extremely rare, but it has been described in association with interstitial deletion of chromosome 17, Aicardi syndrome, and optic nerve hypoplasia (Fig. 3.17). Congenital optic disc pigmentation is compatible with good visual acuity but may be associated with coexistent optic disc anomalies that decrease vision.

The majority of patients with gray optic discs do not have congenital optic disc pigmentation. For reasons that are poorly understood, optic discs of infants with delayed visual maturation and albinism often have a diffuse gray tint when viewed ophthalmoscopically. In these conditions, the gray tint usually disappears within the first year of life without visible pigment migration. It should be noted, however, that gray optic discs may also be seen in normal neonates and are usually a nonspecific finding of little diagnostic value, except when accompanied by other clinical signs of delayed visual maturation or albinism. Myelinated peripapillary nerve fibers may impart a gray cast to the

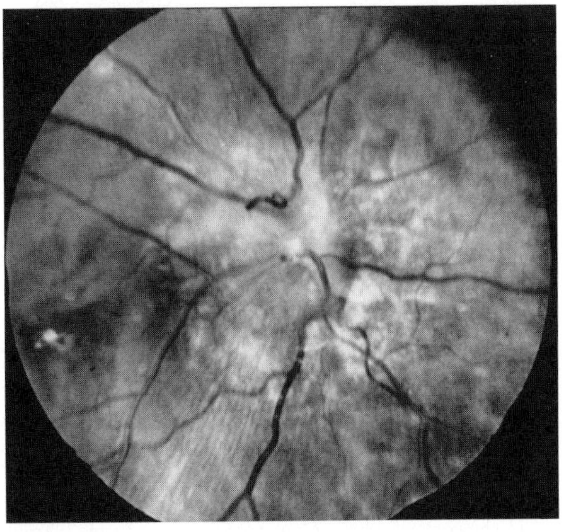

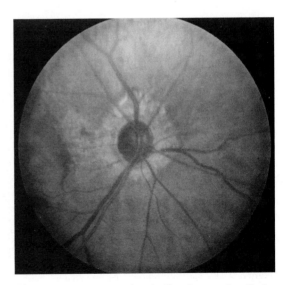

Figure 3.16. Optic disc dysplasia. The optic disc is grossly malformed, and the retinal vessels emerge from the region of the disc in an anomalous pattern.

Figure 3.17. Congenital optic disc pigmentation. Entire disc is gray, and the disc is hypoplastic with a surrounding zone of depigmentation, suggesting migration of peripapillary pigment onto the disc.

optic disc, as may pseudopapilledema associated with buried drusen. A grayish cast to the optic discs was also described in patients with Pelizaeus-Merzbacher disease, with maple syrup urine disease, and with partial trisomy 10q syndrome.

Optically gray optic discs and congenital optic disc pigmentation can usually be distinguished ophthalmoscopically, because melanin deposition in true congenital optic disc pigmentation is often discrete, irregular, and granular in appearance. True optic disc pigmentation may also be acquired, as in cases of melanocytoma or malignant melanoma of the optic nerve head, following scleral buckling procedure, after removal of the retrobulbar optic nerve for optic glioma, and following presumed infectious optic neuritis.

AICARDI SYNDROME

Aicardi syndrome is a congenital cerebroretinal disorder of unknown etiology. This syndrome associates infantile spasms, agenesis of the corpus callosum, a modified form of the electroencephalographic pattern termed hypsarrhythmia, and a pathognomonic optic disc appearance consisting of multiple depigmented "chorioretinal lacunae" clustered around the disc (Fig. 3.18). Histologically, chorioretinal lacunae consist of well-circumscribed, full-thickness defects limited to the retinal pigment epithelium and choroid. The overlying retina remains intact but is often histologically abnormal.

Congenital optic disc anomalies, including optic disc coloboma, optic nerve hypoplasia, and congenital optic disc pigmentation, may accompany chorioretinal lacunae. Other ocular abnormalities include microphthalmos, retrobulbar cyst, pseudoglioma, retinal detachment, macular scar, cataract, pupillary membrane, iris synechiae, iris coloboma, and persistent hyperplastic primary vitreous. The most common systemic findings associated with Aicardi syndrome are vertebral malformations (fused vertebrae, scoliosis, spina bifida) and costal malformations (absent ribs, fused or bifurcated ribs). Other systemic findings in Aicardi syndrome include muscular hypotonia, microcephaly, dysmorphic facies, cleft lip and palate, auditory disturbances, and auricular anomalies. Aicardi syndrome has also been associated with choroid plexus papilloma.

Severe mental retardation is present in almost all cases. Aicardi syndrome is associated with decreased life expectancy, but some patients survive into their teenage years. It has been suggested that the size of the largest chorioretinal lacuna correlates with neurologic outcome, whereas age at presentation, type, and severity of seizures does not. Most children have medically intractable seizures, and 91% attain milestones no higher than 12 months.

Central nervous system anomalies in Aicardi syndrome include agenesis of the corpus callosum, cortical migration anomalies (pachygyria, polymicrogyria, cortical heterotopias), and multiple structural

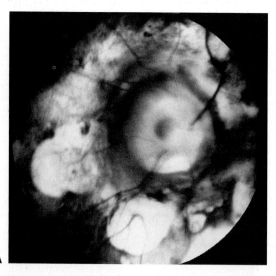
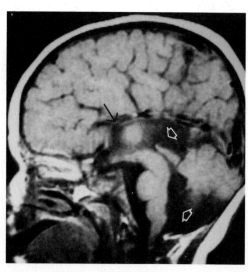

Figure 3.18. Aicardi syndrome. **A:** An enlarged, malformed optic disc is surrounded by numerous, well-circumscribed, chorioretinal lacunae. **B:** Sagittal MR image demonstrating agenesis of the corpus callosum (*upper solid arrow* denotes normal position of the corpus callosum), an arachnoid cyst in the region of the quadrigeminal cistern (*open arrows*) and hypoplasia of the cerebellar vermis with cystic dilatation of the fourth ventricle (Dandy-Walker variant). (**A:** Reprinted from: Carney SH, Brodsky MC, Good WV, et al. Aicardi syndrome: more than meets the eye. *Surv Ophthalmol.* 1993;37:419–424, with permission.)

CNS malformations (cerebral hemispheric asymmetry, Dandy-Walker variant, colpocephaly, midline arachnoid cysts) (Fig. 3.18). Neuropathologic specimens show a characteristic profile, consisting of unlayered polymicrogyria, subcortical or periventricular heterotopias, and agenesis of the corpus callosum. This complex cerebral malformation suggests a problem in nerve cell proliferation and migration. An overlap between Aicardi syndrome and septo-optic dysplasia has been recognized in several patients.

Aicardi syndrome is thought to result from an X-linked mutational event that is lethal in males.

DOUBLING OF THE OPTIC DISC

Doubling of the optic discs is a rare anomaly in which two optic discs are seen ophthalmoscopically and presumed to be associated with a duplication or separation of the distal optic nerve into two fasciculi. Most cases have a "main" disc and a "satellite" disc, each with its own vascular system (Fig. 3.19). Most cases occur unilaterally and are associated with decreased acuity in the affected eye.

Documented separation of the optic nerve into two or more strands is rare in humans but common in some lower vertebrates. More commonly, an apparent doubling of the optic disc results from focal juxtapapillary retinochoroidal colobomas, which may display abnormal vascular anastomoses with the optic disc.

OPTIC NERVE APLASIA

Optic nerve aplasia is a rare nonhereditary malformation seen most often in a unilaterally malformed eye of an otherwise healthy person. The term implies complete absence of the optic nerve (including the optic disc), retinal ganglion and nerve fiber layers, and optic nerve vessels. Histopathologic examination usually demonstrates a vestigial dural sheath entering the sclera in its normal position, as well as retinal dysplasia with rosette formation (Fig. 3.20). Some early reports of optic nerve aplasia actually described patients with severe hypoplasia at a time when the latter entity was not clearly recognized.

Optic nerve aplasia may be diagnosed in the absence of a normally defined optic nerve head or papilla in the ocular fundus, without central blood vessels and with an absence of macular differentiation; when the optic disc appears as a whitish area only, without central vessels or macular differentiation; or when there is a deep avascular cavity surrounded by a whitish annulus in the site corresponding to the optic disc.

Visual fields and fluorescein angiogram are normal in the unaffected eye, while there are no retinal blood vessels in the affected eye. The electroretinographic waveform (ERG) may be flat; if present, the a- and b-waves are diminished. CT scanning may show the globe and bony orbit to be smaller than normal. In addition, MRI may show isolated absence of the optic nerve on the affected side.

The cause of optic nerve aplasia is unknown. Optic nerve aplasia seems to fall within a malformation complex that is fundamentally distinct from that seen with optic nerve hypoplasia, as evidenced by the proclivity of optic nerve aplasia to occur unilaterally

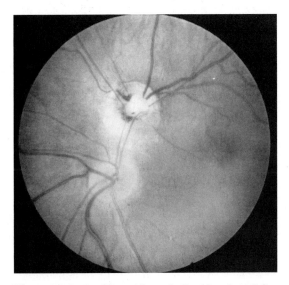

Figure 3.19. Doubling of the optic disc. Note "main" disc and "satellite" disc. (Reprinted from: Donoso LA, Magaragal LE, Eiferman RA. Ocular anomalies simulating double optic discs. *Can J Ophthalmol.* 1981;16:84–87, with permission. Photograph courtesy of Larry A. Donoso.)

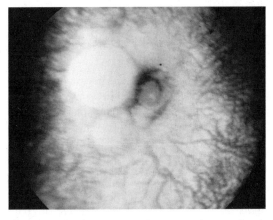

Figure 3.20. Optic nerve aplasia. Note absence of optic disc and retinal vessels (Reprinted from: Little LE, Whitmore PV, Wells TW Jr. Aplasia of the optic nerve. *J Pediatr Ophthalmol.* 1976;13:84–88, with permission).

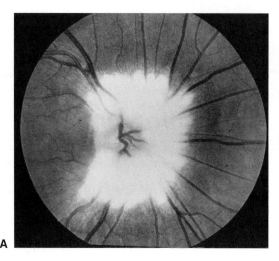
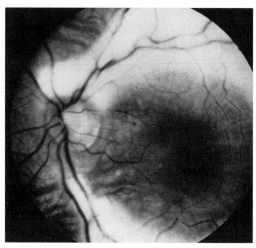

A   B

Figure 3.21. Myelinated nerve fibers. **A:** The optic disc is surrounded by myelinated, feathery nerve fibers. **B:** Myelinated nerve fibers extend superiorly and inferiorly from the optic disc along the arcuate nerve fiber bundles.

and its frequent association with malformations that are otherwise confined to the affected eye (microphthalmia, malformations in the anterior chamber angle, hypoplasia or segmental aplasia of the iris, cataracts, persistent hyperplastic primary vitreous, anterior colobomas, macular staphyloma, retinal dysplasia, or pigmentary disturbance). However, when optic nerve aplasia occurs bilaterally, it is usually associated with severe and widespread congenital CNS malformations.

MYELINATED (MEDULLATED) NERVE FIBERS

Myelination of the anterior visual system begins centrally at the lateral geniculate body at 5 months of gestation. It proceeds distally and reaches the chiasm by 6 to 7 months of gestation, the retrobulbar optic nerve by 8 months, and the lamina cribrosa at term; although in some cases myelination may continue for a short time after birth. Normally, myelin does not extend intraocularly; however, intraocular myelination of retinal nerve fibers occurs in 0.3% to 0.6% of the population by ophthalmoscopy and in 1% by postmortem examinations. In most eyes, myelination is continuous with the optic disc, and the majority of patients had normal visual acuity.

The pathogenesis of myelinated nerve fibers remains largely speculative, but it has been suggested that a defect in the lamina cribrosa may allow oligodendrocytes to gain access to the retina and produce myelin there.

Ophthalmoscopically, myelinated nerve fibers usually appear as white striated patches at the upper and lower poles of the optic disc (Fig. 3.21). In these locations, they may impart a gray appearance to the optic disc, and they may also simulate papilledema, both by elevating the adjacent portions of the disc and by obscuring the disc margin and underlying retinal vessels. Distally, they have an irregular fan-shaped appearance that facilitates their recognition. Small slits or patches of normal-appearing fundus color are occasionally visible within areas of myelination. Myelinated nerve fibers are bilateral in 17% to 20% of cases and, clinically, they are discontinuous with the optic nerve head in 19%. Isolated patches of myelinated nerve fibers are occasionally found in the peripheral retina.

Retinal vascular abnormalities, such as telangiectasia or neovascularization have been described within areas of myelinated nerve fibers. They are sometimes associated with vitreous hemorrhage, suggesting that the retinal vessels within patches of myelinated nerve fibers should be carefully examined for occult microvascular abnormalities.

Myelinated retinal nerve fibers do not usually reduce visual acuity; however, relative scotomas may be charted if a sufficient number of myelinated fibers are present. The scotomas are invariably smaller than the size of the myelinated patch would suggest. Because myelinated fibers are usually adjacent to the optic disc, the blind spot is often enlarged in such patients. When the nerve fibers surround the macula, there may be a ring scotoma, and isolated patches in the retinal periphery may produce isolated peripheral scotomas. If the macula is affected, there may be a central scotoma, but this is rare.

Extensive unilateral (or rarely bilateral) myelination of nerve fibers can be associated with high myopia and severe amblyopia. Unlike other forms of unilateral high myopia that characteristically respond well to occlusion therapy, the amblyopia that occurs in children with myelinated nerve fibers is notoriously refractory to this treatment. In such patients, myelination surrounds most of the disc. Additionally, the macular region (although unmyelinated) usually appears abnormal, showing a dulled reflex or pigment dispersion.

Myelinated nerve fibers may occur in association with the Gorlin syndrome (multiple basal cell nevi). Myelinated nerve fibers may be familial, in which case the trait is usually inherited in an autosomal-dominant fashion. Isolated cases of myelinated nerve fibers may also occur in association with abnormal length of the optic nerve (oxycephaly), defects in the lamina cribrosa (tilted disc), anterior segment dysgenesis, and neurofibromatosis type 2. An autosomal-dominant vitreoretinopathy associated with myelination of the nerve fiber layer is characterized by congenitally poor vision, bilateral extensive myelination of the retinal nerve fiber layer, severe degeneration of the vitreous, high myopia, a retinal dystrophy with night blindness, reduction of the electroretinographic responses, and limb deformities.

Rarely, areas of myelinated nerve fibers may be acquired after infancy and even in adulthood, sometimes after a trauma to the eye. Progression of myelinated nerve fibers has been documented in children. Conversely, myelinated nerve fibers may disappear as a result of an acquired optic neuropathy, central retinal artery occlusion, and branch retinal artery occlusion.

PSEUDOPAPILLEDEMA

Anomalous optic disc elevation (pseudopapilledema) may bear a striking resemblance to true optic disc swelling and therefore represents a primary diagnostic consideration in the patient referred for papilledema. In most instances, a patient is noted to have elevated optic discs or blurred disc margins during the course of a routine examination. The diagnostic uncertainty and alarm created by this finding overshadows the fact that the patient has no other signs or symptoms of increased intracranial pressure. Many patients with pseudopapilledema are referred for neuro-ophthalmologic evaluation only after being subjected to neuroimaging, lumbar puncture, and extensive laboratory studies.

Once the diagnosis of pseudopapilledema is established, pseudopapilledema associated with optic disc drusen must be distinguished from other local causes of pseudopapilledema, such as hyaloid traction on the optic disc, epipapillary glial tissue, myelinated nerve fibers, scleral infiltration, vitreopapillary traction, and high hyperopia. In the patient with additional systemic disorders, consideration must be given to the possibil-

ity that pseudopapilledema may be related to an underlying genetic disorder. Systemic disorders that include pseudopapilledema are Down syndrome, Alagille syndrome (arteriohepatic dysplasia), Kenny syndrome (hypocalcemic dwarfism), linear nevus sebaceous syndrome, and Leber's hereditary optic neuropathy.

PSEUDOPAPILLEDEMA ASSOCIATED WITH OPTIC DISC DRUSEN

The word drusen, of Germanic origin, originally meant tumor, swelling, or tumescence. The word was used in the mining industry approximately 500 years ago to indicate a crystal-filled space in a rock. Other terms for these lesions include **hyaline bodies** and **colloid bodies** of the optic disc.

In Scandinavia, the prevalence of optic drusen in a clinical series was 3.4 per 1,000, and the prevalence increased by a factor of 10 in family members of patients with drusen. The prevalence of drusen in autopsy series is, as might be expected, somewhat higher than the prevalence on clinical studies, varying between 0.41% and 2%. Men and women are equally affected, and bilateral drusen occurs in 67% to 85% of cases. The age at which visible drusen or pseudopapilledema caused by buried drusen is diagnosed varies widely, depending on the population studies. Familial drusen are transmitted as an autosomal-dominant trait. The low prevalence of disc drusen in African Americans may be attributable to racial variation in optic disc size.

The evolution of disc drusen is a dynamic process that continues throughout life. It is rare to see visible drusen or significant optic disc elevation in an infant. During childhood, the affected optic disc begins to appear "full" and acquires a tan, yellow, or straw color. The buried drusen gradually impart a scalloped appearance to the margin of the disc and produce subtle excrescences on the disc surface that tend to predominate nasally. They later enlarge and calcify, and become more visible on the disc surface. As they enlarge they sometimes deflect retinal vessels overlying the disc. In adulthood, the optic disc elevation diminishes, the disc gradually becomes pale, the nerve fiber layer thins, and discrete slits appear. This evolution reflects a slow attrition of optic axons over decades. Despite this progression, most patients remain asymptomatic and retain normal acuity.

Drusen appear as round, slightly irregular excrescences that are present within and occasionally around the disc (Fig. 3.22). Surface drusen may be scattered or form conglomerates that cover the disc. Surface drusen affecting only a portion of the disc are usually concentrated nasally and are most conspicuous at the periphery of the disc. Superficial drusen reflect whitish yellow light, are globular, and vary in size from minute dots to granules 2 or 3 times the diameter of a retinal vessel.

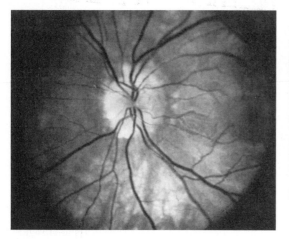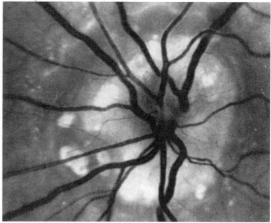

Figure 3.22. Visible disc drusen. Note multiple white nodules lining the periphery of the discs and abnormal branching of retinal vessels.

Deeply situated drusen lack sharp margins, but they may still be illuminated when indirect lighting is used.

Drusen buried within the tissue of the disc produce moderate elevation of the surface of the disc, as well as blurring of its margins (Fig. 3.23): However, the anomalously elevated disc is not hyperemic, and there are no dilated capillaries on its surface; despite extreme elevation of the disc, the surface arteries are not obscured; the physiologic cup is absent in the anomalously elevated disc; anomalously elevated discs are smaller than normal; the most elevated portion of the disc is usually the central area from which the vessels emerge; in a large percentage of cases, there are anomalous vascular patterns on the disc surface, including an increased number of otherwise normal vessels, abnormal arterial and venous branchings, increased tortuosity, vascular loops, and cilioretinal arteries; elevation is confined to the optic disc and does not extend to the peripapillary nerve fiber layer, which may retain its normal linear pattern of light reflexes or show abnormalities indicative of nerve fiber atrophy; the anomalously elevated disc usually has an irregular border with pigment epithelial defects being present.

The distinction between pseudopapilledema associated with buried drusen and papilledema (or other

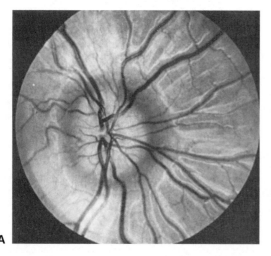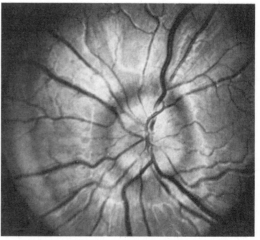

A   B

Figure 3.23. Buried disc drusen. Both optic discs have a similar appearance, with absence of the central cup, and an increased number of retinal vessels with an anomalous branching pattern. The disc elevation does not obscure the overlying vessels. Although no discrete drusen are seen, there is a subtle nodularity of the disc margin.

Table 3.4. *Ophthalmoscopic Features Useful in Differentiating Optic Disc Edema from Pseudopapilledema Associated with Buried Drusen*

Optic Disc Edema	Pseudopapilledema with Buried Drusen
Disc vasculature obscured at disc margins	Disc vasculature remains visible at disc margins
Elevation extends into peripapillary retina	Elevation confined to optic disc
Graying and muddying of peripapillary nerve fiber layer	Sharp peripapillary nerve fiber
Venous congestion ± exudates	No venous congestion No exudates
Loss of optic cup only in moderate to severe disc edema	Small cupless disc
Normal configuration of disc vasculature despite venous congestion	Increased major retinal vessels with early branching
No circumpapillary light reflex	Crescentic circumpapillary light reflex
Absence of spontaneous venous pulsations	Spontaneous venous pulsations may be present or absent

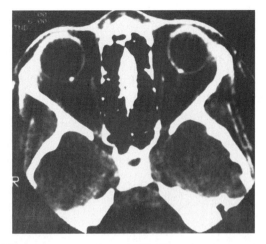

Figure 3.24. Unenhanced axial CT scan showing posterior scleral calcification corresponding to optic disc drusen.

forms of optic disc swelling) can be difficult, but several clinical signs are particularly helpful (Table 3.4).

The differentiation between papilledema and pseudopapilledema caused by buried drusen is frequently aided by ancillary studies. CT scanning (often obtained when papilledema is suspected) and ultrasonography demonstrate calcifications within the elevated optic disc (Figs. 3.24 and 3.25). Special photographic techniques may also be useful in identifying superficial or buried optic disc drusen. Monochromatic (red-free) photography may highlight the glistening drusen against the intact or atrophic nerve fiber layer. Photographs taken with the filters normally used for fluorescein photography in place, but without injection of fluorescein show that superficial disc drusen often demonstrate the phenomenon of autofluorescence (Fig. 3.26). Fluorescein angiography can also facilitate the differentiation between true papilledema and pseudopapilledema. After intravenous fluorescein injection, drusen exhibit a true nodular hyperfluorescence corresponding to the location of the visible drusen. The late phases may be characterized by minimal blurring of the drusen that either fade or maintain fluorescence (i.e., stain). Unlike in papilledema, however, there is no visible leakage along the major

vessels. Fluorescein angiography may also disclose venous anomalies (venous stasis, venous convolutions, and retinociliary venous communications) and staining of the peripapillary vein walls in eyes with optic disc drusen.

Although patients with pseudopapilledema are not immune to the neurologic and ophthalmologic disorders of the general population, there is no significant relationship between drusen and neurologic disorders

Most patients with optic disc drusen are asymptomatic and remain so throughout life. Nevertheless, patients with optic disc drusen occasionally experience acute loss of vision.

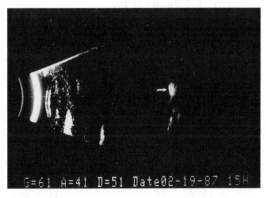

Figure 3.25. B-scan ultrasonography in a patient with deep (buried) optic disc drusen. The area of disc elevation is clearly seen as a focal area of brightness that persists when reflections from the remainder of the posterior segment of the eye are no longer visible (*arrow*). This finding is consistent with the appearance of calcified drusen. (Courtesy of Cathy DiBernardo, RN, RMDS.)

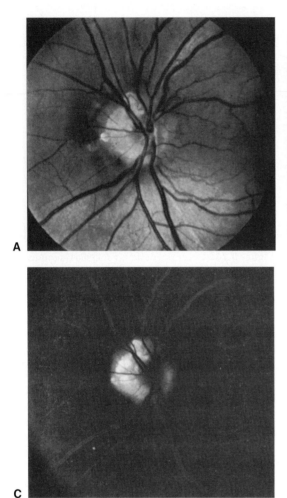

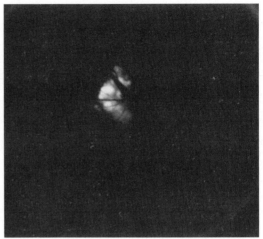

Figure 3.26. Fluorescent characteristics of drusen. **A:** Fundus photograph of optic disc drusen. **B:** Autofluorescence of drusen observed through a fluorescein filter but without injection of fluorescein dye. **C:** Late staining of drusen after fluorescein angiogram.

Peripheral visual field defects develop in up to 75% of eyes with disc drusen. In most cases, the asymptomatic nature of the defects reflects the insidious attrition of optic nerve fibers over decades. Nevertheless, a minority of patients experience episodes of sudden, steplike visual field loss (Fig. 3.27). Visual field defects are more common in eyes with visible drusen than in those with pseudopapilledema. They include nerve fiber bundle defects (inferonasal steps, arcuate defects and sector defects); enlargement of the blind spot; and concentric visual field constriction (Fig. 3.27). Many of these defects are slowly progressive. However, some patients experience sudden severe visual field constriction with and without preservation of central vision. These patients often have no disc swelling or retinal edema to suggest an ischemic process. A relative afferent pupillary defect may result from unilateral or asymmetric visual field loss in the absence of central acuity loss.

The pathogenesis of visual field loss in patients with disc drusen could involve impaired axonal transport in an eye with a small scleral canal leading to gradual attrition of optic nerve fibers, direct compression of prelaminar nerve fibers by drusen, or ischemia within the optic nerve head.

At the heart of the controversy is whether drusen produce damage to nerve fibers through direct axonal or vascular compression, or whether they are merely an epiphenomenon of a chronic low-grade axonal stasis that produces a slowly progressive diminution in optic axons. Several studies have been unable to correlate the location of visible disc drusen with the location of field defects.

Central visual loss is a rare but well-documented complication of disc drusen that should be considered only when no other causes can be identified. In such cases, central visual loss usually follows a series of episodic, steplike events that progressively diminish the peripheral visual field.

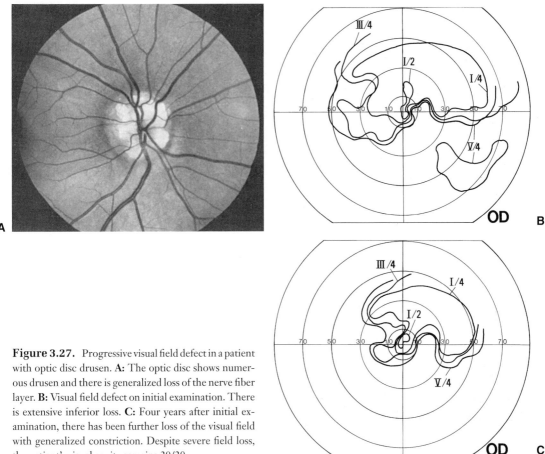

Figure 3.27. Progressive visual field defect in a patient with optic disc drusen. **A:** The optic disc shows numerous drusen and there is generalized loss of the nerve fiber layer. **B:** Visual field defect on initial examination. There is extensive inferior loss. **C:** Four years after initial examination, there has been further loss of the visual field with generalized constriction. Despite severe field loss, the patient's visual acuity remains 20/20.

Prepapillary or peripapillary hemorrhages may develop in eyes with disc drusen, including small superficial hemorrhages on the optic disc, large hemorrhages on the disc, extending into the vitreous; and deep peripapillary hemorrhages extending from the optic disc under the peripapillary retina (Fig. 3.28). Large superficial hemorrhages may rarely extend into the vitreous. Splinter hemorrhages associated with optic disc drusen tend to be single and prepapillary in location, in contrast to the multiple nerve fiber layer hemorrhages that characterize papilledema. Deep peripapillary hemorrhages may be subretinal or subpigment epithelial and are typically circumferentially oriented around the disc (Fig 3.28).

Most patients with optic disc drusen and hemorrhages have a good visual prognosis. Whether or not these hemorrhages can be caused by compression of thin-walled veins by conglomerates of drusen or by erosion of the vessel wall by the sharp edge of the drusen remains unsettled. It is possible that enlarging disc drusen could result in circulatory compromise and local hypoxia, which might stimulate

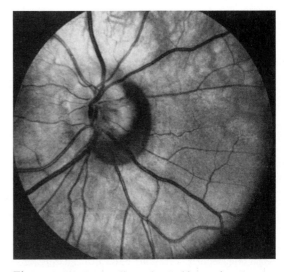

Figure 3.28. Peripapillary subretinal hemorrhage in a patient with intrapapillary drusen. Note the difference between this type of hemorrhage and the superficial nerve fiber layer hemorrhages seen with optic disc swelling.

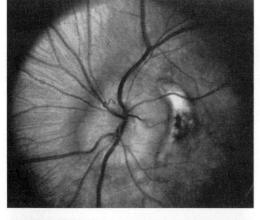

A

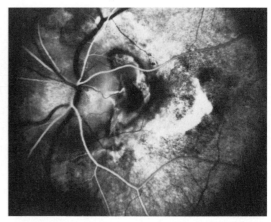

B

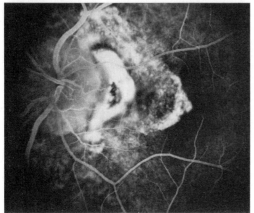

C

Figure 3.29. Subretinal neovascularization in a patient with intrapapillary drusen. **A:** The left optic disc is moderately elevated and has blurred disc margins. Several small drusen were identified in the center of the disc. Temporal to the disc there is a crescent-shaped hyperpigmented area of subretinal neovascularization. **B:** Arterial phase of the fluorescein angiogram shows extensive subretinal and retinal vascular leakage from abnormal vessels. Note that there is no leakage from the disc vessels. **C:** In the arteriovenous phase of the fluorescein angiogram, there is diffuse staining of the optic disc and there is both staining of and leakage of dye from the area of subretinal neovascularization.

the growth of new vessels between the RPE and Bruch's membrane. Peripapillary pigmentary disruption may remain following resolution of subretinal hemorrhage. Subretinal hemorrhage may also occur in severe papilledema, but its occurrence in mild papilledema is rare and should suggest the possibility of disc drusen. A subgroup of patients can develop a serous maculopathy without hemorrhage, which can tent the temporal peripapillary retina into striate folds.

Ischemic optic neuropathy may occur as a single episode or as successive episodes of discrete visual loss over years. The optic neuropathy may develop spontaneously, perhaps from crowding of the optic nerve head by drusen, or it may be precipitated by hypotension, such as during dialysis.

Retinal vascular occlusions can occur in patients with optic disc drusen. Drusen-associated retinal arterial and venous occlusions have all been reported. They tend to occur in young adults, but may rarely be seen in children. Retinal vascular occlusions that occur in eyes with disc drusen could result from vascular crowding secondary to the small scleral canal

size in eyes with drusen, anomalous optic disc vasculature that may make it more susceptible to the effects of disrupted hemodynamics, or mechanical displacement of the prelaminar vasculature by hard, unyielding drusen.

Transient visual loss occurred in 8.6% of the patients with disc drusen in one large study. This phenomenon may occur because of anomalous elevation of the optic disc. Like papilledema, optic disc drusen produce increased interstitial pressure and decreased perfusion pressure in the intraocular portion of the optic nerve. Thus, minor fluctuations in arterial, venous, or cerebrospinal fluid pressure result in brief but critical decrements in perfusion, leading to transient obscurations of vision. Vitreopapillary traction may be an alternative mechanism in some patients. Rarely, transient visual loss may be a harbinger of retinal vascular occlusion in patients with disc drusen.

Peripapillary subretinal neovascularization is a rare but well-documented complication in eyes with disc drusen. Temporary or permanent visual loss can occur in patients with optic disc drusen who develop subpigment epithelial hemorrhages from subretinal neovascularization (Fig. 3.29). Hemorrhages occurring in the absence of choroidal vascularization usually are asymptomatic and resolve without sequelae, whereas hemorrhages arising from choroidal neovascularization commonly produce visual loss. Management remains debated and observation is often recommended for peripapillary choroidal neovascularization associated with disc drusen.

Drusen of the optic disc consist of homogenous, globular concretions, often collected in larger, multilobulated agglomerations. Drusen usually exhibit a concentrically laminated structure that is not encapsulated and contains no cells or cellular debris. Optic disc axons are atrophic adjacent to large accumulations of drusen, whereas axons that are not adjacent to the drusen are normal. Drusen take up calcium salts and must be decalcified before being cut into sections for histopathologic study. According to most investigators, drusen are composed predominantly of a mucoprotein matrix with significant quantities of acid mucopolysaccharides, small quantities of ribonucleic acid and, occasionally, iron. Drusen are insoluble in most of the common solvents.

The primary pathology of optic disc drusen may be an inherited dysplasia of the optic canal, or the optic disc and its vasculature, which predisposes to the formation of optic disc drusen. After formation of the optic stalk is complete, mesenchymal elements from the sclera invade the glial framework of the primitive lamina, reinforcing it with collagen. An abnormal encroachment of sclera, Bruch's membrane, or both, upon the developing optic stalk would narrow the exit space of optic axons from the eye. The small optic disc size and absence of a central cup in affected eyes are consistent with the mechanism of axonal crowding. The clinical and histopathologic observation that drusen are often first detected at the margins of the optic disc suggests that the rigid edge of the scleral canal may be an aggravating factor in producing a relative mechanical interruption of axonal transport. The lower prevalence of optic disc drusen in African Americans, who have a larger disc area with less potential for axonal crowding, is also consistent with the notion that axonal crowding is a fundamental anatomic substrate for disc drusen.

Optic nerve head drusen are occasionally seen in patients with **retinitis pigmentosa.** Such drusen often are located at the disc margin in the superficial retina. In such cases, the disc is not elevated or anomalous but appears waxy yellow.

There is an association between disc drusen and angioid streaks. Using ultrasonography, disc drusen can be detected in about 20% of patients with pseudoxanthoma elasticum and in 25% of patients with angioid streaks with no pseudoxanthoma elasticum.

Optic disc drusen may also occur as part of the **Riley-Smith syndrome** of macrocephaly, multiple hemangiomata, and pseudopapilledema.

Migraine headaches are said to occur with increased frequency in patients with disc drusen. However, the concurrence of migraine and optic disc drusen probably reflects the frequent and often expedited referral of patients with headaches and optic disc elevation.

ANOMALOUS DISC ELEVATION WITHOUT EITHER VISIBLE OR BURIED DRUSEN

Not all anomalously elevated optic discs develop drusen. As noted previously, the morning glory syndrome is associated with disc elevation; the superotemporal portion of a tilted optic disc is usually elevated; and dysplastic discs may show some degree of elevation. In addition, hypoplastic discs may have some elevation that seems out of proportion to the size of the disc. Such discs are often described as "crowded" to distinguish them from discs that are truly swollen. In addition, vitreopapillary traction can produce optic disc elevation. B-scan ultrasonography and optical coherence tomography allow confirmation of vitreopapillary traction.

FOR FURTHER INFORMATION

See *Walsh & Hoyt's Clinical Neuro-Ophthalmology*, 6th edition, Volume 1, Chapter 3, pages 151–195.

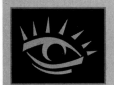

CHAPTER 4

Topical Diagnosis of Acquired Optic Nerve Disorders *

Damage to an optic nerve classically causes an abnormality in visual sensory function, a relative afferent pupillary defect, and, if the damage is irreversible, a change in the appearance of the optic disc. Acquired optic neuropathies can produce any type of visual field defect, including a central scotoma, cecocentral scotoma, arcuate field defect, altitudinal defect, or even a temporal or nasal hemianopic defect. Unless the optic neuropathy is bilateral or the lesion is located near the optic chiasm, the field defect produced by an optic nerve lesion is always monocular.

The visual field defects that occur with various optic neuropathies are not in themselves localizing. Rather, it is the demographics of the patient (age, gender), history of visual loss (rapid vs. slow onset, progressive vs. stable, painful vs. nonpainful), the presence or absence of other neurologic or ocular signs (relative afferent pupillary defect, acquired color deficit, ocular motor paresis, proptosis, optociliary shunt veins, optic disc swelling, optic pallor), and the results of neuroimaging that most often allow the physician to diagnose an optic neuropathy, to localize the pathology along the course of the nerve, and to determine its etiology.

APPEARANCE OF THE DISC

The optic disc has only two ways to respond to the many acquired pathologic processes that may affect the optic nerve. It can swell, or it can remain normal in appearance. If the pathologic process causes irreversible

*Adapted from: Sadun AA, Argarwal MR. Topical diagnosis of acquired optic nerve disorders. In: Miller NR, Newman NJ, Biousse V, Kerrison JB, eds. *Walsh & Hoyt's Clinical Neuro-Ophthalmology.* 6th ed, Vol I. Lippincott Williams & Wilkins: Philadelphia; 2005:197–236.

damage to the optic nerve, the disc will eventually become pale.

OPTIC DISC SWELLING

Swelling of the optic disc occurs when there is obstruction of axon transport at the lamina cribrosa (Fig. 4.1). This may result from compression, ischemia, inflammation, metabolic dysfunction, or toxic damage (Table 4.1). In some cases, infiltration of the proximal portion of the disc by inflammatory or malignant processes causes an appearance that is indistinguishable from true swelling. Anomalies of the optic disc that produce an appearance that mimics true swelling were discussed in Chapter 3 of this text.

Appearance

Useful funduscopic signs of early swelling of the optic disc include blurring of the nerve fiber layer around the disc, especially superiorly and inferiorly, and a tendency for the increasingly swollen and opaque nerve fibers to obscure segments of blood vessels, especially arteries, as they approach or cross the disc edge (Fig. 4.2A) (see Chapter 5). Disc hyperemia and absence of spontaneous venous pulsations may also be noted. When disc swelling is fully developed (Fig. 4.2B), additional funduscopic changes can appear, including intraretinal hemorrhages and infarcts (cotton-wool spots) within the nerve fiber layer, hard exudates (sometimes in a star figure around or on the nasal half of the macula), and subhyaloid hemorrhage, occasionally breaking out into the vitreous cavity.

When disc swelling persists for several months or longer, the hemorrhages and exudates tend to resolve, and the initial hyperemia is replaced by a milky gray appearance that reflects supervening gliosis, often accompanied by the development of "drusen-like" hard exudates in the superficial substance of the disc

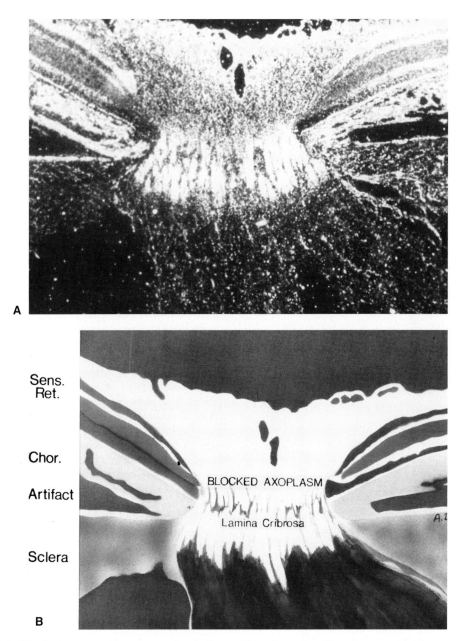

Figure 4.1. The final common denominator of optic disc swelling: obstruction of axon transport. **A:** Phase-contrast photomicrograph of a swollen optic disc in an animal with experimental papilledema shows accumulation of axon products (seen as white material) in the region of the lamina cribrosa. **B:** Artist's drawing of the photomicrograph. *Sens. Ret.:* sensory retina. *Chor.:* choroid. (Reprinted from: Miller NR, Fine SL. *The Ocular Fundus in Neuro-ophthalmologic Diagnosis: Sights and Sounds in Ophthalmology.* Vol. 3. St. Louis: CV Mosby; 1977, with permission.)

itself (Fig. 4.3). Neovascular membranes with subretinal hemorrhages and serous fluid can progressively develop. Optic atrophy with narrowed, often sheathed, retinal vessels may supervene in patients with chronic disc swelling. Optociliary shunt vessels may also appear on the optic disc, presumably secondary to chronic ob-

struction of normal retinal venous drainage through the central retinal vein by chronic disc swelling.

Optic disc swelling may not develop if significant optic atrophy is already present: "dead axons can't swell." This is particularly important to remember when the ophthalmoscopic appearance of an atrophic optic disc is being used to determine recurrence or exacerbation of a condition such as raised intracranial pressure (see Chapter 5).

Specific Etiologies

Patients with increased intracranial pressure may develop optic disc swelling. This condition is called **papilledema.** The symptoms and signs in patients with papilledema generally are those typically associated with raised intracranial pressure, including headache, nausea, vomiting, and pulsatile tinnitus. Visual symptoms in such patients include transient obscurations of vision and diplopia. Loss of central vision, dyschromatopsia, a relative afferent pupillary defect, and visual field defects other than enlargement of the blind spot caused by the swollen disc are uncommon in patients with acute papilledema unless the lesion causing the increased intracranial pressure also directly damages the visual sensory system in some way, or there are hemorrhages or exudates in the macula. The optic disc swelling in papilledema is usually bilateral and symmetric, but it may be asymmetric or even unilateral. It may be very mild or extremely severe (Fig. 4.2). Papilledema is discussed in Chapter 5 of this text.

Inflammation of the proximal portion of the optic nerve produces swelling of the optic disc. This condition, called **anterior optic neuritis** or **papillitis**, is characterized by relatively acute visual loss, usually in one eye; it is almost always associated with pain around or behind the eye. The pain is often exacerbated by eye movement. The appearance of the optic disc ranges from very mild to severe swelling. Vitreous cells may be present, particularly overlying the swollen disc, but peripapillary hemorrhages are rarely seen (Fig. 4.4). In most cases of anterior optic neuritis, vision continues to decline for several hours to several days. It then stabilizes and, after several days to several weeks, begins to improve.

Anterior optic neuritis typically occurs in young adults and is most often caused by demyelination, although it may also develop in patients with a variety of systemic disorders, such as cat-scratch disease, syphilis, Lyme disease, and sarcoidosis. Patients who develop optic neuritis that is unassociated with a systemic inflammatory or infectious disorder have an increased risk of developing clinical evidence of multiple sclerosis (MS) compared with the normal population.

A special form of anterior optic neuritis called **neuroretinitis** is characterized ophthalmoscopically by optic disc swelling associated with a macular star figure composed of lipid (Fig. 4.5). This form of optic neuritis is almost never caused by demyelination and occurs most often in the setting of cat-scratch disease or in association with other systemic infectious diseases, as well as with sarcoidosis. Optic neuritis is discussed in Chapter 6 of this text.

Ischemia that affects the laminar or prelaminar portions of the optic nerve produces swelling of the optic disc. This condition, called **anterior ischemic optic neuropathy** (AION), is characterized by monocular and usually painless visual loss associated with a relative afferent pupillary defect and a visual field defect that is most often altitudinal or arcuate in nature. The loss of vision usually occurs over several hours to several days. It then stabilizes and remains stable in most cases with only mild recovery if any. AION occurs most often in patients over 50 years of age who have underlying systemic vasculopathies, particularly diabetes mellitus, systemic hypertension, and giant cell arteritis.

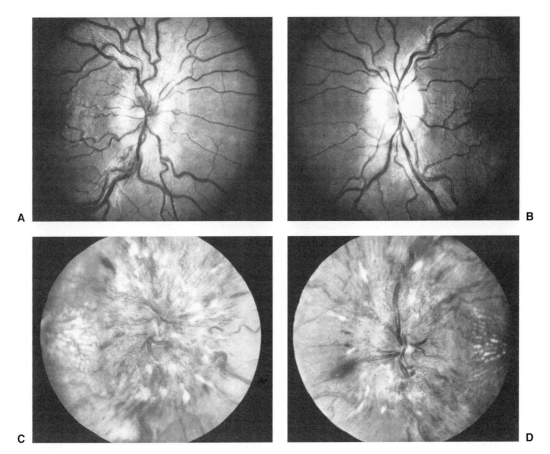

Figure 4.2. Variability in severity of papilledema. **A and B:** Mild papilledema in a 14-year-old boy with hydrocephalus caused by congenital aqueductal stenosis. The right disc **(A)** is somewhat more hyperemic and swollen than the left **(B). C and D:** Severe papilledema in a 32-year-old woman with pseudotumor cerebri. Note numerous hemorrhages and cotton-wool spots surrounding the markedly swollen right **(C)** and left **(D)** optic discs. Also note hard exudates (lipid) in both maculae.

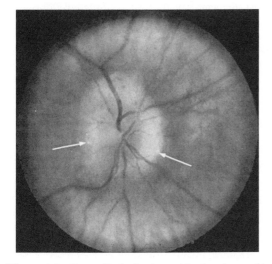

Figure 4.3. Drusenlike bodies (*arrows*) in chronic atrophic papilledema. (Reprinted from: Hoyt WF, Beeston D. *The Ocular Fundus in Neurologic Disease.* St. Louis: CV Mosby; 1966, with permission.)

The optic disc swelling that occurs in AION may be hyperemic or pallid (Fig. 4.6) and is usually accompanied by one or more flame-shaped hemorrhages near the margins of the disc (Fig. 4.7B). Patients with nonarteritic AION invariably have a congenitally small optic disc with an absent or small central cup (Fig. 4.7A), and this congenital abnormality is thought to be the major predisposing factor for the development of the disorder. Patients with arteritic AION, on the other hand, may have any sized optic disc. AION is discussed in Chapter 7 of this text.

Compression of the proximal portion of the optic nerve may produce optic disc swelling. The compression may be caused by a tumor, such as a cavernous hemangioma, meningioma, or schwannoma. In other cases, enlargement of structures normally in the orbit, such as the extraocular muscles in dysthyroid ophthalmopathy, causes optic nerve compression. Patients in whom such compression occurs initially may have no visual complaints and may have few, if any, signs of optic nerve dysfunction other than an enlarged

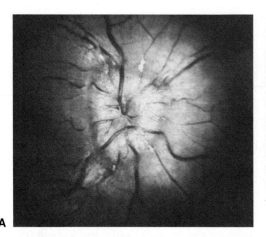
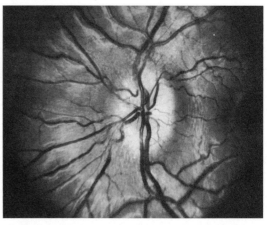

A **B**

Figure 4.4. The appearance of a "choked disc" caused by papilledema compared with a "choked disc" in a patient with anterior optic neuritis. **A:** Right optic disc in a young woman with papilledema. There is moderate swelling of the disc, which is surrounded by several intraretinal hemorrhages and soft exudates. **B:** Left optic disc in a patient with anterior optic neuritis. The disc is moderately swollen, and there are mild circumferential retinal folds temporal to the disc. Note that both optic discs appear similar in appearance. It is impossible to determine the cause of optic disc swelling in most cases unless one obtains a complete medical and ocular history and performs a complete ocular examination (e.g., tests of visual acuity, color vision, visual field).

blind spot on visual field testing. Alternatively, they may complain of insidious and slowly progressive visual loss. In such cases, there is invariably some degree of dyschromatopsia, a relative afferent pupillary defect, and a defect in the visual field of the affected eye. The optic disc is generally only mildly to moderately swollen and hyperemic (Fig. 4.8). Peripapillary hemorrhages are usually absent, but chorioretinal striae are present in some cases, particularly when the compressive lesion is adjacent to the globe. The diagnosis of anterior compressive optic neuropathy is made by neuroimaging of the orbit. Compressive optic neuropathy is discussed in Chapter 8 of this text.

Toxic and metabolic disorders may cause swelling of the optic disc. In such cases, the swelling is usually bilateral and mild (Fig. 4.9). Central vision is often reduced with visual loss progressing slowly over several weeks to months. Color vision is almost always markedly abnormal, regardless of the level of central vision. Bilateral central or cecocentral scotomas are the rule and are associated in some cases with mild to severe constriction of the peripheral visual field. In many but not all cases, eliminating the source of the toxicity or reversing the metabolic abnormality is associated with partial or complete recovery of visual function. Toxic and metabolic optic neuropathies are discussed in Chapter 10 of this text.

Intraocular **hypotony** (low pressure) may induce optic disc swelling. Following a penetrating wound of the eye or following an intraocular operation in which the wound is not tightly closed, there may be development of disc swelling (Fig. 4.10). Blunt trauma to the eye may result in damage to the ciliary body and reduction of aqueous humor formation with subsequent development of hypotony and disc swelling despite an intact globe. In such cases, the hypotony resolves spontaneously as does the disc swelling. Although visual acuity is impaired in such cases, the visual disturbance appears to be related primarily to corneal and retinal

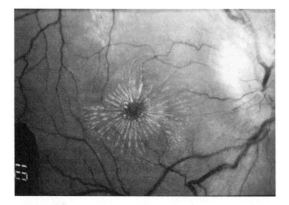

Figure 4.5. Neuroretinitis. The patient was a young woman who developed acute visual loss in the right eye while visiting Connecticut. The right optic disc is swollen, and there is a star figure composed of lipid (hard exudate) in the macula. An evaluation revealed serologic evidence of Lyme disease. Neuroretinitis is not associated with the subsequent development of MS, but is most often caused by an underlying systemic infection, such as cat-scratch disease, Lyme disease, syphilis, or sarcoidosis.

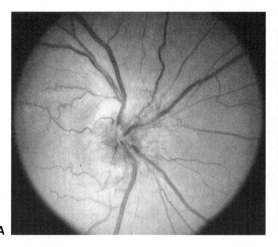 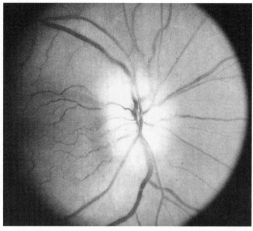

Figure 4.6. Optic disc swelling in anterior ischemic optic neuropathy. **A:** Hyperemic swelling. **B:** Pallid swelling.

changes from the hypotony rather than to a true optic neuropathy. As with other forms of true disc swelling, the pathophysiology of disc swelling in patients with ocular hypotony appears to be blockage of axon transport at the lamina cribrosa.

INFILTRATION OF THE OPTIC DISC

Infiltration of the proximal portion of the optic nerve by tumor or inflammatory cells can produce an appearance similar to true swelling of the optic disc (Fig. 4.11). The disc changes may be asymptomatic or associated with variable visual loss, dyschromatopsia, and a visual field defect. The infiltration may be unilateral or bilateral, and a relative afferent pupillary defect may be present if the infiltration is either unilateral or bilateral but asymmetric. Infiltration of the optic nerve occurs most frequently in patients with malignant tumors, such as leukemia, lymphoma, and various carcinomas that spread to the central nervous system, but it may also occur in patients with systemic inflammatory disorders, including sarcoidosis. Infiltrative optic neuropathies are discussed in Chapter 8 of this text.

OPTIC ATROPHY

Optic atrophy is not a disease. It is a morphologic sequela of disease—any disease—that causes irreversible

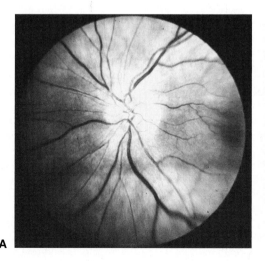 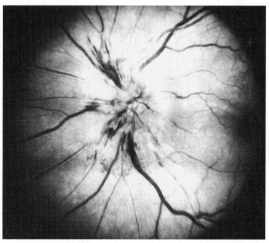

Figure 4.7. The "disc at risk" in nonarteritic anterior ischemic optic neuropathy (NAION). **A:** Small left optic disc with no cup in a patient who had experienced an attack of NAION in the right eye several months earlier. **B:** NAION characterized by hyperemic disc swelling and peripapillary hemorrhages in the same eye several months later.

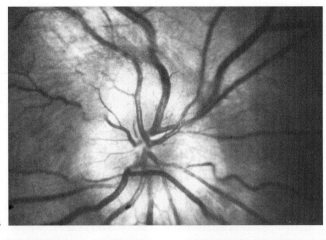

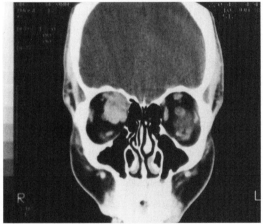

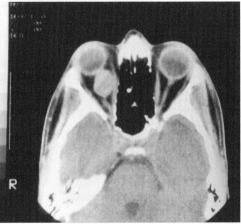

Figure 4.8. Optic disc swelling from compression of the anterior portion of the orbital optic nerve. **A:** Right optic disc of a 25-year-old man who noted mildly decreased vision in the right eye. Visual acuity was 20/25 and there was an ipsilateral relative afferent pupillary defect. The optic disc is moderately swollen. **B:** Noncontrast CT scan, coronal view, shows that the mass compresses the nasal and superior portions of the optic nerve, displacing it downward. **C:** Noncontrast CT scan, axial view, shows a well-circumscribed orbital mass compressing the optic nerve. Note distortion and irregularity of the nerve. The patient's vision returned to normal, and the optic disc swelling resolved after the mass was removed.

damage to ganglion cells and axons of the optic nerve. The term *optic atrophy* is, therefore, a pathologic generalization applied to optic nerve shrinkage from any process that produces degeneration of axons in the anterior visual system (the retinogeniculate pathway), including ischemia, inflammation, compression, infiltration, and trauma. Although the pathologist can make the diagnosis of optic atrophy by direct observation of histopathologic changes in the optic nerve, the clinical diagnosis of atrophy is usually based on (a) ophthalmoscopic abnormalities of color and structure of the optic disc with associated changes in the retinal vessels and nerve fiber layer, and (b) defective visual function that can be localized to the optic nerve.

Nonpathologic Pallor of the Optic Disc

An absolute prerequisite to recognition of the abnormal disc is familiarity with normal disc color. The temporal side of the normal disc usually has less color than the nasal side. The degree of this temporal pallor is primarily related to the size of the physiologic cup, to the thin translucent character of the temporal nerve fiber layer, and possibly to the relative sparseness of capillaries on that side of the disc.

The normal physiologic cup may vary in size. When it extends almost to the temporal edge of the disc, the temporal side of the disc is pale. In addition, the temporal margins of some large physiologic cups are steep-walled. When the margins slope gradually downward from the margin of the disc, the crescent of sclera

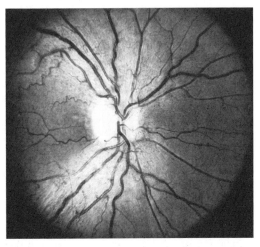
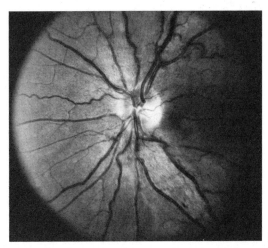

A

B

Figure 4.9. Optic disc swelling in nutritional optic neuropathy. The patient was a 34-year-old alcoholic man who had a poor diet and who developed progressive loss of vision in both eyes. Visual acuity was 20/200 OU, and there were bilateral cecocentral scotomas. The concentration of folic acid in the patient's red blood cells was low. **A:** The right optic disc is pale temporally and hyperemic nasally. There is atrophy of the papillomacular bundle. **B:** The left optic disc is hyperemic and mildly swollen. An assay of the patient's blood for mitochondrial mutations of Leber's optic neuropathy was negative. The patient's vision improved and the disc swelling resolved after he reduced his alcohol intake, improved his diet, and was treated with vitamin supplements that included folic acid.

adjacent to the temporal, and occasionally to the inferior, margin of the disc is visible and appears a mottled grayish white. This crescent, known as a temporal (or sometimes inferior) conus, is exposed by retraction of the dark retinal pigment epithelium from the disc margin. It enhances the whitish appearance of such a disc.

Marked recession or excavation of a physiologic cup makes the center of a disc pale. The retinal vessels at

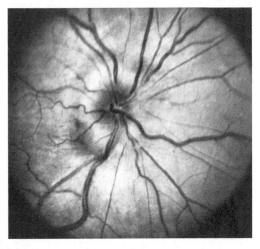

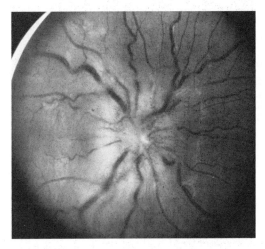

Figure 4.11. Optic disc elevation from infiltration of the orbital portion of the optic nerve. The patient was an 11-year-old boy with acute lymphocytic leukemia that was thought to be in remission when he developed mild blurred vision in the right eye. Note moderate elevation of the right optic disc, associated with dilation of small disc vessels. Malignant cells were detected in the patient's cerebrospinal fluid. The disc elevation resolved and visual acuity improved after radiation therapy.

Figure 4.10. Optic disc swelling in hypotony. The patient was a 43-year-old woman who developed hypotony in the right eye after a glaucoma filtering operation. Note moderate swelling and hyperemia of the right optic disc. The appearance of this disc is similar to that which may occur in papilledema, anterior optic neuritis, and other conditions that produce optic disc swelling.

the base of the cup are partially obscured as they pass through a thin rim of neural tissue that borders the excavation. It may be difficult to distinguish this type of cup from a glaucomatous cup. The pallor of the floor of a physiologic cup is directly related to the glistening whiteness of the lamina cribrosa or cribriform plate, a connective and elastic tissue structure with small sieve-like openings through which transparent nerve fiber bundles pass (see Chapter 2). Because the openings are irregular, direct light entering them is reflected in many directions, and the holes appear as grayish yellow ovals or dots. When this dotting is seen, it signifies that no abnormal opaque connective tissue is present over the surface of the cribriform plate.

Many infants have generally pale fundi; the optic discs in such cases also appear pale. A white-appearing disc is common in an eye with axial myopia. Because the optic nerve enters the globe obliquely, the contents of the disc, including the nerve fibers and the retinal vessels, are displaced nasally. The physiologic cup is shallow, and its extension to the temporal margin produces relative temporal pallor that is often exaggerated by a temporal conus.

An illusory impression of whiteness may be caused merely by fresh batteries or a new bulb in the examiner's ophthalmoscope (thus providing a brighter light source). Conversely, true pallor of an optic disc may be overlooked when the light source is weak. The color of the disc also varies with the color temperature of the light source and the age of the lens. Finally, removal of the natural lens of a patient with cataract extraction causes an illusion of pallor in the aphakic or pseudophakic eye.

Pathology and Pathophysiology of Optic Atrophy

Because the axons in the optic nerve arise from the ganglion cells located in the retina, damage to such axons may occur from numerous sources at several locations:

- From disease within the eye that damages the ganglion cells, the retinal nerve fiber layer, or the optic disc.
- From disease within or surrounding the intraorbital, intracanalicular, or intracranial portions of the optic nerve.
- From disorders that damage the optic chiasm, optic tracts, or lateral geniculate bodies.
- From disorders of the retrogeniculate pathways that produce transsynaptic (transneuronal) degeneration.

A disease may be focal, multifocal, or diffuse. It may destroy axons directly or by its effects on their investing glia or capillary blood supply. Focal disruption anywhere along an axon causes degeneration of the entire axon and its cell body, the retinal ganglion cell. When large numbers of axons undergo such degeneration, gross shrinkage or atrophy of the optic nerve becomes evident.

When an axon is irreversibly damaged, it undergoes two types of degeneration: **anterograde (wallerian)** and **retrograde.** Anterograde degeneration occurs in the distal portion of the axon that has been separated from its cell body, whereas retrograde degeneration occurs in the proximal segment of the nerve that remains in contact with the cell body. Although anterograde degeneration begins and becomes nearly complete within 7 days after injury, the portion of the axon still connected to the cell body, and the cell body itself, remain normal in appearance for 3 to 4 weeks. During this time, orthograde axonal transport continues in a normal manner. After about 3 to 4 weeks, however, the entire remaining structure (the cell body and axon from the point of injury) degenerates rapidly, so that by about 6 to 8 weeks after severe optic nerve injury, no affected ganglion cells remain viable. A most fascinating feature of this retrograde degeneration of the optic nerve (and other nerves as well) is that the time course of this degeneration is apparently independent of the distance of the injury from the ganglion cell body. Damage to the retrobulbar portion of the optic nerve, the optic chiasm, and the optic tract all cause pathologic and visible degeneration of the ganglion cell bodies at about the same time.

Regeneration of axons in the optic nerve in human and nonhuman primates is quite limited and abortive. However, some degree of remyelination does occur after injury. This remyelination results from the activity of uninjured, injured but surviving, and newly generated oligodendroglia.

Transsynaptic (transneuronal) **degeneration** is a secondary degenerative reaction of neurons that occurs in a number of areas of the brain. For example, transneuronal degeneration is a well-established phenomenon in the cells of the lateral geniculate body following destruction of parts of the retina. However, the most profound transsynaptic changes occur following lesions in the immature brain. This type of transsynaptic degeneration occurs most often in patients with occipital lobe damage in utero or during early infancy. Although it has been suggested that transsynaptic degeneration may occur in mature adult human and nonhuman primate visual systems if enough time has elapsed, clinically apparent transsynaptic degeneration probably does not occur after injury in adult humans.

Loss of function within the central nervous system is consistently associated with a reduction of blood supply to the affected tissue, regardless of the primary pathogenetic process. When the optic nerve degenerates, its blood supply is reduced, and small vessels that were once visible in the normal nerve can no longer be seen with an ophthalmoscope. In addition to reduction of blood supply, formation of glial tissue is said to occur with optic atrophy.

Other factors that may account for the normal pink appearance of the optic disc are its thickness and the cytoarchitecture of nerve fiber bundles passing between glial columns containing capillaries. Light entering the disc is normally conducted along the transparent nerve fiber bundles, much like fiberoptic pathways. The light diffuses among adjacent columns of glial cells and capillaries and acquires the pink color of the capillaries. Thus, light rays that exit through the tissue via the nerve fiber bundles are pink and give the disc its characteristic color. The axon bundles of an atrophic optic disc have been destroyed, and the remaining astrocytes are arranged at right angles to the entering light. Thus, little light passes into the disc substance to traverse the capillaries that, although still present, are surrounded by layers of astrocytes. Because the light is reflected from opaque glial cells and does not pass through capillaries, it remains white, and the optic disc thus appears pale. In some areas, loss of tissue also allows light to pass directly to the opaque scleral lamina, and this adds to the pale color of the disc.

Ophthalmoscopic Features of Optic Atrophy

The evaluation of optic disc color is a routine but often challenging problem. The lack of color in an optic disc is difficult to assess, record, compare, and describe. The normal color of the optic disc depends on its composition and the relationship of the components to each other and to the light that is reflected or refracted from the disc surface. Because the neural elements are gray, the pink color of the disc is also related to its blood vessels.

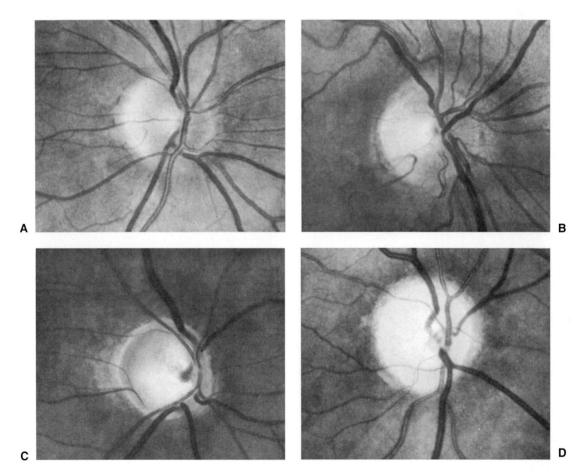

Figure 4.12. Pallor of the optic disc. **A:** Mild temporal pallor in a patient with MS but who denied acute optic neuritis. **B:** Temporal pallor in a patient with toxic amblyopia. **C:** Pallor with glaucomatous cupping. Note preservation of small nasal neuroretinal rim. **D:** Diffuse pallor in a patient with retrograde (descending) optic atrophy from the effects of an intracranial mass. (Reprinted from: Hoyt WF, Beeston D. *The Ocular Fundus in Neurologic Disease.* St. Louis: CV Mosby; 1966. with permission.)

Pallor of the optic disc is often graded as mild, moderate, or severe; however, such distinctions are subjective and unreliable. More objective evaluation of the pale optic disc can be obtained by a detailed observation of its configuration and neural tissue; its veins, arteries, and capillaries; and the peripapillary retinal nerve fiber layer that surrounds it. Pallor of the optic disc may be diffuse or confined to one sector (Fig. 4.12).

In the early stages of atrophy, the optic disc loses its reddish hue, and the substance of the disc slowly disappears, leaving a pale, shallow, concave meniscus: the exposed lamina cribrosa (Fig. 4.13). In the end stages of the atrophic process, retinal vessels of normal caliber still emerge centrally through the otherwise avascular-appearing disc. In many cases, the changes that develop during the progression to atrophy do not result in a significant change in the central cup of the optic disc. In some cases, however, pathologic optic disc cupping develops in patients with normal intraocular pressures and optic atrophy from various causes, including ischemia, compression, inflammation, and trauma (Fig. 4.14).

We would stress that despite the occasional confusion between glaucomatous and nonglaucomatous optic neuropathy that occurs in patients with pathologic cupping and pallor of the optic disc, a careful clinical examination almost always results in the correct diagnosis. Glaucomatous visual field defects occur only after extensive cupping is present, and acuity loss occurs even later. In such cases, there is usually absence

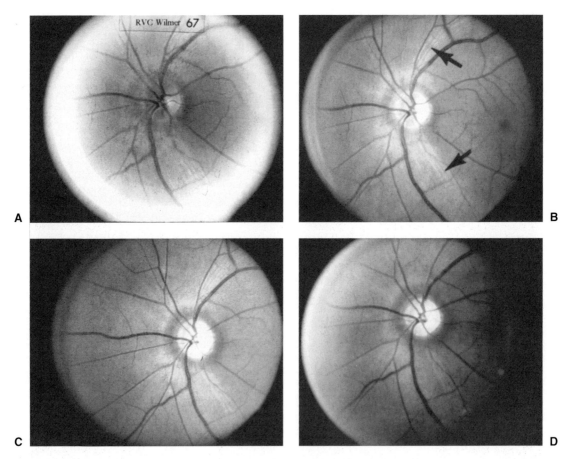

Figure 4.13. Development of pallor of the optic disc in a patient with retrograde (descending) optic atrophy. **A:** The optic disc is normal in the early stage of the process. **B:** With time, the optic disc loses its reddish hue, and the substance of the disc slowly disappears, leaving a pale, shallow concave meniscus, the exposed lamina cribrosa. As these changes occur, the peripapillary retinal nerve fiber layer begins to show defects that appear as dark linear striations (*arrows*). **C:** With more time, the disc becomes more diffusely pale, and the peripapillary nerve fiber layer becomes less visible. **D:** In the end stage of the atrophic process, retinal vessels of normal caliber still emerge centrally through the otherwise avascular-appearing disc, and the peripapillary retinal nerve fiber layer is no longer visible. (Reprinted from: Miller NR, Fine SL. *The Ocular Fundus in Neuro-Ophthalmologic Diagnosis: Sights and Sounds in Ophthalmology.* Vol. 3. St. Louis: CV Mosby; 1977, with permission.)

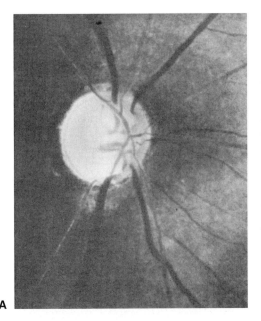
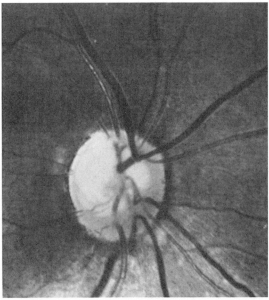

A   B

Figure 4.14. Optic disc cupping in glaucomatous and nonglaucomatous optic atrophy. **A:** Nonglaucomatous cupping. Note pallor and thinning of the neuroretinal rim. **B:** Glaucomatous cupping. Note normal appearance of the remaining neuroretinal rim.

of at least a portion of the neuroretinal rim, and any remaining rim tissue has a normal color (Fig. 4.14B). In nonglaucomatous optic neuropathies, significant loss of visual acuity, color vision, and field may occur in combination with only mild cupping. In addition, the optic discs in such cases rarely have any areas in which the neuroretinal rim is completely absent, and the remaining rim is often pale (Fig. 4.14A). The appearance of the neuroretinal rim is thus a crucial factor in determining if cupping is caused by glaucomatous or nonglaucomatous optic nerve damage. Pallor of the neuroretinal rim is 94% specific for nonglaucomatous atrophy and cupping, whereas focal or diffuse obliteration of the neuroretinal rim with preservation of color of any remaining rim tissue is 87% specific for glaucoma.

Focal destruction of nerve fiber bundles is one of the common pathologic denominators of disease that affects the inner retinal layers, optic disc, retrobulbar optic nerve, or a combination of these structures. The normal appearance of the peripapillary retinal nerve fiber layer consists of fine curvilinear striations that overlie the retinal vessels, causing them to be seen slightly out of focus. Early focal loss of axons is represented by the development of dark slits or wedges in the peripapillary retinal nerve fiber layer. These slits or bands appear darker or redder than the adjacent normal tissue in which the normal linear or curvilinear nerve fiber layer striations can easily be seen (Fig. 4.15A and B). The slit defects are most easily

identified in the superior and inferior arcuate regions where the nerve fiber layer is particularly thick. With increasing distance from the disc, the defects gradually lose contrast and cannot be identified. When only a few nerve fiber bundle defects are present, they can be identified only by the appearance of a dark, linear, arching region among the lighter, linear nerve fiber reflexes; however, when multiple nerve fiber bundle defects are present, they impart a "raked" appearance to the nerve fiber layer.

As nerve fiber bundle defects increase, they may coalesce, producing a large wedge pattern (Fig. 4.15C to E). A similar pattern occurs when a large region of nerve fiber layer is simultaneously damaged (e.g., after ischemic optic neuropathy). Within the wedge, the entire retina takes on a flat granular appearance with no striations being appreciated (Fig. 4.15E and F F). In addition, vessels in this area, having lost their surrounding nerve fiber covering, appear darker than normal and stand out sharply in relief. A prominent light reflex usually emanates from alongside the vessels, presumably as a result of draping of the inner limiting membrane directly over the vessels (Fig. 4.15G).

Clinical detection of nerve fiber layer atrophy is possible in nonhuman primates after loss of 50% of the neural tissue in a given area. The detectability of nerve fiber layer atrophy is directly affected both by the pattern of nerve fiber loss and by the zone of the retina in which the loss has occurred.

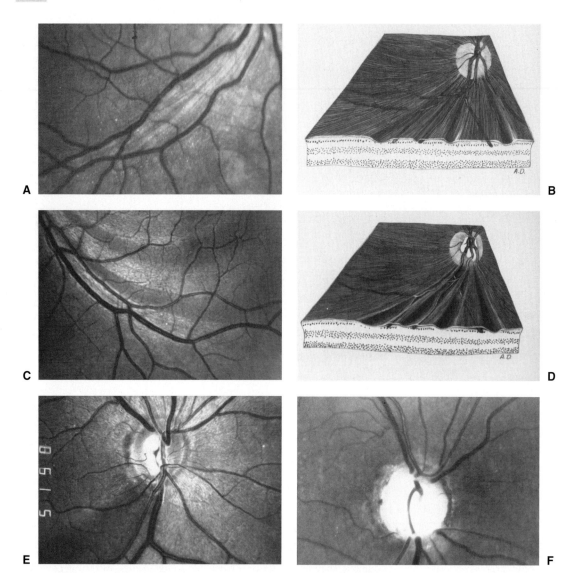

Figure 4.15. Appearance of atrophy of the peripapillary retinal nerve fiber layer. **A:** Monochromatic red-free photograph shows mild nerve fiber bundle defects in the inferior arcuate fiber bundle. They are seen as thin dark streaks interrupting the normal linear light reflexes. **B:** Artist's drawing of the thin defects in the peripapillary retinal nerve fiber layer that occur in patients with mild optic neuropathies. **C:** Monochromatic red-free photograph shows two large defects in the peripapillary retinal nerve fiber layer in the inferior arcuate region of the left eye in a patient with radiation-induced optic neuropathy. Note that compared with **(A)** the defects in this photograph are darker, wider, and more distinct from the surrounding nerve fiber layer. **D:** Artist's drawing of moderate defects in the peripapillary retinal nerve fiber layer. Note that the darker appearance results from both widening and deepening of the defects. **E:** Monochromatic red-free photograph shows a single broad defect in the peripapillary retinal nerve fiber layer in the inferior arcuate region of the right eye in a patient with early glaucoma and inferior extension of the optic cup. The defect is dark and quite distinct from the otherwise normal peripapillary nerve fiber layer. Note the granular appearance of the fundus within the defect. This appearance is caused by loss of the axons. Also note that the vessels crossing the defect are seen more clearly than are other vessels because of loss of the overlying nerve fibers. **F:** Complete loss of the peripapillary retinal nerve fiber layer in a patient with severe glaucoma. No linear striations can be seen, the peripapillary region has a distinct granular appearance, and the retinal vessels are seen clearly because of absence of overlying nerve fibers.

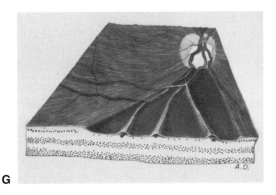

G

Figure 4.15. (*continued*) **G:** Artist's drawing of complete loss of the nerve fiber layer in a large sector. Note draping of the inner limiting membrane over the retinal vessels.

In most cases of optic atrophy, the retinal arteries are narrowed or attenuated. In some instances, the narrowing is minor in nature; in others, such as severe nonarteritic AION, the vessels appear thread-like or are completely obliterated, especially around the edges of the disc (Fig. 4.16). Not all cases of optic atrophy are associated with retinal vascular changes, however. Indeed, in eyes with optic atrophy from damage to the retrolaminar optic nerve, the retinal vessels are often unaffected. Thus, eyes in which significant retinal vascular narrowing is associated with optic atrophy presumably have suffered an additional insult directly affecting the retinal vasculature.

Differential Diagnosis of Optic Atrophy

When optic atrophy is complete, it is often impossible to determine its etiology solely from the appearance

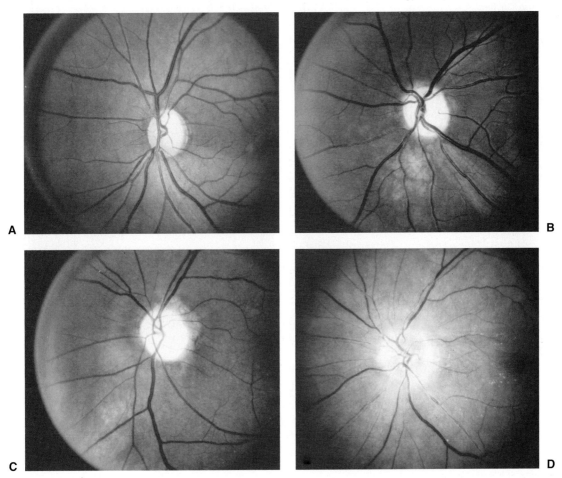

A **B**

C **D**

Figure 4.16. Appearance of retinal arteries in optic atrophy. **A:.** Minimal narrowing of retinal arteries in left eye of a patient with optic atrophy from compression of the intracranial optic nerve by a suprasellar meningioma. **B:** Minimal narrowing of retinal arteries in the left eye of a patient after an episode of severe retrobulbar optic neuritis. **C:** Moderate narrowing of retinal arteries in the left eye of a patient who experienced an attack of nonarteritic anterior ischemic optic neuropathy. **D:** Marked narrowing of retinal arteries in the left eye of another patient who experienced an attack of nonarteritic anterior ischemic optic neuropathy.

of the optic disc. However, the atrophy caused by central retinal artery occlusion and ischemic optic neuropathy can often be differentiated from other entities because of the associated retinal arteriolar attenuation and sheathing.

Acquired temporal pallor is the most common expression of segmental optic atrophy. Sharply demarcated wedge-shaped temporal pallor is a consequence of discrete papillomacular bundle lesions that occur in the retina between the macula and the disc or within the core of the optic nerve. Superior, inferior, or nasal sector-shaped pallor seldom appears as sharply circumscribed as temporal pallor. Acquired temporal pallor is usually caused by optic neuropathies that selectively affect central vision and field, sparing the peripheral field. Such optic neuropathies include toxic and nutritional optic neuropathies, autosomal-dominant and Leber's hereditary optic neuropathies, and optic neuritis (Fig. 4.17). When superior or inferior disc pallor is present, an ischemic etiology is more likely.

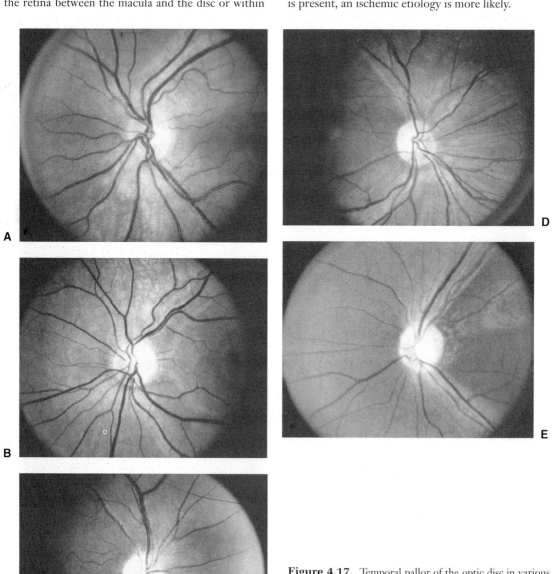

Figure 4.17. Temporal pallor of the optic disc in various optic neuropathies. **A:** After acute retrobulbar optic neuritis. **B:** In a patient with dominant hereditary optic atrophy. **C:** In a patient with Leber's optic neuropathy. **D:** In a patient with toxic optic neuropathy from ethambutol. **E:** In a patient with Cuban epidemic optic neuropathy. Note selective loss of the nerve fiber layer in the papillomacular bundle in several of these photographs.

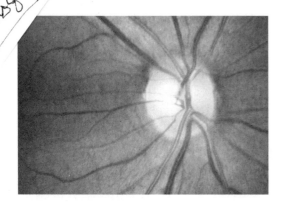

Figure 4.18. "Band" or "bow-tie" atrophy of the right optic disc in a patient with a temporal hemianopia caused by a pituitary adenoma. Note horizontal band of atrophy across the right disc, with preservation of the superior and inferior portions of the disc.

The specific organization of the retinal nerve fiber layer results in specific patterns of nerve fiber layer and optic atrophy in patients with visual loss from optic chiasmal and retrochiasmal-pregeniculate lesions. In patients with chiasmal lesions, for example, temporal field defects are mirrored by loss of fibers from ganglion cells nasal to the fovea. The atrophy is most impressive directly nasal and temporal to the disc, because the superior and inferior arcuate nerve fiber bundles are composed of fibers from ganglion cells both temporal and nasal to the fovea. Thus, the arcuate bundles are relatively spared compared with other areas. The optic pallor is primarily nasal and temporal with sparing superiorly and inferiorly. This "band" or "bow-tie" atrophy is characteristic of temporal field loss (Fig. 4.18). Patients with optic chiasmal syndromes and bitemporal hemianopic field defects ultimately develop "band" optic disc pallor and characteristic nerve fiber layer atrophy in both eyes.

In patients with congenital or neonatally acquired homonymous hemianopia, or in patients with pregeniculate homonymous hemianopias, the eye contralateral to the lesion has temporal field loss and shows the pattern of nerve fiber and optic nerve atrophy described earlier—band atrophy of the optic disc. The eye ipsilateral to the lesion has a complete nasal field loss with loss of ganglion cells temporal to the fovea. Because the nerve fibers from these ganglion cells primarily comprise the superior and inferior arcuate bundles, these regions show extensive loss of nerve fibers, and the disc atrophy is more diffuse. The characteristic features of the fundi of such individuals are thus a bow-tie or band atrophy in the contralateral eye and reduced visibility of the superior and inferior arcuate nerve fiber bundles in the ipsilateral eye compared with the contralateral eye.

Although the presence or absence of pathologic pallor of the optic disc cannot be directly equated with visual function, it should be obvious that no judgment of pallor is meaningful until and unless the pallor is correlated with optic nerve function. The data should be obtained from careful testing of visual acuity and color vision, as well as quantitative perimetry, examination of the pupils, and electrophysiologic studies when appropriate (see Chapter 1). An optic disc may appear to be pale, yet meticulous clinical and electrophysiologic testing of visual function may fail to disclose any abnormality. In such cases, it is most likely that the pallor is physiologic rather than pathologic. Conversely, an optic disc occasionally appears normal despite severe and even long-standing visual acuity or field loss caused by optic nerve dysfunction. In most of these cases, careful evaluation of the optic disc as well as the peripapillary retinal nerve fiber layer will provide evidence of retinal nerve fiber atrophy, either too focal or too mild and diffuse to produce obvious optic pallor.

SYNDROMES OF PRE-CHIASMAL OPTIC NERVE DYSFUNCTION

OPTOCILIARY SHUNTS AND THE SYNDROME OF CHRONIC OPTIC NERVE COMPRESSION

Chronic optic nerve compression may cause a specific syndrome characterized by progressive loss of vision, optic disc swelling that is followed or accompanied by optic atrophy, and the appearance of dilated venous channels called **optociliary shunt veins.** These shunt veins are congenital connections between the retinal and choroidal venous circulations. When there is chronic compression of the optic nerve, particularly when the lesion is within the orbit, these veins enlarge and shunt blood from the retinal to the choroidal venous circulation, thus allowing the retinal venous blood to bypass the obstructed central retinal vein and exit the orbit via the choroidal circulation, vortex veins, and ophthalmic veins (Fig. 4.19). Spheno-orbital meningiomas most commonly cause this syndrome, although it may also be caused by chronic papilledema, optic gliomas, or arachnoid cysts of the optic nerve. Optociliary shunt veins also can appear in patients after chronic central retinal vein occlusion, often without evidence of optic nerve dysfunction.

DISTAL OPTIC NERVE SYNDROME

Where the optic nerve joins the chiasm, at the anterior angle of the chiasm, its particular fiber anatomy provides another opportunity for anatomic diagnosis. The crossed and uncrossed fibers are separated at this level but are quite compact, and a small lesion affecting either the crossed or the uncrossed fibers may produce

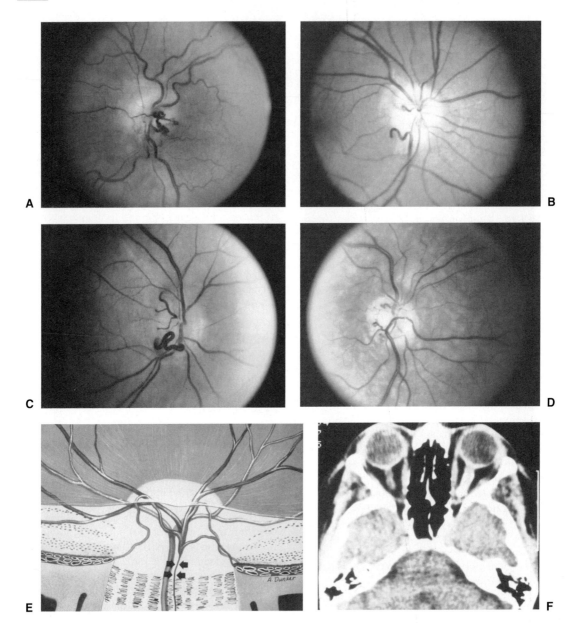

Figure 4.19. Acquired optociliary (retinochoroidal) shunt veins. **A to D:** Four fundus photographs showing optociliary shunt veins in patients with optic atrophy from chronic compression of the optic nerves. Note varying size of the vessels, which are shunting venous blood from the retinal to the choroidal circulation so that it can exit the eye via the vortex veins to the superior and inferior ophthalmic veins rather than via the central retinal vein. **E:** Artist's drawing of acquired retinochoroidal shunt veins that are, in fact, **congenital** structures that simply enlarge in the setting of chronic compression of the optic nerve. **F:** CT scan, axial view, shows the appearance of a left optic nerve sheath meningioma in the patient whose fundus appearance is shown in **(A)**. Note that the nerve is thickened and brighter than the opposite optic nerve. (Schematic drawing reprinted from: Miller NR, Fine SL. *The Ocular Fundus in Neuro-Ophthalmologic Diagnosis: Sights and Sounds in Ophthalmology.* Vol. 3. St. Louis: CV Mosby; 1977, with permission.)

a unilateral hemianopic defect. Such a defect is called a *junctional scotoma*. In such cases, it is not uncommon to find an asymptomatic scotoma in the upper temporal field of the **opposite** eye (Fig. 4.20). This scotoma results from damage to ventrally located fibers

originating from ganglion cells located inferior and nasal to the fovea that, upon reaching the distal end of the optic nerve, were historically thought to loop anteriorly about 1 to 2 mm into the contralateral optic nerve (**Wilbrand's knee**, see Chapter 2). There is some

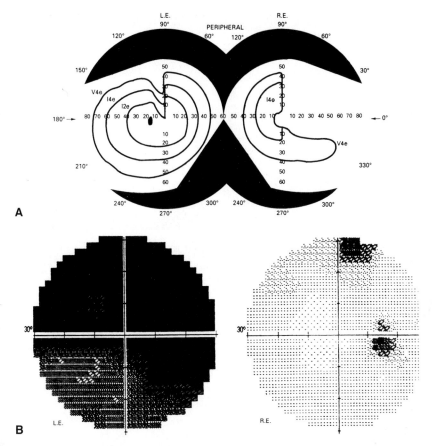

Figure 4.20. Two examples of the syndrome of the distal optic nerve (anterior chiasmal syndrome). **A:** Kinetic perimetry in a patient with decreased vision in the right eye from a pituitary adenoma shows a dense temporal defect with a central scotoma in that eye. In addition, however, there is a superior temporal defect in the visual field of the contralateral eye. **B:** Static perimetry in another patient with loss of vision in the left eye from a pituitary adenoma shows almost complete loss of the central field in that eye as well as a small superior temporal defect in the visual field of the right eye.

evidence that Wilbrand's knee is not a normal anatomic structure but rather an artifact that develops when there is atrophy of the ipsilateral optic nerve. Although this may be true, Wilbrand's knee clearly exists from a clinical standpoint: a patient with evidence of an optic neuropathy in one eye and a superior temporal defect in the visual field of the opposite eye has a lesion of the distal optic nerve at its junction with the optic chiasm.

FOSTER KENNEDY SYNDROME

Intracranial lesions that exert direct pressure on one optic nerve usually produce optic atrophy. As these lesions enlarge, they may eventually produce increased intracranial pressure. When the compressed optic nerve is significantly atrophic by the time intracranial pressure becomes increased, the increased intracranial pressure produces papilledema only in the contralateral eye. Homolateral optic atrophy and con-

tralateral papilledema, when associated with anosmia, are the hallmarks of the so-called **Foster Kennedy syndrome** (Fig 4.21). This syndrome occurs most often with frontal lobe tumors and olfactory groove meningiomas.

In some cases, this syndrome of optic atrophy in one eye and papilledema in the other eye is falsely localizing; that is, the optic atrophy is not on the side ipsilateral to the tumor but on the contralateral side. Additionally, a "Foster Kennedy syndrome" consisting of optic atrophy on one side and optic disc swelling on the other may result from asymmetric optic nerve compression from an intracranial mass in the absence of increased intracranial pressure. Most importantly, a true Foster Kennedy syndrome is extremely rare. It is much more common to see optic atrophy on one side with optic disc swelling on the opposite side in cases of bilateral nonsimultaneous optic neuritis or ischemic optic neuropathy. In such cases, the symptoms

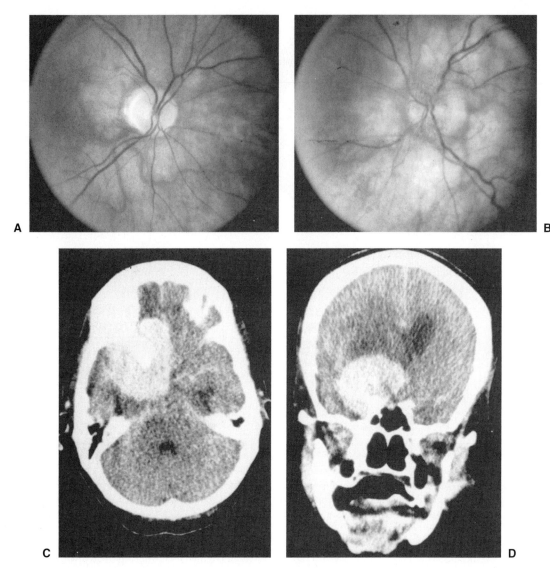

Figure 4.21. Foster Kennedy syndrome of unilateral optic atrophy, contralateral papilledema, and anosmia. The patient was a 34-year-old woman with severe headaches and progressive loss of vision in the right eye. A neurologic examination revealed anosmia and some degree of confusion. Visual acuity was 20/400 OD and 20/25 OS. There was a right relative afferent pupillary defect. **A:** The right optic disc is diffusely pale. **B:** The left optic disc shows chronic swelling. **C:** CT scan, axial view, after intravenous injection of contrast material, reveals a large enhancing mass along the right sphenoid wing, consistent with a meningioma. **D:** CT scan, coronal view, after intravenous injection of contrast material, shows the upward extension of the mass as well as enlargement of the lateral ventricles.

and signs are profoundly different and should cause no difficulty in diagnosis.

BILATERAL SUPERIOR OR INFERIOR (ALTITUDINAL) HEMIANOPIA

The question often arises in a patient with bilateral visual field defects if a single lesion accounts for the field defects or if there are bilateral optic nerve lesions. Bilat-

eral central, cecocentral, and arcuate defects all suggest dysfunction of both optic nerves. A unilateral visual field defect in all or most of the upper or lower portion of the field is always caused by a lesion of the retina or optic nerve. Similarly, bilateral visual field defects of this type usually represent bilateral lesions damaging the retinas or optic nerves. In many of these cases, one eye is affected before the other. In such cases, the cause is typically bilateral nonarteritic anterior ischemic

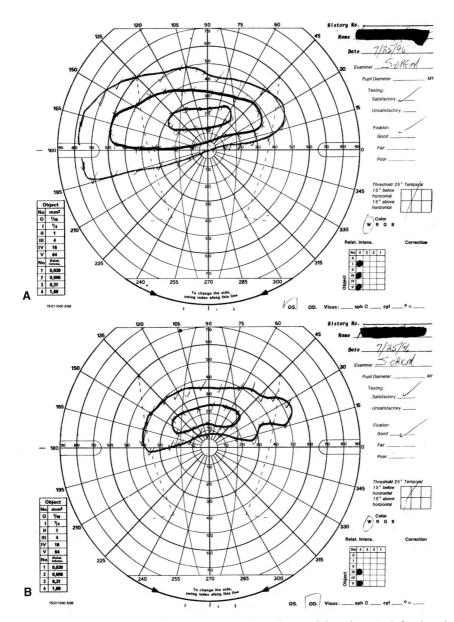

Figure 4.22. Bilateral altitudinal visual field defects in a patient with simultaneous bilateral anterior ischemic optic neuropathy. The patient was a 67-year-old man who awoke from cardiac surgery with loss of vision in both eyes. Visual acuity was 5/200 OD and 20/300 OS. **A:** Kinetic perimetry in the left eye shows complete loss of the inferior field and constriction of the remaining superior field. **B:** Kinetic perimetry in the visual field of the right eye shows almost complete loss of the inferior field with preservation of the superior field.

optic neuropathy. In rare cases, a simultaneous bilateral ischemic optic neuropathy can occur (Fig. 4.22).

Rarely, a large prechiasmal lesion compresses both optic nerves, producing bilateral altitudinal field defects. In most of these cases, the etiology is a pituitary adenoma that compresses the inferior aspects of both optic nerves, producing bilateral superior altitudinal defects. In other cases, however, compression of the optic nerves from below elevates them against the dural shelves extending out from the intracranial end of the optic canals. Pressure from the dura against the superior aspects of the nerves subsequently produces bilateral inferior altitudinal defects.

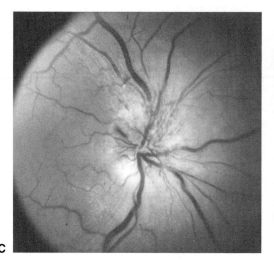
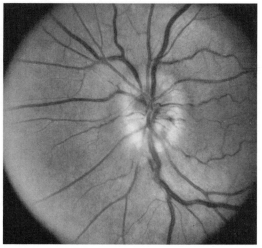

C

D

Figure 4.22. (*continued*) Right (**C**) and left (**D**) optic discs are swollen and hyperemic, and there are flame-shaped hemorrhages at the margins of both discs.

Some patients with bilateral optic neuropathies—particularly those who develop bilateral simultaneous or nonsimultaneous anterior ischemic optic neuropathy—develop a superior altitudinal defect in one eye and an inferior altitudinal defect in the other. In addition to the expected difficulties with visual function that result from loss of visual acuity, color vision, and visual field, such patients may experience binocular diplopia or difficulty reading caused by decompensation of a preexisting vertical or horizontal phoria. The problems encountered by these patients result from loss of the normal partial overlap of the superior or inferior fields of the two eyes. This overlap normally permits fusion of images and helps stabilize ocular alignment in patients with vertical or horizontal phorias. Because their remaining visual fields represent only the superior projection from one eye and the inferior projection from the other, patients with a superior hemianopia in one eye and an inferior hemianopia in the other do not have a physiologic linkage between the two remaining altitudinal hemifields. In such patients, a preexisting asymptomatic phoria becomes a tropia because of vertical or horizontal separation or overlap of the two remaining hemifields. Patients thus complain of diplopia and may have difficulty reading because of doubling or inability to see printed letters or words (Fig. 4.23). This condition, called the **hemifield slide phenomenon,** was initially described in patients with bitemporal hemianopic field defects (see Chapter 12).

NASAL HEMIANOPIA

Most organic nasal visual field defects are actually arcuate in nature and the most common causes are chronic pathology of the optic disc, such as chronic papilledema

and optic nerve head drusen. In some cases, however, a true unilateral hemianopia or bilateral nasal hemianopias occurs, with the defects having no connection to the blind spot and respecting the vertical meridian. Such field defects result from damage to the temporal aspects of one or both optic nerves.

Binasal hemianopia is an exceedingly infrequent visual field defect. Although a "binasal hemianopia" is sometimes said to occur in patients with intracranial tumors that grow between the intracranial optic nerves, pushing them laterally against the anterior cerebral or internal carotid arteries, the field defects in such cases are usually arcuate, not hemianopic, and do not respect the vertical midline. True binasal quadrantic or hemianopic defects occur in rare patients with a variety of intracranial lesions, including pituitary tumors, meningiomas, suprasellar aneurysm, dolichoectatic internal carotid arteries, optochiasmatic arachnoiditis, hydrocephalus with enlargement of the third ventricle, and primary empty sella syndrome (Fig. 4.24).

CHRONIC OPEN-ANGLE GLAUCOMA (GLAUCOMATOUS OPTIC NEUROPATHY)

Chronic open-angle glaucoma requires comment here because the clinical manifestations it produces, particularly the visual field defects, are identical with the field defects produced by other types of optic neuropathy.

Most patients with chronic open-angle glaucoma develop loss of visual field long before they experience loss of central vision. Color vision deficits are typically

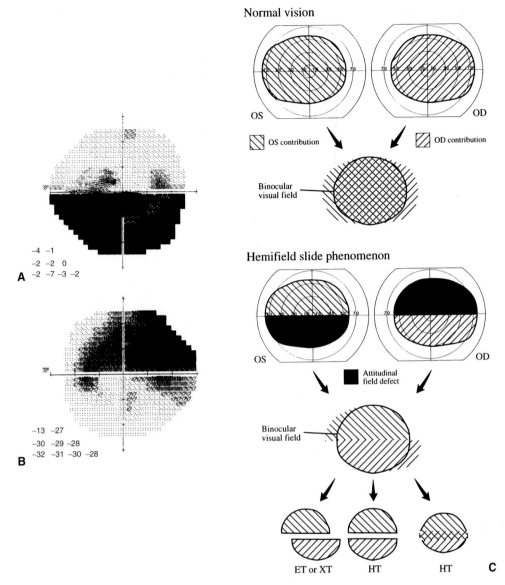

Figure 4.23. Hemifield slide phenomenon from bilateral optic neuropathy. Inferior altitudinal defect in the visual field of the right eye **(A)** and superior altitudinal defect in the visual field of the left eye **(B)** from bilateral ischemic optic neuropathy. **C:** Artist's drawing shows that such defects can produce a vertical or horizontal hemifield slide phenomenon from loss of overlapping portions of the visual fields. Affected patients may complain of vertical, horizontal, or diagonal diplopia.

of the blue-yellow type, but exceptions regularly occur, and red-green deficits are not uncommon. A relative afferent pupillary defect can be present in cases of unilateral or asymmetric glaucoma.

The visual field defects in chronic open-angle glaucoma occur from damage to nerve fiber bundles at the level of the sclera within the optic nerve head. This damage seems to occur focally in its initial stages and is thus expressed in the visual field as isolated scotomas appearing between 5 degrees and 30 degrees from fix-

ation in the arcuate or Bjerrum area (Fig. 4.25). About two thirds of these isolated paracentral or arcuate scotomas are accompanied by a depression in sensitivity in the upper or lower half of the field. This loss of sensitivity appears initially as a step in a plotted isopter, usually at the nasal, horizontal meridian (the nasal step of Rönne). One third of early paracentral scotomas that occur in patients with chronic open-angle glaucoma have no associated nasal step. Even less frequently, a nasal step is present without a paracentral scotoma.

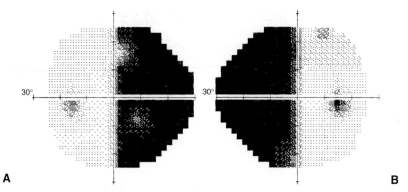

Figure 4.24. Bilateral complete nasal hemianopia in a 34-year-old woman with a suprasellar aneurysm that displaced both optic nerves laterally against the supraclinoid portion of the internal carotid arteries. The field defect resolved after clipping of the aneurysm. **A:** Visual field of the left eye. **B:** Visual field of the right eye.

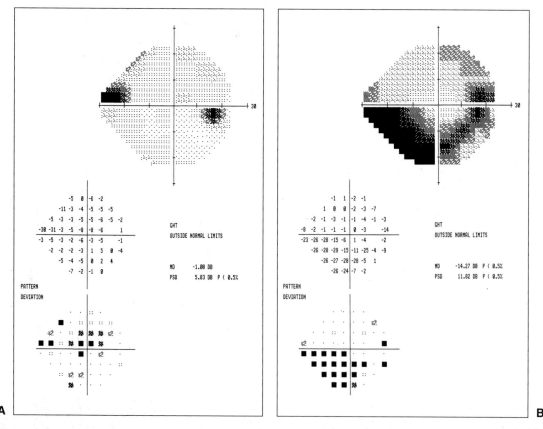

Figure 4.25. Field changes in patients with glaucomatous optic neuropathy. **A:** Superior nasal step in right eye. **B:** Inferior arcuate field defect in right eye.

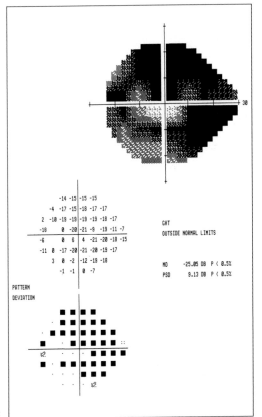

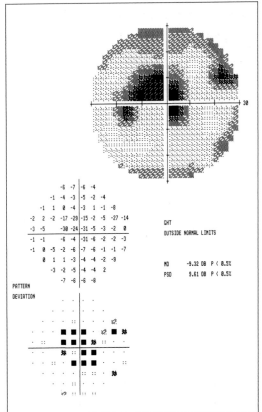

Figure 4.25. (*continued*) **C:** Inferior and superior arcuate defects in left eye. **D:** Central field loss in left eye. In the cases in which central field loss is seen in glaucoma, the horizontal meridian is usually respected.

As damage proceeds, the paracentral scotoma becomes deeper and wider, and new scotomas may develop in the same arcuate region. As these defects coalesce, they take on an arching shape between the nasal horizontal meridian and the blind spot. As arcuate scotomas enlarge and affect both the upper and lower regions, they may meet at the horizontal meridian and produce a ring-shaped scotoma (Fig. 4.25). Further damage results in the breaking out of the scotoma to the peripheral field, so-called "baring" to the periphery. Thus, patients with advanced glaucoma may retain only the central 5 degrees and a temporal island of vision.

Although the visual field defects that occur in chronic open-angle glaucoma are identical with defects that result from various types of nonglaucomatous optic neuropathy, the differentiation between glaucoma and nonglaucomatous optic neuropathy should be easily made by a careful ophthalmoscopic examina-tion. Patients with glaucoma develop visual field defects only after there is extensive damage to the optic disc. The ophthalmoscopic appearance of such a disc is typical (see above). In nearly every case, there is substantial cupping of the disc, with the remaining neuroretinal rim appearing relatively normal, without evidence of pallor (Fig. 4.14). This is in contrast to other types of optic nerve disease producing similar visual field defects in which the optic disc may appear normal, diffusely or sectorially pale without enlargement in the size of the cup, or pale with substantial cupping but also with pallor of the remaining neuroretinal rim.

FOR FURTHER INFORMATION

See *Walsh & Hoyt's Clinical Neuro-Ophthalmology.* 6th ed. Volume 1, Chapter 4, pages 205–236; Volume 2, Chapter 28, pages 1344–1347.

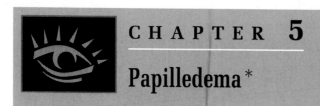

CHAPTER 5

Papilledema*

The term *papilledema* is often mistakenly applied to any type of swelling of the optic disc regardless of the etiology. Although it is true that swelling of the optic papilla can theoretically be denoted as *papilledema*, the term has a particular, ingrained meaning to most clinicians. It should be used *only* for optic disc swelling that results from increased intracranial pressure (ICP). Other forms of disc swelling caused by local or systemic processes should be designated with respect to the presumed etiology—for example, *anterior ischemic optic neuropathy* or *anterior optic neuritis*—or in general terms, such as *optic disc swelling* or *optic nerve head edema*.

MEASUREMENTS OF INTRACRANIAL PRESSURE

Normal cerebrospinal fluid (CSF) pressure in adults, measured by lumbar puncture with the patient in the lateral decubitus position, varies between 80 and 200 mm of water. Contrary to popular belief, CSF pressure is not dependent on weight or height, although pressure readings may be spuriously elevated when the patient coughs, strains, or holds his or her breath during the procedure. Measurements between 201 and 249

mm water are not diagnostic and those greater than 250 mm water are elevated. Normal values have not been well established in children, but are generally accepted to be 200 mm water or less. Additionally, ICP in normal persons and in patients with increased ICP can vary widely overtime. Continuous monitoring of ICP of patients with idiopathic intracranial hypertension (IIH) has shown irregular variations ranging from 50 to 500 mm of water over a 24-hour period. In addition, lumbar CSF pressure is often lower than the true ICP in patients with infratentorial tumors that block communication between the ventricular system and the spinal subarachnoid space.

Lumbar puncture (LP) is generally a safe procedure, but in certain situations it carries significant risk. Except under extraordinary circumstances, a neuroimaging study (computed tomography [CT] or magnetic resonance imaging [MRI]) should always be performed prior to the LP to make sure there is no mass effect in the brain. Removal of fluid from the spinal canal may allow the compressed brain to shift downward and to impact at the tentorial incisura or the foramen magnum, often with fatal results. LP occasionally induces an acquired Chiari malformation that may be reversible. Post-LP headaches may occur in up to 40% of patients after a lumbar tap. These headaches typically worsen when the patient is in the upright position and resolve when in supine position. Other symptoms of having low CSF pressure mimic those of increased ICP with visual disturbances and diplopia from the VIth nerve paresis.

*Adapted from Friedman DI. Papilledema. In: Miller NR, Newman NJ, Biousse V, Kerrison JB, eds. *Walsh & Hoyt's Clinical Neuro-Ophthalmology*. 6th ed. Vol. I. Philadelphia: Lippincott Williams & Wilkins; 2005:237–291.

Table 5.1. *Papilledema Grading System (Frisén Scale)*

Stage 0—Normal Optic Disc

Blurring of nasal, superior and inferior poles in inverse proportion to disc diameter

Radial nerve fiber layer (NFL) without NFL tortuosity

Rare obscuration of a major blood vessel, usually on the upper pole

Stage 1—Very Early Papilledema

Obscuration of the nasal border of the disc

No elevation of the disc borders

Disruption of the normal radial NFL arrangement with grayish opacity accentuating nerve fiber layer bundles

Normal temporal disc margin

Subtle grayish halo with temporal gap (best seen with indirect ophthalmoscopy)

Concentric or radial retrochoroidal folds

Stage 2—Early Papilledema

Obscuration of all borders

Elevation of the nasal border

Complete peripapillary halo

Stage 3—Moderate Papilledema

Obscurations of all borders

Increased diameter of optic nerve head

Obscuration of one or more segments of major blood vessels leaving the disc

Peripapillary halo–irregular outer fringe with finger-like extensions

Stage 4—Marked Papilledema

Elevation of the entire nerve head

Obscuration of all borders

Peripapillary halo

Total obscuration on the disc of a segment of a major blood vessel

Stage 5—Severe Papilledema

Dome-shaped protrusions representing anterior expansion of the optic nerve head

Peripapillary halo is narrow and smoothly demarcated

Total obscuration of a segment of a major blood vessel may or may no be present

Obliteration of the optic cup

OPHTHALMOSCOPIC APPEARANCE OF PAPILLEDEMA

There are several classification systems for papilledema. The disc appearance can be described according to the duration of papilledema (early; fully developed; chronic; and atrophic). However the Frisén grading system (Table 5.1) is most useful as it classifies the papilledema grade by severity.

STAGES OF PAPILLEDEMA

Stereoscopic viewing of a **normal optic disc (Frisén Stage 0)** often reveals mild nasal elevation of the nerve fiber layer. With the direct ophthalmoscope the nasal disc margin may appear indistinct compared to the temporal disc rim. The vessels are generally seen coursing across the optic nerve head, although, rarely, a portion of a major vessel may be obscured in the upper pole.

In very early papilledema **(Frisén Stage 1)**, there is hyperemia of the optic disc, blurring of the peripapillary retinal nerve fiber layer, swelling of the optic disc, blurring of the disc margins, peripapillary flame-shaped hemorrhages, and absent spontaneous venous pulsations (Fig. 5.1A). There may be disruption of the normal radial nerve fiber layer arrangement with grayish opacity accentuating nerve fiber bundles. The absence of spontaneous retinal venous pulsations is thought by some investigators to be an early sign of papilledema. Indeed, pulsations usually cease when ICP exceeds about 200 mm of water. Thus, if spontaneous venous pulsations are present, ICP should be below this figure. However, spontaneous venous pulsations occur in only about 80% of normal subjects. Thus, patients with normal ICP may also lack spontaneous venous pulsations.

Early papilledema (Frisén Stage 2) is characterized by obscuration of the optic disc borders, elevation of the nasal border and a complete peripapillary halo (Fig. 5.1B).

As the severity of papilledema increases to **moderate papilledema (Frisén Stage 3)**, the margins of the optic disc become obscured and elevated. The diameter of the optic nerve head increases, which often results in the enlargement of the physiologic blind spot. The optic cup may still be preserved at this stage. An important finding is that the edematous, opaque nerve fiber layer obscures one or more segments of major blood vessels leaving the disc. The gray peripapillary halo becomes more apparent and may have an irregular outer fringe with finger-like extensions conforming to the nerve fiber layer (Figs. 5.1C, and 5.2A).

Marked papilledema (Frisén Stage 4) is characterized by elevation of the entire optic nerve head. The optic cup is often obliterated. There is obscuration of all the borders of the nerve with a prominent peripapillary halo. Edema and infarction of the nerve fiber layer cause total obscuration on the disc of a segment of a major blood vessel. The retinal veins are often engorged and tortuous (Figs. 5.2B and 5.3).

Severe Papilledema (Frisén Stage 5) is present when the optic nerve protrudes anteriorly with a dome-shaped configuration. The optic cup is obliterated and the peripapillary halo is narrow and smoothly demarcated. Often, there are no appreciable landmarks to

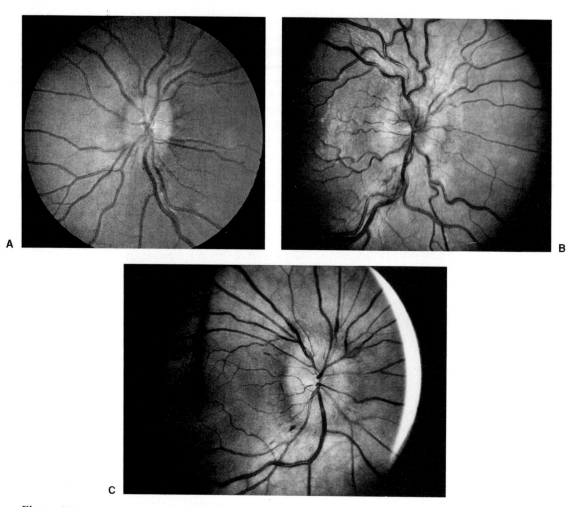

Figure 5.1. A: Very early papilledema (Frisén stage 1). The disc shows slight hyperemia and blurring of the peripapillary nerve fiber layer at the superior and inferior poles of the disc. **B:** Early papilledema (Frisén stage 2). This disc is hyperemic and mildly swollen. Note the inferior peripapillary nerve fiber hemorrhages. **C:** The disc is moderately swollen (Frisén stage 3) with obscuration of all borders, a peripapillary halo, and several small "splinter" hemorrhages adjacent to the disc margins at 7 and 10 o'clock.

distinguish the optic nerve head from the surrounding retina. Obscuration of segments of major blood vessels may or may not be present (Fig. 5.4).

OTHER SIGNS OF PAPILLEDEMA

Other signs of papilledema may contribute to visual impairment but are often not helpful in determining the severity of papilledema. Flame-shaped, nerve fiber layer hemorrhages, cotton wool spots (focal retinal infarcts), and tortuous vessels on or surrounding the disc are common. In severe cases, circumferential retinal folds (Paton's lines) often develop; linear or curvilinear choroidal folds may be observed. Choroidal folds from increased intracranial pressure often result

in acquired, progressive hyperopia. Hard exudates and hemorrhages may occur in the peripapillary region and in the macula, producing decreased central vision (Figs. 5.5 and 5.6). Because nerve fibers in the macula have a radial orientation, hemorrhages and exudates in this region can assume a fan or star shape. Because vascular compromise on and around the optic disc is responsible for these macular changes, the star figure in such cases is usually asymmetric, being more prominent on the nasal side of the fovea toward the disc (Fig. 5.5).

Hemorrhages are frequently present with papilledema, although they are not incorporated into the Frisén staging system. Nerve fiber layer hemorrhages are the most common and indicate that the edema is

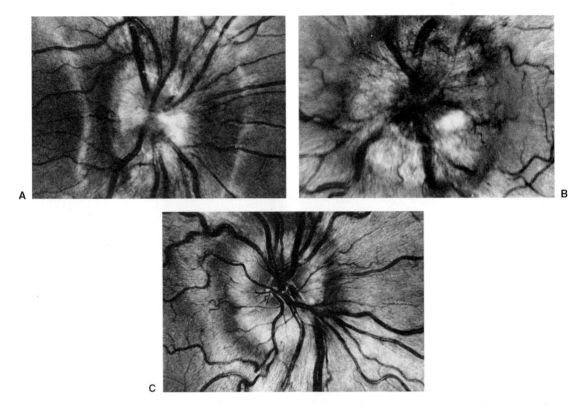

Figure 5.2. Red-free photographs showing nerve fiber layer in papilledema and in pseudopapilledema. **A:** Moderate papilledema (Frisén stage 3). The nerve fiber layer has mild distortion of light reflexes and a "muddy" appearance obscuring small vessels traversing the disc margin. **B:** Marked papilledema (Frisén stage 4). The reflexes from the peripapillary retinal nerve fiber layer are completely distorted and blurred. Note the dilated disc capillaries. **C:** Pseudopapilledema. Although the disc is moderately elevated, the surface vessels appear normal and the nerve fiber layer reflexes are sharply defined. Superficial drusen are visible between 3 and 4 o'clock.

acute to subacute (Figs. 5.4 and 5.5). A small nerve fiber layer hemorrhage in the peripapillary region may be an extremely important sign of early papilledema. Such a hemorrhage appears as a thin, radial streak on the disc or near its margins and is presumably caused by rupture of a distended capillary within or surrounding the disc (Fig. 5.5).

When the increase in ICP is rapid, subhyaloid hemorrhages may be present in addition to the more common intraretinal hemorrhages (Fig. 5.7). These hemorrhages may break into the vitreous in some cases. Rarely patients with papilledema develop macular and peripapillary subretinal neovascularization, especially when the papilledema is chronic (Fig. 5.8). The presence of peripheral retinal hemorrhages in addition to hemorrhages in the posterior pole suggests extensive retinal venous congestion produced by significantly elevated ICP.

CHRONIC PAPILLEDEMA

When papilledema persists, hemorrhages and exudates slowly resolve, and the disc develops a rounded appearance (Fig. 5.9). The central cup, which may be retained in the acute phase of papilledema, ultimately becomes obliterated. Over a period of months, the initial disc hyperemia changes to a milky gray appearance, with hard exudates becoming apparent in the superficial disc substance. These exudates resemble optic disc drusen and may result in a misdiagnosis of pseudopapilledema (Fig. 5.2C).

Most patients with chronic papilledema have evidence of nerve fiber layer atrophy. The appearance of the atrophy ranges from slit-like defects to diffuse loss. Nerve fiber layer atrophy can be best appreciated by viewing through the red-free filter of a direct ophthalmoscope or slit lamp biomicroscope.

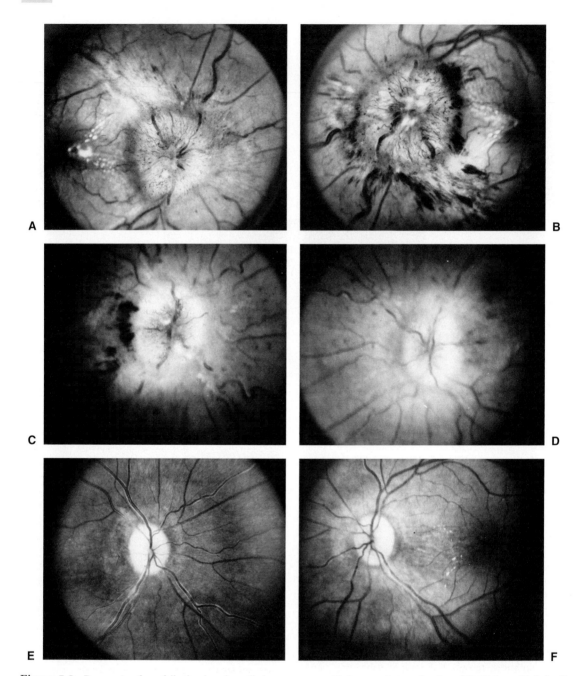

Figure 5.3. Progression from fully developed papilledema to postpapilledema optic atrophy. **A and B:** Right and left fundi showing severe papilledema. Note the obscuration of major vessels traversing the disc margin, and the extensive peripapillary hemorrhages and exudates, including star figure of lipid in the maculae. **C and D:** Two weeks later, both optic discs are less swollen but pale. The hemorrhages and exudates are resolving but the vessels crossing the disc are still partially obscured by the edematous nerve fiber layer. **E and F:** Four months later, both optic discs are diffusely pale; the retinal vessels are sheathed; and the nerve fiber layer is absent.

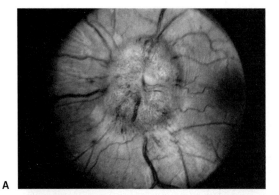

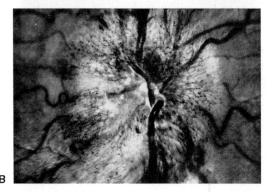

Figure 5.4. Severe papilledema (Frisén stage 5) with marked dilation of disc vessels and formation of micro-aneurysms. **A:** Fundus photograph; **B:** Red-free photograph.

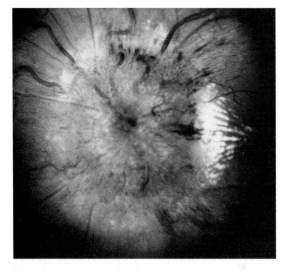

Figure 5.5. Macular star figure in fully developed papilledema. The incomplete star in the papillomacular bundle is characteristic but occasionally a complete star figure is seen.

Occasionally, papilledema persists for a long period of time without significant visual symptoms. This situation occurs primarily in patients with IIH.

POSTPAPILLEDEMA ATROPHY

With time, untreated papilledema subsides, the disc becomes atrophic, and the retinal vessels become narrow and sheathed. Some patients have persistent pigmentary changes or choroidal folds in the maculae (Fig. 5.10). The time required for papilledema to evolve into optic atrophy depends upon many factors, including the severity and constancy of the increased ICP. Atrophic changes can appear within weeks or days following the initial observation of acute papilledema in some cases, particularly if the rise in ICP is rapid, severe, and sustained. In such cases, the disc appearance may rapidly progress to fully developed papilledema and then to postpapilledema optic atrophy without ever having gone through a stage of chronic papilledema. In still other cases, many months or even years may elapse before atrophy develops. In such cases, the appearance of the fundus is typically that of chronic papilledema that gradually melts away into atrophy. In some cases of chronic papilledema, optociliary shunt veins develop. These vessels, which are pre-existing veins that connect the retinal and choroidal venous circulations, enlarge because the increased ICP either directly compresses the central retinal vein or indirectly compresses it by compressing the optic nerve (Fig. 5.11). In either case, the vessels shunt venous blood from the retinal to the choroidal venous circulations. Optociliary shunt veins may disappear after the ICP is surgically lowered or following optic nerve sheath decompression surgery.

Optic atrophy that results from chronic papilledema has a specific pattern of axonal loss. Loss of peripheral axons with sparing of central axons has been demonstrated in several postmortem studies. Good central visual acuity despite severe papilledema and optic atrophy is found in most patients with chronic papilledema.

UNILATERAL OR ASYMMETRIC PAPILLEDEMA

Papilledema is usually bilateral and relatively symmetric in the two eyes. In some instances, it is strictly unilateral or at least much more pronounced in one eye than in the other (Fig. 5.12). Some patients may have had preexisting atrophy before the development of increased ICP (the pseudo-Foster Kennedy syndrome; see the subsequent text and in Chapter 4). If there are not enough viable nerve fibers, papilledema cannot occur ("dead axons don't swell"). However, if sufficient nerve fibers remain, papilledema may develop even though the optic disc is pale. In the Foster Kennedy syndrome, patients with frontal lobe or

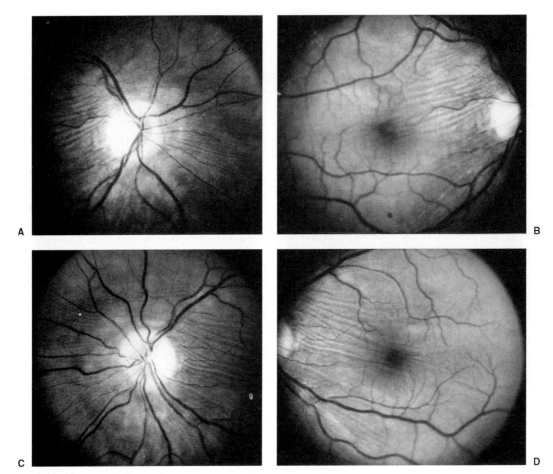

Figure 5.6. Persistent choroidal striae associated with resolving papilledema. **A:** The right optic disc is mildly pale and minimally swollen. Curvilinear striae extend toward the macula. **B:** Striae extend into the right macula. **C:** The left optic disc is also mildly pale and minimally swollen. Striae are present in the papillomacular region. **D:** The striae extend into the left macula.

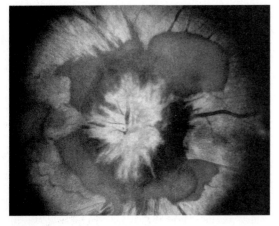

Figure 5.7. Subhyaloid hemorrhage with papilledema. The patient had a severe, subarachnoid hemorrhage from an intracranial aneurysm.

olfactory groove tumors develop the triad of optic atrophy in one eye; papilledema in the other eye; and anosmia. The optic nerve ipsilateral to the tumor is generally atrophic because of compression. A rise in CSF pressure in the optic nerve sheath is a prerequisite condition for development of papilledema. Optic nerve compression prevents elevated intrasheath pressure and produces ipsilateral atrophy of optic nerve fibers. Similarly, patients with unilateral optic disc dysplasia may develop papilledema only on the side of the previously normal disc.

When unilateral papilledema occurs in a patient with an apparently normal optic disc on the opposite side, it often results from some congenital anomaly of the optic nerve sheath or lamina cribrosa that prevents transmission of pressure to the optic nerve head on the side where the papilledema is absent. In most patients with apparent unilateral papilledema, careful

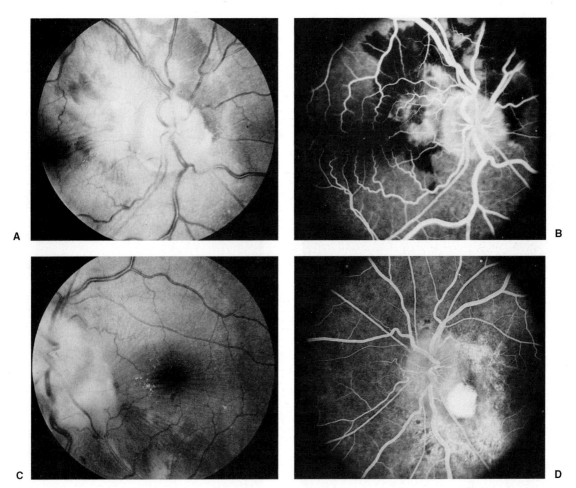

Figure 5.8. Subretinal neovascularization in chronic papilledema. **A:** Right eye shows a marked subretinal neovascular membrane superotemporal to the optic disc with subretinal hemorrhage, serous subretinal fluid, and retinal striae. **B:** Late stage fluorescein angiogram of right eye reveals marked staining of subretinal neovascular membrane and hyperfluorescence of the disc. **C:** Left eye with elevated disc and an inferior-temporal subretinal neovascular membrane with surrounding hemorrhage, hard exudate, and retinal striae. **D:** Fluorescein angiogram of the left eye shows the residual subretinal neovascular membrane with a surrounding area of mottled disruption of the retinal pigment epithelium. (Reprinted from: Morse PH, Leveille AS, Antel JP, et al. Bilateral juxtapapillary subretinal neovascularization associated with pseudotumor cerebri. *Am J Ophthalmol.* 1981;91:312–317, with permission.)

observation of the "normal" optic disc often discloses minimal hyperemia, a blurred nerve fiber layer, or disc swelling that is easily overlooked in the face of significant papilledema on the opposite side (Fig. 5.12). Careful stereoscopic ophthalmoscopy and fluorescein angiography may be necessary to detect subtle papilledema. Nevertheless, purely unilateral papilledema has been described with IIH, cerebral tumors, abscesses, intracranial hemorrhage caused by aneurysm, aqueductal stenosis, and traumatic brain injury.

DIAGNOSIS OF PAPILLEDEMA

The most important method of diagnosing disc edema is careful ophthalmoscopic examination, assessing the features described earlier. An examination that includes red-free ophthalmoscopy and slit lamp biomicroscopy with a handheld lens is usually sufficient to determine whether disc edema is present. After the diagnosis of disc edema is established, the associated clinical features suggest papilledema (i.e., disc edema from increased ICP) versus primary optic neuropathy with disc

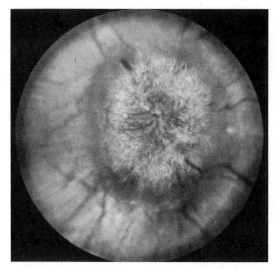

Figure 5.9. Chronic, severe papilledema. Note round compact appearance of the optic disc and lack of hemorrhages.

edema (such as anterior ischemic optic neuropathy, anterior optic neuritis, etc.). Classically, visual acuity is normal until late in papilledema, whereas visual acuity is abnormal in other optic neuropathies. Other symptoms and signs such as headaches, tinnitus, and diplopia may also suggest raised ICP.

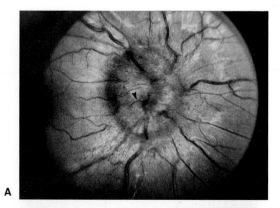

A

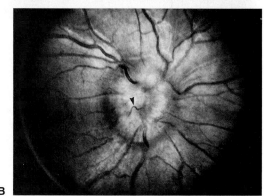

B

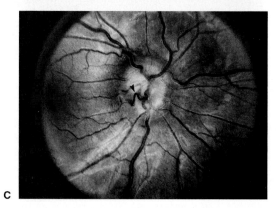

C

Figure 5.11. Development of optociliary shunt veins in a patient with chronic papilledema from pseudotumor cerebri. **A:** Marked (Frisén stage 4) papilledema. Note the small vessel located on the surface of the disc at 8 o'clock (*arrowhead*). **B:** As disc swelling resolves, the previously noted vessel becomes more apparent (*arrowhead*). **C:** Disc swelling has almost completely resolved. The vessel at 8 o'clock appears larger than previously, and clearly represents a retinal-choroidal shunt (*arrowhead*).

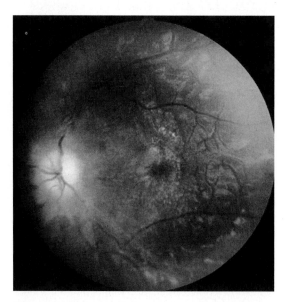

Figure 5.10. Postpapilledema optic atrophy and pigmentary changes in the macula in a patient who previously had severe papilledema. The gliotic changes of the nerve fiber layer give the disc margin a "dirty" appearance. Note pallor of left optic disc, narrowed sheathed retinal vessels, and extensive pigmentary changes in left macula.

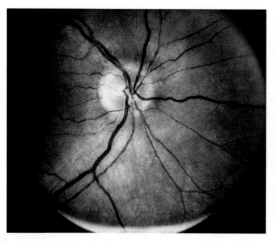
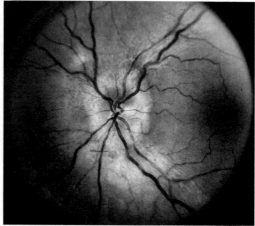

A   B

Figure 5.12. Asymmetric papilledema in a 35-year-old man with pseudotumor cerebri. **A:** The right optic disc is minimally hyperemic and swollen (Frisén stage 1). **B:** Frisén stage 3 papilledema of the left optic disc.

On occasion, the diagnosis of true disc edema remains uncertain and the possibility of pseudo-disc edema is raised (see Chapter 3). In those cases, fluorescein angiography is often used to confirm early papilledema. Typically, the earliest frames of the fluorescein angiogram in patients with early papilledema show disc capillary dilation, dye leakage, and microaneurysms, whereas later frames show leakage of dye beyond the disc margins (Fig. 5.13). Orbital echography can be useful in cases of questionable papilledema. This test can reliably determine if the diameter of the optic nerve is increased and, if so, whether or not the increase is caused by CSF surrounding the nerve. It can also easily detect buried optic disc drusen. Confocal scanning laser tomography (CSLT; Heidelberg Retinal Tomography) and optical coherence tomography (OCT) can also be useful in the diagnosis of disc edema.

Finally, if the diagnosis of papilledema remains uncertain, the ICP can be measured directly by lumbar puncture. This procedure should only be performed after neuroimaging has been performed to determine that no intracranial mass is present.

The differential diagnosis of papilledema includes anomalous elevation of one or both optic discs and true optic disc swelling from a cause other than increased ICP (see Chapter 4). In most cases, the patients have no neurologic or systemic symptoms or signs referable to increased ICP, and this lack of manifestations should help the physician focus on other possibilities.

Anomalous elevation of the optic discs is probably caused most often by buried optic disc drusen; however, hypoplastic discs may be anomalously elevated, and tilted optic discs often show elevation of their superior and nasal portions. In addition, some optic discs are anomalously elevated but do not contain drusen, nor are they small or tilted (see Chapter 3). In all cases, a careful ophthalmoscopic examination combined with ultrasonography or fluorescein angiography should differentiate anomalously elevated optic discs from true optic disc swelling.

True optic disc swelling that mimics papilledema may be caused by local ocular disease, such as intraocular inflammation. Eyes in which optic disc swelling occurs in the setting of inflammation invariably show other evidence of inflammation, particularly aqueous or vitreous cells and, in some cases, sheathing of retinal vessels. Retinal vascular disturbances such as retinal vein occlusion can also produce optic disc swelling. In such cases, there may be no way to determine the cause of the disc swelling without performing appropriate neuroimaging studies and a lumbar puncture. Patients with optic perineuritis (perioptic neuritis) have optic disc swelling that is also indistinguishable from papilledema unless there is associated intraocular inflammation. Nonarteritic anterior ischemic optic neuropathy can mimic papilledema, particularly when it is asymptomatic. Rare patients with anterior optic neuritis have normal central visual acuity; however, such patients invariably complain that they have decreased vision, and other tests of visual function in such patients (e.g., contrast sensitivity, color vision, visual fields) usually reveal an abnormality inconsistent with papilledema. Finally, optic discs infiltrated by inflammatory or neoplastic cells may appear similar to papilledema. The diagnosis in such cases can usually be made by neuroimaging, with or without a lumbar puncture.

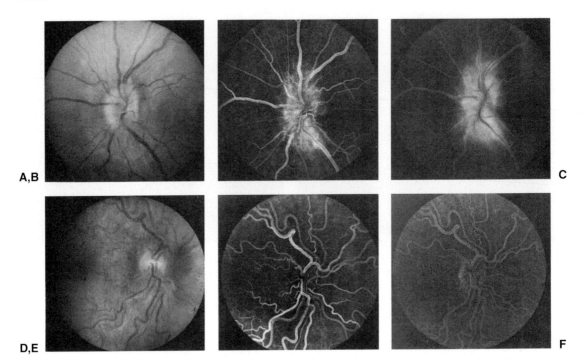

Figure 5.13. Fluorescein angiogram of mild papilledema **(A–C)** and pseudopapilledema **(D–F)**. **A:** Reproduction of color photograph of the left fundus showing indistinct disc margins and an incomplete peripapillary halo (Frisén stage 2). No hemorrhages are visible. **B:** In arteriovenous phase, fluorescein angiogram shows early leakage of dye into peripapillary region. **C:** Ten minutes after fluorescein injection, angiogram shows residual hyperfluorescence of disc and surrounding region. **D:** Optic disc shows tortuous vessels, indistinct disc margins and mild elevation. **E:** Fluorescein angiogram in early arteriovenous phase shows no disc fluorescence or leakage into the peripapillary region. **F:** Eight minutes after fluorescein injection shows no evidence of disc leakage or hyperfluorescence. (Courtesy of Dr. Michael Sanders.)

COURSE OF PAPILLEDEMA

The rapidity with which papilledema can develop depends to a large extent on the etiology of the increased ICP. Papilledema may develop within 2 to 8 hours when there is sudden intracranial or epidural hemorrhage. In addition, minimal papilledema may exist and suddenly become fully developed over several hours in certain settings, such as encephalitis associated with a cerebral abscess. Occasionally, there is the apparently paradoxical development, or increase in the severity, of papilledema several days to a week after normalization of increased ICP.

Fully developed papilledema may disappear completely within hours, days, or weeks, depending on the way in which ICP is lowered (Fig. 5.10). For example, papilledema can resolve 6 to 8 weeks after a successful craniotomy to remove a brain tumor, within 2 to 3 weeks after lumboperitoneal shunting in patients with IIH, and within several days after optic nerve sheath fenestration.

In most cases, retinal venous and disc capillary dilations begin to regress as soon as ICP is lowered to a normal level. During the next few days to weeks, presumably because of the change in hemodynamics at the disc, new hemorrhages may appear; but these are of no significance and disappear within a short time. Gradually, disc hyperemia and elevation resolve. The last abnormalities to disappear are blurring of the disc margins and abnormalities of the peripapillary retinal nerve fiber layer. In some cases, optic atrophy appears as papilledema resolves. There may be extensive sheathing of vessels and gliosis indicating the nature of the etiology in such cases; however, in many cases, the atrophy is indistinguishable from that caused by inflammation, vascular disease, or trauma.

It is difficult to predict the visual prognosis in a patient with papilledema. Generally speaking, the more rapid the development of papilledema, the greater the danger to sight. Similarly, the more severe the papilledema, the worse the visual prognosis. Ominous signs include narrowing of the retinal arteries, often with sheathing, and loss of the peripapillary retinal nerve fiber layer. When these changes are seen, irreversible damage to optic nerve tissue has already occurred. Disc pallor that becomes evident while papilledema is still present is also an indication that the visual prognosis is poor, even if ICP is lowered immediately, because the pallor is caused by loss of axons. Most patients with these changes have clinical evidence of visual dysfunction, including decreased color vision, visual field defects, and abnormal contrast sensitivity. Loss of visual acuity is the last visual parameter to be affected, much as is the case in patients with chronic open-angle glaucoma. Once a patient with papilledema begins to experience, or is found to have, deficits in these parameters, the visual prognosis is extremely tenuous. On the other hand, severe venous engorgement, retinal hemorrhages, and hard and soft exudates have no prognostic significance.

Papilledema may be observed at any age, including in infants and children. This phenomenon is remarkable because we explain the absence of papilledema in most cases of congenital hydrocephalus on the basis of expansibility of the skull. If this were true, one would expect a lower prevalence of papilledema in infants and children with intracranial tumors. Nevertheless, studies have found papilledema or postpapilledema optic atrophy in 56% to 90% of children with brain tumors.

PATHOGENESIS OF PAPILLEDEMA

Although the pathogenesis of papilledema remains unclear, there are some general points of agreement: (a) papilledema occurs only when there is patency of the meningeal spaces surrounding the optic nerve and intracranial structures. Blockage of these spaces by adhesions or tumor prevents papilledema from occurring on the side of the obstruction; (b) papilledema does not occur in an eye in which antecedent optic atrophy has destroyed most or all of the nerve fibers; (c) axon transport is abnormal in patients with papilledema as well as in patients with disc swelling from other causes (ischemia, inflammation, hypotony, etc.). Accumulation of axoplasm results in the swelling of axons.

However, numerous questions still exist regarding the pathogenesis of papilledema: (i) is there a relationship between the severity of axon transport obstruction and the clinical degree of optic disc swelling? Although it is clear that even in early experimental papilledema, disc swelling is due to blockage of axon transport, resulting in secondary axon distention, no studies relating severity of the block to severity of disc swelling have yet been performed; (ii) is obstruction of axon transport compatible with normal conduction of nerve impulses? Transport and conduction are two separate, although related, processes. Abundant evidence suggests that conduction can continue along an axon in which there is partial blockage of axon transport. Nevertheless, it is not clear how long an axon can survive and continue to conduct action potentials when there is sustained, although partial, blockage of axon transport. In addition, although detailed psychophysical testing in patients with papilledema often reveals a variety of deficits in vision not detected on routine visual acuity, color vision, or visual field testing, the marked difference in visual function among patients with optic disc swelling from different causes (e.g., papilledema vs. anterior optic neuritis) suggests that either the degree of axon transport blockage is different in different types of optic disc swelling or that obstruction of axon transport is not, in and of itself, sufficient to cause loss of visual function; (iii) what is the cause of axon transport obstruction in papilledema? This is the critical question that has yet to be answered. Although the direct cause of optic disc swelling is the blockage of axon transport, the cause of the blockage is still unknown. Some investigators believe that the cause is mechanical (i.e., from transmission of raised ICP to retinal ganglion cell axons in the optic nerve). In this scheme, visual loss occurs in the setting of chronic papilledema from prelaminar ischemia secondary to the mechanically induced optic disc swelling. Other investigators believe that ischemia caused by disturbances of autoregulation in the prelaminar, laminar, and retrolaminar regions of the optic nerve head contributes to axon transport obstruction.

SYMPTOMS AND SIGNS OF PAPILLEDEMA

Both nonvisual and visual symptoms occur in patients with papilledema. As a general rule, the nonvisual symptoms are more severe and bothersome to the patient, although visual symptoms can be both distressing and indicative of impending permanent visual dysfunction.

NONVISUAL MANIFESTATIONS

Headache is one of the earliest symptoms of increased ICP, although there may be a considerable increase in ICP without headache. Neither the severity of the headache nor its location has any value in determining whether an intracranial mass is present, and if so, its location. An exception to this rule is the meningioma that infiltrates the dura over the convexity of the cerebral hemispheres and produces a palpable swelling and local pain at the site of the lesion. In some patients, headache associated with increased ICP is increased by coughing, straining, and valsava maneuvers. This is an inconstant phenomenon, but its presence may suggest a ball-valve action of the lesion within the ventricular system. It is believed that headache associated with increased ICP is caused by stretching of the meninges,

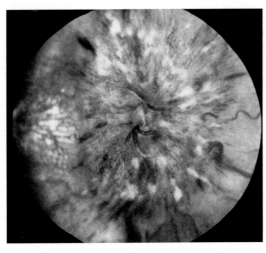
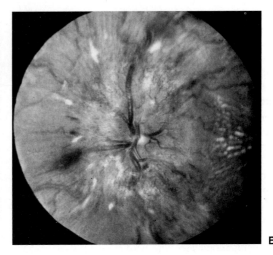

A   B

Figure 5.14. Papilledema associated with bilateral visual loss related to macular hard exudate. The patient was a 35-year-old woman with headaches and decreased vision in both eyes. Visual acuity was 20/50 OU. Visual fields showed marked enlargement of the blind spots. Both optic discs are severely swollen (Frisén stage 5). **A and B:** There are numerous hemorrhages and soft exudates on and surrounding the discs, and there is a star figure composed of hard exudate (lipid) in the maculae.

whereas sharply localized pains in such cases may be explained on the basis of damage to sensory nerves at the base of the skull or localized dysfunction of meningeal nerves.

Nausea and vomiting are frequently associated with significantly increased ICP, although so-called projectile vomiting is rare. Vomiting, bradycardia, difficulty swallowing, and eventual respiratory failure may all be explained by herniation of the medulla into the foramen magnum.

Loss of consciousness, generalized motor rigidity, and pupillary dilation are terminal effects of increased ICP. Loss of consciousness presumably occurs from compression of the cerebral cortex and the reduction of its blood supply. Herniation of the hippocampal gyrus through the tentorium from increased ICP results in crowding of the temporal lobe into the incisura of each side. Tentorial herniation thus places pressure on the crura cerebri, resulting in generalized motor rigidity. Finally, direct pressure on the oculomotor nerves or dorsal midbrain produces bilaterally dilated pupils that do not respond to light stimulation.

Patients with increased ICP may, on occasion, develop spontaneous **CSF rhinorrhea.** In some cases, there is a history of previous trauma; in others, there is a congenital anomaly at the base of the skull. When spontaneous, CSF fistulas are usually located in the region of the cribriform plate.

VISUAL MANIFESTATIONS

Patients with early, and even fully developed, papilledema are usually visually asymptomatic with nei-

ther visual acuity nor color vision being affected. In some of these patients, the only abnormality found on careful testing is mild to moderate enlargement of the physiologic blind spot. Other patients may be aware of the physiologic blind spot, and such patients may complain of a negative scotoma in the field of vision of one or both eyes. Other patients have variable loss of visual acuity, color vision, visual field, or a combination of these visual parameters. Some of these patients have retinal or vitreous hemorrhages or exudates that reduce central acuity (Fig. 5.14). In others, an intracranial mass produces a visual sensory deficit in one or both eyes by one or more mechanisms, including direct compression of a portion of the visual sensory pathway (e.g., compression of the occipital lobe by a meningioma, producing a homonymous field defect), indirect compression of part of the pathway via a secondary effect on surrounding brain (e.g., gyrus rectus compression of the optic nerves producing a bilateral optic neuropathy in a patient with a frontal lobe tumor), and infiltration of a part of the pathway (e.g., infiltration of the optic chiasm by a germinoma, producing a bitemporal hemianopia).

Patients with papilledema may experience **brief, transient obscurations of vision.** During these episodes, vision may vary from mildly blurred to complete blindness. Some patients describe a rapid grayout of vision, whereas others experience positive visual phenomena—such as photopsias, phosphenes, and even scintillating scotomas—that obscure their vision. In all cases, recovery of vision is invariably rapid and complete. The obscurations may affect only one eye, alternate eyes, or both eyes simultaneously. They usually last only a few seconds, although attacks lasting several hours sometimes occur. Some patients experience up to 20 to 30 such episodes a day, with the obscurations often precipitated by changes in posture, particularly from sitting to standing or from lying down to sitting or standing; rare patients experience gaze-evoked amaurosis, a phenomenon much more commonly observed in patients with orbital lesions that compress and deform the optic nerve.

Transient visual obscurations have little prognostic value. Indeed, in many patients with transient obscurations, papilledema resolves completely without producing any detectable visual deficit. Conversely, patients with papilledema may develop permanent visual damage without ever having experienced any transient visual obscurations. The cause of these obscurations is most likely related to transient compression or ischemia of the optic nerve.

Concentric enlargement of the blind spot is the most common—and frequently the only—**visual field defect** in patients with papilledema. Compression, detachment, and lateral displacement of the peripapillary retina appear to be the major reasons that the blind spot increases in size in patients with papilledema; however, the blind spot may be enlarged even when there is no obvious retinal displacement or detachment. In this setting, the enlarged blind spot represents a refractive scotoma caused by acquired peripapillary hyperopia, which in turn results from elevation of the retina by peripapillary subretinal fluid.

Early visual field defects in eyes with papilledema are not uncommon on automated static perimetry and are often present when standard kinetic perimetry gives normal results. These early defects are generally arcuate scotomas or nasal steps, whereas constriction of the visual fields is invariably a late sign of papilledema, occurring during the chronic stage as it progresses to optic atrophy. The field defects are usually worse nasally than temporally (Figs. 5.15 and 5.16). Thus, an eye may have only a temporal island of vision before becoming completely blind.

Loss of visual field in the setting of papilledema is usually slow and progressive. Sudden loss of visual field in this setting suggests a local cause, such as ischemia. Superimposed ischemic optic neuropathy presumably occurs from occlusion of prelaminar disc arterioles caused by increased tissue pressure in the optic disc. These vessels may be more sensitive to increased intraocular pressure than are other vessels in the ocular fundus.

Patients with papilledema caused by intracranial mass lesions or meningitis (septic, aseptic, carcinomatous, lymphomatous) can **lose central vision** acutely or progressively from the effects of the underlying process on the optic nerves. In other cases, permanent loss of central vision results from the nonspecific effects of increased ICP on the optic nerve and begins with visual field constriction that is slowly progressive. In such cases, loss of central acuity is usually a late phenomenon, although it may occur over several weeks in cases with markedly increased ICP.

Acute loss of vision occurs in some patients with papilledema. In most of these cases, local causes are responsible. Some patients lose central vision because they develop hemorrhages or exudates in the maculae. Others develop ischemic optic neuropathy or retinal vascular occlusions that may be related to the underlying process (e.g., a coagulopathy) or to the rapid rate at which the ICP has risen. In addition, rare patients, many of them children, seem to have a fulminant course characterized by a rapid progression from normal vision to profound and permanent visual loss.

As in other types of optic neuropathies, papilledema may be associated with abnormalities of visual sensation that can be detected when specific tests are performed. For example, patients with visual acuity of 20/20, a full visual field, and normal color perception may nevertheless have abnormal contrast sensitivity. Such patients also may have delayed latency of the P100 wave when visual-evoked potentials are measured.

Increased ICP may result in **diplopia** via compression or stretching of the abducens nerve at the base of the skull. The damage may be unilateral or bilateral. Some patients have a comitant esotropia worse for distance than for near, which is often called "divergence insufficiency." Trochlear nerve palsies may rarely occur in patients with increased ICP, presumably from compression of either the dorsal midbrain or the nerves themselves by a ballooned suprapineal recess. Such palsies are often misdiagnosed as skew deviation if quantitative testing of eye movements or a Bielschowsky head tilt test is not performed, although true skew deviation can exceptionally occur in patients with increased ICP.

ETIOLOGY OF PAPILLEDEMA

The craniospinal cavity is an almost rigid bony enclosure completely filled by tissue, CSF, and circulating blood. Within this enclosure, CSF is constantly produced at the rate 500 mL/day, or 0.35 mL/minute. Almost all of the production is by the choroid plexus within the lateral ventricles. The secretion of CSF is dependent on sodium-potassium-activated ATPase as well as the enzyme carbonic anhydrase. CSF flows from the lateral ventricles through the interventricular foramina into the 3rd ventricle and mixes with the CSF produced in that ventricle. The CSF then flows through the cerebral aqueduct (of Sylvius) into the fourth ventricle and out into the subarachnoid space through the foramina of Luschka and Magendie. In the

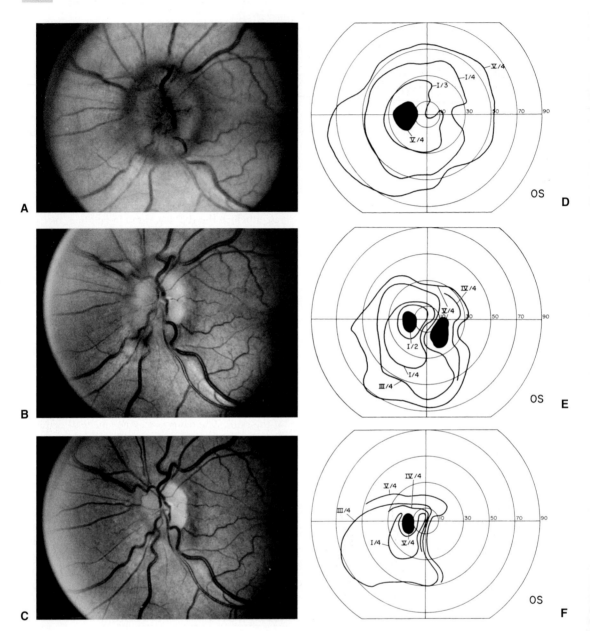

Figure 5.15. Progression of visual field defect in a patient with chronic papilledema. **A–C:** Progression of chronic papilledema to optic atrophy. **D–F:** Progression of the visual field defects. Note progressive loss of nasal and superotemporal fields and associated constriction with preservation of visual acuity.

subarachnoid space, CSF flows rostrally from the posterior fossa through the lower ventral basal cisterns and tentorial notch to reach the interpeduncular and chiasmatic cisterns. The CSF then flows dorsally through the communicating cisterns to reach the dorsal cisterns, and lateral and superiorly from the chiasmatic cistern into the cisterns of the Sylvian fissure. From the cisterns and Sylvian fissures, CSF moves outward and superiorly over the cerebral convexities where it is absorbed.

The main route of absorption of CSF is passively through the arachnoid granulations that protrude into

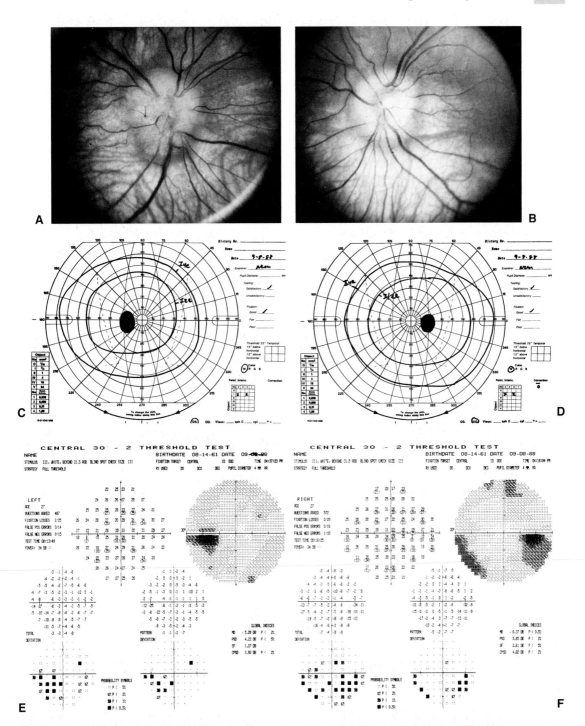

Figure 5.16. Difference in sensitivity of kinetic versus static perimetry in chronic papilledema. **A and B:** Right and left optic discs show chronic papilledema. **C and D:** Kinetic perimetry shows no abnormalities except for mildly enlarged blind spots. **E and F:** Static perimetry in the same patient shows nasal steps, inferior arcuate defects, and reduction in sensitivity in both eyes.

the venous sinuses and diploic veins. These vessels drain to the internal jugular vein and other extracranial veins. CSF is also absorbed in the spinal sac. Many factors influence CSF formation, including toxins, medications, and neurotransmitters, whereas CSF absorption is affected by venous pressure, and meningeal processes that may affect the arachnoid granulations.

The volume of blood, brain and CSF within the cranial cavity must be in equilibrium, suggesting that a change in the volume of one component must be offset by a reciprocal change in another. As little as 80 cc of rapidly added volume (CSF, blood, edema, tissue, etc.) may raise ICP to a level incompatible with life. Table 5.2 details the mechanisms involved in intracranial hypertension.

Table 5.2. *Causes of Increased Intracranial Pressure*

Space-occupying lesions
  Neoplasm
  Abscess
  Inflammatory mass
  Hemorrhage
  Infarction
  Arteriovenous malformation

Focal or diffuse cerebral edema
  Trauma
  Toxic
  Anoxia

Reduction in the size of the cranial vault
  Craniosynostosis
  Thickening of the skull

Blockage of CSF flow
  Non-communicating hydrocephalus

Reduction in CSF resorption
  Communicating hydrocephalus
  Meningeal processes
    Infectious meningitis (bacterial, viral, fungus, parasitic)
    Inflammatory (aseptic) meningitis
    Carcinomatous meningitis
    Elevated CSF protein
      Spinal cord tumors
      Guillain-Barré syndrome
      Chronic inflammatory demyelinating polyneuropathy (CIDP)
  Elevated venous pressure

Increased CSF production

Idiopathic intracranial hypertension (pseudotumor cerebri)

INTRACRANIAL MASSES

Intracranial masses such as tumors produce increased ICP through most of the mechanisms mentioned above. They may act solely as space-occupying lesions; they may produce focal or diffuse cerebral edema, and they may block the outflow of CSF by direct compression of CSF drainage pathways or by infiltration of the arachnoid villi or the cerebral venous sinuses. Other potential mechanisms are the production of increased protein or blood products that secondarily block the arachnoid villi, and by directly producing CSF.

Papilledema does not develop in every patient with a brain tumor. Several large studies found papilledema in 60% to 80% of patients with cerebral tumors. Tumors that are situated below the tentorium (infratentorial), which may obstruct the aqueduct, are more likely to produce papilledema than those situated above it (supratentorial). Associated symptoms and signs usually allow a proper diagnosis; however, tumors in certain locations may produce papilledema without lateralizing or localizing signs, particularly if they are supratentorial and situated within the nondominant hemisphere or within one of the lateral ventricles. This emphasizes the importance of examining the fundus of all patients with chronic or new-onset headaches.

Papilledema may occur with any type of intracranial mass. Neither the type of intracranial tumor nor its rate of growth correlates well with the development of papilledema.

DISORDERS OF CSF FLOW

Aqueductal stenosis often presents in childhood. It may be congenital, in which case it may or may not be associated with a Chiari malformation, or it may be acquired from intracranial infections. Presentation in infancy is accompanied by macrocephaly. Adults may have headaches, dorsal midbrain syndrome, meningitis, hemorrhage, endocrine disturbances from compression of the pituitary gland, seizures, gait disturbances, and CSF rhinorrhea.

Subarachnoid hemorrhage usually produces papilledema either by blocking CSF flow within the ventricular system (obstructive hydrocephalus) or by blocking CSF absorption at the arachnoid granulations. Papilledema occurs in 10% to 24% of the patients with aneurysmal subarachnoid hemorrhage. Papilledema can develop several hours after the hemorrhage or it may develop only after several weeks of increased ICP.

Meningitis and encephalitis produce severe cerebral edema, and resultant raised ICP, although obstructive hydrocephalus and impaired CSF absorption by arachnoid granulations may also occur. However, the reported frequency of papilledema with meningitis is fairly small, and the papilledema tends to be mild and transient. Papilledema is more likely to occur in patients with tuberculous meningitis (25% of cases) and cryptococcal meningitis than in any other type of infectious meningitis. These patients may have fulminant papilledema and severe visual loss from secondary optic atrophy is common. Any type of meningeal process may be associated with papilledema. It is found in about 20% of patients with viral encephalitis. It is also common in non-infectious processes such as sarcoidosis or carcinomatous meningitis. This is why CSF analysis is an essential step in the diagnosis of papilledema. It must be emphasized that in almost all CNS infections and inflammations as well as neoplasms, swelling of the optic nerve may occur without increased ICP, presumably from inflammation or infiltration of the optic nerve or optic nerve sheath. In such cases, differentiating between papilledema and perineuritis is impossible, because in both cases, there is normal visual function. Only when a lumbar puncture is performed in a patient with a meningeal process and disc swelling, and the CSF is found to be under normal pressure with an increased protein and pleocytosis, can the true inflammatory or infiltrative etiology of the disc swelling be ascertained.

SYNDROMES OF ELEVATED VENOUS PRESSURE

Obstruction or impairment of cerebral venous drainage may result in increased ICP and papilledema. Indeed, most of the CSF drainage occurs passively into the cerebral venous sinuses at the level of the arachnoid granulations. When one (or more) cerebral venous sinus is occluded, the venous pressure rises and the CSF is not resorbed properly into the venous sinuses, thereby producing increased ICP.

Although cerebral venous thrombosis often produces neurological symptoms and signs, it can also present with an isolated syndrome of raised ICP indistinguishable from IIH. The venous sinus obstruction is most often caused by compression or thrombosis, with the sinuses most often affected being the superior sagittal and transverse (lateral) sinuses. There are numerous local and systemic causes of cerebral venous sinus obstruction (Table 5.3).

Occlusion of one jugular vein (if it is the principal vein draining the intracranial area) or both jugular veins may also produce increased ICP and papilledema by producing increased venous pressure (Table 5.3).

It is very important to rule-out venous hypertension from cerebral venous thrombosis or internal jugular vein thrombosis when evaluating a patient with isolated raided ICP. Indeed, the prognosis of these disorders is often poor unless a thorough work-up is obtained, and appropriate treatment is rapidly initiated.

Table 5.3. *Etiologies of Obstruction/Impairment of Cerebral Venous Drainage*

Cerebral venous thrombosis
  Primary hematologic
    Antiphospholipid antibody syndrome
    Thrombophilia (antithrombin III deficiency,
      protein S deficiency, antithrombin deficiency,
      resistance to activated protein C,
      prothrombin gene mutation)
    Thrombocythemia
    Polycythemia
    Disseminated intravascular coagulation
    Hyperviscosity syndrome

  Systemic conditions associated with coagulopathy
    Behçet's disease
    Systemic lupus erythematosus
    Neurosarcoidosis
    Cancer
    Pregnancy/postpartum
    Renal disease (nephrotic syndrome)
    Infections
    Post surgery

  Local infections
    Mastoiditis
    Facial/orbital cellulitis
    Meningitis
  Traumatic
  Tumors (compression of a sinus)
  Dural arteriovenous Fistula

Transverse sinus stenosis

Occlusion of internal jugular vein
  Iatrogenic
  Indwelling catheter
  Surgery
  Traumatic
  Tumors (extravascular)

Increased venous pressure
  Right cardiac insufficiency
  Superior vena cava syndrome
  Morbid obesity
  Hyperviscosity syndrome

TRAUMA

Papilledema occurs in 20% to 30% of persons who have suffered severe cranial injuries, both with and without an associated skull fracture. In most of these cases, the increased ICP is caused by a severe subarachnoid hemorrhage or a significant intracerebral, subdural, or epidural hematoma. In other cases, the increased ICP is caused by cerebral venous thrombosis or by diffuse or localized cerebral edema.

Papilledema that develops in patients after head trauma is usually mild and may develop immediately, several days after the injury, or up to 2 weeks later. A sudden, severe, but transient increase in ICP is usually responsible for the immediate development of papilledema, whereas sustained but mild to moderately elevated ICP accounts for papilledema that appears during the first week after injury. Papilledema in the second week or later results from impaired CSF absorption and consequent communicating hydrocephalus or delayed focal or diffuse cerebral swelling.

CRANIOSYNOSTOSES

The intracranial vault may become smaller in certain types of craniosynostoses. Among patients with premature synostosis of the cranial sutures, 12% to 15% eventually develop papilledema. However, simple cranial synostosis (oxycephaly, scaphocephaly, trigonocephaly, or plagiocephaly) is almost never associated with papilledema, whereas about 40% of patients with craniofacial dysostosis (Crouzon's syndrome) or acrocephalosyndactyly (Apert's syndrome) develop papilledema.

If papilledema is going to develop in a patient with a craniosynostosis, it usually does so before the age of 10 years. It is often chronic by the time it is detected, possibly because such patients may not undergo a careful examination of the ocular fundi unless they complain of visual disturbances. However, papilledema may develop at any age.

EXTRACRANIAL LESIONS

The association of increased ICP and papilledema with **tumors in the spinal canal** is an unusual but well-documented phenomenon. Most of these tumors are intradural; however, extradural spinal tumors can also cause increased ICP associated with papilledema. In some cases, the tumors are located in the high cervical region, and the explanation for the increased ICP in such cases is thought to be upward swelling of the tumor with compression of the cerebellum and obstruction of CSF flow through the foramen magnum. This mechanism seems unlikely to be the explanation in the majority of cases, however, because over 50% of spinal cord lesions associated with papilledema are ependymomas or neurofibromas that are usually located in the thoracic and lumbar regions. These tumors can produce extremely high concentrations of protein in the CSF, and it is therefore likely that increased ICP and papilledema in such cases is caused by the decreased CSF absorption that results from blockage of the arachnoid granulations by protein. In other cases, recurrent subarachnoid hemorrhage, which occurs commonly from bleeding from the surface of ependymomas, may also cause reduced CSF absorption from blockage of the arachnoid villi by blood or blood products.

Papilledema is an uncommon complication of **Guillain-Barré syndrome** (GBS). Its pathogenesis remains uncertain, although it is postulated that protein in the arachnoid villi and granulations alters cerebral venous dynamics or causes partial venous thrombosis, leading to increased ICP. Increased ICP, often associated with papilledema, occurs more often in patients with **chronic inflammatory demyelinating polyneuropathy (CIDP)** than in patients with acute GBS. It seems to be caused in most cases by the markedly increased protein concentration that is one of the laboratory hallmarks of the disease; however, patients with CIDP can develop papilledema even with only a mildly increased concentration of protein in the CSF.

The **POEMS syndrome** is an unusual multisystem disorder that is characterized by polyneuropathy (*P*), organomegaly (*O*), endocrinopathy (*E*), monoclonal gammopathy (*M*), and skin changes (*S*). Patients with POEMS syndrome not infrequently develop ICP associated with papilledema. In addition, optic disc swelling may occasionally occur in patients without evidence of increased ICP. The POEMS syndrome may be a variant of multiple myeloma, and the associated monoclonal immunoglobulin may mediate the multiple systemic manifestations. Patients with multiple myeloma can also develop increased ICP and papilledema, but the mechanism is unknown.

IDIOPATHIC INTRACRANIAL HYPERTENSION (PSEUDOTUMOR CEREBRI)

Idiopathic intracranial hypertension (IIH), (previously called *pseudotumor cerebri* and *benign intracranial hypertension*), is the term used for a syndrome that is defined by four criteria: (i) increased ICP, (ii) no hydrocephalus on neuroimaging, (iii) no evidence of an intracranial mass lesion or cerebral venous thrombosis, and (iv) normal CSF composition. Most, but not all patients have papilledema. About 10% of the cases of IIH are caused by an identifiable process (see the subsequent text). In the remaining 90% of the cases, no cause is found, although most of these patients are obese young women, suggesting an endocrinologic disturbance.

The pseudotumor cerebri syndrome was first described by Quincke in 1897. The terminology used historically in the literature gives a sense of the various conditions previously described under the term *pseudotumor cerebri*: toxic hydrocephalus, otitic hydrocephalus, hypertensive meningeal hydrops, pseudoabscess, ICP without brain tumor, brain swelling of unknown cause, and papilledema of indeterminate etiology. The most popular and enduring term *pseudotumor cerebri* was first used in 1914. Noting that the condition was not caused by a tumor or malignancy, Foley introduced the term *benign intracranial hypertension* in 1955. However, the term *benign* also implies a favorable process or the absence of harm. As significant visual morbidity may result from PTC, the use of the prefix "benign" was challenged and is no longer considered acceptable terminology. The disorder is most correctly termed *IIH* or intracranial hypertension from a secondary cause, depending upon whether or not an etiology is identified. The older term, *pseudotumor cerebri*, describes the clinical syndrome without reference to the underlying cause.

The overall incidence of IIH is unknown and varies throughout the world. It approaches zero in countries in which the incidence of obesity is low, and it is common in countries or regions within countries with an increased incidence of obesity. In Iowa, the incidence is 0.9 per 100,000 in the general population; 3.5 per 100,000 in women aged 20 to 44 years; 13 per 100,000 in women who are 10% over ideal weight; and 19 per 100,000 in women who are 20% over ideal weight. There is a similar incidence in Louisiana. The incidence of IIH in Rochester, Minnesota, is 1 per 100,000 in the general population; 1.6 in the female population; and 7.9 per 100,000 in obese women (defined as body mass index greater than 26). The annual incidence of IIH in Benghazi, Libya, is 2.2 per 100,000 in the general population; 4.3 per 100,000 in women; and 21.4 per 100,000 in women aged 15 to 44 years who are 20% over ideal weight. In Israel, whose population is a mixture of people originating from various Eastern and Western countries, the incidence is similar to that in western populations, with a preponderance of obese women.

The age range in patients with PTC in general and IIH in particular is broad. Children and even infants are not infrequently affected, and such patients may have a higher incidence of permanent visual loss. The peak incidence of the disease, however, seems to occur in the third decade of life with a female preponderance that ranges from 2 to 1 in some studies and to 8 to 1 in others.

The occurrence of IIH in family members is uncommon, but well recognized. No common metabolic or endocrinologic abnormalities have been found in such patients.

DIAGNOSIS OF IIH

The diagnostic criteria for IIH are: (a) symptoms and signs solely attributable to increased ICP; (b) elevated CSF pressure; (c) normal CSF composition; (d) normal neuroimaging studies; and (e) no other etiology of intracranial hypertension identified. Each of these criteria is discussed below.

Clinical Manifestations

The most common presenting symptom in patients with IIH is headache, occurring in more than 90% of cases. The headache is usually generalized, worse in the morning, and aggravated when cerebral venous pressure is increased by some type of Valsalva maneuver (coughing, sneezing, etc.). Headaches improve dramatically or resolve after lumbar puncture, which confirms that they are directly related to intracranial hypertension. Other common nonvisual manifestations of IIH include nausea, vomiting, dizziness, and pulsatile tinnitus. Pulsatile tinnitus is often described as a "whooshing sound," which may be uni- or bilateral and is usually relieved after lumbar puncture. Focal neurologic deficits in patients with IIH are extremely uncommon, and their occurrence should make one consider alternative diagnoses. Patients with chronic IIH may occasionally develop persistent disturbances in cognition and depression.

Visual manifestations of IIH are usually preceded by headache and occur in 35% to 70% of patients. These symptoms are identical with those described by patients with increased ICP from other causes, including transient visual obscurations, loss of vision from macular hemorrhages, exudates, pigment epithelial changes, retina striae, choroidal folds, subretinal neovascularization, or optic atrophy, horizontal diplopia from unilateral or bilateral abducens nerve paresis. Other ocular motor deficits have been rarely reported and should suggest cerebral thrombosis or a meningeal process rather than IIH.

The papilledema that occurs in over 90% of patients with IIH is identical with that which occurs in patients with other causes of increased ICP. There is no correlation between severity of optic disc swelling and age, race, or body weight in patients with IIH, although men may have worse swelling than women. Postpapilledema optic atrophy occurs in untreated or inadequately treated patients after a variable period of time, usually over several months, but occasionally within weeks of the onset of symptoms. Some patients have persistent chronic papilledema without development of atrophy. Postpapilledema optic atrophy in patients with IIH usually develops symmetrically; but just as papilledema may be asymmetric, so postpapilledema optic atrophy can be asymmetric, and some patients develop a pseudo-Foster Kennedy syndrome characterized by postpapilledema optic atrophy on one side and papilledema on the other. Rarely, IIH is asymptomatic and papilledema is discovered during a routine ophthalmic examination.

Ancillary Testing

To satisfy the criteria required to diagnose IIH, a patient must undergo neuroimaging studies followed by a lumbar puncture. It is inappropriate to diagnose IIH without a lumbar puncture or in the setting of abnormal CSF.

Neuroimaging Studies   Brain CT is often the first test performed in patients with papilledema and is appropriate to detect most intracranial lesions that could produce raised ICP and to rule-out obstructive hydrocephalus. However, this study is insufficient to exclude Chiari malformations, posterior fossa abnormalities, isodense lesions not associated with ventriculomegaly, gliomatosis cerebri, meningeal abnormalities or cerebral venous thrombosis. Thus, MRI with contrast is required to diagnose IIH. In some cases, MR venography or CT venography should also be considered. Rarely, a patient's body habitus exceeds the capacity of the MR gantry, and a brain CT with contrast with CT venogram should be obtained; catheter angiography with venous phase is only very rarely required to definitely rule-out cerebral venous thrombosis.

The brain MRI is normal in IIH. An asymptomatic empty sella which results from chronically increased ICP is present in over half of cases. Other radiographic evidence of increased ICP, best visualized on orbital images, includes dilation of the perineuronal subarachnoid space surrounding the optic nerves, protrusion of the optic papilla into the posterior aspect of the globe and flattening of the posterior sclerae.

Cerebrospinal Fluid Examination   CSF examination is required for the diagnosis of IIH to confirm an elevated opening pressure and exclude a meningeal process that might simulate IIH. Lumbar puncture should be performed in the lateral decubitus position, relaxed with the legs partially extended. The pressure may be artifactually elevated if the patient is crying, performing a Valsalva maneuver or is in severe pain. The opening pressure should be measured with a manometer, and adequate CSF should be obtained for assessment of cellular content, concentrations of protein and glucose, and any other tests deemed appropriate by the treating physician. In obese patients, lumbar puncture is more easily performed with fluoroscopic guidance. For the diagnosis of IIH, the CSF opening pressure should be 250 mm (25 cm) of water or greater. In prepubertal children, a value over 200 mm water is likely abnormal. Because CSF pressure normally fluctuates, multiple CSF pressure measurements or prolonged CSF pressure monitoring is sometimes required, depending on the clinical circumstance. The CSF contents are always normal in IIH; the protein is generally in the normal to low-normal range.

Once a diagnosis of IIH is made by CT scanning or MRI followed by lumbar puncture, the physician should attempt to determine if a cause can be found. This is particularly important in nonobese women and in men, regardless of age or body habitus, because such patients are much less likely to have IIH. A particularly careful history is necessary in such patients, with special attention given to any underlying systemic inflammatory or infectious disease, associated disorders such as anemia or sleep apnea, or ingestion or exposure to an inciting agent. Cerebral venous thrombosis should be carefully ruled-out.

ETIOLOGY OF IIH

IIH occurs primarily in young obese women, and occasionally men, with no evidence of any underlying disease. In about 10% of patients, particularly in men and nonobese women, a pseudotumor syndrome develops in a number of different settings, including obstruction or impairment of cerebral venous drainage, endocrine and metabolic dysfunction, exposure to exogenous drugs and other substances, withdrawal of certain drugs, and systemic illnesses. Tables 5.4 and 5.5 list some of these purported associations. Except for those cases in which venous occlusive disease can be demonstrated, the exact mechanisms of increased ICP in these settings remain undetermined and a definite causal association unproven.

As noted previously, uncompensated **obstruction of cerebral venous drainage** may cause increased ICP and may mimic IIH. Such patients may be thought to have IIH unless the cerebral veins and venous sinuses are imaged using standard MRI, MR angiography, or CT angiography. Some patients with IIH are found to have a uni- or bilateral stenosis of the transverse venous sinus. It results in increased venous pressure and

Table 5.4. *Exogenous Substances Most Classically Associated with Idiopathic Intracranial Hypertension*

Antibiotics
  Tetracycline
  Minocycline
  Doxycycline
  Nalidixic acid
Beta-human chorionic gonadotropin hormone
  withdrawal
Chlordecone (Kepone)
Corticosteroids withdrawal
Cyclosporine
Danazol administration or withdrawal
Growth hormone
Leuprolide acetate (Lupron)
Levonorgesterol implants (Norplant)
Lithium carbonate (533,534)
Retinoids:
  Vitamin A
  Isotretinoin
  All-*trans*-retinoic acid

Table 5.5. *Systemic Illnesses Associated with Idiopathic Intracranial Hypertension*

Obesity
Hyperthyroidism
Anemia
Chronic respiratory insufficiency
Pickwickian syndrome
Obstructive sleep apnea
Renal disease (nephrotic syndrome)
Sarcoidosis
Systemic lupus erythematosus
Systemic hypertension

subsequent CSF drainage impairment. Whether these transverse sinus stenoses are a primary phenomenon leading to the syndrome of IIH, or whether it occurs secondary to raised ICP, which compresses the lateral sinus, remains controversial. Some authors have suggested that endovascular stenting of such stenotic venous sinuses may relieve symptoms of intracranial pressure.

Patients with **endocrine and metabolic dysfunction** can also develop IIH (Table 5.5). Obesity is the most common finding in patients with IIH, and recent weight gain has been associated with worsening of vision in such patients. In many of these patients, there is also a history of menstrual irregularity. However, attempts to uncover specific underlying endocrinologic disturbances in patients with this form of IIH have been unsuccessful. IIH not infrequently occurs during **pregnancy.**

Patients who are exposed to, or ingest, a variety of **exogenous substances** can develop PTC (Table 5.4). For some of these substances, a causative relationship is supported by only a single case report and is tenuous at best. For other drugs, such as tetracyclines, vitamin A, or cyclosporine, the association between exposure or ingestion and the development of increased ICP is well documented in numerous reports and investigations.

We have already commented on increased ICP with papilledema in patients with meningitis and encephalitis. In many of these cases, the ventricular system is blocked in some location and is thus dilated, and the CSF contains white blood cells or an elevated protein content. Such cases are not, by definition, examples of IIH. In other cases, such as meningeal carcinomatosis and lymphomatosis, Whipple's disease, neuroborreliosis, and neurosarcoidosis, the ventricular system appears normal, although the CSF contains white blood cells, malignant cells, an increased protein content, or a combination of these. These cases also are not examples of IIH because the CSF content is abnormal. Nevertheless, some **systemic diseases** produce increased ICP, papilledema, normal-sized ventricles, and normal CSF content—a clinical picture consistent with IIH

(Table 5.5). Anemia and sleep apnea need to be looked for as they may be associated with increased ICP and papilledema.

Optic disc swelling occurs in some patients with severe systemic hypertension and is not always associated with other funduscopic signs of hypertensive retinopathy. This emphasizes that blood pressure should be carefully checked in patients with papilledema and headaches.

Rarely, a syndrome resembling IIH has been reported with systemic inflammatory disorders such as **sarcoidosis** or **systemic lupus erythematosus.** Such as diagnosis should be made with caution as most patients have an inflammatory meningeal process or cerebral venous thrombosis.

PATHOPHYSIOLOGY OF IIH NOT ASSOCIATED WITH OTHER FACTORS

The pathogenesis of IIH remains unknown. A number of hypotheses have been suggested but none explain all IIH syndromes. It is logical to think that diminished absorption of CSF and cerebral edema may produce IIH. Indeed, patients with IIH may have both a defect in CSF resorption and an increased cerebral volume associated with a noncompliant ventricular system that resists dilation. Venous hypertension has long been proposed as one of the main mechanisms of IIH. Indeed, venous hypertension is common in obese patients with IIH especially those with sleep apnea. In addition, cerebral transverse venous sinus stenoses sometimes found in these patients may also produce venous hypertension. Because this disorder is more common in young obese women, it has been suggested that hormonal changes (excess of estrone) may increase the secretion of CSF by the choroid plexus. Vitamin A and retinol are also thought to play a role in IIH.

COMPLICATIONS

The natural history of IIH is variable. In some cases it is a self-limited condition; in others, the ICP remains elevated for many years. The feared complication of IIH is permanent visual loss, which is severe in up to 25% of patients. IIH may recur years after successful treatment, and most patients need to be followed-up for many years. Depression is common in IIH patients who often develop chronic tension headaches.

TREATMENT

The primary goals of treatment are to preserve vision and alleviate symptoms. The treatment of IIH in adults and children is similar. Both medical and surgical treatments are used, often in combination. Current practice patterns regarding the management of IIH are based largely on case series and clinical experience; there are no randomized trials prospectively assessing the effectiveness of treatment in this disorder. Additionally, IIH is considered an "off label" usage for all medications currently prescribed to treat the disorder.

Most patients with IIH require careful follow-up by a neurologist (who will manage the headaches) and an ophthalmologist (who will monitor the visual function and perform repeated formal visual field testing). Follow-up is decided on a case-by-case basis based on the severity of visual symptoms. Some patients need to be evaluated weekly until vision stabilizes or improves, whereas others who have good visual function may only need to seen every few months. Therapeutic decisions are made individually based on each patient's characteristics. Particularly important to consider are: (a) the presence and severity of headaches; (b) the degree of visual loss at presentation; (c) the rate of progression of visual loss; (d) the presence of an identifiable underlying etiology or aggravating factor (e.g., medication-induced IIH, anemia, sleep apnea, etc.).

Medical Treatment

Medical therapy is always the first line treatment in patients with IIH. It follows the lumbar puncture performed as part of the diagnostic workup (which is the most efficient way to reduce ICP rapidly and improve symptoms and signs). When the primary problem is headache in the setting of good vision, medical treatment is usually sufficient and surgery not necessary. In asymptomatic patients with papilledema, close observation of visual function without specific therapy may be employed once an underlying etiology is excluded. If a secondary cause is identified, it should be treated appropriately. For example, implicated exogenous agents should be discontinued.

Weight loss is advised for obese patients based on retrospective analyses indicating that a modest degree of weight loss (approximately 6% of body weight) correlates with a reduction in papilledema. When weight loss efforts fail, bariatric surgery may be considered. Such surgery is generally successful in producing weight reduction, although significant complications exist.

Obese patients with intracranial hypertension secondary to hypoxia and hypercapnia (i.e., the Pickwickian syndrome, obstructive sleep apnea) may respond not only to weight loss, but also to treatment of obstructive sleep apnea

Carbonic anhydrase inhibitors decrease production of CSF and have a mild diuretic effect. The most commonly used agent is acetazolamide (usually 1 to 2 g per day in adults). High doses are often limited by side effects, which include paresthesias of the extremities, lethargy, and altered taste sensation. Alternatively, methazolamide (Neptazane) may be used and is sometimes better tolerated than acetazolamide. Other diuretics may be used, such as furosemide and chlorthalidone. Spironolactone and triamterene may be considered in patients who are allergic to carbonic anhydrase inhibitors and other sulfonamide containing diuretics. Combining diuretics, or using them with carbonic anhydrase inhibitors, may produce hypokalemia and should be done with extreme caution.

Although systemic corticosteroids may be beneficial in the treatment of isolated raised ICP associated with various systemic inflammatory disorders, such as sarcoidosis and systemic lupus erythematosus, they are not generally recommended for routine use in IIH. Indeed, rebound increase in ICP is common, and weight gain is an undesirable side effect in the obese population most affected by IIH. Corticosteroids should be reserved for the urgent treatment of patients with severe visual loss while arranging a definitive surgical procedure.

Headaches from IIH usually improve dramatically after a lumbar puncture. They most often can be managed medically as for chronic tension headaches. Early experience with topiramate is promising; indeed, it prevents headaches, has mild carbonic anhydrase activity, and commonly produces weight loss. However, many patients with IIH experience other types of headaches unrelated to intracranial hypertension, and analgesic abuse is common in this population.

Lumbar punctures (LP) are extremely helpful to relieve most symptoms of IIH. They can easily be repeated when the vision deteriorates and while waiting for a more definite treatment. The first LP performed for the diagnosis of IIH is the first treatment of IIH. However, repeated LPs are usually poorly tolerated and often technically difficult to perform in obese patients.

Surgical Procedures

Surgery is performed in patients with severe optic neuropathy at initial presentation or when other forms of treatment fail to prevent progressive visual loss. It is rarely performed for the treatment of headaches alone. The decision of whether to proceed with a CSF shunting procedure or an optic nerve sheath decompression (ONSD) depends largely on the local resources available. Although one may argue that shunting treats the primary pathology, the risks and benefits to each procedure must be considered for each patient. There are no studies comparing ONSD and shunting. It is often recommended to choose an ONSD (on the most affected eye first) in patients with severe visual loss associated with disc edema, but mild headaches, and a CSF shunting procedure in patients with visual loss, disc edema and severe headaches. Sometimes more than one type of surgical procedure is necessary.

Ventriculoperitoneal shunting is quite effective in lowering ICP in patients with IIH but this procedure can be difficult unless a stereotactic method is used, because the ventricles in patients with IIH are not enlarged. Thus, many neurosurgeons prefer the **lumboperitoneal shunt**, in which a silicone tube is placed percutaneously between the lumbar subarachnoid space and the peritoneal cavity. Most patients treated with a shunt experience rapid normalization of ICP and resolution of papilledema, often with improvement in visual function after shunting. However, rarely, acute visual loss can occur in patients with severe papilledema when the ICP is normalized rapidly. The shunts tend to obstruct over time, and over half of patients ultimately require one or more shunt revisions, often within months after their initial insertion. Complications of the shunt procedure include spontaneous obstruction of the shunt, usually at the peritoneal end, excessively low pressure, infection, radiculopathy, and migration of the tube, resulting in abdominal pain. Some patients also develop a Chiari malformation after lumboperitoneal shunting that may or may not be symptomatic. Although the risks of shunting are generally minor, fatal tonsillar herniation after shunting in IIH has been reported. Many of the complications from lumboperitoneal shunts can be avoided by using a programmable valve.

Optic Nerve Sheath Decompression (ONSD) is an efficient way to treat papilledema. In this procedure, a window or multiple slits are made in the dural sheath of the optic nerve immediately behind the globe. The procedure immediately reduces pressure on the operated nerve, with resultant improvement in visual function. Occasionally, papilledema and visual function also improve on the other side. However, most patients need bilateral procedures. Although some patients relate that it also improves their headaches, there is probably little effect on ICP in most cases and the decrease in papilledema and visual improvement are related to the local decrease in optic nerve sheath pressure rather than from a generalized decrease in ICP. The mechanism of long-term effectiveness from ONSD may be fibrous scar formation between the dura and optic nerve creating a barrier to protect the anterior optic nerve from the intracranial CSF pressure.

The risks of optic nerve sheath fenestration, although low, are nevertheless significant. They include transient or permanent loss of vision from retinal vascular occlusion or optic nerve ischemia, diplopia, and infection. Some patients require a repeat procedure as vision may worsen months to years later. Nevertheless, most adults and children have stabilization or improvement of vision following optic nerve sheath fenestration.

SPECIAL CIRCUMSTANCES
Pregnancy
Women who develop IIH during pregnancy are diagnosed and treated similarly to nonpregnant women. Most women do well, with little or no permanent visual loss. There is no contraindication to pregnancy in women with a history of IIH and no special provisions are required for delivery unless other medical complications are present. The majority of patients may be managed with careful neuro-ophthalmic follow-up and repeated lumbar punctures. Acetazolamide may be used after 20 weeks gestation. If vision deteriorates, corticosteroids may be used. ONSD or lumboperitoneal shunting may be performed if needed, although there is a theoretical risk of shunt malfunction from peritoneal catheter obstruction as the uterus enlarges. Isolated raised ICP arising in the postpartum period or following fetal loss should raise the suspicion of cerebral venous sinus thrombosis.

Fulminant IIH
There is a small subgroup of patients with IIH who experience a rapid onset of symptoms and precipitous visual decline. They often have significant visual field loss, central visual acuity loss, and marked papilledema at presentation. Macular edema or ophthalmoparesis may also be present. A progressive or "malignant" course requires rapid and aggressive treatment, which often includes a surgical procedure. Intravenous corticosteroids and insertion of a lumbar drain are often used while waiting for a more definite treatment. Cerebral venous sinus thrombosis and a meningeal process are important diagnostic considerations in these patients.

FOR FURTHER INFORMATION

See *Walsh & Hoyt's Clinical Neuro-Ophthalmology*, 6th edition, Volume 1, Chapter 5, pages 237–291, Volume 2, Chapter 45, pages 2427–2465.

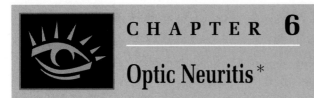

CHAPTER **6**

Optic Neuritis *

*O*ptic neuritis is a term used to refer to inflammation of the optic nerve. When it is associated with a swollen optic disc, it is called *papillitis* or *anterior optic neuritis*. When the optic disc appears normal, the terms *retrobulbar optic neuritis* or *retrobulbar neuritis* are used. In the absence of signs of multiple sclerosis (MS) or other systemic disease, the optic neuritis is referred to as isolated, monosymptomatic, or idiopathic. The pathogenesis of isolated optic neuritis is presumed to be demyelination of the optic nerve, similar to that seen in MS. It is likely that most cases of isolated acute optic neuritis are a forme fruste of MS.

Optic neuritis can be caused by disorders other than MS and related demyelinating diseases. In addition, two variants of optic neuritis occasionally occur. *Neuroretinitis* is a term used to describe inflammatory involvement of both the intraocular optic nerve and the peripapillary retina. *Optic perineuritis*, also called "perioptic neuritis," describes inflammatory involvement of the optic nerve sheath, without inflammation of the nerve itself.

IDIOPATHIC DEMYELINATING OPTIC NEURITIS

Optic neuritis usually is a primary demyelinating process. It almost always occurs as an isolated phenomenon or in patients with MS. Patients in whom optic neuritis occurs as an isolated phenomenon have a higher risk of the subsequent development of MS than the normal population. There are three forms of primary demyelinating optic neuritis: acute, chronic, and subclinical.

ACUTE IDIOPATHIC DEMYELINATING OPTIC NEURITIS

Acute demyelinating optic neuritis is by far the most common type of optic neuritis that occurs throughout the world and is the most frequent cause of optic nerve dysfunction in the young adult population. Much of our knowledge regarding this form of optic neuritis was obtained from the Optic Neuritis Treatment Trial (ONTT). The investigators in this trial enrolled 455 patients with acute unilateral optic neuritis. Although the primary objective of the trial was the assessment of the efficacy of corticosteroids in the treatment of optic neuritis, the trial also provided information about the clinical profile of optic neuritis, its natural history, and its relationship to MS.

Demographics

The annual incidence of acute optic neuritis is estimated in population-based studies to be between 1 and 5 per 100,000. In Olmstead County, Minnesota, where the Mayo Clinic is located, the incidence rate is estimated to be 5.1 per 100,000 person-years and the prevalence rate 115 per 100,000.

The majority of patients with acute optic neuritis are between the ages of 20 and 50 years with a mean age of 30 to 35 years; however, optic neuritis can occur at any age. Females are affected more commonly than males by a ratio of approximately 3:1.

*Adapted from Smith C. Optic neuritis. In: Miller NR, Newman NJ, Biousse V, Kerrison JB, eds. *Walsh & Hoyt's Clinical Neuro-Ophthalmology*. 6th ed. Vol. I. Philadelphia: Lippincott Williams & Wilkins; 2005:293–347.

Clinical Presentation

The two major symptoms in patients with acute optic neuritis are loss of central vision and pain in and around the affected eye.

Loss of central visual acuity is reported by over 90% of patients. Vision loss is typically abrupt, occurring over several hours to several days. Progression over a longer period of time can occur but should make the clinician suspicious of an alternative disorder. The degree of visual loss varies widely from minimal reduction to complete blindness with no perception of light. The majority of patients describe diffuse blurred vision, although some recognize that the blurring is predominantly central. Occasionally, patients complain of a loss of a portion of peripheral field, such as the inferior or superior region, often to one side. The visual loss is monocular in most cases, but in a small percentage, particularly in children, both eyes are simultaneously affected.

Pain in or around the eye is present in more than 90% of patients with acute optic neuritis. It is usually mild, but it may be extremely severe and may even be more debilitating to the patient than the loss of vision. It may precede or occur concurrently with visual loss, usually is exacerbated by eye movement, and generally lasts no more than a few days. The presence of pain is a helpful differentiating feature from other causes of optic neuropathies, such as anterior ischemic optic neuropathy, which typically produces painless visual loss (see Chapter 7).

Up to 30% of the patients with optic neuritis experience positive visual phenomena, called *photopsias*, both at the onset of their visual symptoms and during the course of the disorder. These phenomena are spontaneous flashing black squares, flashes of light, or showers of sparks, sometimes precipitated by eye movement or certain sounds.

Examination of a patient with acute optic neuritis reveals evidence of optic nerve dysfunction. Visual acuity is reduced in most cases, but varies from a mild reduction to no light perception. Contrast sensitivity and color vision are impaired in almost all cases. The reduction in contrast sensitivity often parallels the reduction in visual acuity, although in some cases, it is much worse. The reduction in color vision is often much worse than would be expected from the level of visual acuity. Standard color vision testing with the Ishihara or Hardy-Rand-Rittler pseudoisochromatic plates commonly reveals abnormalities in the affected eye, whereas the more sensitive Farnsworth-Munsell 100-Hues test can reveal more subtle defects. Even when the patient can detect all the pseudoisochromatic figures correctly, careful comparison of the appearance of a single plate by each eye may reveal a striking difference in color and brightness between the two eyes.

Visual field loss can vary from mild to severe, may be diffuse or focal, and can involve the central or peripheral field. Indeed, almost any type of field defect can occur in an eye with optic neuritis. Among 415 patients in the ONTT with baseline visual acuity of hand motions or better, automated perimetry of the central 30 degrees of visual field revealed diffuse visual field loss in 48% of the patients and focal loss in 52%. Focal nerve fiber bundle type defects (altitudinal, arcuate, and nasal step) were present in 20% of the patients; pure central or centrocecal defects in 8%; and hemianopic defects in 5%.

A relative afferent pupillary defect is demonstrable with the swinging flashlight test in all unilateral cases of optic neuritis. When such a defect is not present, either there is a co-existing optic neuropathy in the fellow eye (e.g., from previous or concurrent asymptomatic optic neuritis) or the visual loss in the affected eye is not caused by optic neuritis or any other form of optic neuropathy.

Patients with optic neuritis also can be shown to have a reduced sensation of brightness in the affected eye, either by simply asking them to compare the brightness of a light shined in one eye and then the other, or by more complex tests using polarized lenses or flickering lights of varying frequencies.

About one third of the patients with acute optic neuritis have some degree of disc swelling (Fig. 6.1). The optic disc may be slightly or markedly blurred. At times, the disc swelling is so severe that it mimics the choked disc seen in patients with papilledema (Fig. 6.2). The degree of disc swelling does not correlate with the severity of either visual acuity or visual field loss. Disc or peripapillary hemorrhages and segmental disc swelling are less common in eyes with acute

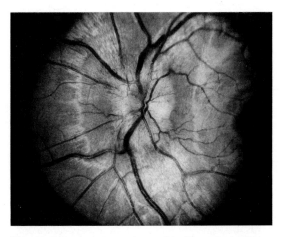

Figure 6.1. Anterior optic neuritis. There is significant swelling and hyperemia of the disc with dilated surface capillaries.

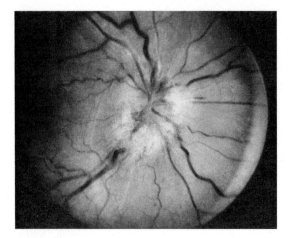

Figure 6.2. Severe anterior optic neuritis mimicking papilledema. Note hyperemia and elevation of the disc and several peripapillary retinal hemorrhages.

optic neuritis than in eyes with anterior ischemic optic neuropathy. The majority of patients with idiopathic acute optic neuritis have a normal optic disc in the affected eye ("the doctor sees nothing when the patient sees nothing"), unless they have had a previous attack of acute or asymptomatic optic neuritis or have ongoing chronic optic neuritis. Over approximately 4 to 6 weeks, the optic disc becomes pale, even as the visual acuity and other parameters of vision improve (Fig. 6.3). The pallor may be diffuse or located to a particular portion of the disc, most often the temporal region.

Slit lamp examination in eyes with demyelinating optic neuritis is almost always normal. In some patients with optic neuritis, anterior or posterior uveitis may be observed. Sheathing of retinal veins may also occur, especially in patients with MS. When the cellular reaction is extensive, etiologies other than demyelination should be considered, including sarcoidosis, syphilis, cat-scratch disease, and Lyme disease (see below).

In adults, bilateral, clinically simultaneous acute optic neuritis is uncommon, although the relative frequency increases when evaluating populations of patients with established MS. The ONTT showed a relatively high percentage of presumably asymptomatic fellow eye deficits at baseline: 14% with visual acuity abnormalities, 22% with color vision abnormalities, and 48% with visual field defects. The majority of the fellow eye deficits resolved over several months, suggesting that such abnormalities may be caused by subclinical but concurrent acute demyelination in the fellow optic nerve. In contrast to adults, acute optic neuritis is often symptomatically bilateral and simultaneous in children. In such cases, the optic neuritis is presumed to be related to infection (see the subsequent text).

Diagnostic Studies

Studies in patients with presumed acute optic neuritis are usually performed for one of three reasons: (a) to determine if the cause of the optic neuropathy is something other than inflammation, particularly a compressive lesion; (b) to determine if a cause other than demyelination is responsible for inflammation of the optic nerve; and (c) to determine the visual and neurologic prognosis of optic neuritis.

With the widespread availability of magnetic resonance imaging (MRI), computed tomographic (CT)

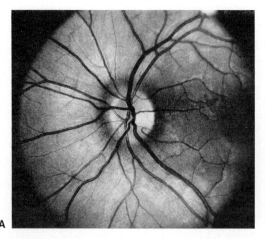

A

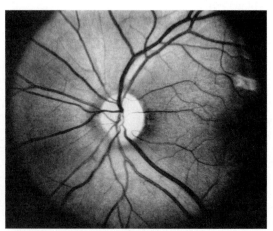

B

Figure 6.3. Optic atrophy after acute, retrobulbar optic neuritis. **A:** In acute phase, visual acuity in the left eye is 20/300 with a central scotoma, but the optic disc is normal. **B:** Three months later, visual acuity has returned to 20/30, but the optic disc is pale, particularly temporally, and there is mild nerve fiber layer atrophy.

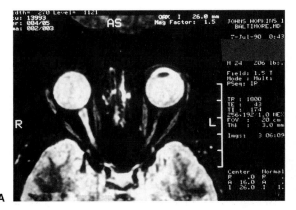

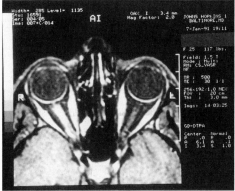

Figure 6.4. Magnetic resonance imaging (MRI) of the optic nerve in acute demyelinating optic neuritis. **A:** Unenhanced proton density-weighted axial MRI in a 24-year-old man with right optic neuritis shows diffuse hyperintensity of the right optic nerve. **B:** T1-weighted axial MRI after intravenous injection of paramagnetic contrast material in a 25-year-old woman with right optic neuritis shows marked thickening and enhancement of the orbital portion of the right optic nerve.

scanning has little or no role in the evaluation of patients with presumed optic neuritis. MRI can detect demyelinating lesions of the optic nerve, manifesting as foci of T2-bright signal, areas of enhancement, and even optic nerve enlargement (Fig. 6.4). These lesions are nonspecific, and a similar appearance can be observed in patients with infectious and other inflammatory optic neuropathies.

The most important application of MRI in patients with optic neuritis is the identification of signal abnormalities in the white matter of the brain, usually in the periventricular region, consistent with demyelination (Fig. 6.5). Two or more brain lesions on MRIs of patients with isolated optic neuritis are reported in 27% to 64% of the cases, depending on the referral population and the timing of the MRI. Finally, studies have shown that MRI is the strongest predictor of MS in patients with acute idiopathic optic neuritis (Fig. 6.6).

Other tests are similarly nonspecific in differentiating acute demyelinating optic neuritis from the less common systemic and local infectious and inflammatory optic neuropathies. The vast majority of patients with optic neuritis caused by such disorders can be identified (or at least suspected) simply by performing a thorough history. Therefore, diagnostic testing should be performed on a case-by-case basis in order to rule out common disorders such as syphilis, sarcoidosis, cat-scratch disease, Lyme disease, or systemic lupus erythematosus.

The role of CSF analysis in the evaluation of patients with acute optic neuritis is not clear. Although the presence of oligoclonal banding in the CSF is associated with the development of MS, the powerful predictive value of brain MRI for MS has reduced the role of lumbar puncture in the evaluation of patients

with optic neuritis. Lumbar puncture can help define a very low risk population for MS if both CSF and MRI are normal. CSF studies in patients with optic neuritis are mostly useful to rule-out another inflammatory or infectious disorder.

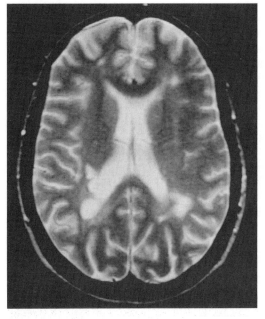

Figure 6.5. Magnetic resonance imaging (MRI) of the brain of a patient with isolated optic neuritis and no previous history of neurologic dysfunction. T2-weighted axial MRI shows multiple ovoid periventricular white-matter lesions in both hemispheres. These lesions are identical with those seen in patients with acute multiple sclerosis

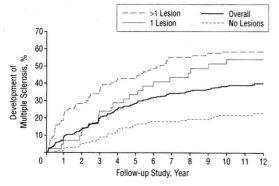

Figure 6.6. The cumulative probability of multiple sclerosis was statistically significantly higher in patients with one or more lesions seen on the baseline MR scan of the brain than in patients with no brain lesions ($p < 0.001$, log rank test) but was not significantly different between patients with a single brain lesion and patients with multiple lesions $p = 0.22$, log-rank test). (Reprinted from: Optic Neuritis Study Group. High- and low-risk profiles for the development of multiple sclerosis within 10 years after optic neuritis: experience of the optic neuritis treatment trial. *Arch Ophthalmol.* 2003;121:944–949, with permission.)

Visual Prognosis

The natural history of acute demyelinating optic neuritis is to worsen over several days to 2 weeks, and then to improve. The improvement initially is fairly rapid. It then levels off, but further improvement can continue to occur 1 year after the onset of visual symptoms. Among patients in the ONTT who received placebo, visual acuity began to improve within 3 weeks of onset in 79% and within 5 weeks in 93%. For most patients in this study, recovery of visual acuity was nearly complete by 5 weeks after onset (Fig. 6.7). The mean visual acuity 1 year after an attack of otherwise uncomplicated optic neuritis is 20/15, and less than 10% of patients have permanent visual acuity less than 20/40. Other parameters of visual function, including contrast sensitivity, color perception, and visual field, improve in conjunction with improvement in visual acuity.

Although the overall prognosis for visual acuity after an attack of acute optic neuritis is extremely good, some patients have persistent severe visual loss after a single episode. Furthermore, even patients with improvement in visual function to "normal" may complain of movement-induced photopsias or transient loss of vision with overheating or exercise (Uhthoff symptom). The Uhthoff symptom is most common in patients with other evidence of MS, but it is also experienced after isolated optic neuritis, by patients with chronic or subclinical optic neuritis, and occasionally by patients with optic neuropathies from other causes. Two major hypotheses regarding the Uhthoff

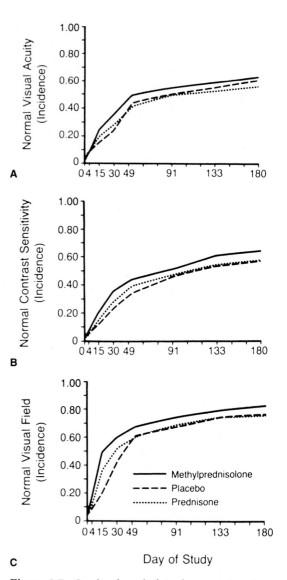

Figure 6.7. Graphs of speed of visual recovery in patients with acute optic neuritis treated with intravenous high-dose methylprednisolone (1 g/day × 3 days) followed by a 2-week course of oral prednisone (1 mg/kg/day) (*solid line*), compared with patients treated with oral prednisone alone (*dotted line*) and untreated patients given placebo (*dashed line*) in the Optic Neuritis Treatment Trial. Note that improvement in **(A)** visual acuity, **(B)** contrast sensitivity, and **(C)** visual field occur more rapidly in patients treated with the intravenous regimen than in patients given either low-dose oral prednisone or untreated patients. (Reprinted from: Beck RW, Cleary PA, Anderson MM Jr, et al. A randomized, controlled trial of corticosteroids in the treatment of acute optic neuritis. *N Engl J Med.* 1992;326:581–588, with permission.)

symptom are that (a) elevation of body temperature interferes directly with axon conduction, and (b) exercise or a rise in body temperature changes the metabolic environment of the axon which, in turn, interferes with conduction.

Subjectively, patients with recovered optic neuritis frequently complain that their vision in the affected eye is "not right" or "remains fuzzy," or that colors are "washed out." One cause of these symptoms is probably related to subtle abnormalities in the visual field in which patients experience abnormally rapid disappearance of focal visual stimuli and abnormally rapid fatigue in sensitivity. These patients typically complain that when they look at something, it appears as if they have "holes" in their vision.

Recurrent attacks of optic neuritis may occur in either eye. The 10-year ONTT recurrence rate was 35%. The risk of recurrence was increased (41%) in the ONTT group treated with prednisone compared with those receiving intravenous steroids or placebo (25%).

Neurologic Prognosis

Optic neuritis occurs in about 50% of patients with MS and is the presenting manifestation in about 20%. Both retrospective and prospective studies have been performed to determine the prognosis for the development of MS in patients who experience an attack of acute optic neuritis. Although retrospective studies provide figures ranging from 11.5% to 85%, most prospective studies support the higher figures. The risk of developing MS is about 30% in patients followed 5 to 7 years after an attack of optic neuritis, and eventually increases to about 75% in women and 34% in men with 15 to 20 years of follow-up. Among 95 incident cases of optic neuritis in Olmstead County, Minnesota, the estimated risk of MS was 39% by 10 years, 49% by 20 years, 54% by 30 years, and 60% by 40 years. The average time interval from an initial attack of optic neuritis until other symptoms and signs of MS develop varies considerably; most studies found that the majority of persons who develop MS after optic neuritis do so within 7 years of the onset of visual symptoms. It therefore seems appropriate to consider most cases of optic neuritis a limited form of MS and to counsel patients appropriately.

There appear to be certain risk factors that increase the likelihood that a patient with isolated optic neuritis will eventually develop MS. Without question, the most highly predictive baseline factor is multiple lesions in the periventricular white matter on an MRI, which is a phenomenon noted in 50% to 70% of the patients with isolated optic neuritis. This was demonstrated by several studies, including the ONTT. Among patients with isolated optic neuritis in the ONTT, the cumulative percentage developing MS within 5 years was 16% in patients with normal MRI and 51% in patients with more than two lesions on the brain MRI. Fifty-six percent of the patients with even one typical MRI lesion at baseline (regardless the number of lesions) had developed MS at 10 years, whereas only 22% of those who had a normal MRI at baseline had developed MS. Other risk factors for the development of MS among ONTT patients were caucasian race, a family history of MS, history of previous ill-defined neurologic complaints, and a previous episode of optic neuritis. However, none of these factors affected the risk of developing MS as much as the results of MRI. Among patients with normal MRI, negative risk factors included male gender, absence of pain, mild visual acuity loss, and optic disc swelling. Although the ONTT did not support any correlation between age of onset and the development of MS, other studies suggest that the younger the age of onset of optic neuritis, the greater the subsequent risk for MS. Winter onset of optic neuritis may also be a risk factor.

The ONTT and the Longitudinal Optic Neuritis Study (LONS) have revealed a particularly low MS-risk group. Among the patients who had a normal brain MRI, none of the patients with severe disc edema, macular star, or disc hemorrhages developed MS at 10 years. These findings emphasize the role of the ophthalmologist in defining the prognosis of optic neuritis.

Treatment

Corticosteroids are the main treatment option for patients with acute idiopathic optic neuritis. The ONTT had three treatment groups: (a) oral prednisone (1 mg/kg/day) for 14 days; (b) intravenous methylprednisolone sodium succinate (250 mg 4 times a day for 3 days) followed by oral prednisone (1 mg/kg/day) for 11 days; and (c) oral placebo for 14 days. Each regimen was followed by a short oral taper (20 mg on day 15, 10 mg on days 16 and 18). Most patients in all three treatment groups had a good recovery of vision with only 10% of patients in each group having a visual acuity of 20/50 or worse in the affected eye at 6 months of follow-up. Among the three groups 1 year after onset of visual symptoms, there was no significant difference in mean visual acuity, contrast sensitivity, color vision, or visual field. However, patients treated with the regimen of intravenous methylprednisolone followed by oral prednisone recovered vision faster than patients in the other two groups. The benefit of this treatment regimen was greatest in the first 15 days of follow-up and decreased subsequently. Patients treated with oral prednisone alone did not recover vision any faster and had no better visual outcome. A meta-analysis of

12 randomized controlled clinical trials of steroid treatment in MS and optic neuritis confirmed these results.

Importantly, ONTT patients treated with oral prednisone alone had an increased rate of recurrent attacks of optic neuritis in the previously affected eye and an increased rate of new attacks of optic neuritis in the fellow eye compared with patients in the other two groups.

The ONTT also evaluated the rate of development of MS in the three treatment groups and found that the patients treated with the intravenous followed by oral corticosteroid regimen had a reduced rate of development of clinically definite MS during the first 2 years. The benefit of treatment was seen only in patients who had abnormal brain MRI at the time of onset of the optic neuritis, and the clinical benefit of the intravenous treatment lessened over time such that by 3 years of follow-up, there was no significant difference in the rate of development of MS among treatment groups.

The question of whether long-term treatment of selected patients with optic neuritis should be initiated in order to decrease the subsequent risk of MS remains debated

The Controlled High MS risk Avonex MS Prevention Study (CHAMPS) was a randomized, double blind, placebo controlled trial that enrolled patients with a first demyelinating event (e.g., optic neuritis) and two or more white matter lesions on a brain MRI. All patients received intravenous steroids per the ONTT protocol. They were then randomized to interferon-beta-1a (Avonex) versus placebo. The group of patients receiving interferon beta-1a had a 44% reduction in the 3 year risk of developing MS when compared to placebo. In addition, patients in the interferon group had fewer new and enhancing brain MRI lesions. The Early Treatment of Multiple Sclerosis study (ETOMS) also found that interferon beta-1a (Rebif) was associated with a short-term reduction in the conversion to MS, although the reduction was weaker (24%) than in CHAMPS. Other studies are currently evaluating whether such treatments should be recommended in patients with optic neuritis who have an abnormal MRI.

Management Recommendations

In a patient with typical features of optic neuritis, a clinical diagnosis can be made with a high degree of certainty without the need for ancillary testing. Patients who have a single attack of optic neuritis are at increased risk of developing MS, particularly those with an abnormal brain MRI. Such patients may be considered for intravenous steroids which may accelerate visual recovery and may delay the onset of MS, but do not change the long-term prognosis. Long-term treatment with interferon beta-1a should be considered in high-risk patients, but this decision should still be made on a case-by-case basis.

CHRONIC DEMYELINATING OPTIC NEURITIS

Chronic optic neuritis is less common than acute optic neuritis. However, numerous patients with MS have no history of acute visual loss (painful or otherwise), but nevertheless complain that their vision is not normal and have evidence of unilateral or bilateral optic nerve dysfunction. Such patients may complain of a static disturbance of vision, a slowly progressive loss of vision in one or both eyes, or, occasionally, a stepwise loss of vision unassociated with periods of recovery.

Most patients with chronic unilateral or bilateral demyelinating optic neuropathies develop visual symptoms after other signs and symptoms of MS have developed, and it is for this reason that the percentage of patients with MS and evidence of chronic progressive optic neuritis increases the longer patients are followed. Nevertheless, slowly progressive visual loss or complaints of blurred or distorted vision in one or both eyes are the first symptoms underlying neurologic disease in some patients.

ASYMPTOMATIC (SUBCLINICAL) OPTIC NEURITIS

A substantial percentage of patients with MS have clinical or laboratory evidence of optic nerve dysfunction even though they have no visual complaints and believe their vision to be normal. This is not surprising given that the anterior visual pathways show damage in up to 100% of patients with MS in autopsy studies. Evidence for optic neuritis in a patient who is visually asymptomatic may be clinical, electrophysiologic, psychophysical, or a combination of these.

A careful clinical examination may reveal that despite having normal visual acuity, the patient has a subtle disturbance of color perception. There may be subtle visual field defects in one or both eyes detected using automated (static) perimetry. A relative afferent pupillary defect may be present, or the patient may have subtle optic nerve fiber layer atrophy. The ONTT found that 48% of the patients with apparently unilateral optic neuritis and no history of previous optic neuritis in the contralateral eye nevertheless had an abnormal visual field unexplained by intraocular pathology in their asymptomatic, fellow eye. A substantial percentage of these eyes also had disturbances of visual acuity, color vision, and contrast sensitivity. In some cases, MRI showed enhancement of the asymptomatic optic nerve.

Visually asymptomatic patients suspected or known to have MS may have disturbances of the visual sensory pathways by electrophysiologic testing. Visual evoked potentials (VEPs) seem to be a particularly sensitive indicator of optic nerve and other visual sensory pathway disturbances in such patients.

OPTIC NEURITIS IN OTHER PRIMARY DEMYELINATING DISEASES

NEUROMYELITIS OPTICA (DEVIC'S DISEASE)

The association of acute or subacute loss of vision in one or both eyes caused by acute optic neuropathy preceded or followed within days to weeks by a transverse or ascending myelopathy is known as neuromyelitis optica or Devic's disease.

Neuromyelitis optica occurs primarily in children and young adults, but all ages may be affected, and the condition has been described in patients over the age of 60 years. Both sexes are equally affected. It represents less than 1% of demyelinating disease in Western countries and may be more prevalent than typical MS in Japan.

Pathology

The brain, optic nerves, and spinal cord are affected by scattered lesions of demyelination that principally affect the white matter, but also may affect the gray matter. In some cases, the cerebrum may be only slightly affected or completely spared, but the optic nerves and the spinal cord are invariably damaged.

Although some investigators believe that neuromyelitis optica is simply a rare and aggressive variant of MS, there are several important differences in the pathologic findings in the two conditions: (a) the cerebellum is almost never affected in patients with neuromyelitis optica, whereas it is frequently affected in MS; (b) excavation of affected tissue with formation of cavities is rare in MS, but it is common in neuromyelitis optica, where there is often liquefaction of tissue; (c) gliosis is characteristic of MS, but is almost never present or is minimal in neuromyelitis optica; and (d) the arcuate fibers located in the cerebral subcortex are relatively unaffected in patients with neuromyelitis optica, but they are severely damaged in most patients with MS. It remains unclear why the lesions of neuromyelitis optica selectively affect the optic nerves, the optic chiasm, and the spinal cord.

Clinical Manifestations

The primary features of neuromyelitis optica are visual loss caused by damage to the anterior visual sensory pathways and paraplegia caused by damage to the spinal cord. Other visual and neurologic manifestations are much less common.

Many patients with neuromyelitis optica develop a mild febrile illness several days or weeks before the onset of visual or neurologic manifestations. Visual loss is almost always bilateral, although unilateral cases occur (Fig. 6.8). One eye is often affected first, but the second eye usually is affected within hours, days, or rarely

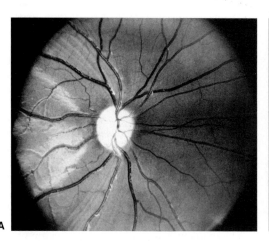
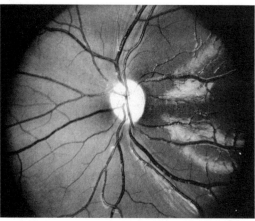

Figure 6.8. Ophthalmoscopic appearance in neuromyelitis optica (Devic's disease). The patient was a 13-year-old girl who developed transverse myelitis, followed several months later by bilateral visual loss. Visual acuity decreased to 20/400 OD and hand motions at 2 feet OS over 72 hours. The pupils were sluggishly reactive to light, and both optic discs appeared normal. The patient was treated with intravenous corticosteroids and gradually recovered both neurologic and visual function. Visual acuity eventually stabilized at 20/40 OD and 20/70 OS associated with small cecocentral scotomas. The ophthalmoscopic appearance of the right and left ocular fundi, **A and B:** respectively, shows symmetric pallor of the optic discs associated with atrophy of the retinal nerve fiber layer, especially in the papillomacular bundles.

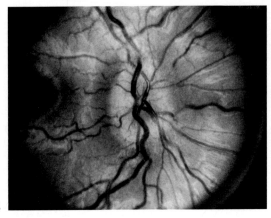
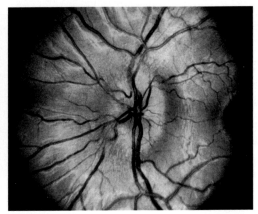

A   B

Figure 6.9. Bilateral anterior optic neuritis. The patient is a 19-year-old girl who suffered bilateral visual loss 2 weeks following a flu-like illness. **A and B:** Both optic discs show moderate swelling without hemorrhages. Visual acuity is 20/400 in the right eye and 20/300 in the left eye, and there are bilateral central scotomas. Visual acuity returned to normal within 6 weeks, and disc swelling completely resolved.

weeks after onset. The loss of vision is typically rapid and usually severe. It is not uncommon for complete blindness to develop. In such cases, the pupils become dilated and nonreactive to light. When some vision remains, the size of the pupils and their reactivity to light stimulation are related to the severity of visual acuity and visual field loss. The rapid, bilateral loss of vision that occurs in patients with neuromyelitis optica is in sharp contrast to the loss of vision in optic neuritis, which tends to be unilateral and not as severe, and to the loss of vision in Leber's hereditary optic neuropathy, which tends to be more slowly progressive. Pain in or around the eyes precedes the loss of vision in a minority of cases, again distinguishing the condition from typical idiopathic optic neuritis in which pain is an almost universalfeature.

Because the foci of demyelination that affect the optic nerves are irregular and occur in a variety of different locations, the visual field defects that develop in patients with neuromyelitis optica are similarly variable. In many instances, vision is so poor when the patient is first examined that it is impossible to plot the field defect. Nevertheless, central scotomas seem to be the most common defect observed, with some patients developing concentric contraction of one or both fields. The ophthalmoscopic appearance of the optic discs varies considerably. A majority of patients have mild swelling of both optic discs. Some patients, however, have substantial disc swelling that may be associated with dilation of retinal veins and extensive peripapillary exudates, and others have normal-appearing optic discs. With time, most patients develop pallor of the discs regardless of their initial appearance (Fig. 6.9). In some of these cases, there is slight narrowing of retinal vessels.

Some recovery of vision usually occurs in patients with neuromyelitis optica. Visual acuity usually begins to improve within 1 to 2 weeks after visual symptoms begin with maximum improvement occurring within several weeks to months. The peripheral fields usually begin to recover before there is noticeable improvement in the central field defects. Nevertheless, some patients have severe and permanent visual loss in both eyes.

There is some controversy about the relationship of visual loss to the onset of paraplegia. Most studies indicate that the loss of vision precedes the onset of paraplegia in the majority of cases, whereas others find that paraplegia usually precedes the loss of vision. Regardless of which manifestation develops first, the interval between manifestations may be days, weeks, or months. In some cases, the blindness and paraplegia occur simultaneously. The onset of the paraplegia, like that of visual loss, usually is sudden and severe, and it may be associated with a mild fever. There may be severe radicular pain, and urinary retention may be present or develop shortly after the onset of motor weakness. Ascending paralysis may paralyze respiration and cause death at an early stage of the disease. Rarely, there is peripheral nerve involvement. Most patients recover motor function to some extent but have residual paraparesis, some have persistent and complete paralysis, and rare patients have complete recovery.

The mortality rate in patients with neuromyelitis optica was reported in the past to be as high as 50%, but improvement in supportive care have greatly reduced this rate, and we would estimate that death occurs in less than 10% of cases now. The disease tends to occur as a single episode without recurrences, unlike MS. Nevertheless, occasional recurrences of both visual loss and paraplegia, both separate and simultaneous, can occur.

Diagnosis

During the active stage of neuromyelitis optica, the CSF usually shows evidence of an inflammatory process. There often is a mild lymphocytic pleocytosis; the concentration of protein in the CSF may be increased, but intrathecal synthesis of IgG is usually not increased and oligoclonal bands are rarely detected. Neuroimaging rarely shows intracranial lesions, aside from the anterior visual pathways. However, MRI may show abnormal T2-weighted signals and enhancement with gadolinium in the optic nerves, chiasm, and spinal cord. Myelin-specific antigens (NMO-IgG) can be detected in the serum of about 50% of patients with neuromyelitis optica.

It may be impossible to differentiate between neuromyelitis optica and MS on clinical grounds alone, and some investigators believe that they are simply variants of the same disease. Nevertheless, not only are there important pathologic differences and differences in CSF findings between the two diseases (see the previous text), but also there are important clinical differences: (i) neuromyelitis optica is not uncommon in the first decade of life, whereas MS rarely occurs in patients under 10 years of age; (ii) the occurrence of bilateral optic neuritis associated with myelitis is rarely recorded in cases of pathologically proven MS; (iii) bilateral blindness is extremely unusual in MS, but is the rule in neuromyelitis optica; and (iv) some serologic and neuroimaging findings seem specific to NMO.

Treatment

There is no specific treatment for neuromyelitis optica. Supportive care is crucial to ensure survival in patients with severe myelitis. The use of intravenous corticosteroids may lessen the severity of the attack and increase the speed of recovery of both visual and motor function. Administration of immunosuppressive agents or intravenous gamma globulin also may be considered.

MYELINOCLASTIC DIFFUSE SCLEROSIS (ENCEPHALITIS PERIAXIALIS DIFFUSA, SCHILDER'S DISEASE)

Although original descriptions of **Schilder's disease** may have inadvertently included examples of adrenoleukodystrophy and subacute sclerosing panencephalitis, there remains a characteristic group of patients with a noninherited demyelinating disease related to MS that is most commonly referred to now as **myelinoclastic diffuse sclerosis.** The character-

istic lesion in these patients is a large, sharply outlined, asymmetric focus of demyelination with severe, selective myelinoclasia that often affects an entire lobe or cerebral hemisphere. There is typically extension across the corpus callosum and damage to the opposite hemisphere. Both hemispheres are symmetrically affected in some cases. Careful examination of the optic nerves, brainstem, cerebellum, and spinal cord often discloses typical discrete lesions consistent with MS, and histopathologic examination of both large and small foci reveals the characteristic features reminiscent of MS, including fibrillary gliosis with formation of giant multinucleated or swollen astrocytes and perivascular cuffing with inflammatory infiltrates containing plasma cells. The axons themselves may show little damage. Indeed, both the clinical and histopathologic features of myelinoclastic diffuse sclerosis disease suggest that it is closely related to MS and probably is a variant of it.

Myelinoclastic diffuse sclerosis occurs most often in children and young adults. It is characterized by a progressive course that may be steady and unremitting or punctuated by a series of rapid worsening. A change in personality may be the first evidence of the disease. Cerebral blindness may be an early feature of the disease, particularly in adults. Central deafness may also occur. Other manifestations include dementia, homonymous visual field defect, varying degrees of hemiparesis and quadriparesis often culminating in plegia, and pseudobulbar palsy. The brainstem and cerebellum are affected in some cases, resulting in nystagmus, intention tremor, scanning speech, and spastic paraplegia.

Visual loss occurs in approximately 60% of the cases, which is most often a result of damage to the postchiasmal visual pathways, producing homonymous hemianopic or quadrantic visual field defects or cerebral blindness. Involvement of the visual association areas may also cause visual difficulties. Occasional patients develop demyelination in the optic chiasm, producing bitemporal field defects. Optic neuritis occurs less frequently than in patients with MS, although the true incidence is not known. Rarely, papilledema occurs.

The CSF may show changes similar to those seen in typical MS. The intracranial pressure is usually normal, but in some patients the pressure is elevated. The protein concentration of the CSF is usually slightly increased, and there may be a mild lymphocytic pleocytosis. The IgG content is often increased, as is the CSF IgG index. Oligoclonal bands may be present, and myelin basic protein may be extremely elevated. Neuroimaging studies show large, multifocal areas of extensive demyelination. In some cases, these lesions are similar in appearance to tumors or abscesses.

The diagnosis of myelinoclastic diffuse sclerosis may be suspected when a child or young adult develops evidence of a subacute or chronic progressive neurologic disease with neuroimaging and laboratory evidence of focal hemispheric demyelinating disease but without adrenal dysfunction or abnormal long-chain fatty-acids.

Most patients with myelinoclastic diffuse sclerosis follow a progressive unremitting course that ends in death within a few months or years. A few cases have been reported in which there was temporary or permanent spontaneous improvement, and rare patients survive for a decade or longer. Some patients improve after being treated with corticosteroids or immunosuppressants. Patients who improve clinically generally show disappearance or shrinkage of the lesions seen on neuroimaging studies.

ENCEPHALITIS PERIAXIALIS CONCENTRICA (CONCENTRIC SCLEROSIS OF BALÓ)

Encephalitis periaxialis concentrica clinically resembles myelinoclastic diffuse sclerosis but differs from it pathologically. Patients rapidly develop a variety of neurologic symptoms and signs separated in time and space, including visual loss and diplopia. The visual loss is usually caused by damage to postgeniculate visual pathways and is characterized by homonymous field defects or cerebral blindness, although optic nerve involvement can occur.

The pathologic changes consist of alternating bands of demyelination and preserved myelin in a series of concentric rings in the cerebral white matter. The predominant feature of the bands of myelin is remyelination. The lesion likely originates as a small focus of acute demyelination around a perivascular inflammatory cuff, and the concentric bands are actually alternating areas of demyelination and remyelination. Some patients not only have pathologic changes consistent with encephalitis periaxialis concentrica but also have lesions typical of acute MS, suggesting that the former disease may actually be a variant of the latter.

Neuroimaging studies initially may be normal in patients with encephalitis periaxialis concentrica; however, eventually both CT scanning and MRI show multiple lesions consistent with demyelination. Similarly, analysis of the CSF at an early stage of the disease may reveal normal findings, but later analysis may show mild to moderate pleocytosis, increased protein, an increased IgG index, and multiple oligoclonal bands. The diagnosis can only be made conclusively by pathologic examination, either by biopsy or on postmortem studies.

Without treatment, encephalitis periaxialis concentrica usually progresses inexorably and is invariably fatal within a few weeks to a year. Treatment with systemic corticosteroids, however, may result in both immediate and long-term improvement in neurologic symptoms and signs. Early diagnosis thus is extremely important.

CAUSES OF OPTIC NEURITIS OTHER THAN PRIMARY DEMYELINATION

In a small percentage of cases, a primary demyelinating process in the optic nerve or the central nervous system is not the cause of unilateral or bilateral anterior or retrobulbar optic neuritis. Instead, the condition develops in the setting of, or as the presenting manifestation of, an underlying or recent systemic infection, vaccination, or systemic inflammatory disease.

INFECTIOUS AND PARAINFECTIOUS OPTIC NEURITIS

Inflammation of the optic nerve can result from direct infection of the nerve by a variety of infectious agents such as viruses and bacteria. In addition, systemic or central nervous system infections can trigger an immune response that results in inflammation of the optic nerve.

Parainfectious optic neuritis typically follows the onset of a viral, or less often a bacterial, infection by 1 to 3 weeks. It is more common in children than in adults and is thought to occur most often on an immunologic basis, producing demyelination of the optic nerve. The optic neuritis may be unilateral, but it is often bilateral (Fig. 6.10). The optic discs may appear normal or swollen. Swelling of the peripapillary retina may be observed in patients with anterior optic neuritis. If a star figure composed of lipid and exudate develops in the macula of the affected eye, the condition is called *neuroretinitis* (see below). If there is evidence of optic nerve dysfunction and the intracranial pressure is normal, the inflammation is assumed to be affecting the periphery of the nerve and is called *perioptic neuritis* or *optic perineuritis* (see below). Parainfectious optic neuritis, whether viral or bacterial, may occur in patients with no evidence of neurologic dysfunction or in association with a meningitis, meningoencephalitis, or encephalomyelitis—so-called acute disseminated encephalomyelitis (ADEM). When neurologic manifestations are present, patients have typical abnormalities in the CSF, such as a lymphocytic pleocytosis and an elevated protein concentration. Patients with encephalitis usually have disturbances on electroencephalography, and they may also have lesions on brain imaging, whereas patients with encephalomyelitis may show lesions in both the brain and spinal cord. Both enlargement and enhancement of the optic nerves may be demonstrated on MRI.

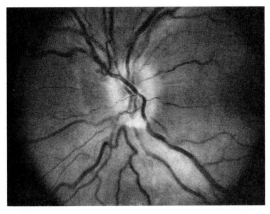
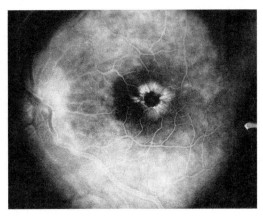

A   B

Figure 6.10. Optic disc swelling in a patient with pars planitis (chronic cyclitis). The patient was initially believed to have papilledema. **A:** The left optic disc is hyperemic and slightly swollen. The hazy appearance is due to the presence of vitreous cells. **B:** Fluorescein angiogram of the left macula shows cystoid macular edema, characteristic of this disorder. The opposite eye had a similar ophthalmoscopic appearance.

Visual recovery following parainfectious optic neuritis is usually excellent without treatment. Whether corticosteroids hasten recovery in patients with postviral optic neuritis is unknown, but this treatment is reasonable to consider, particularly in cases in which visual loss is bilateral and severe.

Optic neuritis may occur in association with **infections** by a large number of both deoxyribonucleic (DNA) and ribonucleic (RNA) viruses including adenovirus, coxsackievirus, cytomegalovirus, hepatitis A virus, human herpes virus 4 (Epstein-Barr virus), human immunodeficiency virus (HIV) type 1, and the measles, mumps, rubeola, rubella, and varicella-zoster (in both chicken pox and herpes zoster) viruses. Bacterial infections can also produce optic neuritis and include syphilis, Lyme disease, cat-scratch disease, anthrax, β-hemolytic streptococcal infection, brucellosis, meningococcal infection, tuberculosis, typhoid fever, and Whipple's disease.

Optic neuritis in **syphilis** is not rare, and it is particularly common in patients also infected with HIV. The optic neuritis of syphilis can be unilateral or bilateral and anterior or retrobulbar. When the condition is anterior, there is usually some cellular reaction in the vitreous, which serves to distinguish it (and other systemic inflammatory diseases that cause anterior optic neuritis) from demyelinating optic neuritis in which the vitreous is usually clear. The diagnosis of syphilis is established using a variety of serologic and CSF assays. Treatment with intravenous penicillin produces visual recovery in many cases; however, the disease may be difficult to cure, particularly in patients who are HIV-positive or who have the acquired immune deficiency syndrome (AIDS). Syphilis can also cause both neuroretinitis and optic perineuritis (see below).

Optic neuritis can occur in patients with Lyme borreliosis (**Lyme disease**). This disorder is a spirochetal infection that is transmitted through the bite of a tick infected with the etiologic agent, *Borrelia burgdorferi.* It can produce a multitude of ocular and neurologic findings, including both anterior and retrobulbar optic neuritis. The diagnosis of Lyme disease is made by serologic detection of infection or by finding the organism or its nucleic acid in the serum, CSF, or both. Treatment with antibiotics is usually effective, particularly in the early stages of the disease. As is the case with other systemic infectious processes that can cause optic neuritis, Lyme disease can also cause neuroretinitis or optic perineuritis (see below).

Many infectious agents that do not normally cause optic neuritis can do so in patients who are immunocompromised from drugs or disease. Such optic neuritis is particularly common in patients who are infected with **HIV** and in patients with AIDS. Optic neuritis, both anterior and retrobulbar can develop in HIV-infected patients with cryptococcal meningitis, cytomegalovirus infection, herpesvirus infections, syphilis, tuberculous meningitis, and a variety of fungal infections. Rare patients with toxoplasmosis also develop optic neuritis. In some cases, such infections cause neuroretinitis, whereas in others, optic perineuritis occurs. Some patients with AIDS develop optic neuritis that is probably caused by infection with HIV itself, although it is not clear if the pathogenesis is direct infection or an immune-mediated parainfectious process.

In the pre-antibiotic era, spread of infection from the paranasal sinuses to the optic nerve was not unusual. However, this is now a rare occurrence, and most cases of **sinusitis** in patients with optic neuritis are fortuitous. Nevertheless, some patients with acute severe sinusitis develop a secondary optic neuritis from spread of infection. Spread of infection from the sphenoid sinus to the posterior optic nerve in the apex of the orbit or within the optic canal can produce isolated loss of vision. Aspergillosis and other fungal infections such as mucormycosis (especially in diabetic patients) should be considered in this clinical setting.

POSTVACCINATION OPTIC NEURITIS

Optic neuritis can occur after vaccinations against both bacterial and virus infections. Most cases are bilateral, and both anterior and retrobulbar forms of optic neuritis may occur. Optic neuritis may develop after vaccinations with *Bacille Calmette-Guérin* (BCG), hepatitis B virus, rabies virus, tetanus toxoid, and variola virus; combined smallpox, and diphtheria vaccine; and combined measles, mumps, and rubella vaccine. Influenza vaccine is commonly associated with the development of optic neuritis. Most cases of postvaccination optic neuritis appear to be of the anterior variety and typically occur within 1 to 3 weeks of the vaccination. Visual recovery is common but may occur over several months.

INFLAMMATORY OPTIC NEURITIS

Granulomatous inflammation of the optic nerve may occur in **sarcoidosis,** producing a typical anterior or retrobulbar optic neuritis. In some cases, the optic neuritis occurs during the course of the disease, whereas in others it is the presenting manifestation. Clinical findings may be indistinguishable from those of demyelinating optic neuritis. However, the optic disc may have a characteristic lumpy, white appearance that suggests a granulomatous etiology, and there may be an inflammatory reaction in the vitreous or even the anterior chamber. The optic neuritis associated with sarcoidosis is usually extremely sensitive to steroids. In most cases, recovery of vision is rapid after treatment is instituted, although vision may decline again once steroids are tapered or stopped. It must be emphasized that rapid recovery of vision with corticosteroid treatment and subsequent worsening when the steroids are tapered is atypical for demyelinating optic neuritis and suggests an infiltrative or nondemyelinating inflammatory process, such as sarcoidosis.

Patients with **systemic lupus erythematosus, polyarteritis nodosa, and other vasculitides** can experience an attack of what seems clinically to be typical acute optic neuritis. This phenomenon occurs in about 1% of the patients with SLE. In rare cases, the optic neuropathy is the presenting sign of the disease. The pathogenesis is most likely related to ischemia from vasculitis. The clinical profile of optic neuropathy in SLE and other vasculitides can be an acute anterior or retrobulbar optic neuropathy associated with pain or a slowly progressive loss of vision that mimics a compressive lesion.

Autoimmune optic neuropathy is a distinct variety of optic nerve inflammation. It is usually associated without any neurologic or systemic symptom or sign suggesting an underlying inflammatory disorder. Patients present recurrent episodes of visual loss which are usually very sensitive to steroids. Most patients become steroid-dependent and their visual function tends to deteriorate overtime. Long-term immunosuppressive agents are usually required to limit to side effects of steroids. Although workup for evidence of a connective tissue disease remains negative, some patients have abnormal skin biopsies with perivascular infiltrate and immune complex deposition within the dermis.

MISCELLANEOUS CAUSES OF OPTIC NEURITIS

Optic neuritis can rarely occur in a large variety of conditions including almost all infections, and systemic inflammatory disorders. In most cases, associated symptoms and signs suggest the diagnosis and isolated optic neuritis is only rarely the first sign of a systemic disease. Work-up is usually obtained to rule-out the most common causes of optic neuritis; subsequent tests are decided on a case-by-case basis.

Intraocular inflammation alone may cause optic disc swelling; however, in such cases, visual acuity is usually not significantly affected from damage to the optic nerve. In such patients, visual acuity is limited only by the degree of vitreous inflammation or by secondary changes that occur in the macula (e.g., cystoid edema).

OPTIC NEURITIS IN CHILDREN

Optic neuritis in children has several unique characteristics that distinguish it from optic neuritis in adults: (a) it is more often anterior, with disc swelling in more than 70% of cases; (b) it is more often a bilateral simultaneous condition (up to 60% of cases); (c) it often seems to occur within 1 to 2 weeks after a known or presumed viral infection or vaccination; (d) it is less often associated with the development of MS (15 to 44% of cases); and (e) it is often steroid-sensitive and steroid-dependent. The visual prognosis in children with optic neuritis appears to be quite good, but not all children achieve a good visual result. All children with optic neuritis should be evaluated with MRI and a lumbar puncture. An infectious and inflammatory work-up should also be obtained.

NEURORETINITIS

Neuroretinitis is characterized by acute unilateral visual loss in the setting of optic disc swelling and hard

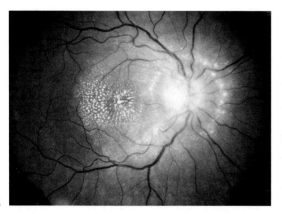
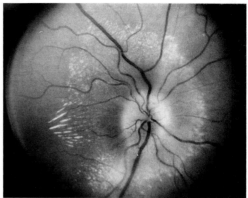

A B

Figure 6.11. Neuroretinitis. **A:** The right optic disc is swollen, there is peripapillary edema, and there is a star figure composed of hard exudate in the macula. This is a form of optic neuritis that is *not* associated with multiple sclerosis. **B:** In another case, the star figure is incomplete and located nasal but not temporal to the fovea. Note the extensive exudate surrounding the swollen optic disc. (Courtesy of Dr. J.M. Christiansen.)

exudate arranged in a star figure around the fovea (Fig. 6.11). Some cases of neuroretinitis are associated with particular infectious diseases, whereas others occur as apparently isolated phenomena, designated "Leber's idiopathic stellate neuroretinitis."

Neuroretinitis affects persons of all ages, although it occurs most often in the third and fourth decades of life, with no gender predilection. The condition is usually painless, but some patients complain of an eye ache that may worsen with eye movements. Visual acuity at the time of initial examination can range from 20/20 to light perception. The degree of color deficit is usually worse than the degree of visual loss would suggest. The most common field defect is a cecocentral scotoma, but central scotomas, arcuate defects, and even altitudinal defects may be present, and the peripheral field may be nonspecifically constricted. A relative afferent pupillary defect is present in most patients, unless the condition is bilateral. The degree of optic disc swelling ranges from mild to severe, depending in part on the timing of the first examination. In severe cases, splinter hemorrhages may be present. A macular star figure composed of lipid (hard exudates) may not be present when the patient is examined soon after visual symptoms begin, but it becomes apparent within days to weeks and tends to become more prominent even as the optic disc swelling resolves (Fig. 6.11). Small, discrete, usually white, chorioretinal lesions may occur in both the symptomatic and asymptomatic eyes. Posterior inflammatory signs consisting of vitreous cells and venous sheathing, as well as occasional anterior chamber cell and flare may occur. Fluorescein angiography in patients with acute neuroretinitis demonstrates diffuse disc swelling and leakage of dye from vessels on the surface of the discs. The retinal vessels may show slight staining in the peripapillary

region; however, the macular vasculature is entirely normal.

Neuroretinitis is usually a self-limited disorder with a good visual prognosis. Typically over 6 to 8 weeks, the optic disc swelling resolves and the appearance of the disc becomes normal or mildly pale. The macular exudate progresses over about 7 to 10 days and then remains stable for several weeks before gradual resolution occurs over 6 to 12 months. Most patients ultimately recover good visual acuity, although some complain of persistent metamorphopsia or nonspecific blurred vision from mild disruption of the macular architecture. Most patients do not experience a subsequent attack in the same eye, and only a small percentage of patients develop a similar attack in the fellow eye.

In many cases, neuroretinitis is related to an infectious or parainfectious (i.e., immune-mediated) process that may be precipitated by a number of different agents. Cat-scratch disease, a systemic infection caused by the pleomorphic gram-negative bacillus *Bartonella henselae*, is the most common infectious process associated with neuroretinitis. Patients with cat-scratch fever usually have a history of contact with a cat, especially a kitten. They complain of malaise, fever, muscle aches, and headache. Examination typically reveals local lymphadenopathy. Some patients also have symptoms of arthritis, hepatitis, meningitis, or encephalitis; others are systemically and neurologically asymptomatic.

Other common infections that cause neuroretinitis are the spirochetoses, especially syphilis, Lyme disease, and leptospirosis. Neuroretinitis frequently occurs in patients with secondary and tertiary (late) syphilis. There is usually a history of previous sexual contact, a chancre, or prior treatment for syphilis or other sexually transmitted diseases. Neuroretinitis may de-velop in patients with secondary syphilis as part of the syndrome of syphilitic meningitis. In such cases, it is usually bilateral and associated with evidence of meningeal irritation and multiple cranial neuropathies. It may also occur as an isolated phenomenon in pa-tients with secondary syphilis, in which case it is often associated with uveitis and may be either unilateral or bilateral. Neuroretinitis occasionally occurs in patients with late syphilis, usually in patients with meningovas-cular neurosyphilis. Neuroretinitis is commonly asso-ciated with an antecedent viral syndrome, suggesting a possible viral etiology for up to 50% of cases; how-ever, viruses are rarely cultured from the CSF of such patients, and serologic evidence of a concomitant vi-ral infection is usually lacking. Proposed causative vi-ral agents include herpes simplex, hepatitis B, mumps, and the herpes viruses associated with the acute retinal necrosis (ARN) syndrome. Other presumed etiologies for neuroretinitis include toxoplasmosis, toxocariasis, and histoplasmosis.

Noninfectious systemic inflammatory disorders may also produce neuroretinitis such as sarcoidosis. One condition that is *not* associated with neuroretini-tis is MS. Although the rate of development of MS

after an attack of typical optic neuritis is substantial (see the previous text), there is no increased tendency for patients who experience an attack of neuroretinitis to develop MS. Thus, the designation of an attack of acute optic neuropathy as an episode of neuroretinitis rather than anterior optic neuritis substantially alters the neurologic prognosis in the patient being evalu-ated.

Treatment of neuroretinitis depends on whether there is an underlying infectious or inflammatory con-dition that requires therapy. The prognosis for most cases of idiopathic neuroretinitis is excellent.

OPTIC PERINEURITIS

Optic perineuritis, also called perioptic neuritis, is a condition in which only the periphery of the op-tic nerve is inflamed (Fig. 6.12). Optic perineuri-tis is a form of orbital inflammatory pseudotumor; it may develop in isolation or it may be associated with other signs of orbital pseudotumor such as scle-ritis and myositis. In many cases of optic perineuri-tis, there are neither ocular symptoms nor signs other than disc swelling that is usually bilateral. The absence of visual dysfunction is explained by the absence of

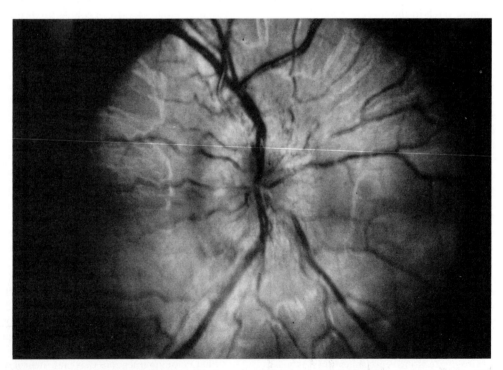

Figure 6.12. Optic perineuritis. The optic disc is hyperemic and swollen (as was the left disc). The patient was a 15-year-old boy complaining of a headache and stiff neck. He had a moderate fever. Visual acuity was 20/15 in both eyes, color vision was normal, and visual fields were full. The patient was believed to have papilledema. A lumbar puncture, however, revealed normal intracranial pressure, an increased concentration of protein in the cerebrospinal fluid (CSF), and a significant CSF lymphocytosis. (Specimen courtesy of Dr. S.T. Orion.)

inflammation of the optic nerve itself. When perineuritis is bilateral, the differentiation from papilledema is often difficult, and it may be necessary to perform neuroimaging and lumbar puncture for diagnosis. Finally, enlargement of the optic nerve sheath on neuroimaging may simulate optic nerve sheath meningioma. As or neuroretinitis, optic perineuritis is *not* associated with MS. It occurs most often in association with an infectious process, such as syphilis, or a systemic inflammatory disorder, such as sarcoidosis or Wegener's granulomatosis.

FOR FURTHER INFORMATION

See *Walsh & Hoyt's Clinical Neuro-Ophthalmology*, 6th edition, Volume 1, Chapter 6, pages 293–347; Volume 3, Chapter 48, pages 2551–2646; Volume 3, Chapter 59, pages 3369–3427, Chapter 60, pages 3429–3525.

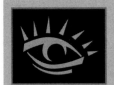

CHAPTER 7

Ischemic Optic Neuropathies*

I schemic syndromes of the optic nerve (ischemic optic neuropathy [ION]) are classified according to (a) the location of the ischemic damage of the nerve and (b) the etiologic factor, if known, for the ischemia. **Anterior** ischemic optic neuropathy (AION) includes syndromes involving the optic nerve head with visible optic disc edema. **Posterior** ischemic optic neuropathy (PION) incorporates those conditions involving the intraorbital, intracanalicular, or intracranial portions of the optic nerve with no visible edema of the optic disc. Although several specific etiologic factors have been identified in ION, the most critical for initial management is the vasculitis of giant cell, or temporal, arteritis (GCA); therefore, ION is typically classified as either **arteritic** (usually due to GCA) or **nonarteritic** (Table 7.1). Nonarteritic ION is most often idiopathic, but specific etiologies such as systemic hypotension and radiation injury have been identified. Finally, several syndromes of optic disc edema with relatively mild dysfunction, including preinfarct optic disc edema and diabetic papillopathy, are presumed to represent optic nerve ischemic edema with dysfunction that is not detectable, mild, or reversible.

ANTERIOR ISCHEMIC OPTIC NEUROPATHY (AION)

AION typically presents with the rapid onset of painless unilateral visual loss developing over hours to days. An altitudinal visual field defect (typically inferior) is the most common pattern of loss (Fig. 7.1) but arcuate scotomas, cecocentral defects, and generalized depression are also frequently seen. Visual acuity is decreased if the field defect involves fixation but may be normal

if an arcuate pattern spares the central region. The pupil in the affected eye has a relative afferent pupillary defect present unless pre-existing or concurrent optic neuropathy in the fellow eye makes its pupillary response equally sluggish. The optic disc is edematous at onset; the edema may be pallid, but it is not uncommon to see disc hyperemia, particularly in the nonarteritic form (Fig. 7.2). The disc most often is diffusely swollen, but a segment of more prominent edema is frequently present (Fig. 7.3). Flame hemorrhages are commonly located adjacent to the disc, and peripapillary retinal arteriolar narrowing may occur (Fig. 7.4).

ARTERITIC ANTERIOR ISCHEMIC OPTIC NEUROPATHY (AAION)

Although it often produces a severe and devastating optic neuropathy, GCA is the cause for AION in a relatively small minority (5.7%) of cases, with an estimated annual incidence in the United States of 0.57 per 100,000 over age 60. AION is, however, the most common cause of visual loss in GCA, accounting for 71% to 83% of cases, with retinal artery occlusion, choroidal ischemia, and PION less common. The mean age of onset for AAION is 70 years, with only rare occurrence under age 60. GCA occurs more frequently in women and with increasing age. It is most common in Caucasians and is unusual in African-American and Hispanic patients.

Clinical Manifestations

AAION usually occurs in association with other systemic symptoms of the disease. Headache is the most common symptom, while jaw claudication and temporal artery or scalp tenderness are the most specific for the disorder. The syndrome of polymyalgia rheumatica (PMR), including malaise, anorexia, weight loss, fever, proximal joint arthralgia and myalgia, is frequently reported. So-called occult GCA, without overt systemic symptoms and sometimes without abnormal

---

*Adapted from Arnold AC. Ischemic optic neuropathy. In: Miller NR, Newman NJ, Biousse V, Kerrison JB, eds. *Walsh & Hoyt's Clinical Neuro-Ophthalmology.* 6th ed. Vol. I. Philadelphia: Lippincott Williams & Wilkins; 2005:349–384.

Table 7.1. *Disorders and Drugs Associated with the Occurrence of Anterior Ischemic Optic Neuropathies*

Arteritic anterior ischemic optic neuropathy
  Giant cell arteritis + + +
  Periarteritis nodosa
  Churg-Strauss syndrome
  Wegener's granulomatosis
  Connective tissue diseases such as systemic lupus
    erythematosus
  Rheumatoid arthritis
  Relapsing polychondritis

Nonarteritic anterior ischemic optic neuropathy
  Anomalous optic nerve:
    "Disc-at-risk": small crowded optic nerve
    Papilledema
    Optic nerve head drusen
  Elevated intraocular pressure (acute glaucoma,
    ocular surgery)
  Radiation-induced optic neuropathy
  Diabetes mellitus
  Other vascular risk factors (atherosclerosis)
  Hypercoagulable states*
  Acute systemic hypotension/anemia:
    Bleeding
    Cardiac arrest
    Peri-operative (especially cardiac and spine
      surgeries)
    Dialysis
  Sleep apnea
  Drugs:
    Amiodarone
    Interferon-alpha
    Vasoconstrictor agents (such as nasal
      decongestants)
    Erectile dysfunction drugs

*Hypercoagulable states are rarely responsible for AION and should only be tested in younger patients without other risk factors for AION.

blood testing, occurs in about 20% of patients with GCA and visual loss.

In addition to systemic symptoms, certain associated local signs may aid in the diagnosis of AAION. Induration of the temporal region, decreased or absent temporal artery pulse, and cordlike firmness or nodularity of the temporal artery all may be seen. Ischemic scalp necrosis has been documented in GCA, and it may masquerade as herpes zoster dermatitis with facial pain and even a vesicular reaction of the affected skin. Rarely, vasculitic ischemia of the central nervous system occurs, including mental status alterations, brain stem and cerebellar syndromes, and damage to the retrochiasmal afferent visual pathways.

AAION typically presents with severe visual loss (visual acuity less than 20/200 in 57.8% to 76.5% of cases, frequently hand motion or worse) developing rapidly over hours to days (Table 7.2). While the initial presentation is often unilateral, bilateral simultaneous AION is more commonly arteritic than nonarteritic, and its occurrence raises suspicion for GCA. The persistent visual loss of AAION is preceded in 7% to 18% of the cases by transient visual loss similar to that of carotid artery disease, although the episodes may be of shorter duration. The pallid type of optic disc edema (Fig. 7.5) is seen more frequently in the arteritic than in the nonarteritic form. Cotton-wool patches (Fig. 7.6) indicative of concurrent retinal ischemia may be seen. Retinal arterial occlusion may occur simultaneously with the optic neuropathy, especially cilioretinal artery occlusion (Fig. 7.7). Peripapillary choroidal ischemia may be associated with the optic neuropathy, exacerbating the visual loss. The optic disc of the fellow eye in AAION most frequently is of normal diameter with a normal physiologic cup as opposed to that in NAION, which tends to be small in diameter with little or no physiologic cup (see below).

If untreated, AAION results in severe damage of the affected optic nerve. Recovery of useful vision after initial involvement is unusual, even with prompt therapy. In cases with unilateral presentation, estimates for development of AAION in the fellow eye without therapy range from 54% to 95%. Time to second eye involvement varies greatly, but it may occur within hours to days. The optic disc edema typically resolves over 4 to 8 weeks with resultant optic atrophy and generalized attenuation of retinal arterioles. Excavation of the optic disc (Fig. 7.6) occurs frequently after AAION but is unusual in NAION.

Diagnostic Confirmation

The most important initial step in the management of AION is the assessment for evidence of GCA. A tentative diagnosis may be made on the basis of advanced age and typical clinical symptoms in conjunction with elevation of the erythrocyte sedimentation rate (ESR). Most cases of active GCA show markedly elevated ESRs (mean 70 mm/hour, often above 100 mm/hour). When the level is not extremely high, however, interpretation of the value becomes more difficult, because normative data are imprecise. As a rule, we recommend the clinically useful guideline that the upper level of normal, in mm/hour, is calculated by dividing patient age by 2 in males and patient age plus 10 by 2 in females. However, by these criteria, the level may be normal in up to 22% of patients with GCA. Conversely, the ESR rises with age, and levels above the listed upper limit of normal for the laboratory are common (up to 40% over 60 mm/hour) in patients over

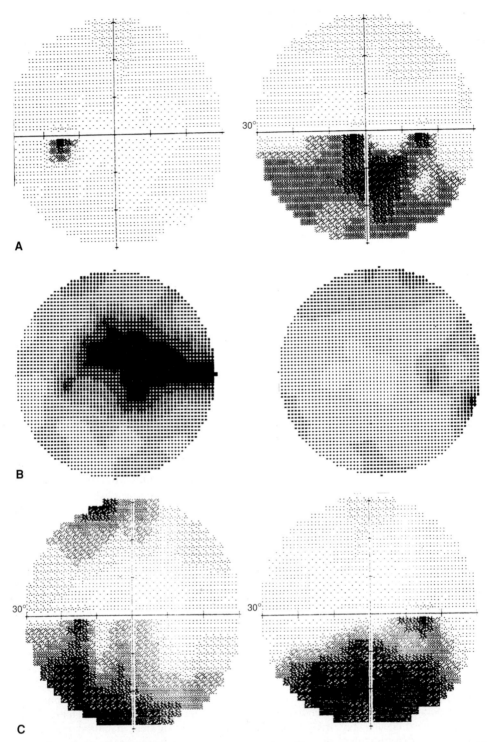

Figure 7.1. Automated quantitative perimetry in AION. Broad arcuate (altitudinal) defect (*A*) is most common, with central (*B*) and less severe arcuate (*C*) defects also frequently noted.

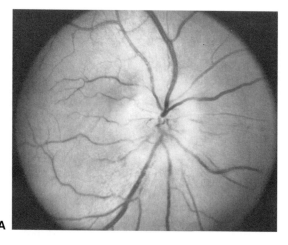 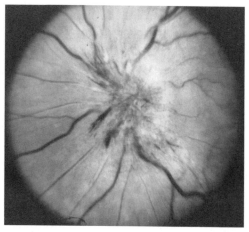

A   B

Figure 7.2. Ophthalmoscopic appearance of nonarteritic anterior ischemic optic neuropathy. **A:** Pallid swelling of the optic disc associated with a few small flame-shaped hemorrhages at the disc margin. **B:** Hyperemic swelling of the optic disc associated with numerous hemorrhages and a few soft exudates.

70 without arteritis. Moreover, the test is nonspecific, elevation confirming only the presence of any active inflammatory process or other disorder affecting red cell aggregation. In studies of temporal artery biopsy-negative cases with such elevation, the most common associated diseases have been occult malignancy (most frequently lymphoma) in 18% to 22%, other inflammatory disease in 17% to 21%, and diabetes in 15% to 20%.

Additional blood abnormalities are common in GCA and may have prognostic value. Measurement of C-reactive protein, levels of which do not rise with age or anemia, increases diagnostic accuracy and is currently recommended in conjunction with the ESR. In one study, specificity of 97% for GCA was attained for AION patients with ESR levels above 47 mm/hour

and C-reactive protein above 2.45 mg/dL (normal less than 0.5). Fibrinogen is commonly elevated and may supplement C-reactive protein levels in increasing accuracy over the use of ESR alone. Thrombocytosis is seen in up to 50% of patients with GCA; its presence has been shown to be a marker for positive temporal artery biopsy and may be a predictor of visual loss.

Histopathologic studies in AAION demonstrate vasculitis of the short posterior ciliary vessels supplying the optic nerve head, in addition to variable involvement of the superficial temporal, ophthalmic, choroidal, and central retinal arteries. Fluorescein angiographic data support involvement of the short posterior ciliary arteries in AAION. Delayed filling of the

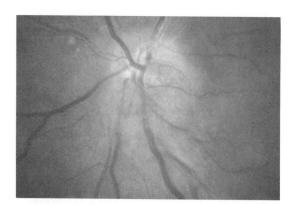 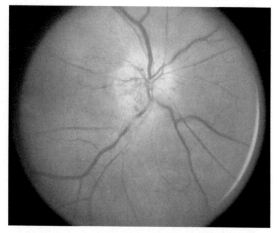

Figure 7.3. Segmental optic disc edema in AION. The optic disc is edematous with more prominent involvement inferiorly.

Figure 7.4. Parapapillary retinal arteriolar narrowing in AION. The vessels are focally attenuated overlying the disc, widening as they course toward the retinal periphery.

Table 7.2. *Ischemic Optic Neuropathies*

	Arteritic	Nonarteritic	Diabetic Papillopathy	Posterior
Age	Mean 70 yr	Mean 60 yr	Variable (<50)	Variable
Gender	F>M	F = M	F = M	F = M
Associated symptoms	Headache, jaw claudication, transient visual loss	Usually none	Usually none	None unless arteritic or postoperative
Visual acuity	<20/200 in >60%	>.20/60 in >50%	>.20/40 in >75%	Usually poor
Disc	Pale swelling common	Pale or hyperemic	Hyperemia, telangiectasia	Normal
	Cup normal + choroid ischemia	Cup small	Cup small	Variable
ESR	Mean 70 mm/hr	Usually normal	Usually normal	Elevated if arteritic
FA	Disc delay	Disc delay	Disc delay	Not studied
	Choroid delay			
Natural history	Rarely improve	16% to 42.7% improve	Resolves 2 to 10 mo	Rarely improves
	Fellow eye 54% to 95%	Fellow eye 12% to 19%	Bilateral 40%	Bilateral >60%
Treatment	Systemic steroids	None proven	None proven	Steroids if arteritic

optic disc and adjacent choroid (Fig. 7.8) is consistently noted and has been suggested as one useful factor in distinguishing arteritic from nonarteritic AION.

Giant cell arteritis is confirmed by a positive temporal artery biopsy, which is strongly recommended in any case of suspected arteritic AION. The certainty of biopsy-proven GCA provides support for long-term systemic corticosteroid therapy, which often is required for up to a year and may be associated with severe systemic complications. It also makes later decisions regarding the risk/benefit ratio of prolonged therapy more clearcut. A negative biopsy, however, does not rule out GCA. A false-negative biopsy may result from (a) discontinuous arterial involvement

("skip lesions"), undetected in 4% to 5% due to insufficient length (minimum 3 to 6 cm recommended) of specimen or insufficiently detailed step-sectioning; (b) unilateral involvement with biopsy of the uninvolved temporal artery; (c) improper handling of specimens; or (d) review by a pathologist inexperienced in the diagnosis of acute and healed arteritis.

The false-negative error rate for unilateral temporal artery biopsy has been estimated at 5% to 11%. Although the overall discordance rate for bilateral biopsies is low (1% to 3% in the largest series), there is substantial variation, even in major academic institutions with experienced pathologists, with rates as high as 13.4%. Considering the severe consequences of

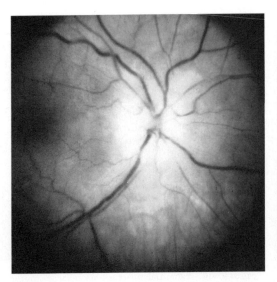 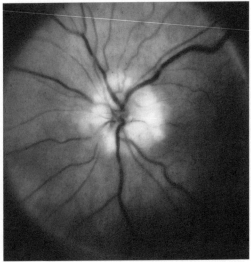

Figure 7.5. Bilateral simultaneous anterior ischemic optic neuropathy in a patient with GCA and no light perception in either eye. The right and left optic discs show markedly pale swelling.

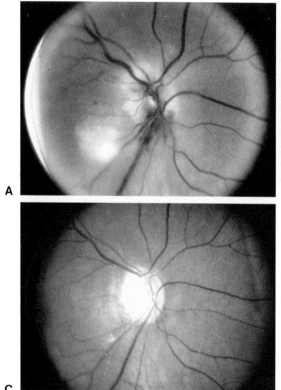

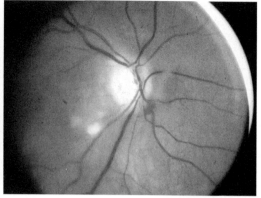

Figure 7.6. Progressive optic atrophy and pseudoglauco-matous cupping after an attack of AAION. **A:** Right optic disc at the time of initial visual loss. Note pale optic disc swelling, peripapillary hemorrhage, and cotton-wool spot. **B:** Eight weeks after visual loss, the optic disc swelling has re-solved, and both the hemorrhage and the cotton-wool spot are resolving. Note narrowing of retinal vessels. **C:** Four months after visual loss, the optic disc is pale and now has a large cup. The retinal vessels, especially the arteries, are markedly narrowed.

missed diagnosis, the relatively low risk of procedural complications, and the benefit of biopsy proof in the long-term management of these patients, we consider bilateral biopsy in all clinically suspicious cases.

Therapy

If GCA is suspected, therapy should be instituted im-mediately, as patients are at high risk for further vi-sual loss in the affected eye, involvement of the fellow eye, and systemic complications of vasculitis, includ-ing stroke and myocardial infarction. Initial treatment should not await diagnostic confirmation by tempo-ral artery biopsy. A delay of 7 to 10 days has no sig-nificant effect on the results. High-dose intravenous

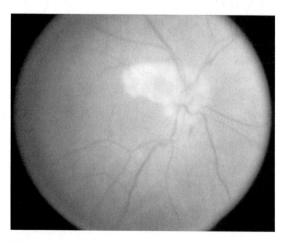

Figure 7.7. AAION with associated cilioretinal artery oc-clusion. In addition to the optic disc edema, there is a focus of retinal edema in the distribution of the cilioretinal artery.

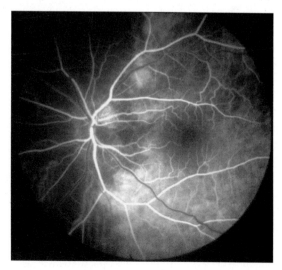

Figure 7.8. Fluorescein angiography in AAION. The optic disc and adjacent choroid show marked filling delay.

methylprednisolone at 1 g/day for the first 3 to 5 days is most often recommended, particularly when the patient is seen in the acute phase, because this mode of therapy produces higher blood levels of medication more rapidly than oral therapy. Because these patients are often elderly with multiple and complex medical problems, we routinely provide inpatient therapy under the supervision of an internist. Oral prednisone at doses of at least 1 mg/kg/day is recommended after intravenous therapy (or initially if the intravenous route is not used) and is tapered slowly, monitoring for control of systemic symptoms and ESR and CRP levels; therapy is usually maintained for at least 4 to 6 months, often up to a year.

Systemic symptoms typically subside within a week, a response so characteristic that if it is absent, an alternate disease process should be strongly considered. Alternate-day corticosteroid therapy is inadequate for GCA. Some degree of visual recovery in the affected eye may be obtained on therapy but is not generally anticipated. However, the major goal of therapy, other than prevention of systemic vascular complications, is to prevent contralateral visual loss. Thrombocytosis in GCA and its possible predisposition to visual loss suggests the possibility that antiplatelet therapy may be of benefit in conjunction with corticosteroids.

NONARTERITIC ANTERIOR ISCHEMIC OPTIC NEUROPATHY (NAION)

Most cases (95%) of AION are nonarteritic. NAION is the most common acute optic neuropathy in patients over 50 years of age with an estimated annual incidence in the United States of 2.3 to 10.2 per 100,000 population, which accounts for at least 6,000 new cases annually. The disease occurs with significantly higher frequency in the white population than in black or Hispanic individuals. There is no gender predisposition. The mean age at onset in most studies ranges from 57 to 65 years. In the Ischemic Optic Neuropathy Decompression Trial (IONDT), a multicenter prospective study of newly diagnosed patients with NAION begun in 1992, the mean age was 66 years and was probably somewhat biased by the exclusion criterion for patients under 50.

Clinical Presentation

NAION presents with loss of vision occurring over hours to days. Although some authors have proposed that visual loss from NAION is most frequently reported upon awakening, this was not confirmed in the IONDT. NAION typically presents without pain, although some form of periocular discomfort has been reported in 8% to 12%; in the IONDT, 10% reported minor ocular discomfort. In contrast to patients with optic neuritis, those with NAION usually do not report pain with eye movement. Headache and other symptoms associated with GCA are absent. Episodes of transient visual loss as seen in GCA are rare, but vague intermittent symptoms of blurring, shadows, or spots were reported in 5% of the patients in the IONDT. The initial course may be static with little or no fluctuation of visual level after initial loss or progressive with either episodic, stepwise decrements, or steady decline of vision over weeks prior to eventual stabilization. The progressive form has been reported in 22% to 37% of nonarteritic cases.

NAION usually presents with less severe visual loss than AAION, with visual acuity better than 20/200 in 58% to 66% of patients (Table 7.2). In the IONDT, 49% had initial visual acuity of at least 20/64, 66% better than 20/200. Color vision loss in NAION tends to parallel visual acuity loss, as opposed to that in optic neuritis, in which color loss is often disproportionately greater than visual acuity loss. Visual field defects in NAION may follow any pattern related to optic nerve damage, but altitudinal loss, usually inferior, occurs in the majority, ranging from 55% to 80% of reported cases.

The optic disc edema in NAION may be diffuse or segmental, hyperemic or pale, but pallor occurs less frequently than in the arteritic form. A focal region of more severe swelling is often seen and may display an altitudinal distribution, but it does not consistently correlate with the sector of visual field loss. In the IONDT, 25% of patients demonstrated sectoral disc edema. Focal hyperemic telangiectatic vessels may appear on the optic disc of an eye with NAION within days to weeks after the onset of symptoms. This phenomenon has been interpreted as luxury perfusion, which is a vascular autoregulatory response to ischemia characterized by dilation of blood vessels and increased perfusion of tissues in a region surrounding an infarct. It is associated with focal early disc hyperfluorescence and corresponds to a spared region of the visual field. In some instances, this vascular response is so impressive that it is misinterpreted as a capillary hemangioma or neovascularization of the disc. Peripapillary retinal hemorrhages are common (Fig. 7.9), seen in 72% in the IONDT. Retinal exudates are unusual, but both soft and hard exudates may occur (7% in the IONDT). The retinal arterioles are focally narrowed in the peripapillary region (Fig. 7.4) in up to 68% of the cases. The optic disc in the contralateral eye is typically small in diameter and demonstrates a small or absent physiologic cup (Fig. 7.9A). The disc appearance in such eyes has been described as the "disc at risk," referring to structural crowding of the axons at the level of the cribriform plate, associated mild

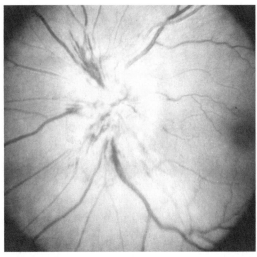

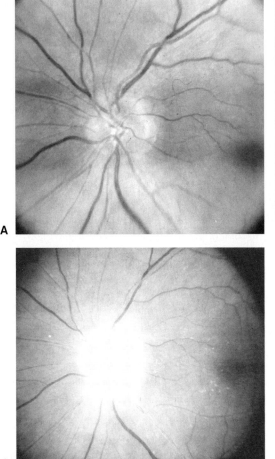

Figure 7.9. Development of optic atrophy after AION. **A:** Appearance of the left optic disc before visual symptoms in the left eye. The patient subsequently developed decreased vision in the left eye associated with an inferior altitudinal field defect. **B:** The left optic disc is swollen and hyperemic. There are numerous flame-shaped, peripapillary, intraretinal hemorrhages. **C:** Two months later, the left optic disc is diffusely pale, the retinal arteries are narrowed, and the nerve fiber layer is no longer visible.

disc elevation, and disc margin blurring without overt edema.

Histopathology and Pathophysiology

NAION is presumed to result from circulatory insufficiency within the optic nerve head, but the specific location of the vasculopathy and its pathogenetic mechanism remain unproven. Indeed, there has been no definite histopathologic documentation of the vasculopathy resulting in NAION. Implication of both the posterior ciliary arteries and the choroid has been based on indirect evidence. Recent data suggest that vasculopathy within the paroptic branches of the short posterior ciliary arteries may play a major role with resultant infarctions predominantly located in the retrolaminar region of the optic nerve head. Although carotid occlusive disease occasionally results in optic nerve ischemia, most often in the setting of more general ocular ischemia and occasionally with associated cerebral ischemia, the vast majority of cases of NAION are unrelated to carotid disease.

The mechanisms involved in the development of optic disc ischemia in NAION similarly remain unclear. Whether ischemia results from local arteriosclerosis with or without thrombosis, embolization from a remote source, generalized hypoperfusion, vasospasm, failure of autoregulation, or some combination of these processes is not known. Although structurally small, "crowded" optic discs are associated with NAION, the mechanism by which this contributes to ischemia (perhaps via a compartment syndrome) has not been fully elucidated. The role of additional factors such as nocturnal hypotension and sleep apnea is unproven. Multiple risk factors for vasculopathy and coagulopathy have been associated with NAION, but conclusive large-scale epidemiologic studies have not been performed (Table 7.1). Whatever the cause for impaired blood flow in the optic nerve vasculature, persistent hypoperfusion may require impairment in the normal autoregulatory mechanisms of the optic nerve head.

NAION has been reported in association with many conditions that may predispose to decreased optic nerve head perfusion via microvascular occlusion. Several cross-sectional case series have estimated the prevalence of systemic diseases that might predispose to vasculopathy in patients with NAION. Systemic hypertension was documented in 34% to 50% of patients (47% in the IONDT). Diabetes was reported in 5% to 25% (24% in the IONDT), with statistically significant increased prevalence in all ages in all but one study. Diabetes was associated with the development of NAION at a younger age in most series as well. The association of NAION with other vascular events, such as stroke and myocardial infarction, and with other vascular risk factors, such as smoking, hypercholesterolemia, hypertriglyceridemia, hyperhomocysteinemia and prothrombotic factors, is inconsistent.

NAION has been associated infrequently with a multitude of additional factors and disorders that may be causative, either due to optic disc structure or other features that might affect optic disc perfusion pressure, including hyperopia, optic disc drusen, elevated intraocular pressure, cataract surgery, and migraine. Two medications have been associated with the development of NAION (interferon-alpha and sildenafil), although the number of cases is insufficient to confirm a definite causative effect. Amiodarone may produce a toxic optic neuropathy that mimics NAION or may trigger NAION in the susceptible individual (see Chapter 10).

Clinical Course

Untreated, NAION generally remains stable; most cases show no significant improvement or deterioration over time. Even in the so-called progressive form, further deterioration after reaching the low point of visual function within 1 to 2 months is rare. Some spontaneous improvement of visual acuity, however, is not unusual. In the IONDT, recovery of at least 3 Snellen acuity lines was found in 42.7% of patients who had initial visual acuity worse than 20/64. Visual acuity at 6 months was 20/200 or worse in 52% of the randomized (initial visual acuity 20/64 or worse) patients in the IONDT. Other studies, which included patients with better initial acuity, reported 31% to 41% of patients with final visual acuity 20/200 or worse and 21% to 53% of patients having vision 20/200 or better. After stabilization of vision, usually within 2 months, recurrent or progressive visual loss in an affected eye is extremely unusual and should prompt evaluation for another cause of optic neuropathy.

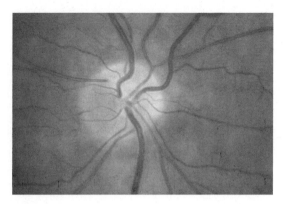

Figure 7.10. Sectoral optic atrophy after NAION.

The optic disc becomes visibly atrophic, either in a sectoral (Fig. 7.10) or diffuse pattern (see Fig. 7.9*C*), usually within 4 to 6 weeks. Persistence of edema past this point should prompt consideration of an alternate diagnosis. Eventual involvement of the contralateral eye was reported in 14.7% of patients in the IONDT after a median follow-up of 5 years. A history of diabetes and baseline visual acuity of 20/200 or worse in the study eye, but not age, sex, aspirin use, or smoking were significantly associated with new NAION in the fellow eye. The IONDT found second-eye visual acuity within three lines of the first in approximately half of patients.

Occurrence in the second eye produces the clinical appearance of the "pseudo-Foster Kennedy syndrome," in which the previously affected disc is atrophic and the currently involved nerve head is edematous. Significantly impaired visual function in the eye with disc edema distinguishes this condition from the true Foster Kennedy syndrome, in which disc edema is due to elevated intracranial pressure and therefore does not produce visual loss acutely in the edematous eye.

Diagnosis

NAION must be differentiated from idiopathic optic neuritis, syphilitic or sarcoid-related optic nerve inflammation, particularly in patients under 50 years of age; infiltrative optic neuropathies, anterior orbital lesions producing optic nerve compression; and idiopathic forms of optic disc edema, including diabetic papillopathy.

In patients with a typical presentation of NAION, without symptoms or signs to suggest GCA, and with normal ESR and C-reactive protein levels, we do not routinely perform additional testing. Evaluation by a primary care physician for evidence and control of risk factors, such as hypertension, diabetes, and hyperlipidemia, is essential. Neuroimaging is not performed unless the patient presents with substantial pain or follows an atypical course, such as prolonged optic disc edema or continued progressive or recurrent visual loss more than 2 months after initial presentation. The value of additional testing for vasculopathic and prothrombotic risk factors remains unclear. Carotid studies are not routinely performed unless prominent pain or other signs of orbital ischemia are present. For NAION in the typical age group, we do not routinely assess homocysteine levels, but in patients under 50, we proceed with this testing because elevated levels are amenable to therapy. We do not test for prothrombotic risk factors unless there is other evidence of personal or familial thrombosis, and we do not screen for vasculitides other than GCA unless there is clinical evidence for them.

Therapy

There is no proven effective therapy for NAION. No medications have been proven useful in the acute phase, and in the IONDT, optic nerve sheath decompression surgery for NAION was not beneficial and was potentially harmful. Similarly, there is no proven prophylactic measure for NAION. Although aspirin has a proven effect in reducing stroke and myocardial infarction in patients at risk, published data regarding its role in decreasing the severity of optic neuropathy and the incidence of fellow-eye involvement after the initial episode show no consistent positive effect. However, many experts recommend the use of aspirin after an initial episode of NAION, if only for its role in decreasing risk for stroke and myocardial infarction in this vasculopathic population group. The risk for subsequent stroke, myocardial infarction, and death in patients with NAION has been incompletely studied.

POSTERIOR ISCHEMIC OPTIC NEUROPATHY

Although the anterior form of ION is far more common than the posterior variety, ischemia of the retrobulbar portions of the optic nerve occurs in many settings, both arteritic and nonarteritic. Ischemia can independently affect the posterior portion of the optic nerve because of the distinct and separate arterial supplies of the anterior and posterior portions of the optic nerve. The anterior optic nerve is supplied by the short posterior ciliary artery and choroidal circulations, while the retrobulbar optic nerve is supplied intraorbitally by a pial plexus arising from the ophthalmic artery and intracranially by branches of the ipsilateral internal carotid, anterior cerebral, and anterior communicating arteries.

Posterior ischemic optic neuropathy (PION) is a syndrome of acute visual loss with characteristics of optic neuropathy without initial disc edema and marked by the subsequent development of optic atrophy. Occasionally, a small amount of disc edema appears within the first week or so after acute visual loss, presumably as a result of propagation of swelling forward along the course of the optic nerve from the point of original ischemia. The diagnosis of PION is most often made in one of the following settings:

1. GCA or rarely other vasculitides such as herpes zoster, polyarteritis nodosa, or lupus erythematosus. Indeed, evaluation for GCA is essential in cases without other apparent cause and should be the primary consideration with this presentation in the elderly, with urgent ancillary testing as described earlier for AION (see above).
2. Nonarteritic PION in a population of patients with similar demographics to those patients with NAION.
3. Related to surgery (coronary artery bypass and lumbar spine procedures most frequently reported), or severe bleeding, or hypotension (as seen in cases of gastrointestinal hemorrhage or trauma; see below).

The differential diagnosis includes compressive and infiltrative optic neuropathies, although the onset in PION is typically more abrupt. In all cases, neuroimaging is indicated to rule out these possibilities. NAION typically shows no enhancement of the optic nerves on magnetic resonance (MR), presumably due to limitation to the optic nerve head. PION also typically shows no abnormalities of the optic nerves, except in cases of GCA PION in which enhancement has been demonstrated and must be differentiated from other causes, such as inflammation and infiltration.

In a recent multicenter, retrospective review covering 22 years, 72 patients with PION were classified into the three groups: perioperative PION, arteritic PION, and nonarteritic PION. The nonarteritic group accounted for 38 of the 72 patients, exhibited similar risk factors, and followed a clinical course precisely like that of NAION. In contrast to perioperative and arteritic PION, which were characterized by severe visual loss with little or no recovery, nonarteritic PION was less severe and showed improvement in 34% of the patients. It is important to recognize this nonarteritic form in patients with acute optic neuropathy but no optic disc edema, a scenario that may be mistaken for optic neuritis. Such patients, as in some patients with AION and disc edema, particularly those with ischemic white matter lesions on MR imaging, might be incorrectly started on immunomodulatory therapy to reduce the risk of multiple sclerosis. PION differs from optic neuritis by its occurrence in older age groups and its lack of pain on eye movements.

ISCHEMIC OPTIC NEUROPATHY IN SETTINGS OF HEMODYNAMIC COMPROMISE

Systemic hypotension, blood loss, and anemia may produce optic nerve ischemia. The most commonly reported causes of blood loss associated with ION are (a) spontaneous gastrointestinal or uterine bleeding and (b) surgically induced hemorrhage, related most frequently to cardiac bypass or lumbar spine procedures. Less often, hypotensive episodes in the setting of chronic anemia without blood loss (as in chronic hemodialysis) may result in ION.

The optic neuropathy that occurs in these settings is typically bilateral, although unilateral cases occur. Visual loss is often severe. AION (with optic disc edema) accounts for the majority of cases, although PION is not infrequent. Visual loss may occur immediately after the episode or may be delayed as much as 2 to 3 weeks in cases of AION. It has been postulated that delayed visual loss is caused by vasoconstriction in the ciliary artery system secondary to activation of the renin-angiotensin pathway as a late response to blood loss.

Patients in whom visual loss occurs after **spontaneous hemorrhage** are usually 40- to 60-years-old and debilitated. Most of these patients have experienced repeated episodes of bleeding, but cases following a single episode of massive hemorrhage with secondary hypotension have been reported. The visual loss is usually bilateral, but it may affect both eyes asymmetrically or be unilateral, and any degree of visual loss is possible. Both AION and PION have been reported in this setting, although AION is more common. The most frequent sites are the gastrointestinal tract in men and the uterus in women. A combination of both anemia and hypotension is frequently present when visual loss occurs in this setting (Fig. 7.11).

ION occurs in the setting of various surgical interventions, most commonly cardiopulmonary bypass, and lumbar spine surgery. Indeed, lumbar spine surgery may carry an increased risk for postoperative ION, usually PION, compared with other surgeries. Proposed risk factors for **perioperative ION** include prolonged surgeries in the prone position with orbitofacial vascular congestion, anemia, blood loss, hypotension, hemodilution, hypovolemia, hypoxia, and use of vasoconstricting agents. The purposeful maintenance of relative systemic hypotension to control intraoperative hemorrhage and the prolonged prone position may be significant features in the development of some cases of perioperative ION, although it remains a rare occurrence in a common surgical procedure.

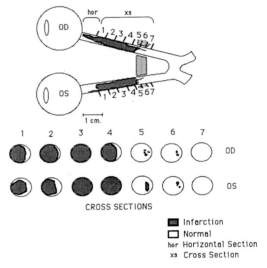

Figure 7.11. Schematic illustration of extent of optic nerve infarction in a patient with chronic anemia and massive intraoperative hemorrhage with hypotension. Note that the main region of infarction in both nerves is in the midorbital portion. (Reprinted from: Johnson MW, Kincaid MC, Trobe JD. Bilateral retrobulbar optic nerve infarctions after blood loss and hypotension. *Ophthalmology.* 1987;94:1577–1584, with permission.)

Although aggressive fluid replacement and transfusion of blood products seem appropriate in cases where deficiencies are detected, there are no controlled studies of these interventions, and no therapy has been proven to significantly improve visual outcome in perioperative ION. To help understand the multiple and likely complicated interacting factors underlying perioperative ION, the American Society of Anesthesiologists (ASA) established the international ASA Postoperative Visual Loss (POVL) Registry in 1999 with the goal of acquiring a large database with detailed information on patient characteristics and perioperative conditions. Preliminary results confirm that at least two thirds of cases are associated with spine surgery and that ION can occur even with the head suspended in Mayfield tongs with no external compression of the eyes and face. Indeed, perioperative ION can occur in young patients, with relatively short prone durations, with little blood loss, a normal hematocrit, and without hypotension. Clearly there is more we need to learn regarding the cause of this potentially devastating disorder.

It is important to distinguish visual loss from postoperative ION with associated facial edema from the prolonged prone position from those cases of visual loss secondary to direct compression of the eye from malpositioning. In the latter cases, which have been termed the *headrest syndrome,*, direct compression results in ocular ischemia, with severe orbital congestion, ecchymoses, and most often central retinal artery occlusion.

ION related to **hypotension** most often presents in patients with chronic renal failure and dialysis. The hypotension may be acute, temporally associated with the dialysis procedure, or it may be chronic. Most patients also are chronically anemic. The accelerated diffuse vasculopathy that occurs in this disease may predispose to the development of ION, as may previous chronic hypertension, with possible arteriosclerosis and impaired autoregulation of the optic disc vascular supply. Visual loss from hypotension-induced ischemia in this setting may respond to rapid volume replacement and restoration of normotension.

RADIATION OPTIC NEUROPATHY

Radiation optic neuropathy (RON) is thought to be an ischemic disorder of the optic nerve that usually results in irreversible severe visual loss months to years after radiation therapy to the brain and orbit. It is most often a retrobulbar process. RON occurs most frequently after irradiation of paranasal sinus and other skull base malignancies, but it may develop after radiation treatment for pituitary adenomas, parasellar meningiomas, craniopharyngiomas, frontal and temporal gliomas, and intraocular tumors. It has also been reported after low-dose radiation therapy for dysthyroid orbitopathy, although only in patients with diabetes mellitus. Pathologic specimens of optic nerves with RON show ischemic demyelination, reactive astrocytosis, endothelial hyperplasia, obliterative endarteritis, and fibrinoid necrosis, reflecting the presumed pathogenesis of both direct effects to replicating glial tissue and secondary effects from damage to vascular endothelial cells. The risk of RON appears to increase significantly at doses over 50 Gy, but both the total dose of radiation given and the daily fractionation size are important factors in determining the risk of delayed radiation necrosis in the central nervous system. However, RON should be considered even in situations where "safe" doses of radiation therapy have supposedly been administered, especially in optic nerves already compromised by tumor compression or chemotherapy.

The syndrome typically presents with acute, painless visual loss in one or both eyes. Visual loss in one eye may be rapidly followed by visual loss in the fellow eye. Episodes of transient visual loss may precede the onset of RON by several weeks. The onset of visual symptoms associated with RON may be as short as 3 months or as long as 8 years after radiation therapy, but most cases occur within 3 years after radiation

with a peak at 1.5 years. Visual acuity loss ranges widely and progression of visual loss over weeks to months is common. Spontaneous visual recovery is unusual. Final vision is no light perception in 45% with a total of 85% of reported eyes with RON having final visual acuity of 20/200 or worse.

The affected optic disc is often pale initially, which is related to prior damage from the tumor with possible superimposed radiation injury; less frequently it is edematous. Cases with disc edema at onset often have associated radiation retinopathy, with cotton-wool patches, hard exudates, and retinal hemorrhages, secondary to irradiation of intraocular or orbital structures. The visual field may show altitudinal loss or a central scotoma. A junctional syndrome with an optic neuropathy and contralateral temporal hemianopia may occur in patients with damage to the distal optic nerve. Patients with radionecrosis of the optic chiasm typically develop a bitemporal hemianopia that initially may suggest recurrence of the tumor for which the patient was initially irradiated, but superimposed optic neuropathy may involve the nasal visual fields as well.

The differential diagnosis of RON includes recurrence of the primary tumor, secondary empty sella syndrome with optic nerve and chiasmal prolapse, arachnoiditis, and radiation-induced parasellar tumor. These conditions typically present with slowly progressive visual loss rather than the rapid onset of RON. MRI (magnetic resonance imaging) is the diagnostic procedure of choice to distinguish tumor recurrence from RON. In RON, the unenhanced T1- and T2-weighted images may show no abnormality, but on T1-weighted enhanced images (Fig. 7.12), there is marked enhancement of the optic nerves, optic chiasm, and even the optic tracts in some cases. The enhancement usually resolves in several months, at which time visual function usually stabilizes. Occasionally, enhancement may even precede visual loss.

Treatment for RON is controversial. Although delayed radionecrosis in the central nervous system can be treated with some success with systemic corticosteroids, which are effective in reducing tissue edema and may have some beneficial effect on demyelination, their use in RON, in oral or intravenous form, has produced disappointing results. Similarly, the use of anticoagulation to reverse or stabilize central nervous system radionecrosis does not appear to provide significant benefit in patients with RON. To the extent that RON is an ischemic process, hyperbaric oxygen therapy has a theoretical basis for effectiveness, but clinical results are not uniform. Visual improvement has been documented with therapy only in those treated within 72 hours; after 2 weeks, therapy is most likely ineffective.

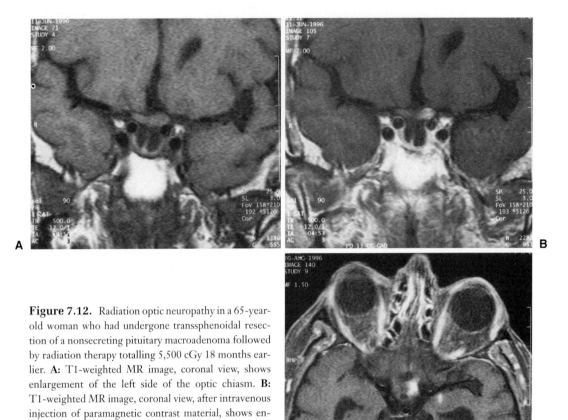

Figure 7.12. Radiation optic neuropathy in a 65-year-old woman who had undergone transsphenoidal resection of a nonsecreting pituitary macroadenoma followed by radiation therapy totalling 5,500 cGy 18 months earlier. **A:** T1-weighted MR image, coronal view, shows enlargement of the left side of the optic chiasm. **B:** T1-weighted MR image, coronal view, after intravenous injection of paramagnetic contrast material, shows enhancement of the enlarged region. **C:** T1-weighted MR image, axial view, after intravenous injection of paramagnetic contrast material, shows enhancement and enlargement of the distal portion of the left optic nerve and the left side of the optic chiasm.

ISCHEMIC OPTIC DISC EDEMA WITH MINIMAL DYSFUNCTION

Patients may develop **disc swelling from NAION before** they have **any visual symptoms.** In such cases, the patient may be thought to have papilledema or a compressive optic neuropathy from an orbital mass. Often, however, the asymptomatic disc swelling is noted in the fellow eye of a patient with a history of a previous attack of NAION, and the diagnosis is less confusing. On the basis of vasculopathic risk factors, lack of evidence for other causes of disc edema, evidence of AION in the fellow eye, and the later development in some patients of AION in the asymptomatically edematous eye, the disc edema has been presumed ischemic in origin.

An atypical form of NAION called **diabetic papillopathy** occurs most commonly in young diabetic patients. In most instances, transient unilateral or bilateral disc swelling develops in a juvenile diabetic who has minimal if any visual symptoms, and the swelling resolves spontaneously within several weeks. In some cases, there is a transient arcuate field defect; in others, the field defect persists. In most cases, however, there is only enlargement of the blind spot. When visual acuity is initially affected, it usually recovers as the disc swelling resolves. Eyes with diabetic papillopathy usually show prominent, dilated, telangiectatic vessels over the disc that mimic optic disc neovascularization (Fig. 7.13) but do not share the same fluorescein angiographic features. This phenomenon is akin to the luxury perfusion phenomenon described after typical NAION. As disc swelling resolves, these vessels usually disappear, although they may occasionally persist. Diabetic papillopathy may develop in eyes with evidence of both preproliferative and proliferative diabetic retinopathy as well as in eyes with no evidence of retinopathy.

Patients with juvenile diabetes mellitus may also develop typical NAION, with persistent decrease in visual acuity and permanent visual field defects. In

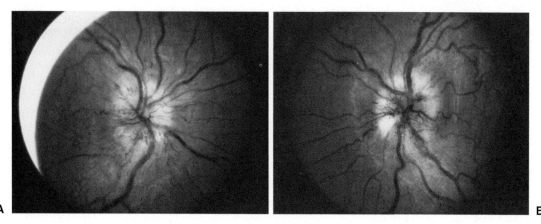

A   B

Figure 7.13. Appearance of diabetic papillopathy. The patient was an 18-year-old man with juvenile diabetes mellitus who was noted to have optic disc swelling during a routine eye examination. He had no visual complaints. Note dilated telangiectatic vessels mimicking neovascularization on the surface of both the right **(A)** and left **(B)** optic discs.

some patients, true disc neovascularization develops after resolution of visual symptoms and disc swelling. Although diabetic papillopathy was initially described in juvenile diabetics, the condition also may occur in patients with adult-onset diabetes mellitus. Patients with diabetic papillopathy, like patients with typical NAION, have a disc at risk. Thus, although the clinical features of diabetic papillopathy are different from those of typical NAION, this condi-tion probably is a variant of NAION with a similar pathogenesis.

FOR FURTHER INFORMATION

See *Walsh & Hoyt's Clinical Neuro-Ophthalmology*, 6th edition, Volume 1, Chapter 7, pages 349–384; Volume 2, Chapter 40, pages 2052–2053; and Chapter 44, pages 2347–2365.

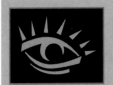

CHAPTER 8

Compressive and Infiltrative Optic Neuropathies*

COMPRESSIVE OPTIC NEUROPATHIES

COMPRESSIVE OPTIC NEUROPATHIES WITH OPTIC DISC SWELLING (ANTERIOR COMPRESSIVE OPTIC NEUROPATHIES)

Lesions within the orbit, occasionally within the optic canal, and extremely rarely intracranially, may compress the optic nerve, resulting in optic disc swelling (Fig. 8.1). Such lesions include tumors, infections, inflammations, and even adnexal structures that have become swollen or enlarged by disease. Specific orbital disorders include optic gliomas, meningiomas, hamartomas (e.g., hemangiomas, lymphangiomas), choristomas (e.g., dermoid cysts), and other malignancies (e.g., carcinoma, lymphoma, sarcoma, multiple myeloma), as well as inflammatory orbital pseudotumor and thyroid ophthalmopathy.

In most cases of anterior compressive optic neuropathy, there is progressive visual loss associated with proptosis; however, in many patients, visual acuity remains normal or near normal, and there is almost no external evidence of orbital disease despite obvious disc swelling. This clinical picture occurs particularly in patients with orbital hemangiomas adjacent to the optic nerve and in patients with primary optic nerve sheath meningiomas. In such patients, careful testing of color vision may reveal subtle defects, and there may occasionally be a relative afferent pupillary defect despite retention of normal acuity. The visual field of the affected eye generally shows only enlargement of the

blind spot or minimal reduction in the mean deviation on automated perimetry. When other signs of orbital disease are not present (e.g., proptosis, limitation of ocular motility, orbital congestion), these patients may be thought to have unilateral papilledema from increased intracranial pressure. Although it is obvious that patients with slowly progressive, unilateral visual loss and proptosis associated with disc swelling should undergo evaluation for a possible orbital lesion, patients with unilateral optic disc swelling without signs of intraocular inflammation and *without* visual loss or other evidence of an optic neuropathy should also undergo such an evaluation, particularly when there are no systemic or neurologic symptoms or signs of increased intracranial pressure. Orbital disease is the most common cause of unilateral disc swelling without visual loss.

In addition to proptosis, congestion, and limitation of ocular motility, patients with orbital disease may develop various folds or striae that occur at the posterior pole, adjacent to the optic disc (Fig. 8.2). These folds may be horizontal or vertical. Transient monocular visual loss can occur in patients with orbital lesions. The visual loss usually occurs only in certain positions of gaze, and vision immediately clears when the direction of gaze is changed. It is assumed that either direct pressure on the optic nerve or interruption of blood supply is responsible for this phenomenon.

Computed tomographic (CT) scanning, magnetic resonance imaging (MRI) offer superb topographic depiction (size, shape, and location) of lesions, and standardized echography provides supplementary information that often helps in refinement of the differential diagnosis. CT scanning is particularly useful for imaging bone, calcium, and metallic foreign bodies (suspicion of the latter being a contraindication for the use of MRI), whereas MRI excels at defining inflammatory and intrinsic disease of the visual pathway and parasellar area. MRI is particularly suited to imaging

---

*Adapted from Volpe NJ. Compressive and infiltrative optic neuropathies. In: Miller NR, Newman NJ, Biousse V, Kerrison JB, eds. *Walsh & Hoyt's Clinical Neuro-Ophthalmology.* 6th ed. Vol. I. Philadelphia: Lippincott Williams & Wilkins; 2005:385–429.

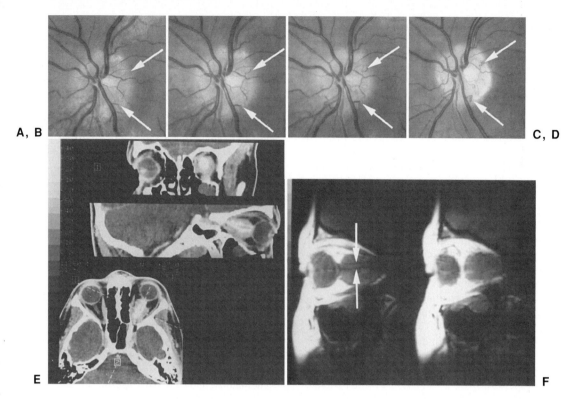

Figure 8.1. Optociliary shunt veins in a patient with optic nerve sheath meningioma. **A–D:** Progressive development of optociliary shunt veins (*arrows*) from the stage of chronic disc swelling **(A)**, through intermediate stages of shunt vein formation **(B and C)**, to the final stage of optic atrophy with fully formed optociliary shunts **(D)**. Neuroimaging with computed tomographic (CT) scanning and magnetic resonance imaging (MRI) provides complementary information. Calcified psammoma bodies in the tumor produce a well-delineated "tram-track" sign in the contrast-enhanced, reconstructed CT images **(E)**, whereas MRI with surface coil (T1-weighted, without fat suppression or enhancement) **(F)** clearly defines the nerve surrounded by tumor (*arrows*).

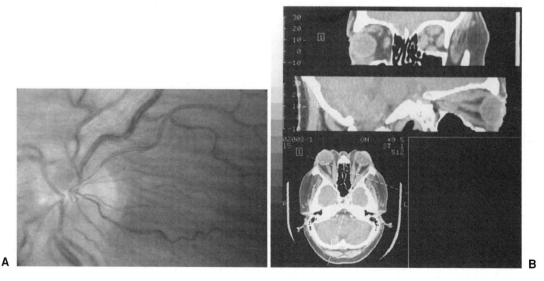

Figure 8.2. Optic disc swelling and choroidal folds in thyroid eye disease. **A:** The left optic disc shows mild hyperemia, swelling, and blurring of the peripapillary retinal nerve fiber layer at the upper and lower poles. Horizontal chorioretinal folds extend across the posterior pole toward the macula. **B:** Coronal and off-axis sagittal reconstructed CT scans show greatly enlarged extraocular muscles surrounding the optic nerve within the orbit. Note that the muscles actually appear to be in contact with the nerve.

the intracanalicular optic nerve. With the use of fat-saturation techniques and gadolinium, demarcation of optic nerve sheath meningiomas can be optimized.

When inflammatory conditions involve the orbit, especially the nonspecific condition called **"idiopathic inflammatory pseudotumor,"** the optic nerve may be compressed with secondary disc swelling. Affected patients usually experience visual loss, pain, proptosis, and congestion, and the presence of an orbital process is rarely in question. Infrequently, meningiomas of the orbital apex produce a similar clinical picture.

Patients with **thyroid eye disease** may develop evidence of a compressive optic neuropathy associated with optic disc swelling (Fig. 8.2). In such patients, congestive symptoms almost always precede visual loss, which is usually bilateral, symmetric, and gradual in onset. Presenting visual acuities are usually 20/60 or worse, with central scotomas often combined with arcuate defects. The compressive etiology of the optic neuropathy in dysthyroid optic neuropathy can be seen on CT which demonstrates moderate to severe enlargement of the extraocular muscles at the orbital apex (Fig. 8.2). Treatment options for thyroid-associated compressive optic neuropathy include intravenous or oral steroids and orbital decompression. Radiation therapy may also be effective, but its effects are often delayed and therefore more acutely effective treatments with steroids or surgery should be given in conjunction with radiation.

Anterior compressive optic neuropathy may result from primary **optic nerve sheath meningioma** (ONSM). Optic nerve sheath meningiomas surround the optic nerve and result in impaired axonal transport (leading to disc swelling) and also interfere with the pial blood supply to the optic nerve. The tumor occurs most commonly in middle-aged women and is usually unilateral. Patients present with slowly progressive vision loss, mild proptosis, double vision, transient visual obscurations, and gaze-evoked amaurosis. Examination reveals a color vision defect, afferent pupillary defect, and visual field defects including central scotomas, enlarged blind spots, and generalized constriction. The optic nerve appears abnormal with either optic atrophy and/or disc edema. Optociliary collateral vessels may be present and are seen in both swollen and atrophic nerves (Fig. 8.1) (see Chapter 4).

Neuroimaging demonstrates focal or diffuse, tubular or fusiform, optic nerve enlargement (Fig. 8.1). MRI is often diagnostic, showing the tumor to be separate from the optic nerve proper on coronal views, allowing distinction from gliomas. MRI is particularly good at imaging the intracanalicular optic nerve and delineating the extent of intracranial extension of the ONSM. On CT, calcification can be seen in one third of patients as linear bright lines extending over the length of the optic nerve (tram track sign). Clinical findings and neuroimaging generally establish the diagnosis and biopsy is almost never needed. In the rare equivocal case, biopsy is only recommended in an eye with poor vision, after a systemic work-up and serial lumbar punctures exclude inflammatory disorders and neoplasms, and after steroids fail to improve vision.

Natural history data suggest that ONSMs can remain stable or improve over several years. If progression is documented, radiation therapy is the best treatment available. Surgical excision of these lesions to improve vision is usually not possible because of the tumor involvement of the pial blood supply to the optic nerve. Portions of the tumor are occasionally removed to treat blind or uncomfortable eyes (proptosis), to decompress associated mass effect, or reduce the risk of intracranial extension.

Patients with meningiomas confined entirely to the optic canal may occasionally present with blurred vision and optic disc swelling (112). The mechanism by which disc swelling occurs in such cases is not clear, but it presumably results from direct compression of the optic nerve with blockage of axonal transport. Less common than optic disc swelling from an intracanalicular lesion is optic disc swelling from compression of the *intracranial portion* of the optic nerve.

Intracranial lesions, particularly sphenoid wing meningiomas, not infrequently extend through the optic canal, compressing the intracranial, intracanalicular, and intraorbital optic nerve in the process. Optic disc changes, from swelling to pallor, may be minimal in such cases, even when the lesion is quite large (Fig. 8.3).

COMPRESSIVE OPTIC NEUROPATHIES WITHOUT OPTIC DISC SWELLING (RETROBULBAR COMPRESSIVE OPTIC NEUROPATHIES)

The importance of early diagnosis of compressive lesions that affect the retrobulbar portions of the optic nerve and do not cause optic disc swelling cannot be overemphasized. Early decompression of the optic nerves or chiasm may result in significant return of visual function, whereas delayed diagnosis may result in progressive visual failure and irreversible visual loss, neurologic dysfunction, or death. Intracranial, intracanalicular, and occasionally posterior orbital compressive lesions usually do not produce disc swelling or significant neurologic or systemic manifestations. Thus, by the time such lesions cause visible optic pallor, significant damage to the optic nerve has often already occurred, preventing return of visual function even with otherwise successful decompression. The physician managing a patient with unexplained unilateral visual loss must be aware of the characteristic history and early findings in patients with a retrobulbar compressive optic neuropathy.

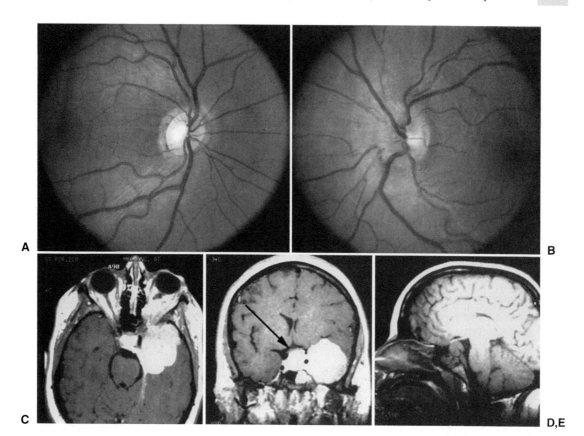

Figure 8.3. Optic disc swelling in a patient with a large meningioma with intraorbital, intracanalicular, and intracranial components. The patient was a 21-year-old woman who experienced reduced vision in the left eye during pregnancy. **A:** Normal right optic disc. **B:** Mild swelling of left optic disc. **C:** T1-weighted MRI, axial view, obtained after intravenous injection with gadolinium-DTPA shows a large mass involving the left sphenoid wing and posterior orbit. Although both coronal (**D**) and sagittal (**E**) images clearly show compression of the optic chiasm by the tumor (*arrow*), the resulting visual field defect was purely unilateral, affecting only the left eye.

In cases of prechiasmal optic nerve compression, progressive, painless dimming of vision is noted at an early stage. Although these patients may read the 20/25 or even 20/20 Snellen letters with the affected eye, they do so slowly and with great difficulty compared with the ease with which they read the 20/15 line with the opposite eye. There is usually some type of visual field defect, particularly when tested with automated perimetry, but the nature of the defect does not, in itself, suggest the etiology of the visual loss. Compression of the optic nerve may produce *any* type of field defect, including an altitudinal, arcuate, hemianopic, central, or cecocentral scotoma. Although a hemianopic field defect or a "junctional" scotoma in the superior temporal field of the opposite eye strongly suggests a compressive lesion, it is the insidious, progressive nature of the symptoms that is most often the critical feature of the compressive process.

Two important abnormalities that are nearly always present in a patient with a retrobulbar compressive optic neuropathy are unilateral dyschromatopsia and an ipsilateral relative afferent pupillary defect. The afferent defect is usually obvious even when visual acuity is minimally reduced and provides the observer with absolute evidence that the visual difficulty is caused by something other than a simple refractive error, incipient cataract, or minimum macular disease. After a relative afferent pupillary defect is detected in a patient with an apparently normal fundus who is complaining of progressive dimming of vision, compression must be ruled out by neuroimaging, preferably MRI. Despite the almost universal availability of neuroimaging, however, it is astonishing that patients with progressive visual loss from compressive optic neuropathy continue to be diagnosed with macular degeneration, cataract, glaucoma, or "chronic optic neuritis."

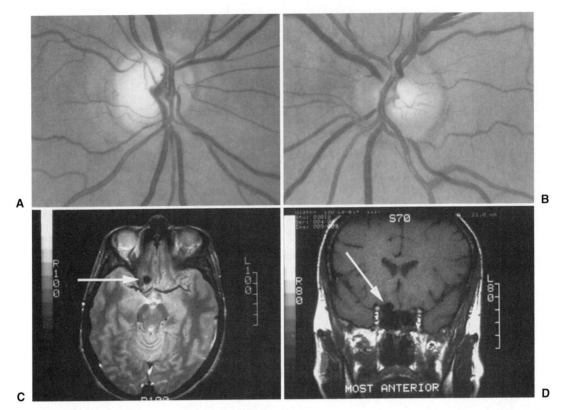

Figure 8.4. Optic disc cupping in a patient with aneurysmal compression. The patient was a 55-year-old woman who suddenly lost the inferior field in the right eye after suffering mild head trauma in a motor vehicle accident 8 days earlier. **A:** Cupped and pale right optic disc. **B:** Normal left optic disc. **C and D:** Magnetic resonance images, axial **(C)** and coronal **(D)** views, revealing flow void (*arrows*) in a carotid-ophthalmic aneurysm that is compressing the right optic nerve.

The optic disc of a patient with a compressive optic neuropathy may appear normal or show a variable degree of pallor. Asymmetric cupping of the optic disc is not usually a prominent feature, but it may occur and be quite prominent in some patients (Fig. 8.4). In such cases, the visual loss may be thought to have resulted from glaucoma, particularly when there is an arcuate defect, but pallor of the neuroretinal rim indicates the nonglaucomatous nature of the lesion. Optic atrophy in one eye and disc swelling in the other may result from asymmetric optic nerve compression or from tumor-induced direct optic nerve compression in one eye and papilledema from increased intracranial pressure in the other (Foster Kennedy syndrome) (see Chapter 4).

Causes of retrobulbar optic nerve compression include: intraorbital and intracranial benign and malignant tumors (most commonly pituitary tumors, meningiomas and craniopharyngiomas); aneurysms (Fig. 8.4); inflammatory lesions (particularly of the paranasal sinuses); primary bone disease (e.g., osteopetrosis, fibrous dysplasia, craniometaphyseal dysplasia, Paget's

disease); orbital fractures; dolichoectatic intracranial vessels; congenital and acquired hydrocephalus; thyroid eye disease; and orbital hemorrhage. Meningiomas arising from the planum sphenoidale or olfactory groove, pituitary tumors, and aneurysms are the most commonly identified lesions causing retrobulbar compressive optic neuropathy without disc swelling.

The **sudden onset of unilateral visual loss,** combined with signs of retrobulbar optic nerve dysfunction, usually suggests a diagnosis of optic neuritis or ischemic optic neuropathy. In rare instances, however, compressive lesions produce acute monocular visual loss, presumably from hemorrhage or from sudden interruption of the vascular supply to the optic nerve. This phenomenon probably occurs most frequently in patients with pituitary apoplexy, but it has also been reported in patients with pituitary tumors and meningiomas during pregnancy and in otherwise healthy patients upon awakening. Sudden onset of monocular visual loss can also occur from a ruptured ophthalmic artery aneurysm, fibrous dysplasia, orbital hemorrhage, subperiosteal abscess, orbital cellulites, and mucocele (particularly of the sphenoid sinus).

VISUAL RECOVERY FOLLOWING DECOMPRESSION

Restoration of visual function is not only possible following surgical decompression, but it can begin within hours to days after surgery, sometimes with full recovery. "Medical decompression" of the optic nerve with bromocriptine in patients with prolactin-secreting pituitary tumors has yielded similar improvements in visual function. Although it is not surprising that prompt decompression may restore visual function in patients rendered suddenly blind by pituitary apoplexy, it is not intuitively obvious that patients who have lost all light perception for days or weeks can occasionally experience dramatic visual recovery following decompression surgery. There is no correlation between the rapidity of visual loss and the rapidity of visual return.

It has been theorized that there are three stages of visual recovery after decompression of the anterior visual pathway:

1. Relief of visual pathway compression is initially followed by **rapid recovery** of some vision within minutes to hours. This recovery can be likened to the relief of conduction block after an arm or leg "goes to sleep."
2. This initial recovery is followed by **delayed recovery** of additional function over weeks to months. This improvement may be related to progressive remyelination of previously compressed demyelinated axons.
3. Finally, there is an even longer period of improvement, taking many months to years. The mechanism by which this **late recovery** occurs is unknown.

INFILTRATIVE OPTIC NEUROPATHIES

The optic nerve can become infiltrated by a variety of different processes, primarily tumors and inflammatory processes (Table 8.1). The most common lesions that infiltrate the optic nerve are tumors and inflammatory or infectious processes. Tumors may be primary or secondary. The most common inflammatory disorder is sarcoidosis; the most common infectious agents are opportunistic fungi. Such processes typically produce one of three clinical pictures: (a) optic disc elevation with evidence of an optic neuropathy, (b) optic disc elevation with no evidence of optic nerve dysfunction, and (c) a normal-appearing optic disc associated with evidence of an optic neuropathy.

Infiltration of the proximal portion of the optic nerve, either anterior or just posterior to the lamina

Table 8.1. *Lesions that Infiltrate the Optic Nerve*

Primary Tumors
 Optic glioma
 Benign/malignant ganglioglioma
 Malignant teratoid medulloepithelioma
 Capillary hemangioma
 Cavernous hemangioblastoma
 Other

Secondary Tumors
 Metastatic carcinoma
 Nasopharyngeal carcinoma and other contiguous
  tumors
 Lymphoreticular tumors
  Lymphoma
  Leukemia
 Other

Infections and Inflammation
 Sarcoidosis
 Idiopathic peri5ptic neuritis
 Bacteria
 Virus
 Fungi

cribrosa, produces elevation of the optic disc. When the prelaminar portion of the nerve is infiltrated, the elevation of the disc is caused by the infiltrative process and is not true disc swelling. When the retrolaminar portion of the nerve is infiltrated, the disc elevation is caused by true swelling of the disc, and the appearance is indistinguishable from the disc swelling caused by such diverse entities as increased intracranial pressure, ischemia, and inflammation.

TUMORS
Primary Tumors

Primary tumors that infiltrate the optic nerve are far more common than are secondary ones, and the most common primary tumor is the **optic nerve glioma** (Fig. 8.5). Optic pathway gliomas represent 1% of all intracranial tumors and 1.5% to 3.5% of all orbital tumors. Gliomas confined to the optic nerve constitute about 25% of all optic pathway gliomas with the remainder infiltrating the optic chiasm and optic tracts in addition to one or both optic nerves. Seventy percent of patients with optic pathway gliomas develop visual symptoms or signs in the first decade of life, and 90% of the lesions are detected by the second decade.

Patients with gliomas confined to the optic nerve have three clinical presentations that are determined in part by the location, size, and extent of the tumor. When the glioma is confined to the orbital portion of the nerve or the bulk of the lesion is within the orbit, the patient typically develops proptosis associated with

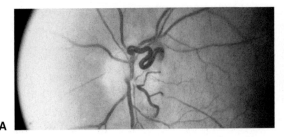
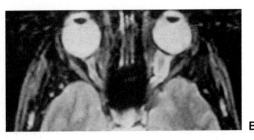

A

B

Figure 8.5.   Optociliary shunt vessels in a patient with an optic nerve glioma. **A:** The left optic disc is pale and mildly swollen. There are optociliary shunt vessels on its surface. **B:** T2-weighted MRI, axial view, shows diffuse enlargement of orbital portion of left optic nerve. The patient was initially thought to have an optic nerve sheath meningioma. Note "pseudo-CSF sign" caused by extension of tumor into subdural space around intraorbital optic nerve.

evidence of an anterior optic neuropathy with a swollen optic disc. Patients with optic nerve gliomas can develop optociliary shunt vessels (Fig. 8.5), although not as commonly as seen with optic nerve sheath meningiomas. Hyperopia may be induced by the increased volume of the optic nerve pressing on the globe, often also causing retinal striae (Fig. 8.6).

When the tumor is located posteriorly in the orbit, and especially when the process begins in, or is limited to, the intracanalicular or intracranial portions of the nerve, the presentation is that of a slowly progressive or relatively stable retrobulbar optic neuropathy. In most of these cases, the optic disc on the affected side is pale and these patients do not typically have proptosis. Sometimes gliomas in these locations are discovered incidentally, often on routine screening MRI in patients with neurofibromatosis type 1 (NF-1). Such

patients have no visual complaints and may or may not have evidence of visual dysfunction.

Many children first come to medical attention because they develop a sensory strabismus. In other patients, the tumor displaces the globe, producing a primary strabismus. Such patients may have variable visual loss that is caused not by the tumor per se but by strabismic amblyopia. The diagnosis in such cases may be suspected when color vision is normal or is less severely affected than is visual acuity.

On neuroimaging, optic nerve gliomas typically appear as fusiform enlargement of the orbital portion of the optic nerve, with or without concomitant enlargement of the optic canal (Figs. 8.5B and 8.7). Although gliomas may show minimal enhancement, the enhancement is not nearly as pronounced as is typically seen with a meningioma. Two important signs help

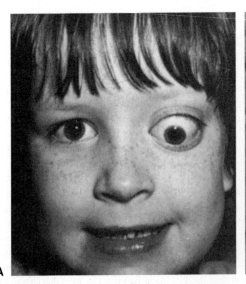
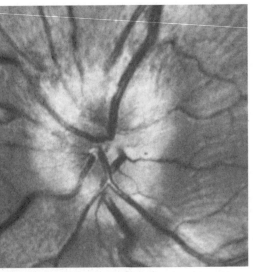

A

B

Figure 8.6.   Optic nerve glioma producing proptosis, optic disc swelling, and chorioretinal striae in a 7-year-old girl. **A:** The left eye is proptotic and displaced inferiorly. **B:** The left optic disc is swollen, and chorioretinal striae are present.

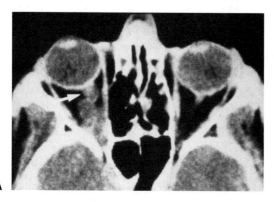 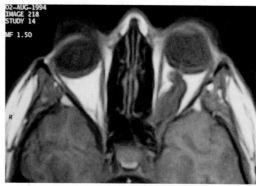

Figure 8.7. Kinking of the optic nerves in patients with neurofibromatosis type 1 and an optic nerve glioma. **A:** Axial CT scan shows "kinking" (*arrow*) of an enlarged optic nerve within the right orbit. **B:** Axial T1 weighted MRI scan demonstrating kinking of the left optic nerve. This sign is pathognomonic of an optic nerve glioma. (**B**, Courtesy of Dr. Grant T. Liu.)

differentiate optic nerve gliomas from other lesions. One is an unusual "kinking" of the optic nerve within the orbit (Fig. 8.7). The other is a double-intensity tubular thickening of the nerve, best seen on MRI. This sign is called the "pseudo-CSF" signal because the increase in T2 signal surrounding the nerve may be misinterpreted as a CSF signal (Fig. 8.8). The genesis of this signal is perineural arachnoidal gliomatosis that occurs in optic nerve gliomas in patients with NF-1.

Approximately 29% of optic pathway gliomas occur in the setting of NF-1. Therefore, any patient found

to harbor an optic pathway glioma should be assessed for evidence of NF-1, and patients with cutaneous lesions consistent with NF-1 should be screened for optic pathway gliomas and other intracranial lesions that occur in patients with neurofibromatosis. Among visually asymptomatic children with NF-1, neuroimaging reveals optic pathway gliomas in about 15% of cases.

The optimum treatment of optic nerve gliomas is unclear. The natural history of these benign lesions is generally good with long-term useful visual function and few, if any, neurologic complications. Most optic

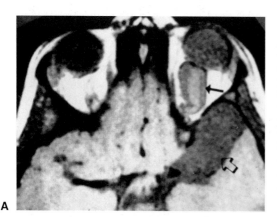 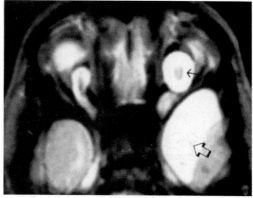

Figure 8.8. The pseudo-CSF sign in a patient with neurofibromatosis type 1 and bilateral optic nerve gliomas. **A:** T1-weighted MRI, axial view, shows that the orbital portion of the left optic nerve consists of a fusiform area of low intensity (*solid arrow*) surrounding a core of high signal intensity. An arachnoid cyst (*hollow arrow*) occupies the left anterior cranial fossa. Note that the peripheral (outer) tumor signal is isointense to the CSF in the cyst. The tumor is kinked posteriorly. The right optic nerve glioma cannot be seen on this image. **B:** T2-weighted MRI, axial view, shows a donut-shaped signal of high intensity (*black arrow*) surrounding an inner circle of low signal intensity in the left orbit. This image represents a tangential cut through the superior aspect of the upwardly kinked tumor. In the right orbit, a linear area of high signal intensity surrounds a central core of low signal intensity. Note that the outer signal within both tumors is isointense to CSF within the arachnoid cyst (*hollow arrow*). (Reprinted from: Brodsky MC. The "pseudo-CSF" signal of orbital optic glioma on magnetic resonance imaging: a signature of neurofibromatosis. *Surv Ophthalmol.* 1993;36:213–218, with permission.)

nerve gliomas do not change substantially in size over many years. Some, however, rapidly enlarge and extend along the nerve to the chiasm and even into the third ventricle. Others suddenly expand from intraneural hemorrhage. Conversely, rare lesions exhibit spontaneous regression. Patients with optic nerve glioma with unequivocal sparing of the chiasm at presentation who later develop chiasmal involvement are exceedingly unusual. However, the possibility of intracranial extension exists in any given patient and for this reason patients are followed with serial neuro-ophthalmic examinations and MRI scanning. The natural history and prognosis may be better in patients with NF-1-associated tumors.

Patients with optic nerve gliomas are generally not treated with either chemotherapy or radiation therapy unless there is clear evidence of progression with the lesion extending into the optic chiasm, opposite optic nerve, or hypothalamus. Radiation therapy is probably effective in improving vision and disease-specific survival probability in gliomas of the anterior visual pathway that are clearly progressing clinically. Because of the risk of radiation to the developing brain, chemotherapy is the first-line treatment in a child under age six, while radiation of the optic nerve tumor would be the primary option in an older child. Surgical resection is generally reserved for those patients who are already blind when first seen; for patients with severe proptosis; and for patients whose lesions seem to be threatening the optic chiasm but that have not yet reached it. No clinical trials have been performed to indicate if removal of an apparently unilateral optic nerve glioma is associated with a better visual and neurologic prognosis than no treatment at all.

Most gliomas that infiltrate the optic nerve or chiasm are benign juvenile pilocytic astrocytomas. Rarely, **malignant optic nerve gliomas** occur, almost always in adults. When the tumor initially affects the intracranial optic nerves or chiasm, there is rapidly progressive visual loss associated with optic discs that initially appear normal but that rapidly become atrophic. The visual loss in these cases is often bilateral and simultaneous, but it may initially begin in one eye and thus may be mistaken for retrobulbar optic neuritis, particularly when there is associated pain. When the malignant glioma initially affects the proximal portion of the intraorbital optic nerve, there is acute loss of vision associated with optic disc swelling and the ophthalmoscopic appearance of a central retinal vein occlusion. The prognosis in almost all cases of malignant optic glioma is poor, regardless of treatment with radiotherapy or chemotherapy. Most patients become completely blind within several months after the onset of symptoms, and most die within 6 to 12 months.

Tumors primarily composed of mature ganglion cells may occur in both the peripheral nervous system and, more rarely, in the central nervous system. Central nervous system **ganglion cell tumors** include ganglioneuromas (also called gangliocytomas), which are composed predominantly of mature ganglion cells supported by a stroma of spindle cells and containing calcospherites, and gangliogliomas, which are composed of a mixture of mature ganglion cells and mature glial cells and thus true mixed neurogliogenic tumors. These tumors occur most frequently in children and young adults and their most common location is the floor of the third ventricle. In rare instances, the gangliogliomas originate within the substance of the optic chiasm or intracranial portion of the optic nerves, and thus may be mistaken for a typical "optic glioma." Most ganglion cell tumors have a good prognosis because they behave biologically as low-grade astrocytomas.

Astrocytic hamartomas can infiltrate the optic disc. In most cases, they protrude above or overlie the surface of the affected disc. They initially have a grayish or grayish-pink appearance, but they later develop a glistening, yellow, mulberry appearance (Fig. 8.9). Although this latter appearance is similar to that of optic disc drusen, drusen are located within the substance of the disc, whereas astrocytic hamartomas overlie the disc (Fig. 8.10). Astrocytic hamartomas are composed almost entirely of acellular laminated calcific concretions, which are often interspersed among areas composed of large glial cells. The visual function in an eye with an astrocytic hamartoma of the optic disc is usually normal. Some eyes, however, develop a serous detachment of the retina or vitreous hemorrhage, resulting in variable loss of vision. Seventy percent of astrocytic hamartomas occur in patients with tuberous sclerosis or NF-1.

Both **capillary and cavernous hemangiomas** can occur within the substance of the optic disc. In addition, cavernous hemangiomas can develop at any location in the optic nerve and in the optic chiasm. Capillary hemangiomas may be endophytic or exophytic. The endophytic type appears as a circular, reddish, slightly elevated mass internal to the disc vasculature and is represented histologically by a capillary hemangioma lying immediately beneath the internal limiting membrane (Fig. 8.11). These lesions may be a manifestation of von Hippel-Lindau disease, or they may occur as an isolated phenomenon. The exophytic type of capillary hemangioma is typically seen as blurring and elevation of the disc margin, often associated with a variable degree of serous detachment of the peripapillary sensory retina and a ring of lipid deposition (Fig. 8.12). This lesion is often misdiagnosed as unilateral papilledema or papillitis, but fluorescein angiography clearly demonstrates the vascular anomaly, as does ultrasonography. These tumors may also occur as part of von Hippel-Lindau disease.

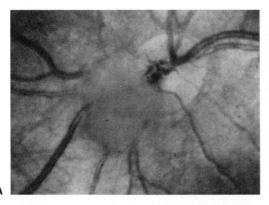
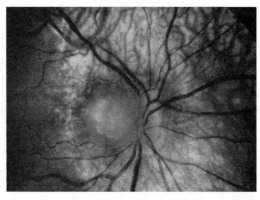

Figure 8.9. Astrocytic hamartoma of the optic disc. **A:** Before significant calcification, lesion appears as a pinkish gray mass rising above the disc. **B:** When calcification occurs, small globular clusters can be observed within the mass. Eventually, the entire mass may become calcified.

Cavernous hemangiomas consist of large-caliber vascular channels. When these lesions occur as isolated masses within the orbit, they are well circumscribed and encapsulated. Within the eye, however, their appearance is that of a cluster of small purple blobs located within and above the substance of the optic disc (Fig. 8.13). The blood flow within the vessels in cavernous hemangiomas is extremely slow, indicating that this lesion is more isolated from the general circulation than its capillary counterpart. Cavernous hemangiomas of the optic disc are usually unilateral, more common in females, and almost always asymptomatic.

Cavernous hemangiomas, unlike capillary hemangiomas, can occur within the retrolaminar, intracanalicular, and intracranial optic nerves, the optic chiasm, or the optic tracts. In some cases, the lesion itself causes slowly progressive loss of vision. In most cases, however, visual loss is rapidly progressive and occurs because of hemorrhage into the surrounding tissue. Up to one third of the patients have episodes of transient visual loss that are erroneously diagnosed as optic neuritis. Cavernous hemangiomas are not associated with von Hippel-Lindau disease, but they are often associated with similar lesions of the skin and brain and may also be associated with anomalies of extracranial and intracranial arteries.

Not all vascular lesions within the substance of the optic nerve are benign. Both the orbital and intracranial portions of the nerve can be infiltrated by a malignant **hemangioblastoma.** The typical patient with an optic nerve hemangioblastoma presents with progressive visual loss and evidence of an optic neuropathy that may be anterior or retrobulbar. The affected portion of the optic nerve is enlarged and has a fusiform appearance that mimics an optic nerve glioma on neuroimaging. Only 30% of these lesions are associated

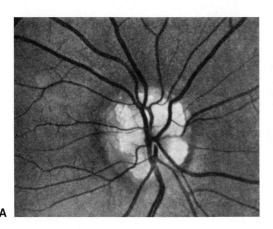
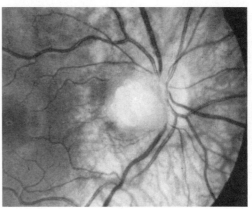

Figure 8.10. Difference in ophthalmoscopic appearance of optic disc drusen and astrocytic hamartoma of the optic disc. **A:** Optic disc drusen are located within the substance of the disc *beneath* the vessels. **B:** Astrocytic hamartomas are located *above* the optic disc, thus obscuring the vessels.

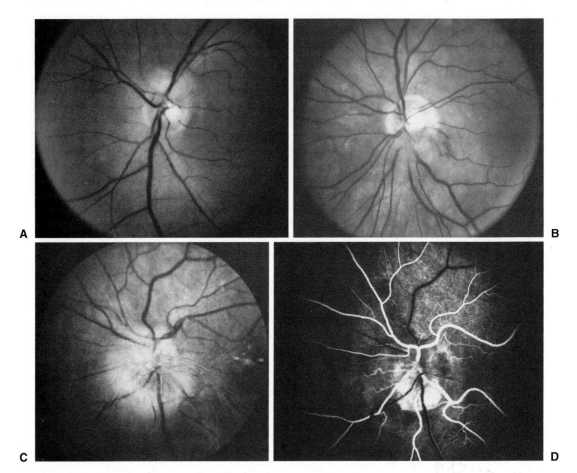

Figure 8.11. Endophytic capillary angioma. **A–C:** The lesions appear as a circular, reddish, slightly elevated mass internal to the disc vasculature. **D:** Fluorescein angiography of lesion seen in **(C)** shows intense staining and leakage from vessels at inferior aspect of disc.

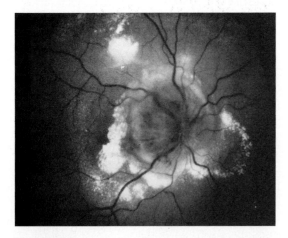

Figure 8.12. Exophytic capillary angioma of the optic disc. This lesion appears as diffuse blurring and elevation of the disc, associated with a variable degree of serous detachment of the peripapillary sensory retina and a ring of lipid deposition. (Courtesy of Dr. Andrew Schachat.)

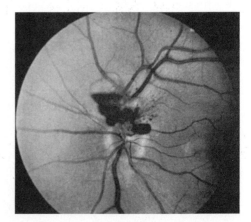

Figure 8.13. Cavernous angioma of the optic disc. Note "cluster of grapes" appearance of lesion. (Reprinted from: Davies WS, Thumin M. Cavernous hemangioma of the optic disc and retina. *Trans Am Acad Ophthalmol Otolaryngol.* 1956;60:217–218. AFIP Acc. 219953, with permission.)

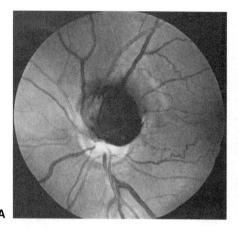 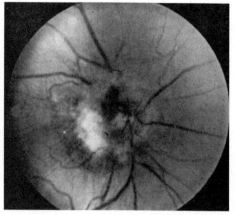

A B

Figure 8.14. A: Melanocytoma of the optic disc. The optic disc is almost completely obscured by an elevated, black mass. The mass is much darker than a malignant melanoma. **B:** Malignant melanoma of the choroid invading the optic disc. The disc tissue is elevated and shows areas of pigmentation with partial obscuration of vessels and blurring of disc margins.

with the von Hippel-Lindau disease; however, partial expression of genetic disorders is being documented with increasing frequency, and many of the other lesions associated with von Hippel-Lindau disease may not become apparent for a number of years.

Melanocytomas are intraocular tumors that typically occur within the substance of the optic disc. Clinically, these lesions are elevated masses that are gray to dark black in color and are located eccentrically on the disc (Fig. 8.14A). About 90% are two disc diameters or less in diameter, and the majority are less than 2 mm in height. Swelling of the disc occurs in about 25% of cases and is thought to be caused by a disturbance of axoplasmic flow secondary to chronic compression. Vascular sheathing may be seen in 30% of eyes, and subretinal fluid is observed in approximately 10% of the patients. A nevus may be seen adjacent to a melanocytoma in up to 50% of cases. Visual acuity remains 20/20 or better in the majority of the patients, and nearly all patients retain visual acuity of 20/50 or better. Although few patients are aware of any visual distortion, most have abnormal visual fields, especially blind spot enlargement, arcuate scotomas, and even generalized constriction. Rarely, patients develop an associated central retinal artery occlusion or ischemic necrosis of the tumor and surrounding neural tissue.

Melanocytomas are benign tumors that do not require therapy. Slight growth may occur over many years in a minority of patients, and malignant transformation is not characteristic. The deep black appearance of melanocytomas generally allows them to be differentiated not only from optic disc swelling but also from other lesions that infiltrate the optic disc, particularly malignant melanomas. Nevertheless, the distinction can be difficult in rare cases, particularly when the lesion is not changing in size or shape (Fig. 8.14B).

Secondary Tumors

The most common secondary tumors that infiltrate the optic nerve are metastatic and locally invasive carcinomas and various lymphoreticular malignancies, particularly lymphoma and leukemia.

The optic nerve may be the site of **metastasis** from distant tumors. Metastases can reach the optic nerve by one of four routes: (i) from the choroid, (ii) by vascular dissemination, (iii) by invasion from the orbit, or (iv) from the CNS. Regardless of the mode of spread, the substance of the nerve is affected more often than the sheath.

Patients with metastases to the optic nerve usually have evidence of an optic neuropathy. The visual loss is usually severe, but relatively normal vision may be present in the early stages. When the metastasis is located in the prelaminar or immediately retrolaminar portion of the optic nerve, the optic disc is usually swollen; a yellow-white mass can be seen to protrude from the surface of the nerve (Fig. 8.15); and clumps of tumor cells can occasionally be seen in the vitreous overlying the disc. A central retinal vein occlusion occurs in up to 50% of eyes. When the metastasis is to the posterior aspect of the orbital portion of the optic nerve or to the intracanalicular or intracranial portions of the nerve, the optic disc initially appears normal.

The most common metastatic tumors to the optic nerve are adenocarcinomas, primarily because these are the most common metastatic tumors to all parts of the body. In women, carcinomas of the breast and lung are the most common tumors, whereas carcinomas of the lung and bowel are most common in men. Other tumors that can metastasize to the optic nerve include carcinomas of the stomach, pancreas, uterus, ovary, prostate, kidney, and tonsillar fossa. Skin cancers, malignant melanoma, and mediastinal tumors also may

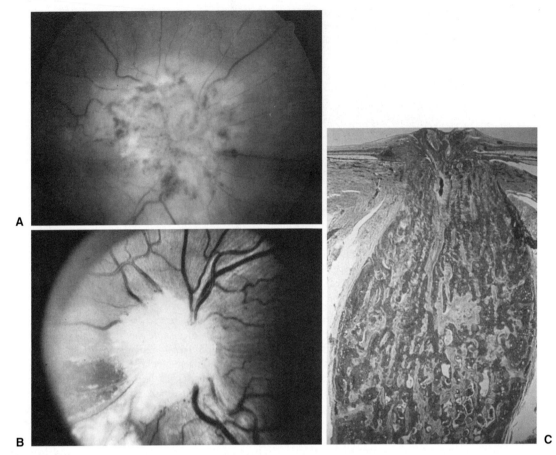

Figure 8.15. Metastatic adenocarcinoma to the optic disc. **A:** Breast carcinoma in a 47-year-old woman. The entire optic disc is infiltrated by a large mass of yellow-white tissue. Note loss of normal disc architecture. There were numerous malignant cells in the vitreous. **B:** Lung carcinoma in a 56-year-old man. Note the white mass protruding from disc surface. **C:** Appearance at autopsy of optic nerve infiltration by adenocarcinoma of the lung.

metastasize to one or both optic nerves. Isolated metastases to the optic nerve of intracranial tumors, such as medulloblastomas, may rarely occur.

Contiguous spread of primary tumors from the paranasal sinuses, brain, and adjacent intraocular structures to the optic nerve occurs much less often than does metastasis to the nerve. Because of its close anatomic association with the paranasal sinuses, the optic nerve can be infiltrated or compressed by cancer that arises in the sinuses or the nasopharynx. In most cases, the tumor invades the posterior orbit or cavernous sinus, producing a syndrome that is characterized by loss of vision, diplopia, ophthalmoparesis, and trigeminal sensory neuropathy.

Most patients with metastatic tumor to the optic nerve already have a known diagnosis of a primary carcinoma with other evidence of metastases at the time that visual loss occurs. This makes the diagnosis relatively straightforward, whereas most patients with a tumor that spreads contiguously to the optic nerve are not known to harbor a tumor when they first experience loss of vision. Any person with known cancer in another part of the body, with or without other evidence of metastases, who develops an optic neuropathy should be suspected of having cancer as the cause until proven otherwise. Similarly, any patient with a basal skull tumor who develops an optic neuropathy should be assumed to have spread of tumor to the optic nerve, unless there has been previous radiation therapy to the region, in which case the possibility of radiation-induced optic neuropathy must also be considered.

Neuroimaging should be performed in all patients suspected of having infiltration of the optic nerve by cancer. Imaging typically shows an enhancing nerve that may or may not be enlarged (Fig. 8.16). Most metastatic optic nerve tumors show at least a temporary response to radiation therapy.

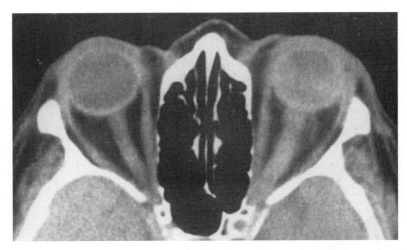

Figure 8.16. Neuroimaging appearance of infiltration of optic nerve by metastatic carcinoma. CT scan, axial view, in a 56-year-old woman with small-cell carcinoma of the lung and progressive loss of vision in the left eye associated with a massive retinal infiltrate with nasal retinal detachment reveals that the orbital portion of the left optic nerve is diffusely enlarged. (Reprinted from: Allaire GS, Corriveau C, Arbour JD. Metastasis to the optic nerve: clinicopathological correlations. *Can J Ophthalmol.* 1995;30:306–311, with permission.)

Rarer than cases of metastatic or locally invasive tumors of the optic nerve are cases of "tumor within a tumor" or so-called "collision tumors." In these cases, one tumor is metastatic to another tumor. Renal cell carcinoma seems to be the best recipient or host tumor to "attract" other cancers, with lung carcinoma being the most common primary tumor to metastasize to the site. In the cases of metastasis to benign optic nerve tumors, the host tumor is usually a benign optic nerve meningioma.

Meningeal tumor cuffing or direct infiltration of the optic nerve can cause loss of vision in the setting of meningeal spread of carcinoma. This phenomenon is called **carcinomatous meningitis** or **meningeal carcinomatosis.** The frequency of optic nerve involvement in patients with carcinomatosis of the meninges ranges from 15% to 40%. Patients who develop meningeal carcinomatosis with visual loss may do so after the primary lesion, usually in the lung or breast, has already been diagnosed. In other cases, visual loss may occur coincident with other signs of chronic meningitis or as an isolated finding as the first sign of disease.

Although blindness may begin in one eye, both eyes are usually affected within a short period of time. The optic neuropathy that occurs in the setting of meningeal carcinomatosis is usually associated with a "diagnostic quartet" that consists of (a) headaches typical of raised intracranial pressure, (b) blindness, (c) sluggish or absent pupillary reflexes, and (d) normal-appearing optic discs. In some cases, there is true histopathologic evidence of infiltration of the optic nerve; in other cases, the lesion is more compressive

than infiltrative, with malignant cells invading the subarachnoid space surrounding the optic nerve.

Lymphoreticular malignancies, such as leukemia and lymphoma, may infiltrate the optic nerve. Central nervous system involvement in non-Hodgkin's lymphoma (NHL) is unusual, but it occurs in about 10% of cases. Of these, 5% (or a total of 0.5% of patients with NHL) will have infiltration of the optic nerve at some time during the course of their disease. Infiltration of the optic nerve in Hodgkin's disease is even less common.

The symptoms and signs of patients with lymphomatous infiltration of the anterior visual system depend on the location and extent of the lesion. In some cases, the visual loss is insidious in onset and slowly progressive, whereas in other cases the visual loss is acute and mimics optic neuritis or ischemic optic neuropathy. The appearance of optic nerve infiltration by lymphoma is nonspecific. The infiltrated structure is enlarged and typically enhances on neuroimaging (Fig. 8.17). **Multiple myeloma, lymphomatoid granulomatosis,** and **Langerhans cell histiocytosis** can all also produce an optic neuropathy, sometimes via infiltration rather than compression of the nerve.

About 4% of children with acute **leukemia** have evidence of optic nerve infiltration. In some of the patients, visual acuity is lost abruptly; in others, there is a gradual progression of visual loss over days, weeks, or months. In still others, the disc appears swollen, but there is no evidence of visual dysfunction. Most patients with leukemic infiltration of the optic nerve are known to have leukemia at the time the visual loss

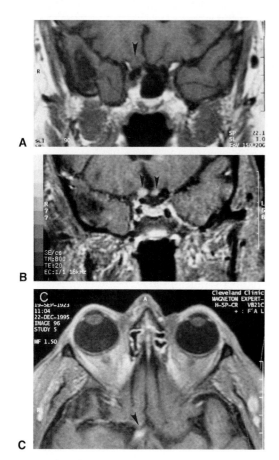

Figure 8.17. Neuroimaging appearance of infiltration of the right optic nerve, chiasm, and tract by a lymphoma. **A:** T1-weighted MRI, coronal view, shows enlarged right optic nerve (*arrowhead*). **B:** T1-weighted MRI, coronal view, after intravenous injection of paramagnetic contrast material shows enhancement of the right optic nerve and, to a lesser extent, the left optic nerve (*arrowheads*) just anterior to the optic chiasm. **C:** T1-weighted MRI, axial view, after intravenous injection of paramagnetic contrast material shows enhancement of anterior portion of the right optic tract (*arrowhead*).

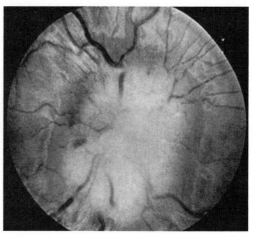

Figure 8.18. Leukemic infiltration of the optic disc mimicking optic disc swelling in a child with acute lymphocytic leukemia. The child was thought to be in remission at the time the abnormality was discovered. The disc is whitish gray and markedly elevated with obscuration of vessels. Visual acuity is 20/25.

occurs or the patient is found to have asymptomatic disc swelling. Patients can have acute lymphocytic leukemia, acute myelogenous leukemia, monocytic leukemia, erythroleukemia, or chronic lymphocytic leukemia

Two distinct clinical patterns of infiltration can occur: (i) infiltration of the optic disc and (ii) infiltration of the immediate retrolaminar portion of the proximal optic nerve. In leukemic infiltration of the optic disc, the features of the disc are obscured by a whitish fluffy infiltrate that is often associated with true disc swelling and peripapillary hemorrhage (Fig. 8.18). The visual acuity in such patients is minimally affected, unless the infiltration or associated edema and hemorrhage extend into the macula. Infiltration of the proximal optic nerve just posterior to the lamina cribrosa usually produces markedly decreased visual acuity associated with true optic disc swelling. Such patients have a variety of visual field defects, and a relative afferent pupillary defect is invariably present unless the infiltration is bilateral and symmetric. In addition, there are often peripapillary and peripheral retinal hemorrhages. Neuroimaging in such cases typically reveals a diffusely enlarged and enhancing optic nerve.

The response of leukemic infiltration of the optic nerve to radiation therapy is usually rapid and dramatic. In almost all cases, visual function returns to normal or near normal, and the disc elevation, if present, resolves.

One must consider a number of pathologic mechanisms in addition to infiltration in any patient with acute leukemia and apparent optic disc swelling. Swelling of the optic disc can occur in patients with acute leukemia when central nervous system involvement by the disease results in increased intracranial pressure. Optic disc swelling and neovascularization also occur as a local phenomenon in the setting of the diffuse retinopathy of acute leukemia.

The acute leukemias are responsible for most of the reported cases of infiltrative optic neuropathies caused by lymphoreticular disorders; however, patients with chronic forms of leukemia may also develop optic nerve infiltration. Autopsy studies reveal a high percentage of asymptomatic central nervous system involvement in patients with chronic lymphocytic leukemia. Patients with optic nerve infiltration in the setting of chronic lymphocytic leukemia and other chronic leukemias have a more indolent clinical course than patients with the acute leukemias. Optic disc swelling is usually present, but visual loss is less severe, and retinal changes of the type seen in acute leukemia are rare.

INFLAMMATORY AND INFECTIOUS INFILTRATIVE OPTIC NEUROPATHIES

The intraocular, intraorbital, intracanalicular and intracranial segments of the optic nerve can all be infiltrated by inflammatory and infectious processes. The most common inflammatory process that produces an infiltrative optic neuropathy is sarcoidosis. The most common infectious processes that produce an infiltrative optic neuropathy are syphilis, tuberculosis, and opportunistic fungal infections, such as cryptococcosis.

Sarcoidosis

Optic nerve dysfunction probably is the most common neuro-ophthalmologic manifestation of sarcoidosis. The optic nerve may be affected at any time during the course of the disease and may be the site of its initial presentation. Sarcoidosis may affect the optic nerve in several different ways. It may produce papilledema, a compressive anterior or retrobulbar optic neuropathy, an ischemic optic neuropathy, or anterior or retrobulbar optic neuritis. The optic neuritis results from granulomatous infiltration of the optic disc, anterior orbital, posterior orbital, intracanalicular, or intracranial portions of the nerve, or a combination of these. In some cases, more than one process is responsible.

Granulomatous infiltration of the optic disc may or may not be associated with evidence by neuroimaging or ultrasonography of diffuse enlargement of the orbital portion of the optic nerve. The optic disc in such cases usually is markedly elevated, either diffusely or sectorially (Fig. 8.19), and it often has a solid or nodular appearance. There may be dilated vessels resembling neovascularization on the surface of the disc.

The appearance of optic disc infiltration by sarcoid granulomas may mimic that of papilledema, except that

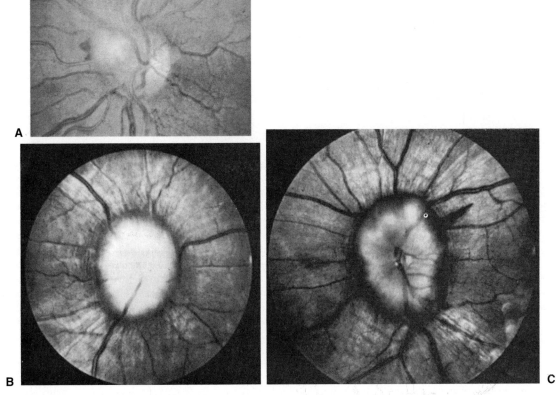

Figure 8.19. Sarcoid granulomas infiltrating the optic disc. **A:** In a 25-year-old woman with visual acuity of 20/20 OU. There is a small elevated yellow-white mass overlying the nasal portion of the left optic disc. A small hemorrhage is just nasal to the mass. (Reprinted from: Laties AM, Scheie HG. Evolution of multiple small tumors in sarcoid granuloma of the optic disk. *Am J Ophthalmol.* 1972;74:60–66, with permission.) **B:** In another patient, the entire disc is infiltrated by granulomas. Note diffuse symmetric elevation of the disc substance. **C:** In a third patient, a multinodular granuloma has infiltrated the left optic disc. (Reprinted from: Jampol LM, Woodfin W, McLean EB. Optic nerve sarcoidosis. *Arch Ophthalmol.* 1972;87:355–360, with permission.)

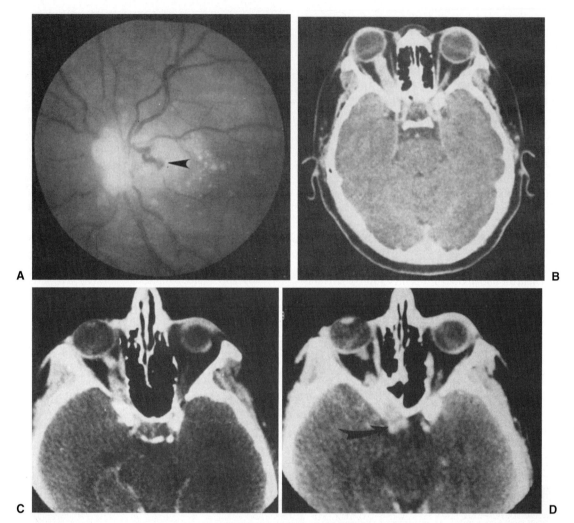

Figure 8.20. CT scanning of optic nerve sarcoidosis. **A:** Bilobed mass projecting from the medial aspect of the left optic disc in a patient with sarcoidosis. Note optociliary shunt vessel (*arrowhead*). **B:** CT scan, axial view, after intravenous injection of contrast material shows diffuse thickening and enhancement of the orbital portion of the left optic nerve. (Reprinted from: Lustgarden JS, Mindel JS, Yablonski ME, et al. An unusual presentation of isolated optic nerve sarcoidosis. *J Clin Neuroophthalmol.* 1983;3:13–18, with permission.) **C:** CT scan, axial view, after intravenous injection of contrast in another patient with painless progressive loss of vision in the right eye and biopsy-proven sarcoidosis shows diffuse enlargement and enhancement of the orbital portion of the right optic nerve. Note the "kinking" of the nerve, similar to that seen in patients with optic nerve glioma in the setting of neurofibromatosis type 1. **D:** CT scan, axial view, after intravenous contrast enhancement at a slightly higher plane in the same patient as *C* shows intracranial extension of the optic nerve lesion (*arrow*). (Reprinted from: Jordan DR, Anderson RL, Nerad JA, et al. Optic nerve involvement as the initial manifestation of sarcoidosis. *Can J Ophthalmol.* 1988;23:232–237, with permission.)

the former condition is more often unilateral than bilateral, and it is usually associated with decreased vision, intraocular inflammation, and/or neuroimaging evidence of an intracranial process affecting the base of the skull.

When the proximal portion of the intraorbital optic nerve is infiltrated by granulomatous inflammation in patients with sarcoidosis, the condition typically presents as an acute, subacute, or rarely chronic optic neuritis, with progressive loss of vision and disc swelling. This condition may be impossible to differentiate clinically from demyelinating optic neuritis and even from certain causes of compressive optic neuropathy, particularly optic nerve sheath meningioma. Even neuroimaging, which shows enlargement and enhancement of the orbital portion of the optic nerve (Fig. 8.20), cannot establish the diagnosis with certainty. In some cases, the diagnosis is made by finding

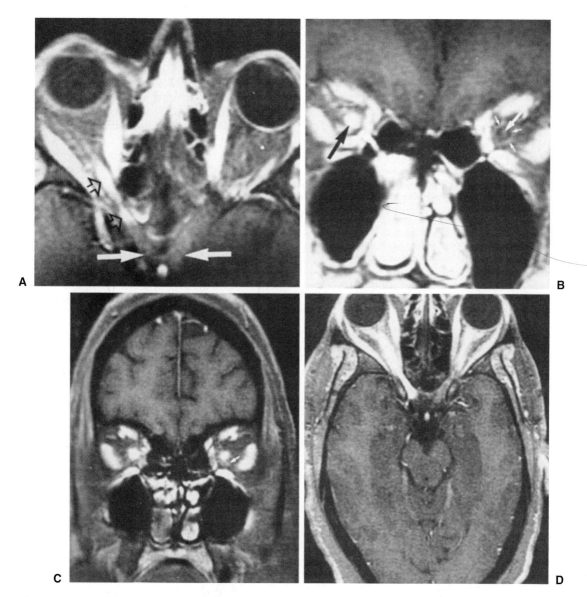

Figure 8.21. MRI in patients with sarcoidosis of the optic nerves. **A:** T1-weighted fat-suppressed MRI, axial view, after intravenous injection of paramagnetic contrast material in a 52-year-old woman with progressive loss of vision in the right eye shows irregular enhancement of the right optic nerve near the apex of the orbit and within the optic canal (*hollow arrows*). The intracranial portions of the optic nerves and the optic chiasm do not enhance and appear normal in size and shape (*solid arrows*). **B:** Enhanced T1-weighted fat-suppressed MRI, coronal view, in the same patient shows enlargement and abnormal enhancement of the orbital portion of the right optic nerve (*black arrow*). The left optic nerve is normal in size and does not enhance (*large white arrow*); however, there is mild enhancement of its leptomeningeal sheath (*small white arrows*). A biopsy of the nerve revealed noncaseating granulomas. **C:** Enhanced T1-weighted fat-suppressed MRI, coronal view, in another patient with sarcoidosis and progressive bilateral loss of vision with evidence of bilateral optic neuropathies reveals enlargement and abnormal enhancement of the orbital portions of both optic nerves. The right optic nerve is slightly larger than the left. Note mild enhancement of the leptomeningeal sheath of the left optic nerve (*arrow*). **D:** Enhanced T1-weighted fat-suppressed MRI, axial view, in the same patient shows enlargement and abnormal enhancement of both optic nerves throughout the orbits, with extension through the optic canal on the right side. (Reprinted from: Engelken JD, Yuh WTC, Carter KD, et al. Optic nerve sarcoidosis: MR findings. *AJNR Am J Neuroradiol.* 1992;13:228–230, with permission.)

clinical, radiographic, or laboratory evidence of sarcoidosis elsewhere. In other cases, the diagnosis is not confirmed until a biopsy of the nerve or other abnormal tissue is performed.

The posterior retrobulbar or intracanalicular portion of the optic nerve can also be affected by sarcoid. In such cases, the patient develops acute or, more often, progressive loss of vision associated with evidence of an optic neuropathy. The optic disc in such cases is normal but gradually becomes pale if no treatment is given. On neuroimaging, the posterior orbital portion of the optic nerve may be enlarged and may enhance (Fig. 8.21). The optic foramen may be enlarged. Because of the predilection of neurosarcoidosis to affect the basal meninges, the intracranial portion of one or both optic nerves and the optic chiasm may occasionally be affected by the disease, producing a variety of patterns of visual loss. In some patients, visual loss is associated with evidence of hypothalamic dysfunction and/or hypothalamic hypopituitarism (particularly gonadotropin failure).

The diagnosis of sarcoidosis depends on a compatible clinical picture combined with appropriate imaging studies and, in some cases, serologic evaluation for elevated levels of angiotensin-converting enzyme (ACE) and histologic evidence of the disease by biopsy of involved tissues. A standard chest radiograph is an essential part of the evaluation, and chest CT may prove useful. Abnormal uptake on gallium scanning, although not specific for sarcoidosis, may reveal areas accessible for biopsy. Conjunctival or lacrimal gland biopsy can establish the diagnosis, especially if the biopsied tissues are clinically affected.

The primary treatment of sarcoidosis is with corticosteroids. Most of the neurologic manifestations, including optic neuropathy, respond promptly to treatment; however, many patients require chronic therapy. Other agents reported beneficial in the treatment of sarcoid optic neuropathy, either separately or in combination with steroids, include immunosuppressive drugs such as cyclosporine, azathioprine, methotrexate, and cyclophosphamide, and radiation therapy.

Infectious Disorders

Tuberculosis can infiltrate the optic nerve. In some cases, the tuberculoma is adjacent to the optic nerve and is part of a dense adhesive arachnoiditis that may or may not be separable from the surrounding structures. In other cases, however, the inflammatory tissue actually invades the nerve, making removal impossible. Rarely, a tuberculoma is completely contained within the optic nerve.

Syphilitic gummas may act in a similar fashion. Retrobulbar optic neuritis occurs in patients with syphilis, and gummas within the optic disc also have been described. Viral diseases, such as cytomegalovirus and some of the herpes viruses, can produce an infiltrative process of the optic nerve.

Invasion of the anterior visual system by cryptococcal organisms in the setting of cryptococcal meningitis is not uncommon, especially in patients with AIDS. Visual loss in such instances may reflect direct optic nerve or chiasmal invasion by the organisms, adhesive constricting arachnoiditis, increased intracranial pressure with papilledema, or a combination of these processes. Visual loss can be sudden, subacute over days, or chronic over a period of months. Presumably, other organisms causing both acute and chronic meningitis cause visual loss in a similar manner.

FOR FURTHER INFORMATION

See *Walsh & Hoyt's Clinical Neuro-Ophthalmology*, 6th edition, Volume 1, Chapter 8, pages 385–429; Volume 2, Chapter 28, pages 1344–1347; Chapter 29, pages 1428–1439; Chapter 30, pages 1502–1508; and Volume 3, Chapter 59, pages 3369–3427.

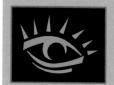

CHAPTER 9

Traumatic Optic Neuropathies*

CLASSIFICATION
EPIDEMIOLOGY
CLINICAL ASSESSMENT
PATHOLOGY

PATHOGENESIS
PHARMACOLOGY
MANAGEMENT

CLASSIFICATION

Traumatic optic neuropathy is classically separated into two types of injury: direct and indirect. **Direct** optic nerve injuries result from orbital or cerebral trauma that transgresses normal tissue planes to disrupt the anatomic and functional integrity of the optic nerve, such as a bullet penetrating the orbit or endoscopic forceps avulsing the optic nerve. **Indirect** injuries are caused by forces transmitted at a distance from the optic nerve. Normal tissue planes are not transgressed in indirect optic nerve injuries. Instead, the anatomy and function of the optic nerve are compromised by energy absorbed by the nerve at the moment of impact. The classic example of an indirect injury to the optic nerve is that which occurs when blunt trauma to the forehead results in a transmission of force through the cranium to the confined intracanalicular portion of the nerve.

The prognosis of an optic nerve injury depends in part on whether it is direct or indirect. Direct injuries tend to produce severe and immediate visual loss with little likelihood of recovery. Indirect optic neuropathies, on the other hand, are not infrequently associated with visual recovery and may also produce delayed visual loss that occurs several hours to days after the injury.

Optic nerve injuries can also be classified anatomically as optic disc trauma (avulsion), anterior optic neuropathy, or posterior optic neuropathy. An avulsion of the optic nerve as it enters the globe produces a distinct ophthalmoscopic appearance, consisting of a partial ring of hemorrhage at the optic nerve head. In some cases, the site of the avulsion can be identified (Fig. 9.1).

Injuries to the proximal portion of the optic nerve within 10 mm of the globe, anterior to where the cen-

tral retinal artery enters and the central retinal vein leaves the nerve, produce a variety of disturbances that are immediately apparent in the ocular fundus, including an ophthalmoscopic picture of a central retinal or branch artery occlusion, central retinal vein occlusion, or anterior ischemic optic neuropathy (Fig. 9.2).

In contrast, injuries to the optic nerve posterior to the entrance of the central retinal artery produce no immediate change in the appearance of the ocular fundus. Specifically, the optic disc remains normal in appearance for at least 3 to 5 weeks, following which it becomes pale. The most common site of posterior indirect optic nerve injury is the optic canal.

The intracranial optic nerve is the next most common site of injury. When the intracranial portion of the optic nerve is injured, the field defect is likely to be hemianopic, and bilateral injury is common, as is associated injury to the optic chiasm.

EPIDEMIOLOGY

The type of trauma that produces a traumatic optic neuropathy is usually a deceleration injury of significant momentum. In cases of isolated traumatic optic neuropathy, the force of the impact is typically directed to the ipsilateral forehead or to the midface region. Motor vehicle and bicycle accidents are the most frequent causes, accounting for 17% to 63% of the cases. Motorcycle accident victims may be particularly vulnerable to traumatic optic neuropathy with up to 18% of such accidents resulting in optic nerve dysfunction. Falls are the next most common cause. Traumatic optic neuropathy can also occur in such diverse settings as frontal impact caused by falling debris, assault, stab wounds, gunshot wounds, skateboarding, and following seemingly trivial head trauma. It may also occur from iatrogenic injury, particularly after endoscopic sinus surgery and orbital surgery.

Optic nerve injury is often associated with multisystem trauma and serious brain injury. Loss of consciousness occurs in 40% to 72% of the patients with traumatic optic neuropathy, and traumatic optic

*Adapted from: Steinsapir KD, Goldberg RA. Traumatic optic neuropathy. In: Miller NR, Newman NJ, Biousse V, Kerrison JB, eds. *Walsh & Hoyt's Clinical Neuro-Ophthalmology.* 6th ed. Vol. I. Lippincott Williams & Wilkins: Philadelphia; 2005:431–446.

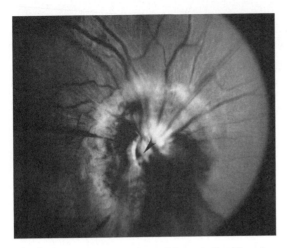

Figure 9.1. Traumatic avulsion of the optic disc. Note ring of hemorrhage around the optic disc. The site of avulsion is clearly visible as a crescentic dark area at the temporal portion of the disc (*arrowhead*).

neuropathy occurs in about 1.6% of head trauma cases and in 2.5% of patients with maxillofacial trauma.

Traumatic optic neuropathy that occurs in the setting of orbital hemorrhage defines an important subset of optic nerve injury that does not fit well into the classic delineation of direct and indirect optic nerve injuries. For example, orbital hemorrhage after retrobulbar block occurs in 0.44% to 3% of the patients. In most cases, the hemorrhage is quickly recognized and readily managed with little impact on visual outcome unless a direct optic nerve injury has occurred from perforation of the nerve by the retrobulbar needle. Thus, the incidence of traumatic optic neuropathy in the setting of iatrogenic orbital hemorrhage is extremely low.

When retrobulbar hemorrhage occurs in association with blunt trauma to the orbit, the risk of visual loss is much greater. In this setting, blood may be dispersed throughout the orbit, in the subperiosteal space, and in the optic nerve sheath. In other cases, a hematic cyst may form, resulting in optic neuropathy from compression of the nerve by the cyst. Imaging studies can help to localize the hemorrhage in such cases. Orbital emphysema is also a rare cause of optic nerve injury. It can follow orbital fractures, usually after vomiting or nose blowing force air into the orbit, compromising the optic nerve.

CLINICAL ASSESSMENT

Traumatic optic neuropathy is a clinical diagnosis typically made when there is evidence of an optic neuropathy that is temporally related to blunt or penetrating head trauma. The head trauma may have been severe,

in which case the patient may be unconscious. There may be a history of transient loss of consciousness, or the trauma may have seemed trivial, and the patient is neurologically intact. In some cases, there is no other evidence of orbital or ocular trauma; in other cases, there is obvious evidence of injury to the eye or orbit, such as periorbital or ocular hemorrhage, ecchymosis, or lacerations.

The clinical evaluation of a patient with visual loss following trauma should begin with a complete history, usually obtained from family, friends, or witnesses to the trauma. It is particularly important, for both medical and legal purposes, to determine if the patient with evidence of visual loss had any visual deficits before the injury. The examination of a patient with a possible traumatic optic neuropathy is limited by numerous patient factors, including the presence or absence of other injuries, the patient's level of consciousness, and the patient's ability or willingness to cooperate with the examiner.

Whenever possible, the **visual acuity** should first be determined using a Snellen chart or a hand-held near card, using the patient's refraction or a +3.00 sphere in the presbyopic age range. The severity of initial visual loss in patients with traumatic optic neuropathy varies dramatically, from no light perception to 20/20 with an associated field defect. The prevalence of severe initial visual loss from traumatic optic neuropathy probably ranges from 43% to 56%. Visual loss is more likely to be severe in patients with neuroimaging evidence of a fracture of the optic canal. Delayed visual loss is reported to be as high as 10% in some series. **Color vision,** an excellent test of optic nerve function, can be assessed at bedside by using comparison techniques with a red test object viewed by each eye.

In cases of unilateral traumatic optic neuropathy a **relative afferent pupillary defect** (RAPD) must be present on the side of the presumed optic nerve injury. A patient with a presumed traumatic optic neuropathy who does not have a RAPD either does not have an optic neuropathy at all or has a bilateral optic neuropathy. Furthermore, because patients with 20/20 vision in the setting of an optic neuropathy can have a RAPD, the presence of a RAPD in a comatose or semicomatose patient whose visual acuity cannot be measured cannot be taken as evidence that there is little or no vision in the eye. Only when the pupil does not react at all to direct light but reacts consensually (indicating intact efferent function) can one be certain that the patient has no light perception.

A complete and thorough examination of the eye and ocular adnexa is essential following trauma. Palpation of the orbital rim can identify step-off fractures. Periorbital swelling may mask the presence of proptosis. Resistance to retropulsion of the globe followed by tonometry can rapidly identify an orbit that is tense

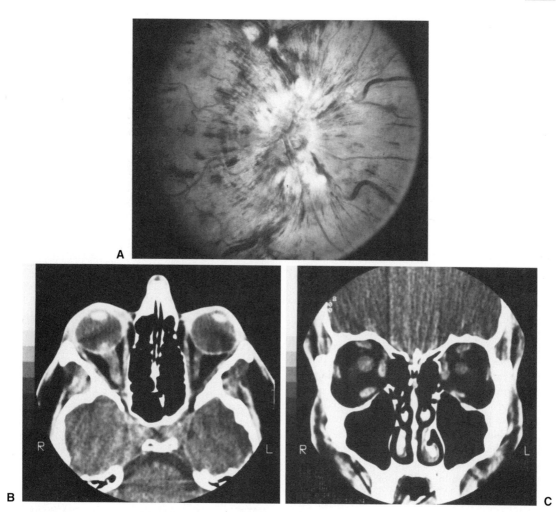

Figure 9.2. Central retinal vein occlusion in a case of anterior (proximal) optic neuropathy. The patient was a 24-year-old man who was struck in the left eye while playing basketball and who immediately noted loss of vision in the eye. Visual acuity was light perception OD and 20/15 OS. **A:** Ophthalmoscopic appearance of right ocular fundus reveals moderate swelling of the optic disc. The disc is surrounded by hemorrhage and soft exudates. The retinal veins are dilated and tortuous. **B:** Computed tomographic (CT) scan, axial view, shows moderate enlargement of the orbital portion of the right optic nerve. **C:** CT scan, coronal view, shows enlargement of right optic nerve compared with left nerve. Note small areas of increased density, consistent with hemorrhage, within the enlarged nerve.

from a retro-orbital hemorrhage. Evidence of a penetrating ocular injury should be sought. Blunt injury to the iris may result in a hyphema or angle recession. The force of trauma may dislocate the lens.

Posteriorly, blood in the vitreous may obscure the fundus. If the patient is neurologically unstable, the treating neurosurgeon or trauma surgeon should be consulted prior to dilating the eyes. If a dilated examination is performed, proper documentation must occur and only short-acting agents should be used. An adequate **fundus examination** will include assessment of abnormalities of the retinal circulation. Partial and complete avulsion of the optic nerve head produces a

ring of hemorrhage at the site of injury or the appearance of a deep round pit (Fig. 9.1). Anterior injuries between the globe and where the central retinal vessels enter the optic nerve produce disturbances in the retinal circulation including venous obstruction and traumatic anterior ischemic optic neuropathy (Fig. 9.2). Hemorrhages in the optic nerve sheath posterior to the origin of the central retinal vessels may leave the circulation of the retina intact, but produce optic nerve head swelling. Frank papilledema may be seen in the setting of raised intracranial pressure in addition to the presence of traumatic optic neuropathy. The presence of choroidal rupture or *commotio retinae* may explain visual loss. Clinical judgment must be exercised to decide if these conditions are consistent with a RAPD.

The presence of decreased visual acuity and a RAPD in the absence of intraocular pathology should suggest a posterior orbital, intracanalicular or intracranial optic nerve injury. The optic disc in these cases will appear normal for 3 to 5 weeks, after which the disc becomes progressively pale and atrophic. The observation of optic atrophy in a patient with acute head trauma and evidence of an optic neuropathy absolutely indicates that at least some disturbance of the optic nerve was present *before* the trauma and was not caused by it, although patients with a mild asymptomatic compressive optic neuropathy from a slowly expanding intracranial mass can occasionally experience acute loss of vision after seemingly trivial trauma from the effects of the trauma on an already compromised optic nerve.

Whenever possible, some type of **visual field testing** should be performed in the awake cooperative patient with possible traumatic optic neuropathy. The visual field may provide limited information regarding the possible location of optic nerve damage. Within the optic canal, for example, the pial penetrating vessels that provide blood to the optic nerve are subject to shearing forces at the moment of injury. Because the superior portion of the optic nerve is most tightly bound within the canal, the superior pial vessels are thought to be the most susceptible to shearing forces. If this concept is correct, patients with injuries to the intracanalicular portion of the optic nerve that spare some vision should have a visual field defect that is worse inferiorly than superiorly. However, there is no pathognomonic visual field defect that is diagnostic of optic nerve trauma. Altitudinal, central, paracentral, cecocentral, and hemianopic defects can all occur, as can generalized field constriction.

The **visual-evoked potential** (VEP) may be helpful in the assessment of optic nerve function in an unresponsive patient suspected of having a traumatic optic neuropathy. This is especially true in possible bilateral cases where a RAPD may not be present. The VEP is useful only when it is not recordable, in which case it may be assumed that there is complete loss of vision in the affected eye and that the chance of visual recovery is low.

CT scanning permits visualization not only of the optic nerve and adjacent soft tissue in the orbit and neural and vascular structures in the brain, but also of the bony anatomy of the optic canals and paranasal sinuses. CT evidence of a fracture through the optic canal on the side of a traumatic optic neuropathy occurs in about 36% to 67% of the cases (Fig. 9.3). The fracture in such cases may injure the optic nerve directly or it may serve as a marker of the severity of force transferred into the optic nerve.

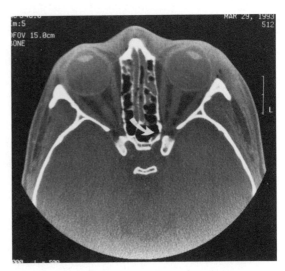

Figure 9.3. CT scan appearance (axial view) of an optic canal fracture (*arrow*) in a patient with a traumatic left optic neuropathy.

Although CT scanning is clearly superior to MRI in delineating fractures of bone, MRI is superior to CT scanning in its ability to image soft tissue. The role of MRI in traumatic optic neuropathy has yet to be fully defined. Certainly, MRI is more sensitive in the detection and the evaluation of associated intracranial abnormalities, and it may indeed prove useful in the detection of subtle hemorrhage of the optic nerve or sheath, especially within the optic canal (Fig. 9.4). In

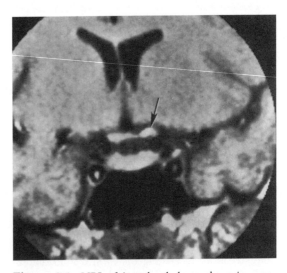

Figure 9.4. MRI of intrasheath hemorrhage in a patient with a traumatic optic neuropathy. The MRI, coronal view, shows hemorrhage in the optic nerve sheaths (*arrow*). (Reprinted from: Crowe NW, Nickles TP, Troost T, et al. Intrachiasmal hemorrhage: a cause of delayed post-traumatic blindness. *Neurology.* 1989;39:863–865, with permission.)

general, MRI should be performed only after a metallic intracranial, intraorbital, or intraocular foreign body has been ruled out by CT scanning or conventional radiographs.

PATHOLOGY

Pathologic examination of the optic nerves from autopsies performed soon after closed head trauma has revealed optic nerve dural sheath hemorrhages in 83% of the cases, interstitial optic nerve hemorrhages in 36% of the cases (with the hemorrhage being present in the optic canal in two thirds of these cases), and shearing lesions and ischemic necrosis in 44% of the cases (with the intracanalicular optic nerve and the intracranial optic nerves affected 81% and 54% of the time, respectively).

The not uncommon finding of fractures of the sphenoid bone in patients with traumatic optic neuropathy after blunt head trauma is one indication of the substantial force that is transmitted to the optic nerve in such cases. Studies using CT scanning suggest that over 50% of the cases of traumatic optic neuropathy are associated with a fracture of the sphenoid bone. Studies using laser interferometry suggest that, whether or not there is a fracture of the optic canal, the forces applied to the frontal bone during a deceleration injury are transmitted to and concentrated in the region of the optic canal. Indeed, the entire force of deceleration is applied to the facial bones over several milliseconds, whereupon elastic deformation of the sphenoid

bone results in the direct transfer of force into the intracanalicular portion of the optic nerve. Because the nerve sheath is tightly adherent to the bony canal, the forces cause immediate contusion necrosis of the nerve by disrupting axons and vasculature. The development and location of a fracture in such cases is determined by the elastic limits of the affected bone. Thin bone is more likely to deform, whereas thick bone is inelastic and more likely to fracture. Although fractures of the optic canal are not uncommon in patients with traumatic optic neuropathy, direct injury to the nerve by displaced bone fragments is infrequent.

The intracranial optic nerve can also be injured against the falciform dural fold which overlies the sphenoid plane or where the nerve becomes fixed entering the intracranial opening of the optic foramen (Fig. 9.5). It has been hypothesized that swelling of the optic nerve within the bony canal may make the intracanalicular portion of the nerve susceptible to ischemic injury. However, there is evidence that astrocytic swelling in the optic nerve is less significant than in brain injury, and optic nerve swelling may be less significant than previously thought.

Partial and complete avulsions of the optic nerve from the globe result from violent rotations of the globe. Traumatic avulsion of the optic nerve can follow self-inflicted injury, so-called autoenucleation or oedipism, or other types of penetrating orbital injury. The transfer of damaging force to the optic nerve following direct injury does not imply that the nerve has been severed or precludes visual recovery. A direct

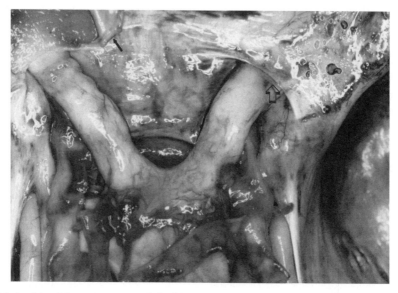

Figure 9.5. Relationship of the optic nerves and the falciform dural folds. The falciform dural fold in close association to the optic nerve as it enters the optic canal (*hollow arrow*). The falciform dural fold has been reflected, exposing the underlying sphenoid bone (*solid arrow*). (Reprinted from: Gossman MD, Roberts DM, Barr CC. Ophthalmic aspects of orbital injury. *Clin Plast Surg.* 1992;19:71–85, with permission.)

optic nerve injury may irreversibly injure a portion of the involved nerve, but leave other areas with the potential for visual recovery.

PATHOGENESIS

Whether direct or indirect, optic nerve injury results in both mechanical and ischemic damage. This damage can result from both primary and secondary mechanisms. **Primary mechanisms** cause permanent injury to the optic nerve axons at the moment of impact. Thus, the primary injury may be caused by laceration of the optic nerve or by shearing forces of deceleration that are transferred to the nerve, particularly within the optic canal, where the nerve is tightly bound.

Secondary mechanisms cause damage to the optic nerve subsequent to the force of impact. These mechanisms include vasoconstriction and swelling of the optic nerve within the confines of the nonexpansile optic canal, leading to worsening ischemia and irreversible damage to axons that may have been spared at the time of the initial injury or that were injured but possessed the potential for recovery immediately following impact. The implication in this concept is that immediate and appropriate intervention after an initial optic nerve injury has the potential to stop secondary injury and preserve vision by salvaging the axons that survived the initial insult.

Ischemia is perhaps the most important feature of secondary injury following trauma. The mechanism of injury is not simply cessation of blood flow. Partial ischemia and reperfusion of transiently ischemic regions generate **oxygen free radicals** resulting in reperfusion damage. **Bradykinin** initiates the release of arachidonic acid from neurons, and the resulting prostaglandins, oxygen free radicals, and lipid peroxides produce a loss of cerebrovascular autoregulation. Other potential mechanisms of injury include thromboxane-induced platelet adhesion and microvascular sludging, other triggers of free radical production, release of excitatory amino acids, and disruption of normal calcium metabolism. Additionally, the early phases of CNS injury are characterized by the release of mediators of **inflammation** with resultant acute and chronic inflammatory damage.

PHARMACOLOGY

Research in acute spinal cord trauma demonstrates that the pharmacologic actions of very high doses of corticosteroids in this setting are separate and distinct from the actions of steroids in the doses more typically encountered in clinical practice. Experimental studies have demonstrated a biphasic dose response to methylprednisolone in a range of doses much higher than the usual clinical usage. Specifically, in animals with exper-

imental CNS injury and ischemia, there appears to be a distinct pharmacologic benefit of doses of methylprednisolone in the range of 30 mg/kg—15 to 30 times the standard clinical dose. The most important of these effects appears to be as an antioxidant that limits tissue damage caused by oxygen free radicals.

The second National Acute Spinal Cord Injury Study (NASCIS II) was a multicenter, randomized, double-blind, placebo-controlled study. Patients enrolled in the study were randomized to one of three treatment arms within 12 hours of injury. The treatment arms consisted of placebo, naloxone, and methylprednisolone. Naloxone, an opiate receptor partial agonist that is effective in limiting neurologic injury in animals, was administered in an initial bolus of 5.4 mg/kg and then at a continuous infusion rate of 4.0 mg/kg/hour for 24 hours. Methylprednisolone was administered as an initial dose of 30 mg/kg followed by a continuous infusion of 5.4 mg/kg/hour for 24 hours (i.e., about 160 mg/kg or 10 grams total over 24 hours). This study showed that treatment with methylprednisolone within 8 hours of injury at the dose described above resulted in a significant improvement in motor and sensory function compared with either patients who received the placebo or patients treated with naloxone. Patients treated with methylprednisolone more than 8 hours after injury did not demonstrate an improvement in neurologic scores when compared with patients given the placebo. Indeed, subsequent analysis of the NASCIS II data suggested that methylprednisolone treatment given in the manner and dose described above and begun more than 8 hours after injury **was detrimental.**

MANAGEMENT

The management of traumatic optic neuropathy should be guided by the Hippocratic adage to do no harm. There is very little help from the published literature on this subject. For example, it is very difficult to use the retrospective data in the literature to characterize the natural history of traumatic optic neuropathy, in part because older series tend to report cases with severe visual loss, whereas contemporary studies contain larger numbers of patients with mild visual loss. In addition, traumatic optic neuropathy is a complex injury that often has both direct and indirect components and both primary and secondary intracellular and extracellular mechanisms of damage. Without an accurate knowledge of the natural history of traumatic optic neuropathy, determining the beneficial effect of a medical, surgical, or combined approach is very difficult.

At present, no studies validate a particular approach to the management of traumatic optic neuropathy. However, the use of systemic corticosteroids in the management of this condition has become commonplace. The beneficial clinical effect of these agents in the treatment of spinal cord injury provides a rationale for the use of these agents in traumatic optic neuropathy, although the doses used by most authors do not approach those used in the NASCIS II study. In addition, there are fundamental differences between the spinal cord and the optic nerve, so the successful application of high-dose corticosteroids in the treatment of spinal cord injury may not fully generalize to the treatment of optic nerve trauma. To date, no clinical studies have considered the possibility that corticosteroids may actually have a harmful effect on a traumatized optic nerve.

In the International Optic Nerve Trauma Study, recruitment was insufficient for a randomized trial, and it was converted to a comparative, nonrandomized interventional study. A total of 133 patients met criteria for inclusion and analysis. There were three treatment arms: untreated patients, steroid treatment, and surgery with or without steroids. There was no clear benefit for either corticosteroid therapy or optic canal decompression. Indeed, critical review of the traumatic optic neuropathy literature does not provide statistical evidence to conclude that surgery, corticosteroids, or a combination of corticosteroids and surgery is more beneficial than no treatment.

Mounting evidence, including the International Optic Nerve Trauma Study, raises significant questions regarding the potential benefits of corticosteroids in the treatment of traumatic optic neuropathy. First, there are no statistically valid studies supporting the use of corticosteroids in the treatment of traumatic optic neuropathy. The value of corticosteroids in the treatment of CNS injury varies by anatomic region and injury circumstance. Indeed, analysis of the NASCIS II data demonstrated that methylprednisolone treatment initiated more than 8 hours after spinal cord injury is detrimental.

Additionally, there are at least two lines of experimental evidence that suggest methylprednisolone is harmful for injured optic nerves. In one study using a rat optic nerve crush injury, there was a dose dependent decline in residual axons with increasing doses of methylprednisolone. Secondly, in an experimental model of multiple sclerosis, high dose methylprednisolone significantly increased apoptotic retinal ganglion cell loss. Given the lack of clinical evidence that corticosteroids are beneficial in the treatment of traumatic optic neuropathy, combined with these two lines of experimental evidence that methylprednisolone may be harmful to the injured optic nerve, clinicians should consider abandoning the routine use of megadose corticosteroids for the treatment of traumatic optic neuropathy.

Surgical intervention for traumatic optic neuropathy also remains empirical. A large percentage of intracanalicular injuries take place at the falciform dural fold, and this is a location that will not benefit from optic canal decompression. However, it is possible that subsets of injuries might benefit from surgical intervention. For example, reduction of bone fragments impinging on the optic nerve is a compelling reason for surgical intervention, especially in cases of delayed visual loss, although these may represent untreatable injuries. The hypothesis that reducing the canal fracture benefits the injured nerve remains untested. The fracture may just be residual evidence of the forces imparted into the nerve at the moment of impact; lifting these fragments of bone may not provide any therapeutic benefit.

Case reports and small series demonstrate visual improvement following evacuation of intraoptic nerve sheath hematomas, or subperiosteal hematomas causing optic nerve embarrassment. These examples provide only limited experience on which to base recommendations for surgery for individual patients. Intracanalicular optic nerve injury is the most common form of traumatic optic neuropathy. Not surprisingly, decompression of the optic canal is the most commonly reported surgical intervention. Theoretically, opening the canal to provide room for the optic nerve to swell into should be beneficial. However, the International Optic Nerve Trauma Study failed to demonstrate a beneficial effect for surgical decompression. This study had significant limitations and it is possible that the study did not have the power to identify a small beneficial effect for a subsets of patients. Consequently, it is difficult to advocate a set of best practices based on this study. Certainly in the case of orbital hemorrhage causing optic nerve compromise, there is little controversy regarding the need to provide immediate surgical relief of the compressive orbitopathy.

It is reasonable to expect that if surgery is to be of benefit, then performing it earlier may decrease secondary axonal loss. An orbitotomy provides the best access for the evacuation of an optic nerve sheath hematoma, reduction of a depressed lateral orbital wall fracture that compromises the optic nerve, or drainage of a subperiosteal hematoma with posterior compression of the optic nerve. An accurate anatomical diagnosis must be made to plan appropriate surgical intervention. Avoidance of surgical intervention on the unconscious patient continues to be a reasonable recommendation until such time as there is clear evidence establishing the value of surgical intervention.

FOR FURTHER INFORMATION

See *Walsh & Hoyt's Clinical Neuro-Ophthalmology*, 6th edition, Volume 1, Chapter 9, pages 431–446.

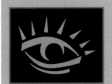

CHAPTER 10

Toxic and Deficiency Optic Neuropathies*

Physicians have known for centuries that the anterior visual pathway is vulnerable to damage from nutritional deficiency and chemicals. The resulting disorders share many signs and symptoms, and several appear to have a multifactorial etiology in which both undernutrition and toxicity play a role. In light of these facts, it is reasonable to group them together. Although evidence for the localization of the primary lesions is lacking in many of the so-called toxic and nutritional "amblyopias," they are generally assumed to be optic neuropathies and that is the rubric under which they are considered here.

ETIOLOGIC CRITERIA

Although certain optic neuropathies have an obvious toxic or nutritional etiology, the toxic or nutritional basis of others is merely presumptive, and the attribution may ultimately prove false. It is also likely that a few of the optic neuropathies now considered idiopathic or ascribed to some other etiology actually result from toxicity or nutritional deficiency. The proliferation of drugs and the introduction of new chemicals into the workplace and environment guarantee that additional toxic optic neuropathies will be identified. For medical and legal reasons, physicians must be alert to the possibility, both in sporadic cases of visual loss and in epidemics of visual loss, that intoxication or nutritional deficiency are factors.

NUTRITIONAL OPTIC NEUROPATHIES

Proving a nutritional basis for an optic neuropathy is by no means a simple task. The first criterion is that

the patient be nutritionally deficient and has been so sufficiently long to deplete nutrients. Evidence from epidemics indicates that this requires months (see below). The reports of large numbers of cases of visual loss after economic and political upheavals suggest the possibility of a nutritional etiology. The patient should show evidence of undernutrition, usually manifested in such obvious forms as weight loss and wasting. Victims of nutritional optic neuropathy, however, are not necessarily emaciated. Other signs such as peripheral neuropathy, keratitis, or the cutaneous and mucous membrane stigmata of the avitaminoses are useful, when present.

There is an important exception to the foregoing statements. The optic neuropathy of pernicious anemia or dietary vitamin B_{12} deficiency can occur in seemingly healthy individuals without obvious symptoms or signs of nutritional deficiency (see below).

The symptoms and signs should be those typical of nutritional optic neuropathy, and other disorders should be considered and eliminated by appropriate investigations. Both in individual cases and in epidemics it is especially important to establish if the patient has been exposed to substances toxic to the visual pathway. In such cases, intoxication may be the alternative explanation or be a cofactor. The absence of an optic neuropathy in well-nourished individuals in the same environment and recovery of vision in patients with restitution of an improved diet strongly support, but do not prove, a nutritional basis. Supporting laboratory evidence for the diagnosis of nutritional optic neuropathy can be obtained in the form of direct or indirect vitamin assays, serum protein concentrations, and antioxidant levels.

Identifying the specific nutritional deficiency responsible for an optic neuropathy is very difficult. Undernourished individuals are rarely deficient in only

*Adapted from Phillips PH. Toxic and deficiency optic neuropathies. In: Miller NR, Newman NJ, Biousse V, Kerrison JB, eds. *Walsh & Hoyt's Clinical Neuro-Ophthalmology.* 6th ed. Vol. I. Lippincott Williams & Wilkins: Philadelphia; 2005:447–463.

one nutrient; multiple deficiencies are the rule. Even if a specific deficiency is identified in a patient with loss of vision, it does not prove that the deficiency caused the visual loss. Nor does recovery when the deficient nutrient is resupplied establish that the resupplied nutrient affected the cure. With the exception of vitamin B_{12} (which only rarely becomes deficient for dietary reasons), no specific nutrient deficiency has been conclusively proved to cause optic neuropathy in humans. At the present state of knowledge, one can only speculate about which specific deficiencies can cause or contribute to nutritional optic neuropathy.

TOXIC OPTIC NEUROPATHIES

The primary issue in patients suspected of having a toxic amblyopia is whether they were exposed to a substance that has been proved to damage the optic nerve by the same route of exposure. Visual loss may occur from either acute or chronic intoxication depending upon the agent, but there should not be a long interval between the cessation of the exposure and the onset of symptoms. The patient must have symptoms and signs that are compatible with a toxic optic neuropathy and typical of those in other patients proved to have suffered loss of vision from the same agent. Of course, the symptoms cannot have preceded the exposure.

The response of patients to rechallenge is helpful in evaluating the validity of presumed intoxications and in helping to establish the cause of the patient's optic neuropathy. If a patient who has recovered vision following cessation of exposure to a drug or chemical loses vision again when reexposed, the recurrent loss of vision tends to verify the neurotoxic nature of the agent and the toxic etiology of the visual loss. Epidemiologic data, especially those showing correlation of changing disease incidence when and where specific drugs or chemicals are introduced or withdrawn, can also prove quite useful.

Confirmatory evidence of exposure from laboratory tests or from associated nonvisual symptoms is desirable. Nontoxic disorders must be considered in the diagnosis of these patients and should be ruled out with appropriate investigations. Animal models can help to validate the optic nerve toxicity of putative intoxicants, despite such problems as species variation in susceptibility and difficulty in measuring visual function.

CLINICAL CHARACTERISTICS OF NUTRITIONAL AND TOXIC OPTIC NEUROPATHIES

Persons of all ages, races, places, and economic strata are vulnerable to the toxic and nutritional optic neuropathies. Certain groups are at higher risk because they are under treatment with drugs, have occupa-

tional exposure, or practice habits such as smoking and alcohol consumption. Nutritional optic neuropathy is more likely to occur in the economically disadvantaged and during times of war and famine. The value of taking a thorough history, including dietary intake, exposure to drugs, use of tobacco, and social and occupational background, is obvious.

The symptoms and signs of nutritional and toxic optic neuropathy are similar and resemble those of most of the other optic neuropathies, primarily those that occur bilaterally and simultaneously. No single characteristic or combination of characteristics is pathognomonic.

Toxic and nutritional amblyopias are not painful. Thus, one should inquire carefully about this symptom because associated ocular or orbital pain suggests some other diagnosis.

Dyschromatopsia is present early and may be the initial symptom in observant patients. Some patients notice that certain colors, such as red, are no longer as bright and vivid as previously. Others experience a general loss of color perception.

Patients with nutritional or toxic optic neuropathies often initially notice a blur, fog, or cloud at the point of fixation, following which the visual acuity progressively declines. The rate of decline can be quite rapid. Although vision can decrease to any level, total blindness or vision limited to light perception is unusual in cases of nutritional optic neuropathy even if the patient is neglected. With the exception of methanol, which typically produces complete or nearly complete blindness, visual loss less than 20/400 is unusual in the toxic optic neuropathies. Bilaterality is the rule, although in the early stages one eye may be affected before the other becomes symptomatic. Profound loss of vision in one eye with completely normal findings in the other eye should cast doubt on the diagnosis of a toxic or nutritional optic neuropathy.

Patients with toxic or nutritional optic neuropathies typically have central or cecocentral scotomas with sparing of the peripheral visual field (Fig. 10.1). Peripheral constriction and altitudinal visual field loss are rare. Because of the symmetric and bilateral visual impairment in toxic and nutritional optic neuropathies, a relative afferent pupillary defect is not a common finding in affected patients. When the patient is bilaterally blind (e.g., as a consequence of methanol poisoning) the pupillary light response will be absent or weak and the pupils will be dilated. However, in most cases, the pupils have relatively normal responses to light and near stimulation.

In the early stages of nutritional optic neuropathy, the disc is normal or slightly hyperemic. Disc hemorrhages may be present in eyes with hyperemic discs, but they are usually small. Optic atrophy supervenes rather late. Most patients in the acute stages of toxic optic

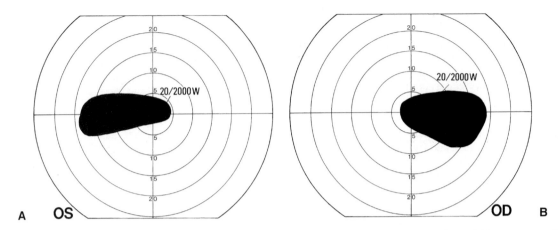

Figure 10.1. Visual fields of a patient with a bilateral toxic optic neuropathy caused by chloramphenicol. Note cecocentral scotomas in the visual fields of the left (**A**) and right (**B**) eyes. The peripheral fields were normal.

neuropathy also have normal discs, but disc swelling may be seen in some intoxications (Fig. 10.2). Optic atrophy develops after a variable interval, most pronounced in the distribution of the papillomacular bundle (Fig. 10.3).

DIFFERENTIAL DIAGNOSIS

When an individual complains of bilateral visual loss that refraction cannot correct and has an otherwise normal examination, there are many diagnostic possibilities in addition to the toxic and nutritional optic neuropathies. Certain maculopathies can present in this guise (see Chapter 2). With time, the fundus will show abnormalities, but until then, fluorescein angiography or focal electroretinography may be the only means of establishing the nature of the lesion. Full-field electroretinography may not reveal the defect.

One should be alert to the possibility of nonorganic visual loss. The absence of optic atrophy is an important clue when the visual loss is longstanding. In the acute phase, the visual field defects in the toxic and nutritional optic neuropathies are typically central or cecocentral. Such defects are exceptional in patients with nonorganic visual loss; in these patients, visual fields are usually constricted and may show spiraling or have a tubular configuration (see Chapter 23).

Dominantly-inherited (Kjer's) and mitochondrially-inherited (Leber's) optic neuropathies can be confused with nutritional optic neuropathy if no other family members are known to be affected. The confusion is most likely to occur in patients who are first evaluated late in their course. Kjer's disease progresses more slowly than the nutritional and toxic optic neuropathies, and optic atrophy is an early finding. In Leber's optic neuropathy, the onset of visual loss is not

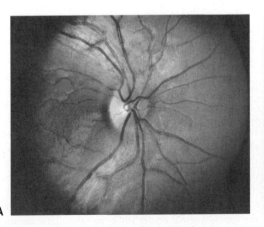
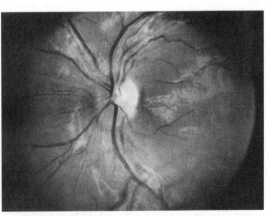

Figure 10.2. Appearance of optic discs in a patient with bilateral toxic optic neuropathy from chloramphenicol. Note that right (**A**) and left (**B**) discs are hyperemic and somewhat swollen nasally. There is already mild pallor of the temporal portions of both optic discs, associated with early loss of the nerve fiber layer in the papillomacular bundle of both eyes.

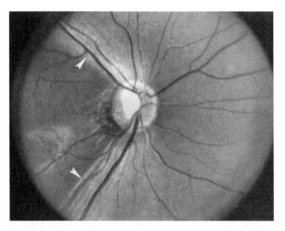 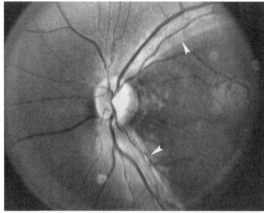

Figure 10.3. Appearance of optic discs in a patient with bilateral optic neuropathy in the setting of poor nutrition and alcohol abuse. Note extent of loss of nerve fiber layer from the papillomacular bundle (*arrowheads*) and marked temporal disc pallor. Visual acuity was 20/400 in both eyes, and there were bilateral central scotomas.

infrequently symmetric or nearly so, and this disorder must therefore be considered in any patient in whom a toxic or nutritional optic neuropathy is thought to be present. Appropriate genetic testing may be required in some cases (see Chapter 11).

It can be tragic to mistake a compressive or infiltrative lesion of the optic chiasm for nutritional or toxic optic neuropathy. There are few instances in which one should be so confident of the diagnosis of toxic or nutritional optic neuropathy that neuroimaging is omitted. Cecocentral scotomas and the bitemporal visual field defects of chiasmal disease resemble each other, and there are many examples of bilateral central and even cecocentral scotomas from tumors.

If a demyelinating, inflammatory, or infectious optic neuritis begins simultaneously in both eyes, there may be confusion with the toxic and nutritional optic neuropathies. The visual field defects are similar, but there is pain or disc swelling in greater than 90% of cases of optic neuritis (see Chapter 6). In some cases, MRI will indicate the nature of the lesion. In others, it may be necessary to examine the cerebrospinal fluid and perform specific testing for systemic infections and inflammations.

In most cases, analysis of the symptoms and signs obtained from a detailed history and physical examination will establish the diagnosis of a toxic or nutritional optic neuropathy. It is prudent to obtain neuroimaging unless one is absolutely confident of the diagnosis. MRI with contrast and special attention to the optic nerves and optic chiasm is the optimum investigation in most cases. A vitamin B$_{12}$ level should be determined to identify pernicious anemia, and red blood cell folate levels provide one marker of general nutritional status.

When a specific intoxicant is suspected, one should try to identify the toxin or its metabolites in the pa-

tient's tissues or fluids. The advice of a toxicologist is invaluable in such instances. In cases of suspected intoxication, one should attempt to evaluate or obtain information about other persons who have had similar exposure. The resulting information has potential public health implications and can help to validate the toxicity of chemicals not previously recognized as dangerous to the human optic nerve.

SPECIFIC NUTRITIONAL OPTIC NEUROPATHIES

EPIDEMIC NUTRITIONAL OPTIC NEUROPATHY

The most useful observations regarding nutritional amblyopia have come not from sporadic cases encountered in practice, but rather from epidemics during war and famine. Two well-documented epidemics were those that afflicted Allied prisoners of war of the Japanese during World War II and Cubans in the early 1990s.

The symptoms developed in an undernourished population after 4 months or more of food deprivation. Among the prisoners of war, vision loss occurred sooner in those who were undernourished at the time they were first incarcerated. Only a minority of people at risk developed loss of vision, and the occurrence of visual loss did not appear to correlate very well with the severity of malnutrition. In some cases, a superficial keratopathy was a prelude to the visual loss, but visual loss developed both with and without a preceding keratopathy. The visual loss was symmetric and often appeared suddenly. In up to one quarter of the cases, the visual nadir was reached in 1 day. Vision plateaued after 1 month in the remainder. At the time of visual loss,

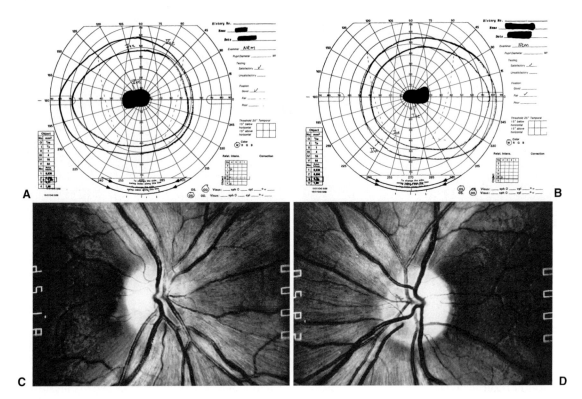

Figure 10.4. Visual fields and appearance of ocular fundi in a patient with Cuban epidemic optic neuropathy. The patient was a 23-year-old Cuban man who developed progressive loss of vision in both eyes associated with a peripheral neuropathy in 1993. Examination revealed visual acuity of 20/200 OU. Visual fields performed by kinetic perimetry reveal a cecocentral scotoma in the field of both the left (**A**) and right (**B**) eyes. Photographs of the right (**C**) and left (**D**) optic fundi show temporal pallor of the optic discs associated with marked loss of the retinal nerve fiber layer in the papillomacular bundle.

many victims also had pain or sensory loss in their extremities. There was a high incidence of bilateral sensorineural hearing loss. The fundi were usually normal at first, but a minority had peripapillary hemorrhages associated with mild optic disc hyperemia and swelling. Optic atrophy was a late development. The visual field defects were central or cecocentral. Most abnormalities could be reversed with improved nutrition. Postmortem examinations on repatriated Allied prisoners found atrophy of the papillomacular bundle and lesions in the fasciculus gracilis of the spinal cord.

In 1992 and 1993, an epidemic of optic neuropathy and peripheral neuropathy similar to that reported among the WW II prisoners of war occurred in Cuba. More than 50,000 persons were affected with bilateral optic neuropathy, sensory and dysautonomic peripheral neuropathy, sensory myelopathy, spastic paraparesis, or sensorineural deafness in various combinations. Slightly more than half of the affected persons had evidence of optic neuropathy, which occurred as a painless rapid loss of vision in both eyes associated with marked dyschromatopsia, central or cecocentral scotomas, and

normal appearing optic discs. Patients who did not recover vision developed temporal pallor of the optic discs, associated with marked loss of the nerve fiber layer in the papillomacular bundle (Fig. 10.4). The majority of cases occurred in people between 25 to 64 years of age with a predominance of males being among those with optic nerve disease. Partial and complete recovery occurred following treatment with parenteral and oral vitamins. In addition, subsequent supplementation of the general population with B-complex vitamins and vitamin A coincided with a dramatic decrease in new cases of the condition.

Although the loss of vision in the epidemic cases was undoubtedly caused by malnutrition, it is impossible to identify a specific deficient nutrient that caused either of the epidemics. Malnourished individuals have multiple deficiencies. Clinical and laboratory data make it unlikely that vitamin deficiency was the sole factor. Systematic investigation of Cuban epidemic optic neuropathy patients and controls showed an increased risk associated with cassava consumption and a decreased risk associated with high serum levels of antioxidant carotenoids, ingestion of B vitamins, and ingestion of animal products.

Factors additional to malnutrition must explain the visual loss in these cases and in similar cases in other countries such as Tanzania. Tobacco use, especially cigar use, was a risk factor in Cuba. Physical labor also seemed to be a risk factor among the prisoners of war. In any case, the conclusion that epidemic cases of nutritional optic neuropathy (and probably sporadic cases as well) are the result of some multifactorial etiology is inescapable.

The treatment of nutritional optic neuropathy is improved nutrition. Unless the vision loss is extensive, there is an excellent prospect for recovery or at least improvement with such treatment.

VITAMIN B_{12} DEFICIENCY

Although the role of vitamin B_{12} in the maintenance and function of the nervous system has yet to be explained, depletion of this nutrient almost invariably leads to neurologic dysfunction. The body's nutritional requirements must be met entirely by food (particularly meat and dairy products). The abundant stores, particularly in the liver, are redistributed so gradually that it takes years for poor intake to cause disease. Indeed, a poor diet is rarely the cause of vitamin B_{12} deficiency, and when it is, it is found only in strict vegans. Impaired absorption because of diphyllobothriasis, intestinal disease, or gastrointestinal surgery accounts for only a few cases.

Pernicious anemia is by far the most common condition in which vitamin B_{12} deficiency and its complications are encountered. This presumably autoimmune disorder results from impaired absorption of the vitamin from the ileum, because the patient lacks the intrinsic factor elaborated by the parietal cells of the gastric mucosa. Pernicious anemia is most often found in, but is not limited to, middle-aged and elderly whites of northern European extraction. The anemia is megaloblastic. It develops slowly and can be severe. Unless treatment is instituted early, most patients with pernicious anemia develop neurologic manifestations. The pathologic substrate is a white-matter lesion that affects both myelin and axons initially in the posterior columns of the upper thoracic and lower cervical portions of the spinal cord ("subacute combined degeneration"). The process subsequently affects other white-matter tracts and other levels of the spinal cord. Paresthesias and weakness in the extremities are heralding symptoms. With time, vibration sense is lost, and the patient develops spasticity with hyperactive knee and ankle jerks, as well as extensor plantar responses. Dementia may also develop.

Deficiency of vitamin B_{12}, whether from inadequate diet or interference with absorption, can cause an optic neuropathy. Lesions in the optic nerves and optic chiasm have been demonstrated in postmortem examinations of patients with pernicious anemia. There are also primate models of the disease. Severe optic nerve degeneration is found in experimental vitamin B_{12} deficiency in monkeys even before there is anemia or a spinal cord lesion. Hence, it is not surprising that in humans, an optic neuropathy may be the first symptom of pernicious anemia and may precede the hematologic disturbance. Indeed, abnormal VEPs can be recorded in patients with pernicious anemia who have no visual symptoms, suggesting that there may also be subclinical damage to the visual pathways in this disease.

The optic neuropathy that results from vitamin B_{12} deficiency resembles other nutritional optic neuropathies. The visual loss is symmetric, painless, and progressive. Central and cecocentral scotomas are the rule, and the optic disc appears normal in the early stages of the condition. Unless optic atrophy becomes well established, one can expect recovery of vision with intramuscular injections of hydroxocobalamin. It is important to obtain a serum vitamin B_{12} level in all cases of unexplained bilateral optic neuropathy.

OTHER VITAMIN DEFICIENCIES

Although there are some experimental, biochemical, and clinical data that suggest that vitamin B_1 (thiamine) deficiency may cause an optic neuropathy, the results of these experiments are not conclusive. Additionally, when chronic thiamine deficiency was produced in human volunteers, their vision did not suffer. Finally, observational studies among prisoners of war present strong evidence against a primary role for thiamine deficiency in nutritional optic neuropathy. Specifically, beriberi was as prevalent among those with normal vision as it was among those with loss of vision, optic neuropathy could not be cured with injections of thiamine, and some prisoners developed visual loss while being treated with thiamine. Indeed, the disorder consequent to thiamine depletion is Wernicke's encephalopathy, in which visual loss is uncommon, and a primate model of this disorder shows no pathologic changes in the optic nerves. These observations cast doubt on a primary role for thiamine deficiency in human nutritional optic neuropathy.

The roles of pyridoxine, niacin, folic acid, and riboflavin deficiency in causing an optic neuropathy are also controversial. As with thiamine, these vitamins are apt to be depleted in patients who are generally malnourished, but there is no definitive evidence indicating that such deficiencies play a primary etiological role in nutritional optic neuropathy. Although low folate levels have been documented in the red blood cells and occasionally in the serum of patients with nutritional optic neuropathy, and some malnourished patients with optic neuropathy recover when treated with folic acid supplements, this does not prove that the folate deficiency caused the loss of vision or that the folic acid supplements affected the recovery. However, it makes sense to enrich the diet of patients with loss of vision and evidence of poor nutrition with all of the water-soluble vitamins in which they might be deficient.

TROPICAL OPTIC NEUROPATHY

There are optic neuropathies endemic to tropical regions for which a nutritional etiology has been invoked. An early report by Strachan from Jamaica appeared in 1897. The clinical features of his patients resemble in some ways those of the epidemic cases described above. There was numbness and cramps in the hands and feet. The visual loss was bilateral and was sometimes accompanied by hearing loss. Unusual features included muscle wasting, severe pain, and a dermatopathy. Strachan made no claim for a nutritional etiology. When the disorder was subsequently reevaluated by others, they concluded that this was not a nutritional disease. Despite that, some authors inappropriately use "Strachan's syndrome" to designate nutritional optic neuropathy.

There is an otherwise unexplained bilateral optic neuropathy called "West Indian amblyopia" found in black expatriates from the West Indies. The history is typically that of bilateral, painless progressive visual decline in a well-nourished adult. The visual field defects tend to be central or cecocentral, but annular scotomas and peripheral constriction have been reported. Optic atrophy develops. Deafness is also present in some of the patients. No treatment, including various vitamin regimens, is effective in reversing either the visual or the nonvisual manifestations of the disorder. Although a toxic basis ("bush tea") has been postulated, there is no good evidence for either a toxic or nutritional etiology.

A disorder similar to so-called Strachan's syndrome has been described in Nigerians, but it differs in that the majority of patients have constricted visual fields and total blindness can occur. Poor diet is said to be the common denominator in the African cases, but investigators have also suggested that exogenous cyanide from an excess of cassava in the diet is an etiologic factor. However, the evidence that cyanide plays a role in causing any optic neuropathy is tenuous at best (see the subsequent text). The endemic tropical neuropathy in Nigeria might result from nutritional deficiency, but this has not been proved.

SPECIFIC TOXIC OPTIC NEUROPATHIES

Table 10.1 lists substances that are suggested or presumed to be toxic to the human optic nerve. It is not always clear if the association of ingestion of, or ex-

Table 10.1. *Substances Known or Believed to Cause Toxic Optic Neuropathy*

Amantadine hydrochloride	Halogenated hydroxyquinolines
Amiodarone	Hexachlorophene
Amoproxan	Infliximab
Arsenicals	Interferon-alpha
Aspidium (male fern)	Iodoform
Cafergot	Iodoquinol
Carbon disulfide	Isoniazid
Carbon tetrachloride	Lead
Catha edulis	Linezolid
Chlorambucil	Methanol (methyl alcohol)
Chloramphenicol	Methyl acetate
Chlorodinitrobenzene	Methyl bromide
Chlorpromazine	Octamoxin
Chlorpropamide	Organic solvents
Cisplatin	Penicillamine
Clioquinol	Pheniprazine
Clomiphene	Plasmocid
Cobalt chloride	Quinine
Cyclosporine	Sildenafil
Dapsone	Streptomycin
Desferrioxamine	Styrene (vinyl benzene)
Dinitrobenzene	Sulfonamides
Dinitrochlorobenzene	Tacrolimus
Disulfiram	Tamoxifen
Elcatonin	Thallium
Emetine	Tobacco
Ergot	Toluene
Ethambutol	Triethyltin
Ethchlorvynol	Trichloroethylene
Ethylene glycol	Vincristine
5-Fluorouracil	

posure to, a particular substance and the subsequent visual loss is fortuitous or cause and effect. The literature is uneven in this regard, and several of the agents are of academic interest only because they are no longer in use. Furthermore, it is often difficult to determine whether the underlying disease or its treatment is responsible for the visual loss. In addition, the suspected toxin may not be the only agent to which the patient has been exposed, further confounding the issue of causation.

METHANOL

Methanol ingestion is the most widely recognized cause of a toxic optic neuropathy, and methanol toxic neuropathy is also the best characterized pathologically and clinically. However, methanol intoxication is not an ideal paradigm for the toxic neuropathies because of its combination of severe irreversible visual loss with acute onset, life-threatening systemic symptoms.

The victim almost always has consumed the poison accidentally because it was mistaken for, substituted for, or added to ethyl alcohol, the taste and smell of which it closely resembles. Although blindness can result from drinking an ounce or less of pure methanol, the toxic effect is ameliorated if it is ingested together with ethyl alcohol.

In the primate model of methanol intoxication, there is optic disc swelling, but the lesion is retrobulbar. The evidence from human postmortem examinations also favors a retrobulbar locus. The early lesion is demyelinating; the later lesion is necrotic.

Initially, the patient has nausea and vomiting. After 18 to 48 hours, the patient begins to experience respiratory distress, headache, and visual loss. Abdominal pain, generalized weakness, confusion, and drowsiness are commonly present at this stage. Coma and death from respiratory failure may follow. Metabolic acidosis is one of the hallmarks of methanol intoxication, and it is consequent to the accumulation of formate.

Methanol intoxication can reduce vision to any level, including total irrevocable blindness. Central and cecocentral scotomas predominate in cases of partial visual loss. The optic disc is often hyperemic, with blurred margins in the acute stage, and there may be some edema of the peripapillary retina. The reaction of the pupils to light is reduced, and when the patient is blind, the pupils are dilated and nonreactive to light. Patients may regain vision, usually within a week, but occasionally later. In some cases, vision fails again weeks after first improving. The optic discs gradually become pale, and there is often cupping of the optic disc and thinning of retinal arteries.

The diagnosis of methanol poisoning can be substantiated by demonstrating a serum methanol level of greater than 20 mg/dL. Other biochemical findings include a large anion gap, a high serum formate level, and a reduced serum bicarbonate level. Treatment must be instituted promptly. Ethanol should be given, because it interferes with the metabolism of methanol. The metabolic acidosis responds to bicarbonate, and hemodialysis can help eliminate the toxin.

ETHYLENE GLYCOL

Ethylene glycol is the active ingredient in automobile antifreeze and may be consumed accidentally or in a suicide attempt. This poison is toxic to the optic nerve, and the metabolic consequences resemble those of methanol poisoning.

The victim initially has nausea, vomiting, and abdominal pain, followed by stupor and coma, then cardiac failure within a few days. There is a high incidence of renal failure. The outcome can be fatal, or recovery can occur, sometimes with permanent residual neurologic and ophthalmologic deficits.

Despite the metabolic similarities to methanol intoxication, the frequency of visual loss seems to be much lower in patients poisoned by ethylene glycol. Nevertheless, profound visual loss can occur. True papilledema, caused by cerebral edema, may occur, or the optic discs can initially appear normal, only to become pale with time. Unlike the situation in methanol intoxication, patients with ethylene glycol intoxication may also develop nystagmus and ophthalmoplegia.

One clue to the cause of the intoxication is the presence of oxalate crystals in the urine. The accumulation of glycolate causes a metabolic acidosis and a large anion gap. Treatment is essentially the same as the treatment of methanol intoxication.

ETHAMBUTOL

Of all the drugs in wide use, ethambutol is undoubtedly the one most often implicated in toxic optic neuropathy. Experiments in monkeys and rats show that ethambutol intoxication causes an axonal neuropathy with a special predilection for the optic chiasm. Ethambutol is metabolized to a chelating agent, and this has been suggested as somehow responsible for the optic neuropathy. It is interesting in this regard that two other chelators—disulfiram and DL-penicillamine—have been implicated in toxic optic neuropathies.

Human ethambutol intoxication is dose-related, with loss of vision most likely to occur in patients receiving 25 mg/kg/day or more. However, vision loss may occur in patients receiving much lower doses. Visual loss rarely occurs until the patient has been receiving the drug for at least 2 months, with 7 months being the average. There is evidence that there is greater susceptibility to intoxication and more severe visual impairment in patients with renal tuberculosis, perhaps because ethambutol depends on the kidneys for excretion.

The loss of vision is bilaterally symmetric and begins insidiously with dyschromatopsia often the earliest symptom. Central scotomas are the rule, but patients may also develop bitemporal defects or peripheral constriction. The fundi are initially normal, but if the drug is not stopped, vision continues to worsen and optic atrophy develops. Visual acuity, color vision, and visual field usually improve slowly once ethambutol is discontinued; however, some patients, particularly but not exclusively those in whom optic atrophy has already developed, do not experience an improvement in visual function.

Beyond stopping the drug, there is no specific therapy for the toxic optic neuropathy caused by ethambutol. Recommendations regarding the appropriate screening strategy are controversial. Certainly, discontinuation of the drug is indicated at the onset of any symptoms or signs of optic neuropathy.

HALOGENATED HYDROXYQUINOLINES

The halogenated hydroxyquinolines are amebacidal drugs. One of these (iodochlorhydroxyquin) was promoted in some parts of the world for preventing or treating travelers' diarrhea and chronic diarrheas. In that setting, it caused a syndrome of optic neuropathy (about 25% of the patients), myelopathy, and peripheral neuropathy (subacute myelo-optic neuropathy or SMON). The irony is that there is no evidence that the halogenated hydroxyquinolines actually prevent traveler's diarrhea. The impact on public health was significant; over 10,000 cases were documented in Japan between 1956 and 1970. SMON virtually disappeared in Japan when the use of these drugs was stopped.

AMIODARONE

Amiodarone is an antiarrhythmic agent primarily used to treat atrial or ventricular tachyarrhythmias. The most common ocular side effect is the formation of verticillate, pigmented, corneal epithelial deposits that eventually occur in most patients treated with the drug. Amiodarone has been associated with an optic neuropathy that in many cases is indistinguishable from nonarteritic anterior ischemic optic neuropathy. Indeed, the association of optic neuropathy and amiodarone treatment is controversial. Several features proposed as suggestive of an amiodarone effect are insidious bilateral visual loss, protracted bilateral disc edema, and potential for recovery when the drug is discontinued.

Amiodarone binds phospholipids and forms complexes that accumulate within many tissues, including the cornea, vascular endothelial cells, retinal ganglion cells, and optic nerve axons. Optic neuropathy may result from direct involvement of neural tissues or from vascular compromise (and hence be a form of ischemic optic neuropathy).

The available data are insufficient to make firm recommendations regarding a screening protocol for patients treated with amiodarone. Certainly, any patient with visual symptoms during treatment should be promptly evaluated. Amiodarone may be a life-saving treatment and the occurrence of an optic neuropathy is therefore not an absolute contraindication to further treatment. However, in patients who have an optic neuropathy while on amiodarone, discontinuation of amiodarone and treatment with an alternative drug should be considered.

TOBACCO

The mechanism, nature, nosology, semiology, and existence of a toxic optic neuropathy caused by tobacco have been debated for many years. The designation *tobacco-alcohol amblyopia* has obfuscated these issues. It is our opinion that although tobacco probably can cause or contribute to a toxic optic neuropathy, alcohol is not a primary or contributing factor, and the two do not exert any toxic effect in concert. If ever a medical term deserved to be expunged, it is *tobacco-alcohol amblyopia*.

Tobacco amblyopia occurs primarily in middle-aged or elderly persons. It is overwhelmingly a disease of men, perhaps because the victims are overwhelmingly pipe and cigar smokers. Why cigarette smokers should be less vulnerable is unknown. The disorder is painless and characterized by slowly progressive, bilateral dyschromatopsia and visual loss. The characteristic visual field defect is a cecocentral scotoma. The optic discs initially appear normal with pallor being a late feature.

The mechanism by which tobacco damages the optic nerves is unclear. One possibility relates to concurrent malnutrition. The Cuban experience suggests that tobacco may be a secondary factor in patients predisposed to an optic neuropathy by malnutrition. During the Nazi occupation of Belgium when there was widespread malnutrition, the incidence of tobacco amblyopia increased dramatically. Vitamin B_{12} deficiency may also play a role in some cases of tobacco amblyopia. Tobacco itself may actually interfere with the absorption of the vitamin. In most cases of tobacco amblyopia, however, there is no defect in vitamin B_{12} metabolism, and blood levels of the vitamin are within normal limits. Patients with tobacco amblyopia slowly improve if they stop smoking, or if they are treated with injections of hydroxocobalamin.

Cyanide is present in tobacco smoke, and this has led to a suspicion that tobacco amblyopia is a limited form of cyanide poisoning. However, attempts to produce a cyanide optic neuropathy in nonhuman primates have failed on numerous occasions. Chronic cyanide injections caused an optic neuropathy in rats, but the characteristics were not those of human tobacco amblyopia; the optic neuropathy only occurred when extensive brain lesions were already present. As with the nutritional amblyopias, it seems likely that the etiology of tobacco amblyopia in many cases is multifactorial.

FOR FURTHER INFORMATION

See *Walsh & Hoyt's Clinical Neuro-Ophthalmology*, 6th edition, Volume 1, Chapter 10, pages 447–463.

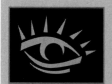

CHAPTER 11

Hereditary Optic Neuropathies*

The hereditary optic neuropathies comprise a group of disorders in which the cause of optic nerve dysfunction appears to be hereditable as demonstrated or suggested by familial expression or genetic analysis. Clinical variability, both within and among families with the same disease, often makes recognition and classification difficult. Traditionally, classification has relied on the recognition of similar characteristics and similar patterns of transmission, but genetic analysis now permits diagnosis of the hereditary optic neuropathies in the absence of family history or in the setting of unusual clinical presentations. As a result, the clinical phenotypes of each disease are broader, and it is easier to recognize unusual cases.

The inherited optic neuropathies typically manifest as symmetric, bilateral, central visual loss. In many of these disorders, the papillomacular nerve fiber bundle is affected with resultant central or cecocentral scotomas. The exact location of initial pathology along the ganglion cell and its axon, and the pathophysiologic mechanisms of optic nerve injury remain unknown. Optic nerve damage is usually permanent and, in many diseases, may be progressive. When optic atrophy is observed, substantial nerve injury has already occurred.

In classifying the hereditary optic neuropathies, it is important to exclude the primary retinal degenerations that may masquerade as primary optic neuropathies because of the common finding of optic disc pallor

(see Chapter 2). At times, there may be co-existent pathology.

Customary classification of the inherited optic neuropathies is by pattern of transmission. The most common patterns of inheritance are autosomal dominant, autosomal recessive, and maternal (i.e., mitochondrial). The same genetic defect may not be responsible for all pedigrees with optic neuropathy inherited in a similar fashion. Similarly, different genetic defects may cause identical or similar phenotypes—some inherited in the same manner, others not. Alternatively, the same genetic defect may result in different clinical expression, although the pattern of inheritance should be consistent.

In some of the hereditary optic neuropathies, optic nerve dysfunction is the only manifestation of the disease. In others, various neurologic and systemic abnormalities are regularly observed. Furthermore, inherited diseases with primarily neurologic or systemic manifestations, such as the multisystem degenerations, can include optic atrophy.

MONOSYMPTOMATIC HEREDITARY OPTIC NEUROPATHIES

LEBER'S HEREDITARY OPTIC NEUROPATHY

Clinical Features

The prevalence of the disease has not been adequately studied, but in Northeast England, there was a minimal prevalence of visual loss from Leber's hereditary optic neuropathy (LHON) of 3.22 per 100,000 individuals. LHON accounts for about 2% of legal blindness in persons under 65 years of age in Australia. Men

* Adapted from Newman NJ. Hereditary optic neuropathies. In: Miller NR, Newman NJ, Biousse V, Kerrison JB, eds. *Walsh & Hoyt's Clinical Neuro-Ophthalmology.* 6th ed. Vol. I. Philadelphia: Lippincott Williams & Wilkins; 2005: 465–501.

become symptomatic more frequently than women. There is a male predominance of 80% to 90% in most pedigrees. Approximately 20% to 60% of men at risk for LHON experience visual loss. Among women at risk, the occurrence rate ranges from 4% to 32%. Affected females are more likely to have affected children, especially daughters, than unaffected female carriers.

The onset of visual loss typically occurs between the ages of 15 and 35 years, but otherwise classic LHON occurs in many individuals both younger and older with a range of onset as broad as 1 to 80 years. This age variability occurs even among members of the same pedigree.

Visual loss typically begins painlessly in one eye. Indeed, the absence of pain is a major feature that differentiates LHON from other optic neuropathies, particularly optic neuritis, which occurs in the same general age group. Uhthoff's symptom (a transient worsening of vision with exercise or warming) may occur in patients with LHON, as it does in patients with other optic neuropathies. The second eye is usually affected weeks to months later. Reports of simultaneous onset are numerous and likely reflect both instances of true simultaneous bilateral visual loss and cases in which initial involvement of the first eye went unrecognized. Rarely, loss of vision in the second eye occurs after a prolonged interval (8 years or longer). Even more infrequently, involvement remains monocular (up to 16 years) or subclinical. The duration of progression of visual loss in each eye also varies and may be difficult to document accurately. Usually, the course is characterized as acute or subacute with deterioration of visual function stabilizing after about 3 to 4 months. However, sudden and complete visual loss or slowly progressive disease over years can occur.

Visual acuities at the point of maximum visual loss range from no light perception to 20/20, but most patients deteriorate to acuities worse than 20/200. Color vision is severely affected, often early in the course, but rarely before there is significant visual loss. Pupillary light responses may be relatively preserved when compared with the responses in patients with optic neuropathies from other causes. Visual field defects are typically central or cecocentral. The scotomas may be relative during the early stages of visual loss but rapidly become large and absolute. Rarely, field abnormalities mimicking the bitemporal configuration of chiasmal defects occur.

Hyperemia of the optic disc, obscuration of the disc margins, and dilation and tortuosity of retinal vessels, and rarely retinal and disc hemorrhages, macular edema, exudates, and retinal striations, may be seen, especially during the acute phase of visual loss. A "classic triad" of signs is seen in many cases of LHON: (a) circumpapillary telangiectatic microangiopathy, (b) swelling of the nerve fiber layer around the disc (pseu-

doedema), and (c) absence of leakage from the disc or papillary region on fluorescein angiography (distinguishing the LHON optic disc from truly swollen optic discs) (Fig. 11.1). These funduscopic changes may be seen in symptomatic patients, some "presymptomatic" cases, and in asymptomatic maternal relatives. However, having abnormalities of the peripapillary nerve fiber layer does not necessarily predict visual loss. Furthermore, many patients with LHON never exhibit the characteristic ophthalmoscopic appearance, even if examined at the time of acute visual loss. The "classic" LHON ophthalmoscopic appearance may be helpful in suggesting the diagnosis if it is recognized in patients or their maternal relatives, but its absence—even during the period of acute visual loss—does not exclude the diagnosis of LHON. Indeed, some patients with LHON have absolutely normal appearing optic discs at the time they become symptomatic.

As visual loss progresses in patients with LHON who have the typical fundus appearance described earlier, the telangiectatic vessels disappear, and the pseudoedema of the disc resolves. Perhaps because of the initial hyperemia, the optic discs of patients with LHON may not appear pale for some time. This feature, coupled with the relatively preserved pupillary responses and the lack of pain, can result in the misdiagnosis of nonorganic visual loss in some LHON patients. Eventually, however, optic atrophy—with nerve fiber layer dropout most pronounced in the papillomacular bundle—supervenes (Fig. 11.2). Nonglaucomatous cupping of the optic discs or arteriolar attenuation may also be seen.

In most patients, visual loss remains profound and permanent. However, not uncommonly, recovery of central vision occurs years after visual deterioration. Spontaneous improvement may occur gradually over 6 months to 1 year after initial visual loss or it may suddenly occur 2 to 10 years after onset. It may take the form of a gradual clearing of central vision or be restricted to a few central degrees, resulting in a small island of vision within a large central scotoma. Recovery is usually bilateral and symmetric, but it may be asymmetric or even occur only in one eye. Patients in whom vision improves substantially have a lower mean age at the time of initial visual loss, usually less than 20 years. Furthermore, the particular mtDNA mutation also influences prognosis. The 11778 mutation carries the worst prognosis for vision and the 14484 mutation the best (see below). After visual recovery occurs, recurrent visual loss is extremely rare.

Associated Findings

In the majority of patients with LHON, visual dysfunction is the only significant manifestation of the disease. However, some pedigrees have members with

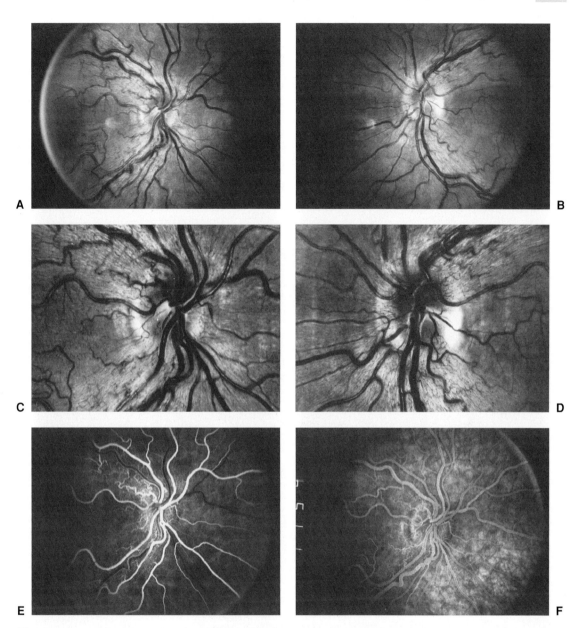

Figure 11.1. Leber's optic neuropathy. **A and B:** Both optic discs in the acute phase of the disorder. Note hyperemic appearance of discs. Peripapillary telangiectatic vessels are present. **C and D:** Both optic discs photographed with red-free (540 nm) light. Note marked hyperemia of the discs with dilation of small vessels both on the surface of the disc and in the peripapillary region. **E and F:** Fluorescein angiogram in arteriovenous (**E**) and late (**F**) phases shows dilation of right disc and peripapillary vessels but no leakage of fluorescein dye.

associated cardiac conduction abnormalities, such as the pre-excitation syndromes (specifically Wolff-Parkinson-White and Lown-Ganong-Levine) and prolongation of the corrected QT interval. Rarely, patients experience palpitations, syncope, or sudden death. Minor neurologic abnormalities, such as exaggerated or pathologic reflexes, mild cerebellar ataxia, tremor, movement disorders, muscle wasting, or distal sensory neuropathy, are present in some patients with LHON. In addition, some patients with molecularly confirmed LHON, predominantly women, exhibit symptoms and signs consistent with multiple sclerosis (MS) at the time they begin to experience the progressive, nonremitting visual loss typical of LHON. Cerebrospinal fluid (CSF) and magnetic resonance imaging (MRI) findings are also characteristic of MS in these

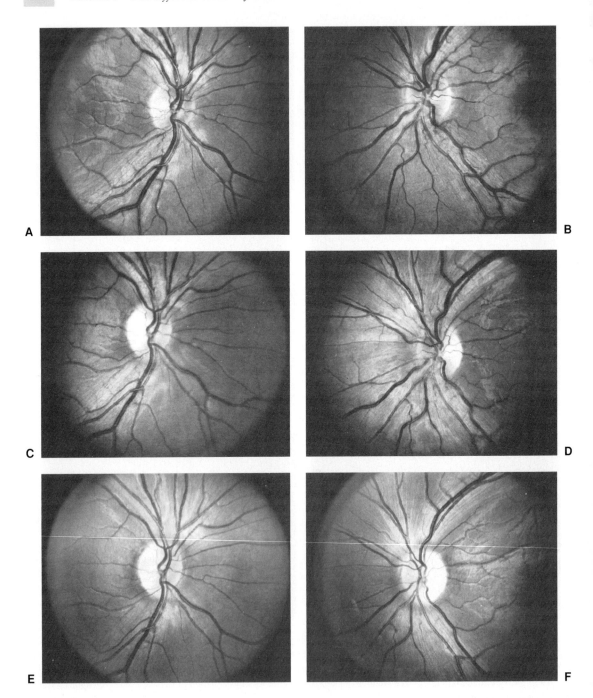

Figure 11.2. Progression to optic atrophy in a patient with Leber's optic neuropathy. **A and B:** Both discs in acute phase of the disease. Visual acuity is 20/100 in both eyes with large cecocentral scotomas. Telangiectatic vessels are evident adjacent to the inferior margin of both discs. The right disc is already pale temporally, and there is atrophy of the papillomacular nerve fiber layer. **C and D:** Two months after onset of visual loss, visual acuity is 5/200 in the right eye and 8/200 in the left eye. Both discs show moderate pallor, particularly temporally, with loss of nerve fiber layer that is especially evident in the papillomacular region. Previously seen telangiectatic vessels are disappearing. **E and F:** Six months after onset of visual loss, visual acuity remains 5/200 in the right eye and 8/200 in the left eye. Both discs are pale, particularly temporally. The telangiectatic vessels have completely disappeared. One year after these photographs were obtained, the patient noted gradual, partial return of visual acuity in both eyes to 20/50. Subsequent genetic testing showed evidence of a mutation in the mitochondrial DNA at position 14484.

patients. It is likely that this apparent association of LHON and MS is no greater than the prevalence of the two diseases, but that an underlying LHON mutation, however, may worsen the prognosis of optic neuritis in patients with MS.

Some pedigrees have been described in which multiple members exhibit the clinical features of LHON in addition to more severe neurologic abnormalities, the so-called "Leber's plus" syndromes. These syndromes include: optic neuropathy, movement disorders, spasticity, psychiatric disturbances, skeletal abnormalities, and acute infantile encephalopathic episodes; optic neuropathy, dystonia, and lesions of the basal ganglia by neuroimaging; optic neuropathy and myelopathy; optic neuropathy and fatal encephalopathy in early childhood. Most of these pedigrees are genetically distinct from those with more classic LHON.

Inheritance and Genetics

All pedigrees clinically designated as LHON have a maternal inheritance pattern. In maternal inheritance, all offspring of a woman carrying the trait will inherit the trait, but only the females can pass the trait on to the subsequent generation. Both the father and the mother contribute to the nuclear portion of the zygote, but the mother's egg is essentially the sole provider of the cytoplasmic contents of the zygote. Therefore, a cytoplasmic determinant is necessary for maternal inheritance. The only source of extranuclear DNA in the cell is the intracytoplasmic mitochondria.

Every cell contains several hundred intracytoplasmic mitochondria that generate the cellular energy necessary for normal cellular function and maintenance. Those cells in tissues particularly reliant on mitochondrial energy production, such as the central nervous system (CNS), contain more mitochondria than cells with low energy requirements. Each mitochondrion contains 2 to 10 double-stranded circles of DNA. Each circle of mtDNA contains only 16,500 base pairs compared with the 3×10^9 base pairs contained within the nuclear genome. However, given that there are several mtDNAs in each mitochondrion and hundreds of mitochondria per cell, the mtDNA comprises approximately 0.3% of the cell's total DNA. Mitochondrial DNA codes for all the transfer ribonucleic acids (RNAs) and ribosomal RNAs required for intramitochondrial protein production, and for 13 proteins essential to the oxidative phosphorylation system. The majority of proteins crucial to normal oxidative phosphorylation function are encoded on nuclear genes, manufactured in the cytoplasm, and transported into the mitochondria. Hence "mitochondrial disease" can theoretically result from genetic defects in either the nuclear or mitochondrial genomes. Over 100 mtDNA point mutations and countless mtDNA re-arrangements have been proposed as etiologic factors in human disease. Expression of these diseases reflects complex genotypic-phenotypic interactions that likely involve nuclear modifying or susceptibility factors.

If a new mutation occurs in the mtDNA, there will be a period of coexistence of mutant and normal mtDNA within the same cell (**heteroplasmy**). At each cell division, the mitochondrial genotype may drift toward pure normal or pure mutant, or it may remain mixed (**replicative segregation**). The phenotype of the cell (and the tissue the cells comprise) depends on the proportional mixture of mtDNA genotypes and the intrinsic energy needs of the cell. The mutant phenotype may only become apparent when the amount of normal mtDNA can no longer provide sufficient mitochondrial function for cell and tissue maintenance (**threshold effect**). Because of the cytoplasmic location of mtDNA, mitochondrial diseases secondary to point mutations in the mtDNA follow a pattern of maternal inheritance.

The first point mutation in mtDNA to be linked to LHON was a single nucleotide substitution at position 11778 in the mtDNA (Fig. 11.3). This region codes for subunit 4 (designated ND4) of complex I (NADH dehydrogenase) in the respiratory chain. The 11778 mutation is present in many racially divergent pedigrees with LHON, suggesting that the 11778 mutation has arisen independently on multiple occasions. Whereas 31% to 89% of European, North American, and Australian LHON pedigrees have the 11778 mutation, greater than 90% of Asian LHON patients are 11778 positive.

Several other mutations have since been deemed causal in LHON (Fig. 11.3). The majority are located within genes that also code for proteins comprising complex 1, but most within subunits other than ND4. A point mutation at mtDNA position 3460 within the gene coding for subunit ND1 of complex I accounts for 8% to 15% of LHON worldwide, and a point mutation at position 14484 in the gene coding for the subunit ND6 of complex I accounts for 10% to 15% of LHON pedigrees. The mutations at sites 11778, 3460, and 14484 are designated "primary" mutations for Leber's disease in that they (a) confer a genetic risk for LHON expression individually; (b) change the coding for evolutionarily conserved amino acids in essential proteins; (c) are found in multiple, different, ethnically divergent pedigrees; and (d) are absent or rare among control pedigrees. In total, they account for about 90% of LHON worldwide. Several other mtDNA mutations may be *primary*, but they each account for only a few reported pedigrees. Still other mtDNA mutations have been termed *secondary mutations*, because they are found with more frequency among LHON patients, but their pathogenetic significance remains unclear (Fig. 11.3).

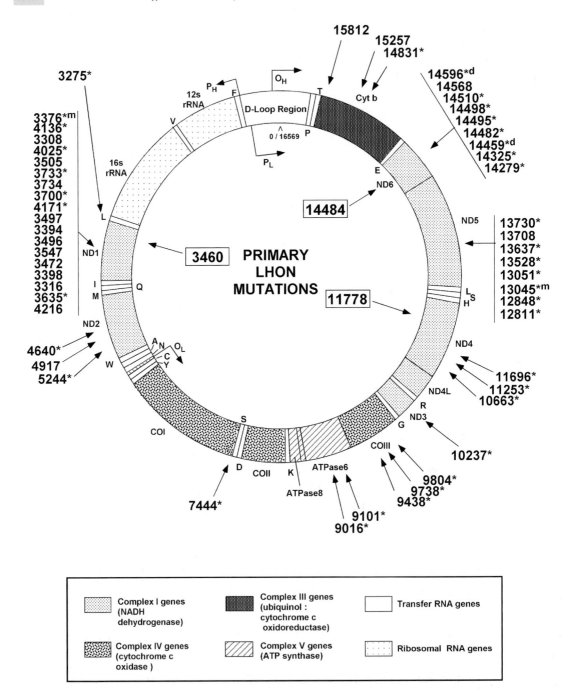

Figure 11.3. Mitochondrial genome showing the point mutations associated with Leber's hereditary optic neuropathy (LHON). Over 90% of all cases of LHON are associated with the three primary mutations located inside the genome, and the other mutations are shown outside the genome. These other mutations vary markedly in their prevalence, degree of evolutionary conservation of the encoded amino acids altered, and frequency among controls. Mutations marked* may be primary, but they each account for only one or a few pedigrees worldwide. Mutations marked*d are primary mutations associated with LHON and dystonia. Mutations marked*m are primary mutations associated with LHON/MELAS overlap syndrome (Adapted from: MITOMAP: A Human Mitochondrial Genome Database. http://www.mitomap.org January 2, 2006 with permission.).

Determinants of Expression

Genetic analysis allows a broader view of what constitutes the clinical profile of LHON. Most striking are the number of patients without a family history of visual loss. Some of these singleton cases are women, some are outside the typical age range for LHON, and some do not have the classic ophthalmoscopic appearance. Clearly, the diagnosis of LHON should be considered in any case of unexplained bilateral optic neuropathy, regardless of age of onset, sex, family history, or funduscopic appearance.

Many questions remain unanswered regarding the determinants of phenotypic expression of LHON. For example, does the specific mtDNA mutation dictate particular clinical features? Although pedigrees with the "Leber's plus" syndromes demonstrate that certain mtDNA mutations may result in specific disease patterns of Leber-like optic neuropathies with other neurologic abnormalities, few significant clinical differences can be demonstrated among patients positive for the 11778 mutation, patients with other mtDNA mutations, and patients as yet genetically unspecified. One major exception is the difference in spontaneous recovery rates among patients with the 11778 mutation and those with the 14484 mutation. Among patients with the 11778 mutation, only about 4% experience spontaneous recovery, compared with 37% to 65% of 14484 patients. Furthermore, the ultimate visual acuities in patients with the 14484 mutation are significantly better than those with the 11778 and 3460 mutations. Cardiac conduction abnormalities occur in 11778 pedigrees, but the 3460 mutation appears to have the highest association with the preexcitation syndromes.

An mtDNA mutation is present in all maternally related family members of patients with LHON, even though most will never become symptomatic. Thus, an mtDNA mutation may be necessary for phenotypic expression, but it may not be sufficient. Does heteroplasmy among individuals in a pedigree play a role in phenotypic expression? In some families, the mutant mtDNA content enriches from one generation to the next and may be at least partially responsible for phenotypic expression of the disease. However, in most large reviews of molecularly confirmed LHON patients, heteroplasmy is documented in the blood of a minority of affected individuals, and once a person becomes symptomatic, there does not appear to be any clinical difference in disease expression among those who are heteroplasmic and those who are homoplasmic.

Assuming that some persons are 100% homoplasmic in all tissues for the causative mtDNA mutation, there is no convincing explanation as to why visual loss should be the sole manifestation of the disease. Vary-ing tissue energy needs may play some role. The CNS is most reliant on mitochondrial adenosine triphosphate (ATP). Histochemical studies of optic nerve in the monkey and rat show a high degree of mitochondrial respiratory activity within the unmyelinated portion of optic nerve fibers located in the most anterior portion of the optic nerve. Ganglion cells and their projections may be especially vulnerable to the energy deficiencies created by mtDNA mutations.

Genetic factors other than the specific mtDNA mutation and the presence and degree of heteroplasmy may play a role in expression. Other mtDNA mutations may be present that modify the expression of the LHON causative mutation or that result in other abnormal proteins involved in mitochondrial function. Nuclear-encoded factors modifying mtDNA expression, mtDNA products, or mitochondrial metabolism may be necessary for phenotypic expression of LHON. The male predominance of visual loss in LHON may be explained by a modifying factor on the X-chromosome. Tissue energy utilization and reserve may also determine the timing and extent of visual loss. Mitochondrial energy production decreases with age, and the timing of visual loss in patients at risk for LHON may reflect the threshold at which already reduced mitochondrial function deteriorates to a critical level.

Environmental factors may also play a role. Both the internal and external environment of the organism must be considered. Systemic illnesses, nutritional deficiencies, and toxins that stress or directly inhibit the body's mitochondrial respiratory capacity may initiate or increase phenotypic expression of the disease. Anecdotal reports suggest a possible role for tobacco and excessive alcohol use in the expression of visual loss, but large studies on the effects of these agents on patients at risk for LHON have yet to be performed.

Treatment

In light of the possibility for spontaneous recovery in some patients with LHON, any anecdotal reports of treatment efficacy must be considered with caution. Attempts to treat or prevent the acute phase of visual loss with systemic steroids, hydroxocobalamin, or cyanide antagonists are ineffective. Other therapies tried are naturally occurring cofactors involved in mitochondrial metabolism or agents with antioxidant capabilities. Therapies tried include coenzyme Q_{10}, idebenone (an analog of coenzyme Q), succinate, vitamin K_1, vitamin K_3, vitamin C, thiamine, and vitamin B_2, but results are not particularly encouraging. A topically applied agent with purported neuroprotective effects was unsuccessful in preventing second eye involvement.

Gene therapy may allow for directed treatment, both in acute LHON and in the protection of eyes at risk.

Nonspecific recommendations to avoid agents that might stress mitochondrial energy production have no proven benefit but are certainly reasonable. We advise our patients at risk for LHON to avoid tobacco use, excessive alcohol intake, and environmental toxins. An electrocardiogram should be obtained and any cardiac abnormalities treated accordingly. Considering the degree of visual acuity loss, it is remarkable that up to 82% of LHON patients are gainfully employed despite their visual handicap. An assessment by a low-vision specialist may be helpful, especially because much peripheral vision may remain intact.

The importance of genetic counseling of patients with this disease and their families cannot be overemphasized. It should be explained to males with an LHON mutation, whether or not they are visually symptomatic, that they **will not** pass the mutation or the disease to their children. On the other hand, women with one of the LHON mutations **will** pass the mutation to all of their children, both male and female, although not all persons with the mutation (indeed, the minority) will become symptomatic.

DOMINANT OPTIC ATROPHY

Autosomal-dominant optic atrophy (DOA), also called Kjer's or juvenile optic atrophy, is the most common of the hereditary optic neuropathies with an estimated disease prevalence in the range of 1:50,000, or as high as 1:10,000 in Denmark.

Dominant optic atrophy is an abiotrophy with onset in the first decade in life. It is difficult for patients and their families to identify a precise onset of reduced vision, but most patients appear to become affected between 4 and 6 years of age. Although some severely affected children develop nystagmus and are found to have decreased vision prior to beginning schooling, the majority of persons with autosomal-dominant optic atrophy are unaware of a visual problem. These persons are discovered to have optic atrophy (a) because there is a family history of the condition, (b) as a direct consequence of examination of another affected family member, (c) because they fail a school vision screening examination, or (d) during a "routine" eye examination. These phenomena attest to the usually insidious onset in childhood, mild degree of visual dysfunction, absence of night blindness, and absence of substantial or dramatic progression.

Visual acuity is usually symmetrically reduced in both eyes. Vision ranges from 20/20 to 20/800 with only about 15% of the patients eventually developing vision of 20/200 or worse; hand motion or light perception vision is extremely rare. Rare patients have a mild or striking asymmetry between the acuities of the two eyes.

Patients with autosomal-dominant optic atrophy nearly always have a disturbance of color perception. Although the tritanopic defect has been deemed classic in this disorder, a generalized dyschromatopsia with both blue-yellow and red-green defects is found most commonly. There is no correlation between the severity of the dyschromatopsia and the visual acuity.

Visual fields in patients with dominant optic atrophy characteristically show central, paracentral, or cecocentral scotomas. A visual field pattern consisting of superobitemporal depression and thus mimicking the field defects of chiasmal compression is not uncommonly demonstrated, especially with automated perimetry.

The optic atrophy in patients with dominantly inherited optic neuropathy may be subtle, temporal only, or may involve the entire disc (Fig. 11.4). The most characteristic change is a triangular (wedge) excavation of the temporal portion of the disc. Other ophthalmoscopic findings reported in these patients include peripapillary atrophy, absent foveal reflex, mild macular pigmentary changes, arterial attenuation, and nonglaucomatous cupping.

Although there are a number of dominantly inherited syndromes in which optic atrophy is associated with neurologic dysfunction (see below), most patients with autosomal-dominant optic atrophy have no additional neurologic deficits. Nystagmus in some patients likely reflects early visual deprivation rather than central neurologic involvement. Hearing loss has been reported in some families.

A mild, slow, insidious progression of visual dysfunction occurs in up to 50% of patients with autosomal-dominant optic atrophy. One study found that, on average, the visual acuity decreases about one line per decade of life. There appears to be no correlation between the rate of visual loss and initial visual acuity nor do members of most pedigrees experience identical rates of progression. Rarely, relatively rapid deterioration of vision occurs after years of stable visual function. Spontaneous recovery of vision is not a feature of this disorder.

Although a linkage study of one large DOA pedigree localized the gene responsible for dominant optic atrophy with the Kidd blood group antigen, subsequently localized to a region on the long arm of chromosome 18 (18q12.2-12.3), most of the pedigrees with DOA have genetic homogeneity in their linkage to the telomeric portion of the long arm of chromosome 3 (3q28-29). Between 30% to 90% of DOA families have been found to harbor over 90 different missence and nonsense mutations, deletions, and insertions in a gene within this region that has been designated the OPA1 gene. The product of the OPA1 gene is targeted to the mitochondria and appears to exert its function in mitochondrial biogenesis and stabilization of mitochondrial

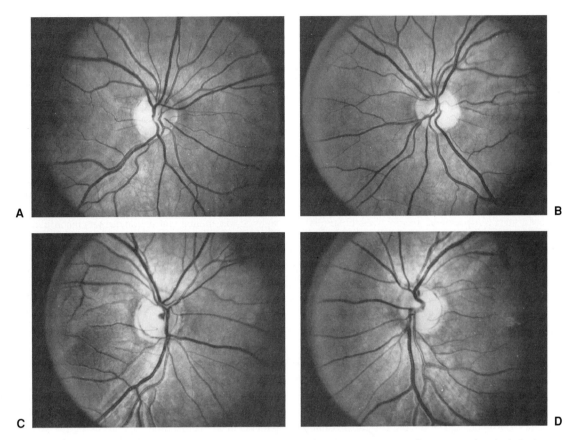

Figure 11.4. Dominant optic atrophy. **A and B:** Right and left optic discs in a patient with 20/40 visual acuity in both eyes, a tritanopic color vision defect, and bilateral, small central scotomas. Note minimal temporal pallor. **C and D:** Right and left discs of the above patient's father. Visual acuity is 20/100 in the right eye and 20/80 in the left eye with severe dyschromatopsia and bilateral central scotomas. The pallor is extensive and is primarily temporal in a "wedge" shape.

membrane integrity. The typical expression of both DOA and LHON as isolated optic neuropathies, emphasizes the crucial role of mitochondria in retinal ganglion cell pathophysiology. There is currently no known treatment for DOA.

OTHER ISOLATED HEREDITARY OPTIC NEUROPATHIES

Other monosymptomatic inherited optic neuropathies are extremely rare. **Congenital recessive optic atrophy** is present at birth or discovered by age 3 to 4 years. Visual loss is severe with near complete blindness and nystagmus. It is presumably nonprogressive and unassociated with neurologic or systemic abnormalities. Its very existence as a distinct entity has been questioned. Similarly, **sex-linked optic atrophy** has been demonstrated in at most two families, with male members demonstrating early childhood optic atrophy with slow progression. In one family in whom affected males manifested subtle neurologic abnormalities, linkage was established at Xp11.4-11.2.

HEREDITARY OPTIC ATROPHY WITH OTHER NEUROLOGIC OR SYSTEMIC SIGNS

PROGRESSIVE OPTIC ATROPHY WITH JUVENILE DIABETES MELLITUS, DIABETES INSIPIDUS, AND HEARING LOSS (WOLFRAM'S SYNDROME, DIDMOAD)

The hallmark of Wolfram's syndrome is the association of juvenile diabetes mellitus and progressive visual loss with optic atrophy, which is almost always associated with diabetes insipidus, and neurosensory hearing loss; hence, the eponym "DIDMOAD," for *d*iabetes *i*nsipidus, *d*iabetes *m*ellitus, *o*ptic *a*trophy, and *d*eafness. Over 300 cases have been reported with a prevalence of 1 in 770,000 in the United Kingdom. The progression and development of this syndrome is variable. Symptoms and signs of diabetes mellitus usually occur within the first or second decade of life and usually precede the development of optic atrophy. In some cases, visual loss associated with optic atrophy is the first evidence of the syndrome. In later stages, visual loss becomes severe. Visual fields show both generalized constriction and central scotomas. Optic atrophy is uniformly severe, and there may be mild to moderate cupping of the disc.

The onsets of hearing loss and diabetes insipidus in this syndrome are, as with the onset of visual loss, quite variable. Both begin in the first or second decade of life and may be severe. Atonia of the efferent urinary tract is present in 46% to 58% of patients and is associated with recurrent urinary tract infections, sometimes with fatal complications. Other systemic and neurologic abnormalities include ataxia, axial rigidity, seizures, startle myoclonus, tremor, vestibular malfunction, central apnea, neurogenic upper airway collapse, anosmia, and gastrointestinal dysmotility. Endocrine manifestations include, but are not limited to, short stature and primary gonadal atrophy. Ophthalmologic and other neuro-ophthalmologic disturbances include ptosis, cataracts, pigmentary retinopathy, iritis, lacrimal hyposecretion, tonic pupils, ophthalmoplegia, convergence insufficiency, vertical gaze palsy, and nystagmus. Mental retardation may occur, as may psychiatric manifestations, which are also seen at an increased frequency among heterozygous carriers. Laboratory abnormalities include megaloblastic and sideroblastic anemia, an abnormal ERG, and elevated CSF protein. Neuroimaging studies and pathologic examinations in some patients with Wolfram's syndrome reveal widespread atrophic changes and suggest a diffuse neurodegenerative disorder, with particular involvement of the midbrain and pons. Median age at death is 30 years, most commonly due to central respiratory failure with brain stem atrophy.

Many of the associated abnormalities reported in Wolfram's syndrome are commonly encountered in patients with presumed mitochondrial diseases, especially those patients with the chronic progressive external ophthalmoplegia (CPEO) syndromes. This has led to speculation that patients with Wolfram's syndrome may have a unifying pathogenesis in underlying mitochondrial dysfunction. Abnormalities of mitochondrial function can result from nuclear or mitochondrial DNA defects, because both genomes code for proteins essential for normal mitochondrial function. Inheritance patterns should help distinguish the location of the underlying genetic defect. Nuclear mutations are transmitted in a mendelian fashion, and primary mtDNA defects are inherited maternally. However, most cases of Wolfram's syndrome have been classified as sporadic or recessively inherited, the latter usually concluded from sibling expression, which we now know could also occur from maternal transmission. Linkage analysis in several families localized the Wolfram's gene to the short arm of chromosome

4 (4p16.1) (WFS1). A phenotypic variant of Wolfram's was subsequently linked to a second locus on chromosome 4q22-24 (WFS2). The Wolfram's phenotype may be nonspecific and may reflect a wide variety of underlying genetic defects in either the nuclear or mitochondrial genomes. When the syndrome is accompanied by anemia, treatment with thiamine may ameliorate the anemia and decrease the insulin requirement.

COMPLICATED HEREDITARY INFANTILE OPTIC ATROPHY (BEHR'S SYNDROME)

In this heredofamilial syndrome, commonly referred to as **Behr's syndrome,** optic atrophy beginning in early childhood is associated with variable pyramidal tract signs, ataxia, mental retardation, urinary incontinence, and pes cavus. Both sexes are affected and the syndrome is usually inherited as an autosomal-recessive trait. Visual loss usually manifests before age 10 years, is moderate to severe, and is frequently accompanied by nystagmus. In most cases, the abnormalities do not progress after childhood. Neuroimaging may demonstrate diffuse, symmetric white-matter abnormalities. In several Iraqi Jewish pedigrees of Behr's syndrome, 3-methylglutaconic aciduria was identified, although the basic enzymatic defect in these families is as yet unknown. These patients have infantile optic atrophy and an early onset extrapyramidal movement disorder dominated by chorea. Approximately half of the patients developed spastic paraparesis by the second decade. The majority of affected individuals are female. Clinical findings in some patients with Behr's syndrome are similar to those in cases of hereditary ataxia; in fact, Behr's syndrome may be a transitional form between simple heredofamilial optic atrophy and the hereditary ataxias. Behr's syndrome is likely heterogeneous, reflecting different etiologic and genetic factors.

OTHER SYNDROMIC HEREDITARY OPTIC NEUROPATHIES

In some other pedigrees, optic atrophy is the main finding in syndromes of inherited specific neurologic or systemic deficits (Table 11.1). Several families have been described with **autosomal dominant optic atrophy and deafness.** There is great inter- and intrafamilial variability in the age of onset of the visual loss and the severity of the hearing loss. It is unclear whether these pedigrees represent a phenotype variant of DOA, a genetically distinct disorder, or a genetically heterogeneous group of disorders with a similar phenotype. For example, two families with **autosomal dominant optic atrophy, deafness and ophthalmoplegia** were found to harbor a common OPA1 mutation associated with DOA. Several of the other syndromes listed in Table 11.1 have been reported in only a few families. Their relationship to the hereditary ataxias

Table 11.1. *Other Syndromic Hereditary Optic Neuropathies*

Autosomal-Dominant Progressive Optic Atrophy and Deafness

Autosomal-Dominant Optic Atrophy, Deafness, and Ophthalmoplegia

Autosomal-Dominant Progressive Optic Atrophy with Progressive Hearing Loss and Ataxia (CAPOS Syndrome)

Hereditary Optic Atrophy with Progressive Hearing Loss and Polyneuropathy

Autosomal-Recessive Optic Atrophy with Progressive Hearing Loss, Spastic Quadriplegia, Mental Deterioration, and Death (Opticocochleodentate Degeneration)

Opticoacoustic Nerve Atrophy with Dementia

Progressive Encephalopathy with Edema, Hypsarrhythmia, and Optic Atrophy (PEHO Syndrome)

and hereditary polyneuropathies (see below) remains unclear.

OPTIC NEUROPATHY AS A MANIFESTATION OF HEREDITARY DEGENERATIVE OR DEVELOPMENTAL DISEASES

HEREDITARY ATAXIAS

The inherited ataxias represent a group of chronic progressive neurodegenerative conditions involving the cerebellum and its connections. The most common classification of the hereditary ataxias is by pattern of inheritance: autosomal dominant (most common), autosomal recessive, X-linked, and maternal (mitochondrial). Advances in biochemical and genetic analysis reveal a wide variability of clinical signs and neuropathology, even within families, and the overlap of clinical and pathologic phenotypes in disorders now known to be caused by different genetic defects makes diagnostic classification by phenotype often inaccurate. A genomic classification by chromosomal location is available for many of these disorders, and the abnormal gene products involved are under investigation. Optic atrophy is not uncommon among individuals with hereditary ataxias.

The prototype of all forms of progressive ataxia is **Friedreich's ataxia.** The onset of the disease is usually between the ages of 8 and 15 years, almost always before age 25. Characteristic clinical features include progressive ataxia of gait and clumsiness in walking and using the hands, dysarthria, loss of joint position and vibratory sensation, absent lower extremity tendon reflexes, and extensor plantar responses. Common findings include scoliosis, foot deformity, diabetes mellitus, and cardiac involvement. Other manifestations include pes cavus, distal wasting, deafness, nystagmus, eye movement abnormalities consistent with abnormal cerebellar function, and optic atrophy. The course is relentlessly progressive, with most patients unable to walk within 15 years of onset, and death from infectious or cardiac causes usually in the fourth or fifth decades. A later-onset, more slowly progressive form has been described.

Friedreich's ataxia is inherited in an autosomal-recessive manner, and the gene defect has been localized to the proximal long arm of the 9th chromosome (9q13–21). The majority of cases are homozygous for an intronic, unstable, GAA trinucleotide expansion in a gene designated FRDA/X25 that codes for a protein known as frataxin. Frataxin is a mitochondrial protein that appears to regulate iron levels in the mitochondria. Its absence leads to mitochondrial iron overload and overproduction of reactive oxygen species and cell death.

Optic atrophy is present in up to 50% of the cases of Friedreich's ataxia, although severe visual loss is uncommon. With electrophysiologic testing, most patients show evidence of visual sensory dysfunction, although visual acuity of less than 20/80 is unusual.

The most common of the hereditary ataxias are inherited in an autosomal-dominant pattern. The majority of these are now designated by the term **spinocerebellar ataxia** (SCA), reflecting their predominant pathology in the spinal cord and the cerebellar pathways. A wide range of clinical and pathologic findings can be seen within and among pedigrees. Although originally classified by clinical descriptions within specific families, they are now defined by the genetic loci and specific mutations in these families. Indeed, the same phenotype can be caused by a multitude of different gene defects.

As of 2003, there were at least 23 different genetic loci for SCAs (SCA 1 to SCA 22). The combination of SCA1 (chromosome 6p), SCA 2 (chromosome 12q), SCA 3 (chromosome 14q and allelic with Machado-Joseph disease), SCA 6 (chromosome 19p), and SCA 7 (chromosome 3p) represents approximately 80% of the autosomal dominant ataxias. Many of the SCAs are caused by mutations involving the expansion of a CAG trinucleotide repeat in the protein coding sequences of specific genes, resulting in a series of glutamines. As with other diseases that involve abnormal repeats, the expanded regions can become larger with each successive generation, resulting in a younger age of onset in each generation (anticipation). Anticipation is seen particularly when the disease is inherited from the father.

Clinically, the SCAs are characterized by signs and symptoms attributable to cerebellar degeneration and sometimes other neurologic dysfunction secondary to neuronal loss. Loss of vision is usually mild but may be a prominent symptom, occurring in association with constricted visual fields and diffuse optic atrophy. However, it is not clear in some cases whether the primary process is retinal with secondary optic atrophy or primary optic nerve. Detailed analysis of the prevalence of optic atrophy among the different genotypes now associated with the spinocerebellar syndromes has not been performed. Prior to genetic analysis, the autosomal-dominant cerebellar ataxias (ADCAs) were categoried into four types, with only the first type having individuals with primary optic atrophy (approximately 30% of cases). We now know that ADCA type I encompasses multiple genetic loci, including those pedigrees now classified genetically as SCA1, SCA2, SCA3, and probably SCA4 and SCA5. Initial studies suggest that patients with the SCA2 genotype do not exhibit optic atrophy, whereas SCA3 patients may have optic atrophy, especially if their ataxia is severe. SCA 7 is the only SCA associated with definite pigmentary retinal degeneration.

HEREDITARY POLYNEUROPATHIES

Charcot-Marie-Tooth disease (CMT) encompasses a group of heredofamilial disorders characterized by progressive muscular weakness and atrophy that begins during the first two decades of life. This group of hereditary polyneuropathies accounts for 90% of all hereditary neuropathies, with the prevalence in the United States being about 40 per 100,000. Most forms of CMT begin between the ages of 2 and 15 years. The first signs are usually pes cavus, foot deformities, or scoliosis. There is slowly progressive weakness and wasting, first of the feet and legs and then of the hands. Motor symptoms predominate over sensory abnormalities.

The most common form of CMT is type 1, a demyelinating neuropathy with autosomal-dominant inheritance, mapped most commonly to the short arm of chromosome 17 (17p11.2) (type 1A), although a few pedigrees with this phenotype are linked to the long arm of chromosome 1 (type 1B). CMT type 2 is clinically similar, but nerve conductions are of normal velocity, suggesting the process is neuronal rather than demyelinating. Type 2 can be inherited in an autosomal-dominant fashion (linked to the short arm of chromosome 1) or autosomal-recessively (linked to the long arm of chromosome 8). Type 3 is the most severe form. When type 3 is inherited in an autosomal-dominant pattern, the linkage is to the same region on chromosome 1 associated with type 1B; when it is autosomal recessive, the linkage is to the same region on chromosome 17 associated with type 1A. There are also X-linked forms of CMT, both X-linked dominant

(linked to defects on the long arm) and X-linked recessive (linked to regions on either the long arm or the short arm). As of 2002, causative mutations for the hereditary peripheral neuropathies had been identified in 17 different genes.

Many patients with CMT have optic atrophy. Associated visual loss is usually mild, and many patients are asymptomatic. In fact, taking into account both electrophysiologic and clinical data, up to 75% of patients with CMT have some afferent visual pathway dysfunction, demonstrating that subclinical optic neuropathy occurs in a high proportion of patients with CMT. Pedigrees specifically designated as CMT type 6 show a regular association of CMT and optic atrophy. This type of CMT is as yet genetically unspecified and may prove genetically heterogeneous.

Familial dysautonomia (Riley-Day syndrome) is an autosomal-recessive disease that almost exclusively affects Ashkenazi Jews. Abnormalities of the peripheral nervous system cause the clinical manifestations of sensory and autonomic dysfunction. The gene responsible has been identified on chromosome 9q31–33.

STORAGE DISEASES AND CEREBRAL DEGENERATIONS OF CHILDHOOD

About 100 inherited **metabolic diseases** with ocular manifestations have been described (Table 11.2). The inheritance pattern in these diseases is almost always recessive, usually autosomal recessive but occasionally X-linked. Optic atrophy may also be a manifestation of quantitative **chromosomal abnormalities.**

Children with **cerebral palsy** have a higher prevalence of ocular defects than normal children. In one study, optic atrophy was found in 10% of children with cerebral palsy. The etiology for the atrophy in these patients was not explained nor was the clinical characteristics of the patients elucidated.

The **subacute necrotizing encephalomyelopathy of Leigh** (Leigh's syndrome) is a degenerative syndrome that can result from multiple different biochemical defects that all impair cerebral oxidative metabolism. This disorder may be inherited in an autosomal-recessive, X-linked, or maternal pattern, depending on the genetic defect. The clinical manifestations of Leigh's syndrome typically begin between the ages of 2 months and 6 years. They consist of progressive deterioration of brainstem functions, ataxia, seizures, peripheral neuropathy, intellectual deterioration, impaired hearing, and poor vision. Visual loss may be secondary to optic atrophy or retinal degeneration. In infants, the onset of the syndrome is insidious, with initial symptoms being failure to thrive, generalized weakness, and hypotonia. Rarely, patients with a familial, adult form of Leigh's syndrome present with bilateral visual loss, dyschromatopsia, central scotomas,

Table 11.2. *Storage Diseases and Cerebral Degenerations of Childhood With Optic Atrophy*

Adrenoleukodystrophy
Allgrove syndrome ("4 A")
Canavan's disease
Cockayne syndrome
COFS
GAPO syndrome
Pantothenate kinase-associated neurodegeneration
(Hallenvorden-Spatz)
Infantile neuroaxonal dystrophy
Krabbe's disease
Lipidoses (infantile and juvenile GM1-1 and GM1-2,
GM2, infantile Niemann-Pick disease)
Menkes syndrome
Metachromatic leukodystrophy
Mucopolysaccharidoses (MPS IH, IS, IHS, IIA, IIB,
IIIA, IIIB, IV, VI)
Pelizaeus-Merzbacher disease
Smith-Lemli-Opits syndrome
Zellweger syndrome

"4A": Alacrine, Achalasia, Autonomic disturbance, and
ACTH insensitivity
COFS: Cerebro-Oculo-Facio-Skeletal syndrome
GAPO: Growth retardation, Alopecia, Pseudoanodontia, and
Optic atrophy
GM1-Gangliosidoses: GM1-1 and GM1-2
GM2-Gangliosidoses: Tay-Sachs disease, Sandhoff disease,
late infantile, juvenile and adult GM2-Gangliosidose
MPS IH: Hurler; MPS IS: Sheie; MPS HIS: Hurler-Sheie;
MPS IIA and IIB: Hunter; MPS IIIA and IIIB: Sanfilippo;
MPS IV: Morquio; MPS VI: Maroteaux-Lamy

and optic atrophy prior to the development of other neurologic symptoms and signs. Typical pathologic alterations consist of spongy necrotizing degeneration of the neuropil, capillary and glial proliferation, and loss of myelin with relative sparing of neurons. The most commonly affected areas are the tegmentum of the brainstem, the optic nerves, basal ganglia, substantia nigra, tectum of the midbrain, cerebellar cortex, dentate nucleus, and inferior olives, with a predisposition for the periaqueductal and periventricular regions of the midbrain, pons, and medulla mimicking the pathology of Wernicke's encephalopathy. In many of the reported cases, the optic nerves show extensive atrophy with varying degrees of demyelination of the optic nerves, tracts, and chiasm.

Leigh's syndrome appears to be a nonspecific phenotypic response to certain abnormalities of mitochondrial energy production. Most of the genetic defects that result in Leigh's syndrome probably occur in nuclear genes encoding proteins essential to mitochondrial oxidative phosphorylation. However, about one-third of Leigh's syndrome cases are associated with a point mutation in the mtDNA at position 8993 within the gene for ATPase 6. This same genetic defect can cause a syndrome of neuropathy, ataxia, and retinitis pigmentosa (NARP) or a condition in which mild pigmentary degeneration of the retina is associated with migraine-like headaches. Visual loss may be caused by retinal or optic nerve degeneration in such cases. The Leigh's phenotype can also occur in patients with the mtDNA point mutations at positions 8344 and 3243—mutations usually associated with the conditions known as myoclonic epilepsy with ragged-red fibers (MERRF) and mitochondrial encephalopathy, lactic acidosis, and stroke-like episodes (MELAS), respectively.

Other presumed mitochondrial disorders of both nuclear and mitochondrial genomic origins may manifest optic atrophy as a secondary clinical feature, often a variable manifestation of the disease. Examples include cases of MERRF, MELAS, and chronic progressive external ophthalmoplegia (CPEO), both with and without the full Kearns-Sayre phenotype.

FOR FURTHER INFORMATION

See *Walsh & Hoyt's Clinical Neuro-Ophthalmology*, 6th ed., Volume 1, Chapter 11, pages 465–501; Volume 3, Chapter 46, pages 2469–2511.

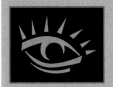

CHAPTER 12

Topical Diagnosis of Chiasmal and Retrochiasmal Lesions *

TOPICAL DIAGNOSIS OF LESIONS OF THE OPTIC CHIASM

The optic chiasm is one of the most important structures in neuro-ophthalmologic diagnosis (Figs. 12.1 and 12.2). The arrangement of visual fibers in the chiasm accounts for characteristic defects in the visual fields caused by such diverse processes as compression, inflammation, demyelination, ischemia, and infiltration. In addition, damage to neurologic and vascular structures adjacent to the chiasm produces typical additional symptoms.

VISUAL FIELD DEFECTS

Although there are many variations in the visual field defects caused by damage to the optic chiasm, the essential feature is some type of bitemporal defect, the hallmark of damage to fibers that cross within the chiasm. The bitemporal defects may be superior, inferior, or complete, and they may be peripheral, central, or both. Many lesions that arise in the region of the chiasm affect not only the entire chiasm but also the intracranial optic nerves. Most visual field defects produced by lesions that damage the optic chiasm seem to result from damage at one of three locations: (a) the anterior angle of the chiasm, (b) the body of the chiasm, or (c) the posterior angle of the chiasm. In addition, a very small number of lesions damage nerve fibers at the lateral aspects of the chiasm. Lesions that damage

*Adapted from Levin LA. Topical diagnosis of chiasmal and retrochiasmal disorders. In: Miller NR, Newman NJ, Biousse V, Kerrison JB, eds. *Walsh & Hoyt's Clinical Neuro-Ophthalmology*. 6th ed. Vol. I. Philadelphia: Lippincott Williams & Wilkins; 2005:503–573.

the **distal portion of one optic nerve at the anterior angle of the optic chiasm,** resulting in the so-called "junctional" scotoma, are discussed in Chapter 4.

Lesions That Damage the Body of the Optic Chiasm

Lesions that damage the body of the optic chiasm characteristically produce a bitemporal defect that may be quadrantic or hemianopic and that may be peripheral, central, or both, with or without so-called "splitting of the macula" (Fig. 12.3). In most cases, visual acuity is normal. In some patients, however, visual acuity is diminished, even though no field defect other than a bitemporal hemianopia is present. When the lesion compresses the chiasm from below, such as occurs with a pituitary adenoma, the field defects are typical. When the peripheral fibers are principally affected, the field defects usually commence in the outer upper quadrants of both eyes (Fig. 12.4). In the field of the right eye, the defect usually progresses in a clockwise direction and in the left eye in a counterclockwise direction. The field defects are often unequal in the two eyes; thus, one eye may become almost or completely blind, whereas the defect in the field of the other eye remains rather mild. In the charting of visual field defects resulting from pituitary adenomas and other tumors, scotomas in the peripheral parts of the visual fields are usually dense and not likely to be overlooked, but small relative paracentral scotomas are frequently missed when only kinetic perimetry is performed. In addition to pituitary adenomas, other suprasellar but infrachiasmal lesions, such as tuberculum sellae and medial sphenoid ridge meningiomas, craniopharyngiomas, and aneurysms can also produce bitemporal field defects that are denser above.

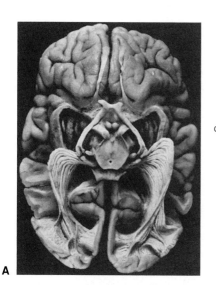

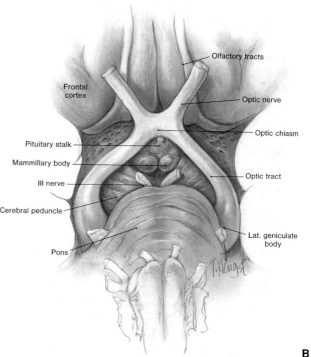

Figure 12.1. Anatomy of the chiasm and postchiasmal visual sensory system. **A:** Appearance of the visual sensory pathway in axial section, viewed from below. Note position of the optic tracts as they originate from the optic chiasm and diverge to end at the lateral geniculate nuclei. (Reprinted from: Ghuhbegovic N, Williams TH. *The Human Brain: A Photographic Guide.* Hagerstown, MD, Harper & Row, 1980, with permission.) **B:** Artist's drawing of the optic chiasm and optic tracts viewed from below. (Redrawn from: Pernkopf E. *Atlas of Topographical and Applied Human Anatomy.* Vol. 1. Philadelphia: WB Saunders, 1963.)

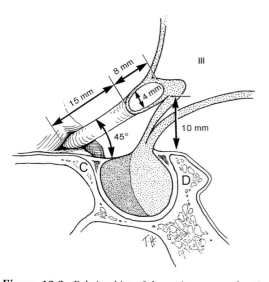

Figure 12.2. Relationships of the optic nerves and optic chiasm to the sellar structures and third ventricle (III). **C,** anterior clinoid. **D,** dorsum sellae. (Redrawn from: Glaser JS. *Neuro-ophthalmology.* 1st ed. Hagerstown, MD: Harper & Row, 1978.)

Alternatively, suprasellar, suprachiasmal compressive lesions—such as tuberculum sellae meningiomas, craniopharyngiomas, aneurysms, and dolichoectatic anterior cerebral arteries—may damage the superior fibers of the optic chiasm, as may infiltrating lesions such as germinomas, benign and malignant gliomas, and cavernous angiomas. The defects in the visual fields in such cases are still bitemporal, but are located in the inferior rather than the superior fields of both eyes (Fig. 12.5). Papilledema, which is quite unusual in patients with suprasellar, infrachiasmal lesions, is somewhat more common in suprachiasmal lesions because such lesions can extend into and occlude the 3rd ventricle.

Infiltrating tumors, such as gliomas and germinomas, as well as inflammatory and demyelinating lesions that affect the optic chiasm, may produce typical bitemporal field defects (Fig. 12.6). However, such lesions may also produce other types of field defects, such as arcuate defects and nonspecific reduction in sensitivity, that do not necessarily correlate with the location, size, or extent of the lesion.

When trauma damages the optic chiasm, the most common field defect is a complete bitemporal

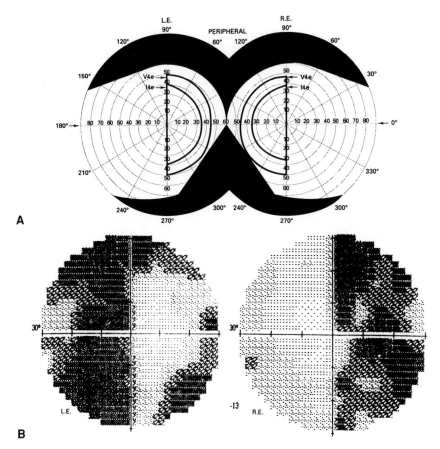

Figure 12.3. Optic chiasmal syndrome. **A:** Kinetic perimetry in a patient with a large pituitary adenoma reveals a complete bitemporal hemianopia. **B:** Static perimetry, using a Humphrey 24–2 Threshold Test, in another patient with a pituitary adenoma, reveals an incomplete bitemporal hemianopia.

hemianopia. Indeed, although most compressive, infiltrative, or inflammatory lesions that damage the body of the chiasm produce defects that are incomplete and that usually have a relative component, complete bitemporal hemianopias can most certainly occur from tumor compression. Successful decompression of the chiasm in such cases not infrequently results in improvement in the visual field, an outcome that might not have been expected from the severity of the visual field defect.

Lesions That Damage the Posterior Angle of the Optic Chiasm

Lesions that damage the posterior aspect of the optic chiasm produce characteristic defects in the visual fields: bitemporal hemianopic scotomas (Fig. 12.7). Such defects occasionally may be mistaken for cecocentral scotomas and attributed to a toxic, metabolic, or even hereditary process rather than to a tumor; however, true bitemporal hemianopic scotomas are almost always associated with normal visual acuity and color

perception, whereas cecocentral scotomas are invariably associated with reduced visual acuity and dyschromatopsia.

Lesions that damage the posterior aspect of the optic chiasm may also damage one of the optic tracts, thus producing an homonymous field defect that is combined with whatever field defect has occurred from damage to the optic chiasm.

Bitemporal homonymous scotomas are particularly important in localizing a lesion, or at least the effects of such a lesion, to the posterior aspect of the optic chiasm. Lesions that produce such defects may be more difficult to treat successfully and, therefore, more likely to be associated with permanent residual field defects after surgical therapy or radiotherapy. Many patients who undergo otherwise successful removal of a lesion that has produced a posterior chiasmal field defect, the chiasmal field defect is replaced by a field defect consistent with damage to the adjacent optic tract (i.e., an incomplete, incongruous homonymous hemianopia or quadrantanopia; see below).

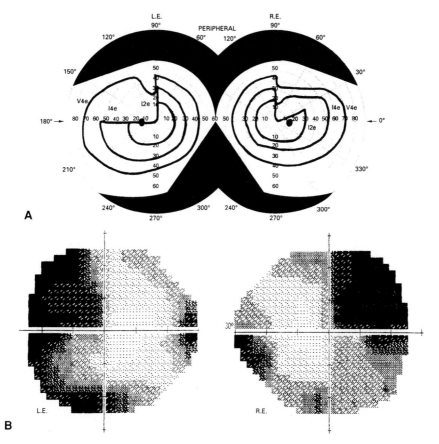

Figure 12.4. Bilateral superior temporal defects in patients with a pituitary adenoma. **A:** Kinetic perimetry in one patient demonstrates defects that are restricted to the superior temporal quadrants of the visual fields of both eyes (a bitemporal superior quadrantanopia). **B:** Static perimetry, using a Humphrey 24–2 Threshold Test, in another patient with a pituitary adenoma demonstrates bitemporal hemianopic defects that are much denser superiorly.

Visual Field Defects Caused by Lesions That Damage the Optic Chiasm after Initially Damaging the Optic Nerve or Optic Tract

If there is extension of a lesion from the optic nerve or the optic tract to the optic chiasm, the blind eye usually is on the side of the lesion. If, for example, a patient with a blind right eye exhibits a defect in the temporal field of the left eye, the lesion obviously is on the right. Similarly, if there has been a left homonymous hemianopia from a right optic tract lesion and if there is extension of the lesion to affect the optic chiasm, blindness develops in the right eye, or if not blindness, an extensive field defect. Conversely, if a lesion of the optic chiasm that has produced a bitemporal hemianopia extends to the right optic nerve, it will eventually produce blindness or near-blindness of the right eye. Similarly, if a chiasmal lesion extends into the right optic tract, there is again blindness or near-blindness of the right eye. In other words, when there is extension of a lesion from an optic nerve or optic tract to the optic chiasm, the blind (or near-blind) eye is always on the side of the original lesion, and when there is extension of a lesion from the optic chiasm to the optic nerve or to the optic tract, the blind (or near-blind) eye is always on the side of the extension of the lesion.

ETIOLOGIES OF THE OPTIC CHIASMAL SYNDROME

Damage to the optic chiasm can occur from the direct or indirect effects of a variety of lesions. The most common causes of an optic chiasmal syndrome are pituitary adenomas, suprasellar meningiomas, craniopharyngiomas, gliomas, and aneurysms originating from the internal carotid artery. In addition, numerous unusual causes of the optic chiasmal syndrome have been reported, including (in alphabetical order) aneurysm of the basilar artery, arachnoid cyst, arteriovenous malformations, cavernous angioma, choristoma, choroid plexus papilloma, cysticercosis, demyelinating disease, dolichoectatic sclerotic intracranial

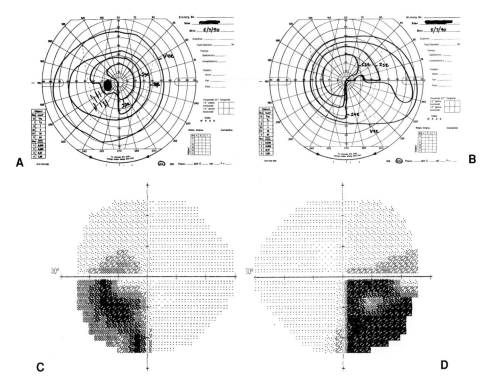

Figure 12.5. Bilateral inferior temporal field defects in a 32-year-old man with a suprasellar mass. **A and B:** Kinetic perimetry reveals inferior temporal quadrantic defects in the visual fields of the left **(A)** and right **(B)** eyes. Note that the defects are scotomatous. Static perimetry, using a Humphrey 24–2 Threshold Test, in the same patient confirms the inferior temporal quadrantic nature of the defects. **C:** Visual field of left eye. **D:** Visual field of right eye. The patient underwent a craniotomy and was found to have a suprasellar suprachiasmatic germinoma.

internal carotid arteries, ependymoma, ethchlorvynol abuse, fibrous dysplasia, ganglioglioma, germinoma, glioblastoma multiforme, granular cell tumor of the neurohypophysis, inflammation (presumed) from Epstein-Barr viral infection, ischemia from small vessel occlusive disease, Langerhans cell histiocytosis, lymphocytic adenohypophysitis, lymphoma, malignant melanoma, medulloblastoma, metastatic carcinoma, multiple myeloma, nasopharyngeal carcinoma, optochiasmatic arachnoiditis, pachymeningitis associated with rheumatoid arthritis, pituitary abscess, plasmacytoma, radiation necrosis, Rathke's cleft cyst, sarcoid granuloma, septum pellucidum cyst, sinus histiocytosis with lymphadenopathy (Rosai-Dorfman), sphenoid sinus mucocele, syphilitic gumma, toxoplasmosis, tuberculoma, varix, vasculitis, venous angioma, and vitamin B_{12} deficiency.

During pregnancy, preexisting intrasellar and suprasellar tumors, most commonly pituitary adenomas, may become symptomatic. In most cases, visual symptoms regress after abortion or delivery. In addition, the pituitary gland itself enlarges during the third trimester of pregnancy and may become sufficiently enlarged that it compresses the chiasm, producing visual manifestations. In such cases, visual symptoms resolve spontaneously following delivery. Another cause of an optic chiasmal syndrome that occurs most often during or shortly after pregnancy is lymphocytic adenohypophysitis, an autoimmune disorder of unknown etiology.

Extension of the subarachnoid space into the sella turcica through a deficient diaphragma sellae results in the "empty sella syndrome." A primary empty sella syndrome occurs spontaneously and may be associated with an arachnoid cyst. It is only rarely associated with any significant visual acuity loss or visual field defects; however, a secondary empty sella syndrome follows surgery or radiation therapy in the sellar region. Patients in whom this syndrome occurs may develop any of the chiasmal syndromes described earlier.

An optic chiasmal syndrome can be produced iatrogenically. Most often, the condition occurs after attempted removal of a lesion compressing or infiltrating the chiasm. In our experience, chiasmal damage occurs most often during surgery to remove a suprasellar meningioma or craniopharyngioma and least often

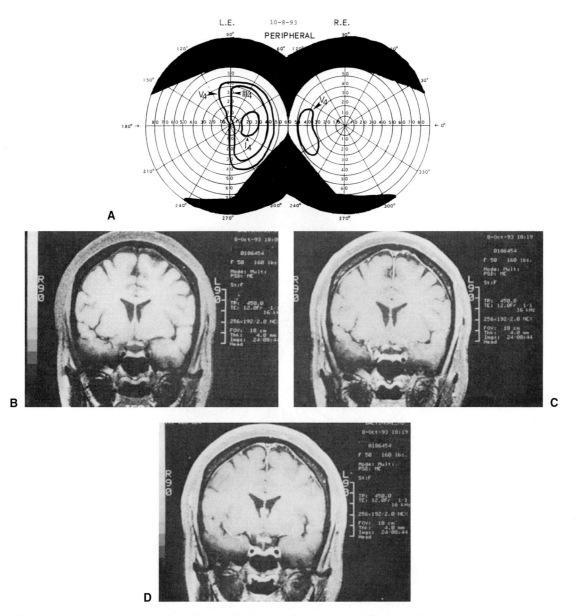

Figure 12.6. Optic chiasmal syndrome in multiple sclerosis. The patient was a 50-year-old woman with a previous history of transient lower extremity weakness who developed progressive loss of vision in both eyes. The patient reported that her vision would worsen considerably whenever she took a steam bath. Visual acuity was counting fingers at 3 feet OD and 20/100 OS. Color vision was diminished in both eyes, and there was a right relative afferent pupillary defect. **A:** Kinetic perimetry at presentation shows a complete temporal hemianopia in the field of vision of the left eye and only a small nasal island in the field of vision of the right eye. **B:** Unenhanced T1-weighted coronal MRI shows an apparently normal optic chiasm. **C and D:** T1-weighted coronal MRI after intravenous injection of contrast material shows enhancement of the intracranial portions of the optic nerves **(C)** and the optic chiasm **(D)**. The patient was treated with intravenous corticosteroids.

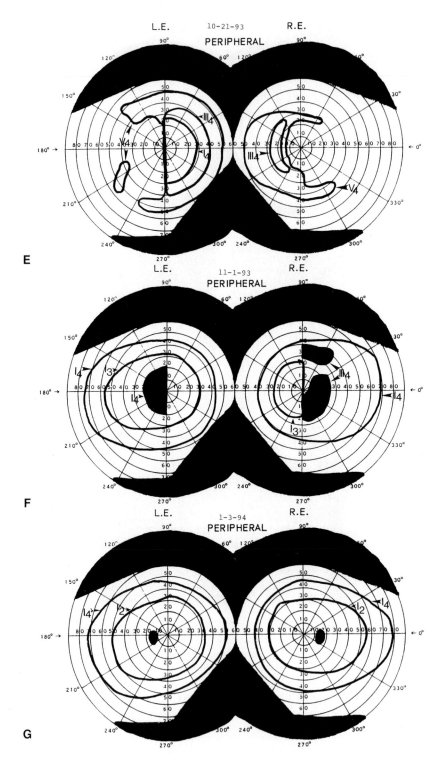

Figure 12.6. (*continued*) **E–G:** Kinetic perimetry shows progressive improvement in visual fields over the subsequent 10 weeks. (Courtesy of Dr. John B. Kerrison.)

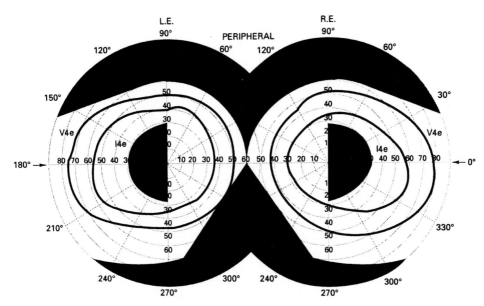

Figure 12.7. Bitemporal hemianopic scotomas in a patient with a pituitary adenoma. Such field defects result from damage to macular fibers in the posterior portion of the optic chiasm.

after surgery to remove a pituitary adenoma or to clip an intracranial aneurysm. Catheters placed to relieve hydrocephalus can inadvertently damage the chiasm, and a chiasmal syndrome can also occur from exuberant packing of the sphenoid sinus with fat following transsphenoidal resection of a pituitary adenoma.

NEURO-OPHTHALMOLOGIC SIGNS AND SYMPTOMS ASSOCIATED WITH THE OPTIC CHIASMAL SYNDROME

The most frequent complaints of patients with lesions that damage the optic chiasm are progressive loss of central acuity and dimming of the visual field, particularly in its temporal portion. In addition, bitemporal field defects, whether complete or scotomatous, may produce two other types of visual symptoms. One type consists of a **disturbance of depth perception.** Patients with this symptom complain of difficulties with near tasks, such as threading needles, sewing, and using precision tools. In such patients, convergence results in crossing of the two blind temporal hemifields. This produces a completely blind triangular area of field with its apex at fixation (Fig. 12.8). The image of an object posterior to fixation falls on blind nasal retinas and thus disappears.

Patients with bitemporal field defects may also experience diplopia or difficulty reading caused by a horizontal or vertical deviation of images unassociated with an ocular motor nerve paresis, the **hemifield slide phenomenon.** Such patients have difficulty reading because of doubling or loss of printed letters or words.

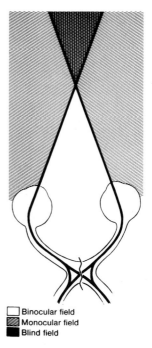

☐ Binocular field
▨ Monocular field
■ Blind field

Figure 12.8. Diagram showing the blind triangular area of the binocular visual field that occurs just beyond fixation in patients with complete bitemporal hemianopia. Such patients have intact binocular vision in the triangular area up to fixation and intact uniocular vision temporal and anterior to the triangular blind region. (Redrawn from: Kirkham TH. The ocular symptomatology of pituitary tumors. *Proc R Soc Med.* 1972;65:517–518.)

The problems encountered by these patients result from loss of the normal partial overlap of the temporal field of one eye and the nasal field of the contralateral eye. This overlap normally permits fusion of images and helps stabilize ocular alignment in patients with vertical or horizontal phorias. Because their remaining visual fields represent only the temporal projection from each eye, patients with bitemporal hemianopia do not have a physiologic linkage between the two remaining hemifields. In such patients, a preexisting minor phoria becomes a tropia because of vertical or horizontal separation or overlap of the two nonoverlapping hemifields, thus causing intermittent sensory difficulties (Fig. 12.9).

Patients with chiasmal syndromes may or may not have ophthalmoscopically apparent nerve fiber layer or optic disc atrophy when first examined. However, when atrophy is present in patients with bitemporal hemianopia, the pattern of atrophy is quite specific. In such cases, degeneration occurs in fibers from peripheral and macular ganglion cells located nasal to the fovea. Axons from peripheral ganglion cells located nasal to the disc (and, thus, nasal to the fovea) attain the disc directly, entering its nasal aspect. Fibers from nasal

macular ganglion cells (i.e., about half the fibers that comprise the papillomacular bundle) also attain the optic disc directly, entering its temporal aspect. Finally, fibers from peripheral ganglion cells located nasal to the fovea but temporal to the optic disc—which make up a small portion of the superior and inferior arcuate bundles along with a larger number of fibers from peripheral temporal ganglion cells—enter the superior and inferior aspects of the disc. Thus, when there is atrophy of nasal fibers, the normal striations of the nerve fiber layer are lost both nasal to the disc and in the papillomacular region. The optic disc shows corresponding atrophy at its nasal and temporal regions with relative sparing of the superior and inferior portions where the majority of spared temporal fibers (subserving nasal field) enter (Fig. 12.10). Thus, the optic atrophy occupies a more or less horizontal band across the disc, wider nasally than temporally, so-called "band" or **"bow-tie" atrophy.**

It is perhaps clinically more useful when atrophy is *absent* in patients with chiasmal (or optic nerve) compression than when it is present. Although patients with significant nerve fiber bundle defects and optic atrophy can still have impressive return of both acuity and field when successful decompression is obtained, patients with normal appearing fundi should have near complete or complete return of visual function with successful decompression. Thus, it is crucial that decompression be carried out as soon as possible in these patients.

Papilledema is more frequently associated with suprachiasmal tumors than with infrachiasmal tumors, because the former lesions can invade or compress the 3rd ventricle, ultimately obstructing the flow of cerebrospinal fluid. In such cases, optic atrophy may result not only from compression of the visual axons in the optic nerves or chiasm but also from the effects of chronic or severe papilledema (i.e., postpapilledema optic atrophy).

Most patients with lesions that affect the optic chiasm have no disturbances of ocular alignment or motility except for the hemifield slide phenomenon. However, patients with lesions that damage the optic chiasm as well as one or more of the ocular motor nerves in the subarachnoid space or within the cavernous sinus almost always complain of double vision. When the ocular motor nerves are damaged within the cavernous sinus, there may also be pain, evidence of a trigeminal sensory neuropathy, or both, in the territory of the first and/or second divisions of the trigeminal nerve. The third division of the nerve, which does not pass through the cavernous sinus, is not affected by such lesions, and a motor neuropathy thus is never present unless the lesion extends posteriorly. The oculosympathetic fibers may also be damaged by a lesion in the chiasmal or parasellar regions, resulting in a

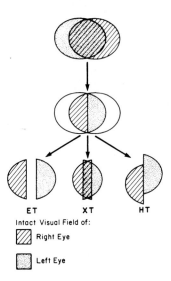

ET   XT   HT

Intact Visual Field of:

▨ Right Eye

▦ Left Eye

Figure 12.9. Diagram showing the "hemifield slide phenomena" experienced by patients with bitemporal hemianopias. Patients with a preexisting exophoria or intermittent exotropia will have overlapping of the intact nasal fields, whereas patients with a preexisting esophoria or intermittent esotropia will have separation of the nasal hemifields, causing a blind area in the center of the field. Patients with pre-existing hyperdeviations will complain of vertical separation of images crossing the vertical meridian. (Redrawn from: Kirkham TH. The ocular symptomatology of pituitary tumors. *Proc R Soc Med.* 1972;65:517–518.)

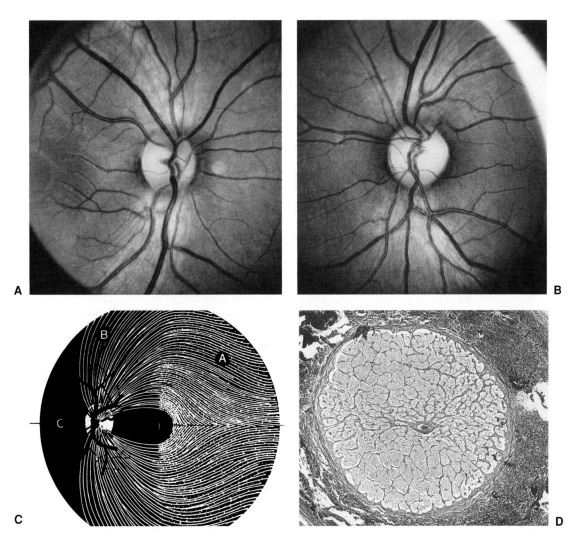

Figure 12.10. Optic chiasmal syndrome. **A and B:** Both right and left optic discs show "band" atrophy with corresponding loss of nerve fibers from ganglion cells located nasal to the fovea. **C:** Diagram of nerve fiber loss in patients with temporal hemianopia. Regions marked **A, B,** and **C** in diagram denote areas of nerve fiber layer preservation, partial loss, and complete loss, respectively. (Reprinted from: Hoyt WF, Kommerell G. Der Fundus oculi bei Homonyer Hemianopia. Klin Monatsbl Augenheilkd. 1973;162:456–464, with permission.) **D:** Transverse section of orbital optic nerve in a patient with a temporal hemianopia shows "band" or "bow-tie" pattern of atrophy with relative sparing of the superior and inferior portions of the nerve. (Reprinted from: Unsöld R, Hoyt WF. Band atrophy of the optic nerve. *Arch Ophthalmol.* 1980;98:1637–1638, with permission.)

postganglionic Horner's syndrome characterized by ipsilateral ptosis and a small reactive pupil (see Chapter 15). Horner's syndrome is often associated with an ipsilateral abducens nerve palsy, because the postganglionic oculosympathetic fibers briefly join the abducens nerve within the cavernous sinus. When both the oculomotor nerve and oculosympathetic fibers are affected, the clinical picture is one of an oculomotor nerve paresis with a small pupil that is normally reactive if the paresis is pupil-sparing or poorly or nonreactive if the paresis involves the pupillomotor fibers. Single or multiple ocular motor nerve pareses in a patient with a bitemporal field defect suggests a process extrinsic to the chiasm rather than an infiltrative intrinsic lesion.

The unusual phenomenon of **seesaw nystagmus** may occur in patients with tumors of the diencephalon and chiasmal regions. This condition is characterized by synchronous alternating elevation and intorsion of one eye and depression and extorsion of the opposite eye. The cause of seesaw nystagmus is unknown, but it may be related to damage to the interstitial nucleus of Cajal or adjacent structures by the tumor.

Lesions causing a chiasmal syndrome may arise from or extend to the hypothalamus. Patients with this presentation may develop diabetes insipidus and hypothalamic hypopituitarism. Prepubertal children may also suffer from both growth retardation and delayed sexual development, and young children and infants may have severe failure to thrive (Russell's syndrome).

TOPICAL DIAGNOSIS OF RETROCHIASMAL VISUAL FIELD DEFECTS

Unilateral lesions of the visual sensory pathway beyond the optic chiasm—the optic tract, lateral geniculate body (LGB), optic radiation, or striate cortex (Fig. 12.1A)—produce homonymous visual field defects without loss of visual acuity. When such defects are complete, they do not, in themselves, allow topical diagnosis. In such instances, the clinician must rely on other symptoms and signs of neurologic disease or on neuroimaging to define both the area of damage and the etiology of the lesion.

Homonymous defects in the visual fields characteristically develop slowly when they are caused by compression and rapidly when they are caused by hemorrhage, ischemia, or inflammation. Compressive lesions generally cause progressive loss of visual field from the periphery of the field to the center. With decompression of the visual system, improvement typically first occurs in the central region and continues toward the periphery. Defects for colored objects invariably appear before disturbances either for form or for black and white objects, a reason to use colored stimuli routinely in the examination of visual fields.

When homonymous visual field defects arise from vascular lesions, the onset of the field defects is sudden. Such defects include complete homonymous quadrantanopsias and hemianopias, incomplete homonymous quadrantanopsias and hemianopias with varying degrees of congruity, and homonymous paracentral scotomas. When and if improvement occurs, the central field clears first and may be followed by gradual enlargement of the peripheral fields if they have been affected.

The location and causes of homonymous hemianopia depend on the age of the patient and the presence or absence of other neurologic findings. In nonisolated cases of homonymous hemianopic defects, 40% to 51% of patients have occipital lobe pathology, 29% to 57% have lesions of the optic radiations, and 3% to 21% have lesions in the region of the optic tract and the LGB (Fig. 12.11). Vascular causes, including infarction, hemorrhage, and arteriovenous

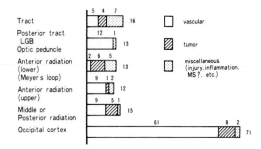

Figure 12.11. Location and causes of homonymous hemianopia in 140 patients. (Reprinted from: Fujino T, Kigazawa K, Yamada R. Homonymous hemianopia: a retrospective study of 140 cases. *Neuro-ophthalmology.* 6;1986:17–21, with permission.)

malformations, account for 42% to 71% of cases; mass lesions account for 19% to 38%. On the other hand, almost 90% of patients with isolated homonymous hemianopia have occipital lobe lesions, usually caused by vascular disease in the territory of the posterior cerebral arteries. Older patients with isolated homonymous hemianopia have an exceedingly high probability of vascular lesions, whereas younger patients may have congenital or acquired nonvascular etiologies, such as neoplasm, abscess, or demyelinating disease. Neuroimaging, preferably MRI, should be the first diagnostic procedure used to determine the location and etiology of an homonymous hemianopia.

TOPICAL DIAGNOSIS OF OPTIC TRACT LESIONS

Although lesions affecting the optic tracts are infrequent, they are of great importance because they are located in the first region beyond the optic chiasm where lesions produce an homonymous visual field defect (Fig. 12.12). Lesions of the optic tract account for about 3% to 11% of cases of homonymous hemianopia. The causes are varied and include tumors, vascular processes, demyelinating disease, and trauma (Figs. 12.13 and 12.14).

Patients with optic tract lesions often have specific findings that permit the recognition of the location of the lesion on clinical grounds alone. All patients with a complete homonymous hemianopia caused by an isolated optic tract lesion have a relative afferent pupillary defect in the eye contralateral to the side of the lesion (i.e., the eye with the temporal field loss). This occurs because (a) the temporal visual field is considerably larger than the nasal field (therefore, there are more crossing nasal fibers than noncrossing temporal fibers); (b) the pupillomotor fibers within the visual sensory pathway hemidecussate in the optic chiasm along with or as part of the visual axons; and (c) the

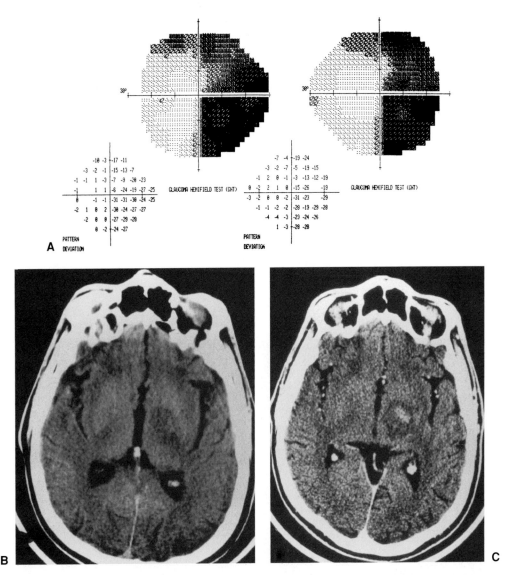

Figure 12.12. A 65-year-old man developed headache, sleepiness, personality changes, memory difficulties, right hemiparesis, and difficulty seeing to the right. **A:** Visual fields reveal an incongruous right homonymous hemianopia. **B–C:** CT scans, axial views, before **(B)** and after **(C)** the administration of intravenous contrast reveal an enhancing lesion with surrounding edema in the region of the left optic tract, diagnosed ultimately as lymphoma.

pupillomotor fibers are present within the optic tract for most of its extent. Because the temporal visual field is 60% to 70% larger than the nasal field, there is a disparity with respect to light input from the two eyes to the mesencephalic pupillary center. A complete lesion of one optic tract thus preferentially reduces input from the contralateral eye.

Another pupillary phenomenon that is sometimes associated with lesions of the optic tract that produce a complete or nearly complete homonymous hemianopia is pupillary hemiakinesia (hemianopic pupillary reaction or Wernicke's pupil). Because the pupillary afferents are present in this section of the visual system, when light is projected onto the "blind" retinal elements (subserving the nasal visual field in the ipsilateral eye and the temporal visual field in the contralateral eye), either no pupillary reaction occurs or the reaction is markedly reduced. However, when light is projected onto the intact retinal elements (subserving the temporal visual field in the ipsilateral eye and the nasal visual field in the contralateral eye), a normal pupillary reaction is observed. This phenomenon is best

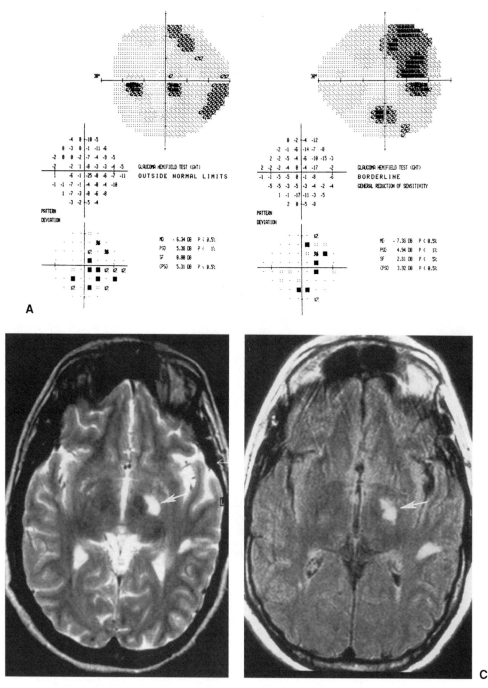

Figure 12.13. A 40-year-old man noted a "black spot" in front of both eyes that gradually worsened over 2 weeks. Visual acuities were normal, but there was a trace right relative afferent pupillary defect. **A:** Visual fields show a highly incongruous right homonymous defect. **B and C:** MRI (**B:** T2-weighted; **C:** Fluid-attenuated inversion-recovery) reveals multiple white-matter lesions consistent with demyelinating disease, including a large plaque in the left optic tract (*arrows*).

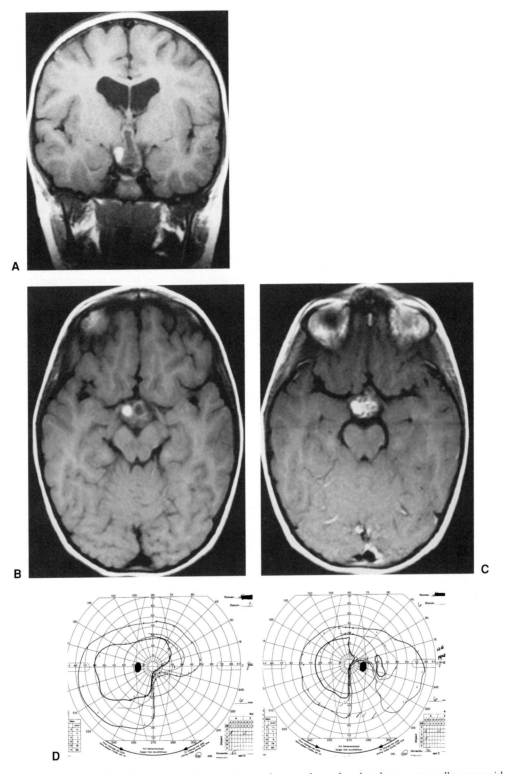

Figure 12.14. A 7-year-old girl presented with precocious puberty and was found to have a suprasellar mass with hydrocephalus. **A:** Coronal, T1-weighted MRI without gadolinium. **B:** Axial, T1-weighted MRI without gadolinium. **C:** Axial, T1-weighted MRI with gadolinium. **D:** Visual field testing reveals an incomplete, incongruous, right homonymous inferior quadrantanopia, consistent with damage to the left optic tract. Biopsy showed findings diagnostic of craniopharyngioma.

observed with a bright, focused beam of light, such as that from a slit lamp biomicroscope or a hand-held transilluminator.

Optic tract lesions do not cause loss of visual acuity nor do they affect color vision unless they also damage the optic chiasm or the intracranial portions of one or both optic nerves. Thus, patients with lesions confined to an optic tract have normal visual acuity and color vision, and they have no sensation of reduced light brightness in the eye with the relative afferent pupillary defect. On the other hand, when lesions of the optic tract also damage the ipsilateral optic nerve or chiasm, reduced visual acuity, abnormal color vision, and a relative afferent pupillary defect occur on the side of the lesion.

Patients with a complete or nearly complete homonymous hemianopia from an optic tract lesion eventually develop a characteristic pattern of optic atrophy. There is a "band" of horizontal pallor of the optic disc in the eye contralateral to the lesion (with temporal field loss) (i.e., "bow-tie atrophy"). This pattern of optic nerve atrophy is caused by atrophy of retinal nerve fibers originating from ganglion cells nasal to the fovea and is identical with that seen in both eyes of patients with bitemporal field loss from chiasmal syndromes. At the same time, there is generalized pallor of the optic disc in the eye on the side of the lesion, associated with significant loss of nerve fiber layer details in the superior and inferior arcuate regions that comprise the majority of fibers subserving the nasal visual field and originating from ganglion cells temporal to the fovea (Fig. 12.15).

Not all patients with optic tract lesions have a complete homonymous hemianopia. Many patients have a complete or incomplete homonymous quadrantanopia or an incomplete hemianopia. Such field defects are quite incongruous and may also be scotomatous (Fig. 12.13). Indeed, the optic tract is one of only two locations in the postchiasmal pathway in which homonymous scotomas routinely occur; the occipital lobe is the other.

Patients with optic tract lesions often have manifestations in addition to homonymous visual field defects, because lesions that damage the optic tract may also damage adjacent neural structures. Neurologic deficits that may occur in patients with lesions of the optic tract include hypothalamic symptoms and signs and contralateral hemiparesis.

TOPICAL DIAGNOSIS OF LESIONS OF THE LATERAL GENICULATE BODY

Lesions affecting the lateral geniculate body are less commonly diagnosed than those of the optic tract but can be caused by a number of different processes, including vascular disease, neoplasms, inflammation, demyelination, and trauma.

Lesions of the LGB may cause incongruous or congruous homonymous field defects. The dorsal region of the LGB subserves macular function, the lateral aspect of the LGB subserves the superior visual field, and the medial aspect subserves the inferior field (Fig. 12.16). Although the intricate retinotopic organization of the LGB may result in the production of relative defects, incongruous defects, and even (theoretically) monocular defects, vascular lesions are more likely to respect specific anatomic boundaries within the LGB and produce homonymous sector defects that are, in fact, quite congruous, with abruptly sloping borders (Figs. 12.17 and 12.18). Two specific patterns of relatively congruous homonymous field defects can occur, most often attributable to focal disease of the LGB caused by infarction in the territory of two specific arteries. Ischemia or other damage in the territory of the lateral choroidal artery typically causes a **congruous homonymous horizontal sectoranopia** (Fig. 12.17A and B). Ischemia in the region of the LGB supplied by the distal portion of the anterior choroidal artery results in loss of the upper and lower homonymous sectors in the visual fields of the two eyes, producing a **congruous homonymous quadruple sectoranopia** (Figs. 12.17C, 12.17D, and 12.18).

Because the pupillomotor fibers leave the optic tract to ascend in the brachium of the superior colliculus, the pupillary reactions in patients with LGB lesions are normal (unless the lesion also damages the optic tract or the brachium)—there is neither a contralateral relative afferent pupillary defect nor a hemianopic pupillary phenomenon. However, the visual axons from retinal ganglion cells first synapse in the LGB. Thus, sectorial or hemianopic atrophy of the retinal nerve fiber layer and optic disc occurs in patients with lesions of the LGB that damage the incoming axons. Such defects, when associated with acquired homonymous field defects, whether congruous or incongruous, must be taken as evidence of optic tract or LGB damage in all cases.

Patients with lesions of the LGB frequently have neurologic symptoms and signs consistent with damage to the ipsilateral thalamus or pyramidal tract. Thalamic damage may result in gross impairment of sensation on the side of the body opposite the lesion, or there may be a complaint of pain of central origin that is referred to the opposite side of the body. Damage to the pyramidal tract causes contralateral hemibody weakness.

TOPICAL DIAGNOSIS OF LESIONS OF THE OPTIC RADIATION

The optic radiation is that part of the postchiasmal visual sensory pathway that begins in the LGB and transmits visual information to the striate cortex. It may be damaged by lesions in several different

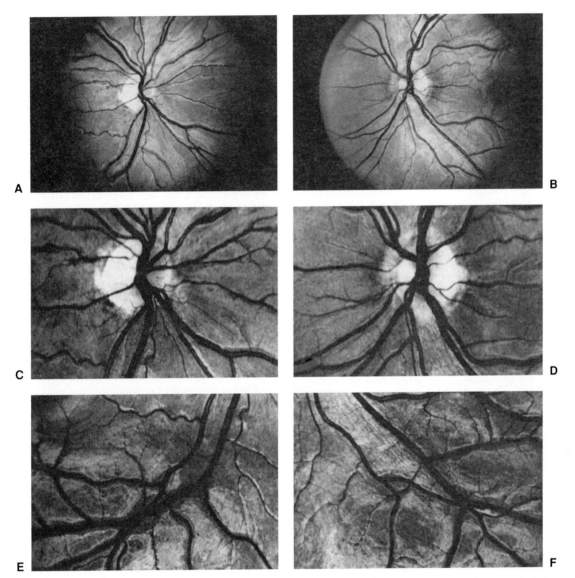

Figure 12.15. Hemianopic optic atrophy in a patient with a left homonymous hemianopia from a right optic tract lesion. **A:** The right optic disc has somewhat diffuse, temporal atrophy from loss of nerve fibers from ganglion cells temporal to the fovea. **B:** The left optic disc shows band atrophy from loss of nerve fibers from ganglion cells nasal to the fovea. **C and D:** Red-free (540 nm) photographs showing atrophy of right and left optic discs. Note band pattern of atrophy of the left disc. **E:** Inferior temporal peripapillary retina of right eye showing relative absence of visible arcuate bundle. **F:** Inferior temporal peripapillary retina of left eye showing relative preservation of arcuate bundle.

locations, including the internal capsule, temporal lobe, and parietal lobe.

Lesions of the Internal Capsule

Efferent projection fibers from and afferent projection fibers to the cerebral cortex traverse the subcortical white matter where they form a radiating mass of fibers, the corona radiata, which converges toward the brainstem (Figs. 12.1A and 12.19). In the rostral brainstem,

the fibers form a broad but compact fiber band, the **internal capsule,** that is bordered medially by the thalamus and caudate nucleus and laterally by the lenticular nucleus. The afferent fibers comprise the thalamocortical radiations in the posterior limb of the internal capsule. The efferent bundles include:

- The corticospinal and corticobulbar tracts in the anterior limb.

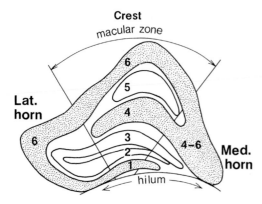

Figure 12.16. Artist's drawing of a coronal section through the lateral geniculate nucleus, viewed from its posterior aspect. Three laminae (white areas, layers 2, 3, and 5) receive input from ipsilateral retinal ganglion cells, and three laminae (stippled layers, 1, 4, and 6) receive input from contralateral retinal ganglion cells.

- The frontopontine tract from the prefrontal and precentral regions of the cerebral cortex in the anterior limb.
- The temporoparietopontine tract from the temporal and parietal lobes in the posterior limb.
- The optic radiation, which begins in the LGB and occupies only a small region of the capsule because it does not proceed to the brainstem.

The internal capsule is thus composed of all fibers, afferent and efferent, that go to, or come from, the cerebral cortex. The most posterior component of the internal capsule is the optic radiation.

Interruption of the optic radiation is characterized by a contralateral, usually complete, homonymous hemianopia that is typically associated with contralateral hemianesthesia from damage to the adjacent thalamocortical fibers in the posterior limb of the internal capsule. Other ocular findings in lesions of the internal capsule include a transient deviation of the eyes to the side of the lesion in many instances and weakness of the frontalis and orbicularis oculi on the contralateral hemiplegic side in a minority of cases. Vascular causes predominate.

Lesions of the Temporal Lobe

Temporal lobe lesions may damage the optic radiation. Such lesions account for about 13% to 24% of homonymous visual field defects, with tumors and abscesses causing the majority of cases. Temporal lobe surgery for epilepsy may also cause such defects, which are often asymptomatic.

The disposition of the visual fibers in the temporal lobe is controversial, and there may be considerable individual variability in the spatial distribution of optic radiation fibers within the temporal lobe. Clearly, the most anterior portion of the temporal lobe may be damaged or removed without the production of any visual field defect. The amount of temporal lobe that may be removed without a resulting field defect is disputed, however. It would appear that up to 4 cm of anterior temporal lobe can be removed in most patients without interruption of visual fibers to the extent that a field defect is produced. Once the lobe is sectioned 4 cm or more posterior to the tip, however, most patients will develop an homonymous field defect. In most cases, the homonymous defect is incomplete and is either confined to the superior quadrants or is denser above, reflecting the anatomy of Meyer's loop—the portion of the optic radiation that courses anteriorly in the temporal lobe around the temporal horn of the lateral ventricle and that consists entirely of axons subserving the superior visual fields of the two eyes. These field defects have other characteristics:

1. They do not affect visual acuity.
2. They do not alter the size of the blind spot.
3. They tend to have sloping inferior margins unless they occur after a temporal lobectomy, in which case they may have sloping superior margins.
4. They may cross the horizontal midline.
5. They are usually incongruous but may be congruous (Fig. 12.20).

Most series report a tendency for macular sparing in patients with partial or complete quadrantic defects from temporal lobe damage. However, the peripheral field, including the monocular crescent, is never spared in these field defects. With temporal lobectomies beyond 8 cm, almost all patients have a complete homonymous hemianopia.

An incongruous homonymous wedge-shaped defect in the upper visual fields, often called a "pie-in-the-sky" defect to emphasize its superior location and wedge shape, almost always indicates damage to the optic radiation in the temporal lobe. Most visual field defects resulting from temporal lobe lesions are incongruous, but the incongruity is usually not as severe as that seen with optic tract and some LGB lesions. A superior homonymous quadrantic defect suggests damage to the inferior fibers of the optic tract, the optic radiation in the temporal lobe, or the inferior occipital cortex. When the defect is congruous, an occipital lobe location is most likely, but the lesion may still be in the temporal lobe (Fig. 12.21). When the defect is incongruous, the lesion is either in the optic tract or the temporal lobe, not in the occipital lobe.

Nonvisual manifestations of lesions of the temporal lobe are common. If there is a mass lesion of the temporal lobe, headache may be a prominent accompaniment. Bilateral lesions of the transverse gyri of

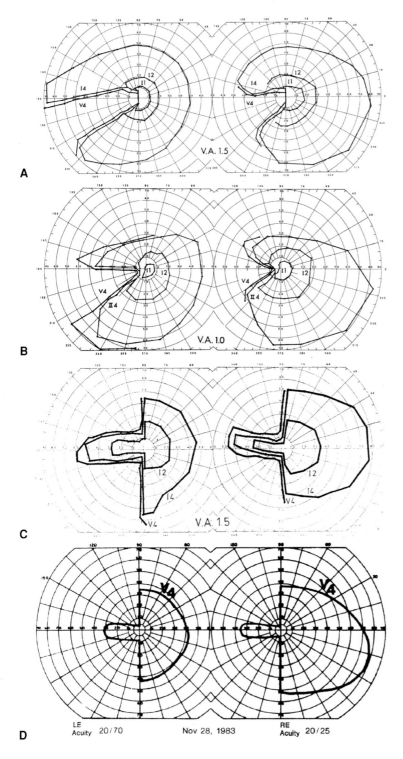

Figure 12.17. Visual field defects in patients with lesions of the lateral geniculate body (LGB). **A and B:** Homonymous horizontal sectoranopia from damage to the LGB in the territory of the lateral choroidal artery. **A:** In a patient with a small arteriovenous malformation. **B:** In a patient with presumed thrombosis of the lateral choroidal artery. Note the relative congruity of the field defect in both cases. (Reprinted from: Frisén L, Holmegaard L, Rosencrantz M. Sectorial optic atrophy and homonymous, horizontal sectoranopia: a lateral choroidal artery syndrome? *J Neurol Neurosurg Psychiatry.* 1978;41:374–380, with permission.) **C and D:** Homonymous quadruple sectoranopia from damage to the LGB in the territory of the distal anterior choroidal artery. **C:** In a patient with occlusion of the distal anterior choroidal artery. (Reprinted from: Frisén L. Quadruple sectoranopia and sectorial optic atrophy: A syndrome of the distal anterior choroidal artery. *J Neurol Neurosurg Psychiatry.* 1979;42:590–594, with permission.) **D:** In another patient with occlusion of the distal anterior choroidal artery. (Reprinted from: Helgason C, Caplan LR, Goodwin J, et al. Anterior choroidal artery-territory infarction. Report of cases and review. *Arch Neurol.* 1986;43:681–686, with permission.)

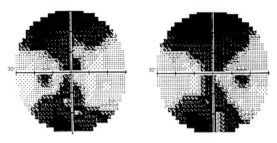

Figure 12.18. A 37-year-old woman had central pontine myelinolysis and complained of bilateral visual loss. Visual acuity was 20/25 OD and 20/30 OS. Automated static perimetry demonstrates fairly congruous defects having an hourglass configuration, with near total depression superior and inferior to fixation. The visual field defects were similar to those reported after anterior choroidal artery infarction, prompting the authors to propose that the cells supplied by the anterior choroidal artery in the lateral geniculate might be particularly susceptible to metabolic insult, such as rapid changes in serum sodium level. (Reprinted from: Donahue SP, Kardon RH, Thompson HS. Hourglass-shaped visual fields as a sign of bilateral lateral geniculate myelinolysis. *Am J Ophthalmol.* 1995;119:378–380, with permission.)

Heschl can cause cortical deafness, usually associated with aphasia; unilateral lesions may cause a disturbance of hearing and sound discrimination contralateral to the lesion. If the lesion is in the dominant temporal lobe, the patient may have difficulty memorizing a series of spoken words, whereas if the lesion is in the nondominant temporal lobe, the patient may exhibit various forms of auditory agnosia. Auditory hallucinations or illusions may occur with lesions of either temporal lobe. Severe disturbances of language can result from lesions in the dominant, usually left, temporal lobe. Disturbances of memory are common in patients with such lesions.

Tumors of the temporal lobe frequently cause seizures. These seizures are typically characterized by transient changes in emotions, mood, and behavior and are associated with motor automatisms—so-called complex partial seizures or psychomotor epilepsy. If the lesion is situated anteriorly and affects the uncinate gyrus, either directly or through pressure, so-called "uncinate fits" occur that are characterized by an aura of unusual taste or smell, followed by abnormal motor activity of the mouth and lips, during which the patient is not in contact with his or her surroundings.

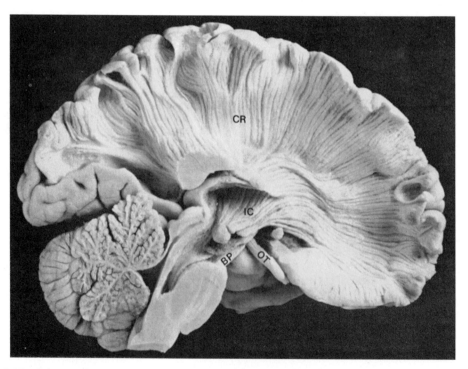

Figure 12.19. Specimen showing the corona radiata and internal capsule, and their relationship to the optic tract. The internal capsule and corona radiata have been exposed by removal of the corpus callosum, caudate nucleus, and diencephalon. Note that the fibers of the basis pedunculi pass adjacent to the optic tract. **CR,** corona radiata. **IC,** internal capsule. **BP,** basis pedunculi. **OT,** optic tract. (Reprinted from: Ghuhbegovic N, Williams TH. *The Human Brain. A Photographic Guide.* Hagerstown, MD: Harper & Row, 1980, with permission.)

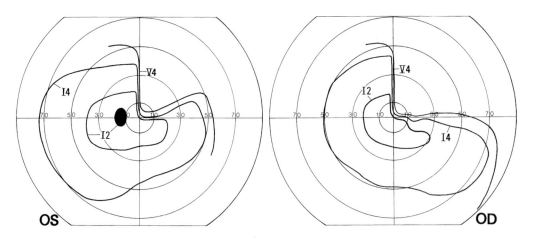

Figure 12.20. Homonymous quadrantanopia in a patient with a glioblastoma of the left temporal lobe. The defects are primarily superior and are moderately incongruous. Note that the greater defect is on the side opposite the lesion.

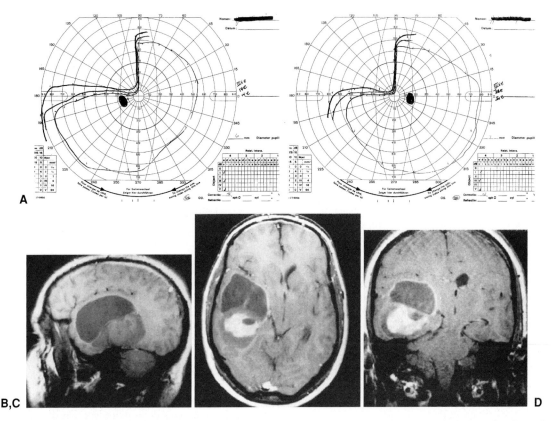

Figure 12.21. A 29-year-old man presented with 2 months of headaches with mood swings and mania and 3 days of intermittent greenish-blue lines appearing in his superior left visual field. Examination was normal except for papilledema and a left homonymous superior quadrantanopia (**A**). T1-weighted MRI (**B:** sagittal pregadolinium. **C:** axial postgadolinium; **D:** coronal postgadolinium) shows an inhomogeneously enhancing, cystic mass in the right temporal lobe. Biopsy was diagnostic of glioblastoma multiforme.

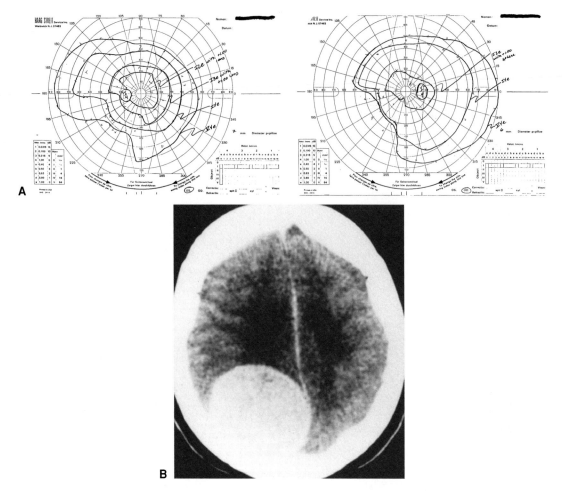

Figure 12.22. A 37-year-old woman complained of intermittent headaches associated with visual hallucinations of "a swirling black circle in the left eye." **A:** Examination was normal except for left homonymous inferior quadrantic visual field defects. **B:** CT scan, axial view, after intravenous injection of iodinated contrast material reveals a large, dural-based homogenously enhancing right parietal lobe tumor with little mass effect, confirmed at surgery to be a meningioma.

Patients with temporal lobe lesions that produce an homonymous visual field defect may also experience visual hallucinations. The hallucinations are typically of the formed type and consist of both animate (e.g., people, animals) and inanimate (e.g., flowers, trees, buildings) objects. They are often seen in color and are always in the affected homonymous hemifield on the side contralateral to the lesion. Visual hallucinations caused by temporal lobe lesions may be pleasurable or frightening to the patient and may be accompanied by auditory hallucinations.

Lesions of the Parietal Lobe

Lesions of the parietal lobe may produce ocular symptoms that have value in topical diagnosis. Homonymous hemianopia affecting primarily the lower fields is caused by damage to the optic radiation in the superior parietal lobe (Fig. 12.22). Such defects are usually more congruous than those produced by lesions of the temporal lobe. Because the entire optic radiation passes through the parietal lobe, large lesions may produce complete homonymous hemianopia with macular splitting.

The optic radiation is a continuous sheet of fibers with no separation of fibers into those ultimately projecting to the superior and inferior visual cortices. Thus, most field defects in patients with lesions of the optic radiation have sloping borders that do not precisely respect the horizontal meridian (Fig. 12.23). Exceptions occur, however, especially when the causative lesion is in the posterior optic radiation where the fascicles approach the calcarine cortex.

Neuro-ophthalmologic features suggesting a lesion in the parietal lobe include an incomplete and

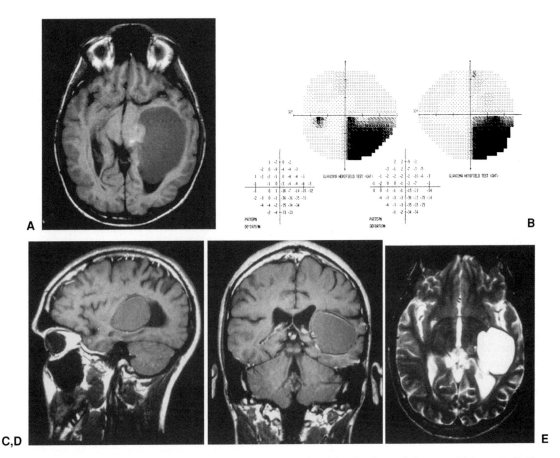

Figure 12.23. A 17-year-old man had a complex partial seizure and was found to have a left temporal lobe cystic fibrillary astrocytoma. **A:** T1-weighted axial MRI shows location of the tumor. The tumor was partially resected and then irradiated. **B:** Visual fields performed 6 years later show a right homonymous inferior quadrantanopia. **C:** T1-weighted sagittal image after gadolinium. **D:** T1-weighted axial image after gadolinium; **E:** T2-weighted axial image now reveals a smaller cystic lesion in the region of the optic radiation. Note that the lesion does not extend into the occipital lobe.

relatively congruous (or mildly incongruous) homonymous hemianopia that is denser below than above, conjugate movements of the eyes to the side opposite the lesion on forced lid closure (Cogan's sign), and an abnormal optokinetic response when the target is moved toward the side of the lesion. A disturbance of fixation reflexes sufficient to interfere with reading ability may develop before the appearance of other symptoms. This disturbance is sometimes manifest during visual field testing, during which the patient cannot maintain central fixation despite repeated instructions to do so, an apparent understanding of the instructions, and an apparent willingness to comply. Other types of visual disturbances caused by lesions in the parietal lobe include visual neglect, visual agnosia, and difficulties with word recognition.

Patients with parietal lobe lesions and homonymous visual field defects are often unaware of their visual deficits. This phenomenon is more likely to occur when the underlying abnormality is in the nondominant cerebral hemisphere (usually the right parietal lobe), but it can also occur in patients with dominant parietal lobe lesions. In other patients, the primary visual pathways may be unaffected or minimally affected, but the patient neglects the contralateral visual field.

The parietal lobe is the principal sensory area of the cerebral cortex, and its postcentral convolution is of particular importance. The patient may complain of numbness but more commonly has complex problems of sensory integration that can be demonstrated using tests of tactile discrimination, position sense, stereognosis, and visual-spatial coordination. Irritative lesions of the postcentral convolution cause sensory Jacksonian seizures that begin contralateral to the lesion at the part of the body that corresponds to the focus of excitation. Tingling or numbness spreads to other adjacent parts of the body according to the order of their representation in the cortex. Lesions in the dominant parietal lobe can cause aphasia (usually fluent), apraxia, agnosia, acalculia, and agraphia. A lesion in the dominant parietal lobe involving the angular gyrus may produce Gerstmann's syndrome (finger agnosia, right-left disorientation, agraphia, and acalculia) in association with a right homonymous hemianopia. Lesions in the nondominant parietal lobe may cause impaired constructional ability, dyscalculia, and, most commonly, inattention or neglect. Indeed, left spatial neglect after a right hemisphere lesion may accentuate the left hemianopia, hemianesthesia, and hemiplegia, and thus contribute to poor recovery.

LESIONS OF THE OCCIPITAL LOBE AND VISUAL CORTEX

Most lesions affecting the occipital lobe are vascular or traumatic in origin, with tumors, abscesses, demyelinating, and toxic disorders of white matter occurring much less frequently. Because of the close anatomic relationship of fibers from corresponding portions of the two retinas, lesions of the occipital lobe cause defects that are almost exclusively homonymous and are also increasingly congruous the more posteriorly situated the lesion.

Unilateral Lesions of the Posterior Occipital Lobe

Defects seen with these lesions are always homonymous. Lesions of the tip of the occipital lobe (occipital pole) produce central homonymous scotomas that are exquisitely congruous. The central 10 degrees of visual field are represented by at least 50% to 60% of the posterior striate cortex, and the central 30 degrees by about 80% of the cortex (Figs. 12.24 and 12.25). Lesions located more anteriorly may produce primarily central field defects that break out into the periphery (Fig. 12.26). Impressive congruity is a feature of such field defects, and the phenomenon of sparing of the macula is often seen in such cases (see below).

Unilateral Lesions of the Anterior Occipital Lobe

Because the temporal field in each eye is larger than the nasal field, the fibers subserving that portion of the peripheral temporal field that has no nasal correlate must be unpaired throughout the postchiasmal portion of the visual sensory pathway. Damage to these unpaired peripheral fibers produces a monocular defect in the extreme temporal visual field. This field defect is crescentic in shape, and its widest extent is in the horizontal meridian, where it extends from 60 degrees out to approximately 90 degrees. Because of the peculiar shape of the defect, patients with the defect are said to have the **temporal crescent (or half-moon) syndrome** (Fig. 12.27). The most anterior portion of the striate cortex harbors the projected monocular temporal crescent of the contralateral eye. Therefore, lesions of the posterior striate cortex tend to spare the temporal crescent (Fig. 12.28), whereas lesions of the anterior striate cortex may selectively produce a defect in the temporal crescent or eliminate it entirely (Fig. 12.27).

Two important, if basic, facts should be kept in mind when considering the temporal crescent syndrome. First, monocular peripheral temporal visual field defects are probably caused most often by *retinal* lesions, not by intracranial ones. Thus, the nasal retinal periphery should be carefully examined ophthalmoscopically in patients with a presumed temporal crescent syndrome. Second, because these defects begin approximately 60 degrees from fixation, central field testing (i.e., that performed using a tangent screen or most automated static perimetry programs) gives normal results and will not detect such defects (Fig. 12.27).

Sparing of the Macula

In homonymous hemianopia, when a portion of the central field of each eye is preserved as a result of deviation of the vertical meridian between the functioning and nonfunctioning halves of the visual fields, there is said to be "sparing of the macula" or "macular sparing." In a majority of such cases, visual acuity is normal, with the zone of preserved visual field ranging from 1 degree or 2 degrees to almost 10 degrees in width (Fig. 12.29). Macular sparing is seen in patients with postgeniculate—usually occipital—lesions, but absence of sparing does not necessarily indicate that the lesion is either noncortical or pregeniculate.

The etiology of macular sparing is controversial. Three theories have been proposed to explain the phenomenon:

1. An artifact of testing.
2. Bilateral representation of the macula.
3. Incomplete damage of the visual sensory pathway.

There is no doubt that some cases of "macular sparing" are caused by inaccurate fixation. It is impossible for even otherwise normal persons to obtain perfect fixation, and physiologic movements of the fixing eye, so slight that they cannot be detected by ordinary means, probably account for at least 1 degree to 2 degrees of deviation of the vertical meridian about the central area.

Histochemical studies demonstrate that, to some extent, a small portion of each macula probably has representation in each occipital lobe. There is a small area of nasotemporal overlap on either side of the vertical meridian in which some axons from ganglion cells temporal to the fovea cross within the chiasm, whereas

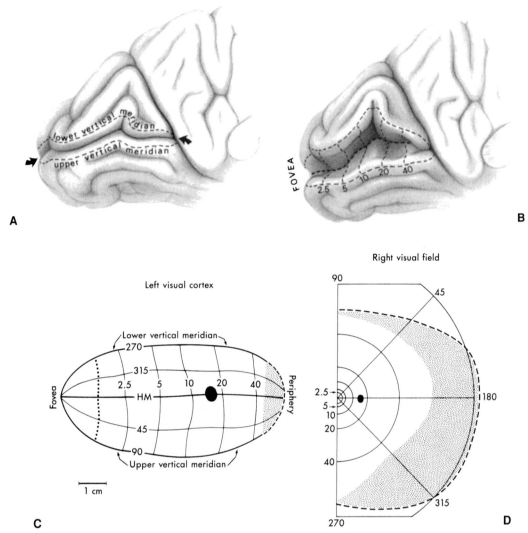

Figure 12.24. The representation of the visual field in the human striate cortex. **A:** Left occipital lobe showing location of striate cortex within the calcarine fissure (*between arrows*). The boundary (*dashed line*) between the striate cortex (area V1) and extrastriate cortex contains the representation of the vertical meridian. **B:** View of striate cortex after opening the lips of the calcarine fissure. The dashed lines indicate the coordinates of the visual field map. The representation of the horizontal meridian runs approximately along the base of the calcarine fissure. The vertical dashed lines mark the iso-eccentricity contours from 2.5° to 40°. Striate cortex wraps around the occipital pole to extend about 1 cm onto the lateral convexity where the fovea is represented. **C:** Schematic map showing the projection of the right visual hemifield upon the left visual cortex by transposing the map illustrated in **(B)** onto a flat surface. The row of dots indicates approximately where striate cortex folds around the tip of the occipital lobe. The black oval marks the region of the striate cortex corresponding to the blind spot of the contralateral eye. *HM,* horizontal meridian. **D:** Right visual hemifield plotted with a Goldmann perimeter. The stippled region corresponds to the monocular temporal crescent, which is mapped within the most anterior 8% to 10% of the striate cortex. (Reprinted from: Horton JC, Hoyt WF. The representation of the visual field in human striate cortex. A revision of the classic Holmes map. *Arch Ophthalmol.* 1991;109:816–824, with permission.)

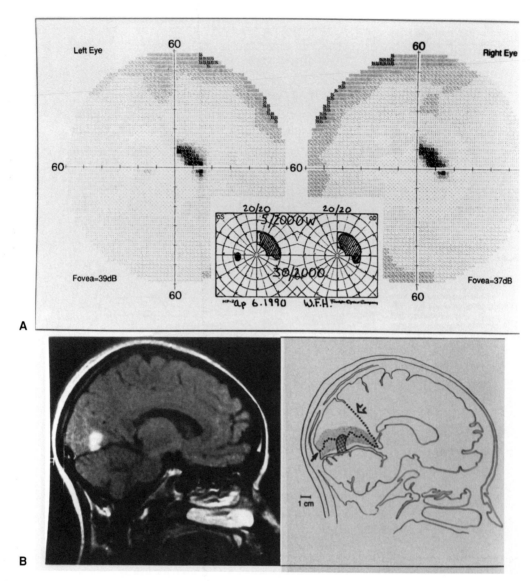

Figure 12.25. A 30-year-old woman reported several episodes of flashing, colored lights in her right upper quadrant of vision. **A:** Merged 30–2 and 60–2 full-threshold visual field tests using a Humphrey Field Analyzer. A homonymous, congruous scotoma was present in the right upper quadrant. In the inset, the visual fields are mapped at the tangent screen. The scotoma extended from 6° to 18°. **B:** Parasagittal magnetic resonance image of the left occipital lobe. The lesion (cross-hatched area in the diagram on the right) is within the visual cortex (stippled area in the diagram on the right). The calcarine sulcus (*solid arrow*) and the parieto-occipital sulcus (*hollow arrow*) are marked by dots. On biopsy, the lesion was a presumed tuberculoma. (Reprinted from: Horton JC, Hoyt WF. The representation of the visual field in human striate cortex. *Arch Ophthalmol.* 1991;109;816–824, with permission.)

some axons from ganglion cells nasal to the fovea remain uncrossed. However, the mere presence of an overlap does not necessarily have any clinical visual consequences.

In fact, most clinically obvious cases of homonymous hemianopia with macular sparing occur in the setting of incomplete damage to the visual sensory pathway, usually the occipital lobe, and appear to be related to a residual intact area of the pathway. The unique dual blood supply of the occipital cortex from the posterior cerebral and middle cerebral arteries provides a mechanism for this partial damage. Thus, in

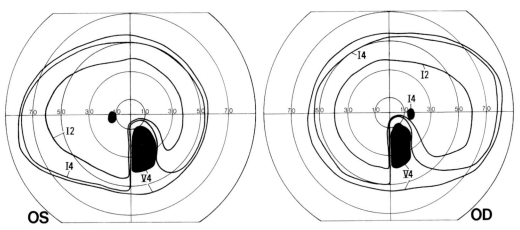

Figure 12.26. Inferior homonymous hemianopic scotomas that break out to the periphery in a patient with an infarct of the left superior occipital cortex.

patients with homonymous hemianopia and substantial macular sparing, not only is the location of the lesion almost always the occipital lobe, but the pathogenesis is almost always posterior cerebral artery territory infarction.

Bilateral Occipital Lobe Lesions

Bilateral lesions of the occipital lobes may occur simultaneously or consecutively. In addition, because such lesions are neurologically asymptomatic except as regards the visual system, patients with unilateral lesions

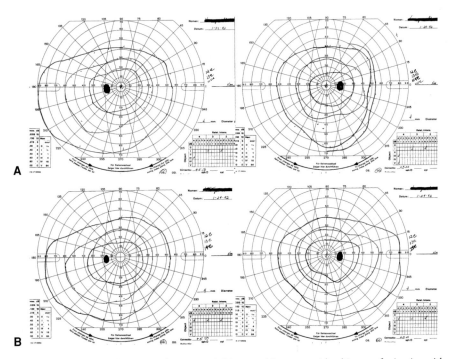

Figure 12.27. Migrainous loss of the temporal crescent. A 31-year-old woman with a history of migraine without aura had the sudden onset of a bright light in the temporal field of vision of the right eye, followed by loss of vision in this same region and subsequent headache. **A:** Kinetic perimetry performed at the time of visual symptoms shows loss of the temporal crescent in the right eye. The field deficit persisted for a few days and then resolved. **B:** Visual fields performed 5 days later are full in both eyes. MRI performed at the time of the initial deficit was completely normal.

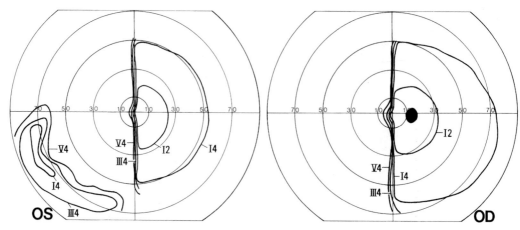

Figure 12.28. Visual field defects in a 56-year-old woman with a right occipital lobe infarction. There is a left homonymous hemianopia with sparing of the inferior portion of the left temporal crescent.

that cause an homonymous field defect may not be aware of the defect until it is called to their attention (e.g., during a routine ocular examination or after the patient is involved in a motor vehicle accident) or until they experience a similar event on the opposite side, producing a more extensive visual deficit.

A double homonymous hemianopia may occur from a single event. In a majority of these cases, there is complete visual loss at the onset (i.e., cortical blindness) that is usually transient, lasting from minutes to days, followed by some degree of clearing in one or both homonymous hemifields. Affected patients have similarly shaped visual field defects on corresponding sides of the vertical midline for each eye, equal visual acuity for each eye that is usually normal, normal pupils and fundi, and full ocular motility unless there is a coexisting brainstem lesion. The majority of these patients have vascular causes of their visual loss.

Much more commonly, bilateral homonymous hemianopia occurs from consecutive events, invariably vascular in nature (Fig. 12.30). In such cases, the patient experiences an acute homonymous hemianopia with retention of normal vision with or without sparing of the macula. At a later time, varying from weeks to years, the patient develops a sudden homonymous hemianopia on the opposite side, again with or without macular sparing. After this second event, the patient is either blind or has only a small central field around the point of fixation.

Whether simultaneous or consecutive, bilateral lesions of the occipital lobes produce bilateral homonymous field defects that are characteristic and vary only in their extent. They may be complete or scotomatous, and they may or may not be accompanied by macular sparing (Figs. 12.31 and 12.32). Occasionally, such sco-

tomas have enough central sparing to produce a "ring" scotoma (Fig. 12.31).

Bilateral occipital lobe disease—whether from infarction, compression, inflammation, infection, or trauma—may result in various types of bilateral homonymous visual field defects. First, there may be complete (cortical or cerebral) blindness. Second, there may be a complete hemianopia on one side and an incomplete, congruous hemianopia on the other. Third, there may be an homonymous hemianopia on one side and a quadrantanopia on the other (Figs. 12.30 and 12.33). Fourth, there may be a bilateral homonymous hemianopia with bilateral macular sparing of a different degree on each side. The remaining visual field thus appears to be severely constricted, and such patients may be thought to have bilateral optic nerve or retinal disease or may even be thought to have nonorganic visual field loss. As with bilateral homonymous hemianopic scotomas, however, careful testing along the vertical midline will establish the bilateral nature of the field defect and its correct origin (Fig. 12.31). Finally, a crossed-quadrant homonymous defect results when patients develop bilateral quadrantic defects that affect the superior occipital lobe above the calcarine fissure on one side and the inferior occipital lobe below the fissure on the other. Such defects are sometimes called "checkerboard" fields and occur quite infrequently, almost always after consecutive rather than simultaneous infarctions (Fig. 12.34).

In addition to the homonymous defects described earlier, trauma, infarction, and, rarely, tumors affecting both occipital lobes may produce bilateral superior or inferior **altitudinal** field defects (Fig. 12.35). Although vascular damage can produce either superior or inferior defects, traumatic injury (most commonly from bullet wounds) usually causes only bilateral inferior

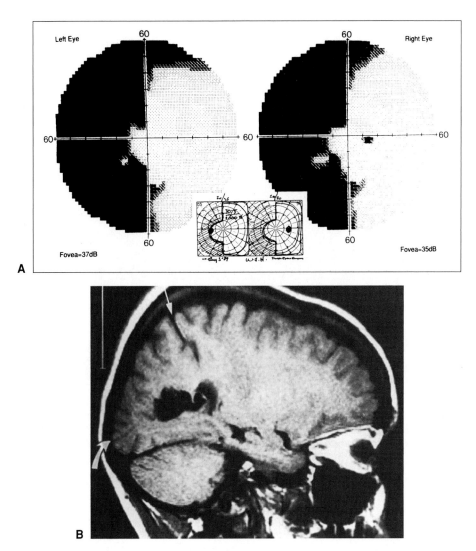

Figure 12.29. A 28-year-old woman suffered a persistent visual field defect after an unusually severe migraine attack. **A:** Full-threshold 60° visual fields using a Humphrey Field Analyzer show that the central 15° of the left hemifield are intact. In the inset, the visual fields mapped at the tangent screen show that the field defect bisects the blind spot representation of the left eye. **B:** T1-weighted parasagittal MRI through the right occipital lobe shows an arteriovenous malformation involving the anterior portion of the right calcarine cortex. The posterior margin of the lesion is situated 31 mm from the occipital tip, marking the approximate location of the representation of the left eye's blind spot. The calcarine (*curved arrow*) and parieto-occipital (*straight arrow*) sulci are indicated. (Reprinted from: Horton JC, Hoyt WF. The representation of the visual field in human striate cortex. *Arch Ophthalmol.* 1991;109:816–824, with permission.)

altitudinal defects. This is probably because damage to the lower portions of the occipital lobes, which would produce bilateral superior altitudinal defects, often results in laceration of the dural sinuses or torcular herophili, with almost uniformly fatal results.

Cortical Blindness and Cerebral Blindness

The term *cortical blindness* indicates loss of vision in both eyes from damage to the striate cortex. *Cerebral*

blindness is a more general term indicating blindness from damage to any portion of both visual pathways posterior to the LGBs. Thus, cortical blindness is a form of cerebral blindness.

The essential features of cerebral (and thus also cortical) blindness are: (a) loss of vision in both eyes; (b) retention of the reflex constriction of the pupils to illumination and to convergence movements (the near response); (c) integrity of the normal structure of the

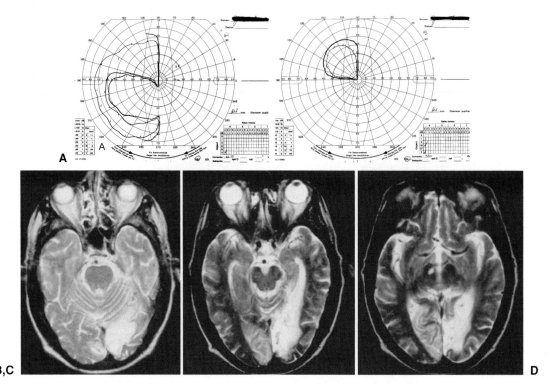

Figure 12.30. Bilateral homonymous hemianopic defects secondary to bilateral posterior cerebral artery infarction. **A:** Kinetic perimetry reveals a dense right homonymous hemianopia combined with a left inferior homonymous quadrantanopia with sparing of the left temporal crescent. **B–D:** Three T2-weighted, axial MRIs demonstrate bilateral posterior cerebral artery infarctions, worse on the left than the right, and extending less inferiorly and less anteriorly on the right.

eyes as verified with the ophthalmoscope (except for patients who are blind from prenatal or perinatal injury); (d) retention of full extraocular movements, unless there is also damage to ocular motor structures.

Some authors stipulate that patients with bilateral postgeniculate visual loss should be said to have cerebral or cortical blindness only if visual acuity is light perception or no light perception. Others modify this definition to add that any level of visual acuity is possible with cerebral blindness, as long as the visual acuity is equal in the two eyes (assuming there is no superimposed abnormality of the anterior visual pathways).

Hypoxia or anoxia involving the occipital lobes is the main etiologic factor producing cerebral blindness. Such damage is, of course, bilateral. Most commonly, an infarction in the posterior cerebral artery territory is initially unrecognized, but this previously silent hemianopia contributes to complete cortical blindness when a contralateral lesion occurs. The most common mechanism for the infarction is cerebral embolism from either the heart or the more proximal vessels of the vertebrobasilar system (Fig. 12.36). Prolonged hypotension can cause cerebral blindness from bilateral watershed infarctions at the parieto-occipital junctions.

Cerebral blindness is observed under many circumstances other than infarction, as shown in Table 12.1. The mechanism of injury underlying the cerebral blindness caused by these events or substances is not always known, but vascular insufficiency plays a role in many of them.

In certain situations, cerebral blindness is transient. This is particularly true in patients who experience temporary vascular insufficiency in the vertebrobasilar system, in hypertensive syndromes following restoration of normal blood pressure, after removal of many of the toxic agents listed in Table 12.1, and after trauma. Children are more likely to experience recovery from cerebral blindness than adults, regardless of the underlying cause. On rare occasions, transient cerebral blindness may follow seizures or be an ictal manifestation. Because focal lesions may be responsible for ictal amaurosis, we believe that MRI should be performed in all cases. We would also emphasize that complete recovery from ictal or postictal blindness can occur even if the blindness lasts for several days.

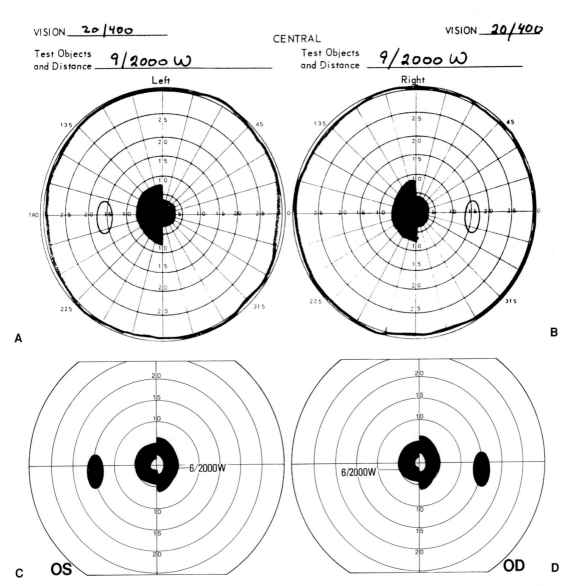

Figure 12.31. Bilateral homonymous hemianopic scotomas. **A and B:** A patient with bilateral nonsimultaneous occipital lobe strokes. Note vertical step that differentiates these defects from a true central scotoma. **C and D:** Macular sparing in a patient who suffered trauma to the occipital region. The tractor on which he was riding overturned, pinning him underneath for several minutes. Initially, he was completely blind, but vision returned within several minutes. He subsequently realized that he had a "ring" of blurred vision around fixation. Note that the homonymous scotomas "respect" the vertical midline.

The relationship between cerebral blindness and the visual-evoked potential (VEP) remains confusing. At least in adults, VEPs do not appear to be useful in establishing the diagnosis or prognosis in patients with cortical or cerebral blindness. The usefulness of VEPs in children with cerebral visual dysfunction also remains controversial, with some studies demonstrating correlation and others not. The variable results from these studies may reflect the many different underlying etiologies of cerebral blindness in children and the many other associated neurologic factors that may contribute to poor recovery.

It is not unusual for patients with cortical blindness to be unaware of their defect. This denial of blindness is called *anosognosia* or **Anton's syndrome.** The syndrome also occurs rarely in patients with blindness

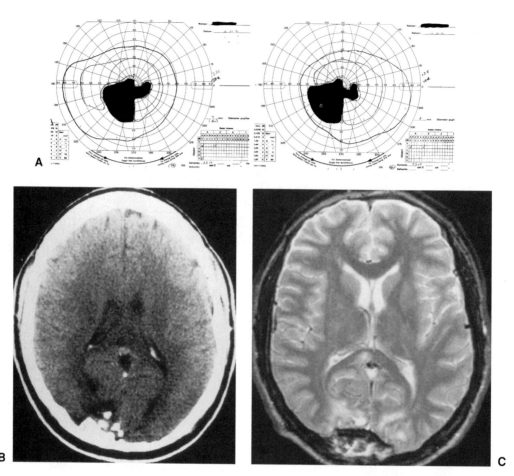

Figure 12.32. A 40-year-old man suffered occipital head trauma with a depressed skull fracture and visual complaints. Visual acuity was 20/20 in both eyes. **A:** Kinetic perimetry reveals exquisitely congruous bilateral homonymous scotomas. **B:** CT scan, axial view, reveals a right occipital pole lesion, but axial MRI **(C)** confirms bilateral occipital pole involvement.

from causes other than occipital lobe disease, such as cataracts, retinopathies, or optic atrophy. The explanation for Anton's syndrome is unclear and may be different in different cases. It is probable that in many patients with cerebral or cortical blindness there are lesions in various areas of the brain responsible for the recognition and interpretation of visual images. In such patients, denial of blindness is caused not by the lesion in the primary visual pathway but by another lesion in another region of the brain. In other patients, denial of visual loss may reflect an emotional or psychiatric response, or it may represent a memory disorder.

Other Visual Features of Occipital Lobe Damage

Although most patients with unilateral lesions of the occipital lobe have visual deficits totally restricted to the contralateral visual field, lesions of the occipital lobe may disrupt not only the striate and extrastriate cortex, but also adjacent underlying white matter. Such damage may alter interhemispheric connections along their presplenial course and disturb the synthesis of visual information from both hemifields. Clinically, these disturbances are subtle compared with the homonymous visual field defect, but they may be responsible for various unexplained complaints of reduced performance in some of these patients, particularly for tasks with high visual information-processing demands such as reading and driving.

Some patients with homonymous hemianopia, especially those with a vascular occlusion in the occipital lobe, report phosphenes in the blind visual field, particularly early in the course of their disorder. Many of the visual field defects in these patients resolve substantially, suggesting that the phosphenes may be viewed

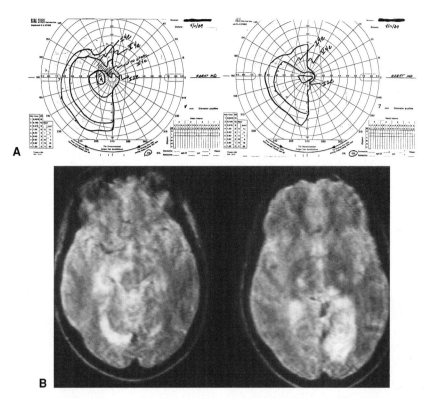

Figure 12.33. After strenuous exercise, a 33-year-old man experienced intermittent confusion, gait disturbances, and right facial weakness, followed by permanent left hemiparesis and difficulties with vision. **A:** Visual fields reveal a right homonymous hemianopia with macular sparing and a left superior homonymous quadrantanopia. **B:** Axial MRIs reveal corresponding infarctions in the occipital lobes bilaterally. Note the involvement of the inferior occipital lobe on the right and the entire calcarine cortex on the left with sparing of the most posterior pole. The patient also had cerebellar and brainstem infarctions, all secondary to artery-to-artery emboli from a vertebral artery dissection.

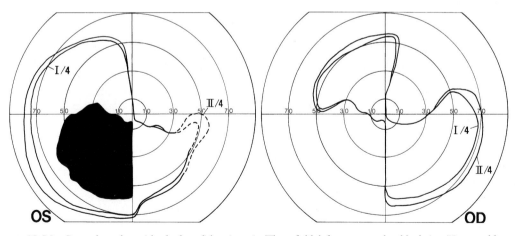

Figure 12.34. Crossed-quadrant (checkerboard) hemianopia. These field defects occurred suddenly in a 70-year-old woman with basilar artery disease. Note the quadrantic defects in the right upper field and the left lower field with the narrow congruous isthmus near fixation. Also note the sparing of the left temporal crescent and the incongruity of the field defects along the upper vertical meridian and the right horizontal meridian. (Courtesy of University of California Hospital, San Francisco.)

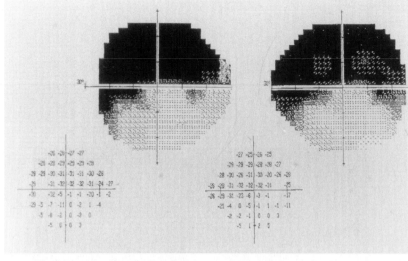

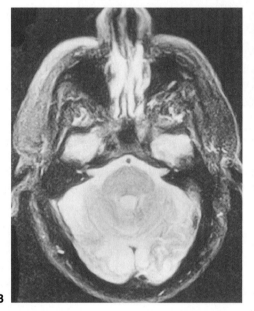

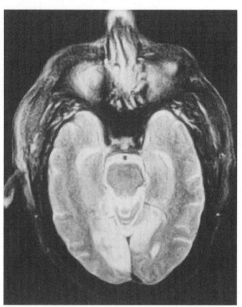

Figure 12.35. A 71-year-old man had the acute onset of complete visual loss, followed by clearing inferiorly. Examination was normal except for visual fields, **A:** which show bilateral superior altitudinal visual field defects (bilateral superior homonymous quadrantanopsias). T2-weighted MRI **B–C:** axial views.

as a prognostically favorable symptom. Visual association areas bordering damaged primary cortex may be the source of these visual symptoms when they are released from normal inhibitory inputs from primary visual cortex.

Lesions of the Extrastriate Cortex with Defects in the Visual Field

The striate cortex (V1, or Brodmann area 17) is the primary visual cortex and the principal recipient of output from the LGB (Fig. 12.37). Surrounding the striate cortex within the occipital lobe are two visual association areas, Brodmann areas 18 and 19, also called the extrastriate visual cortex. Studies from primate electrophysiologic and pathway tracing methods indicate that areas 18 and 19 together represent at least five distinct cortical areas devoted to visual processing. These visual areas are designated V2, V3, V3a, V4, and V5 in the monkey, and corresponding regions are present in the human occipital cortex. Regions V2 and V3 are the major recipient areas for projections from both the magnocellular and parvocellular systems in V1, the primary striate cortex (Fig. 12.38). However, V1 also directly projects to areas V4 and V5, bypassing V2 .

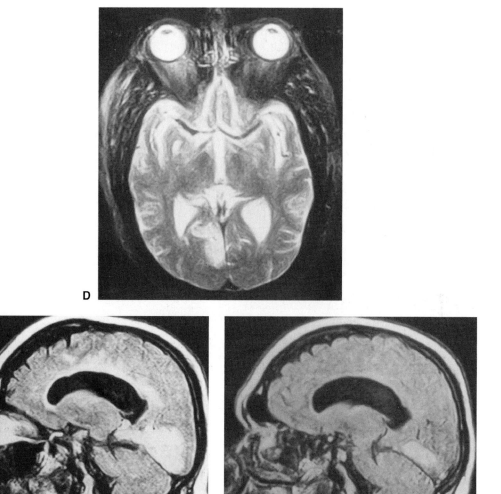

Figure 12.35. (*continued*) (**D:** axial view. **E–F:** coronal views to the right and left of midline, respectively) demonstrates bilateral posterior cerebral artery infarctions involving primarily the inferior occipital lobes.

It has been proposed that a lesion in extrastriate cortex alone can cause an homonymous defect in the visual field. Indeed, not only may a lesion of V2/V3 be sufficient to create a visual field defect, but such lesions may be the principle cause of quadrantic defects that strictly respect the horizontal meridian (Fig. 12.39).

Dissociation of Visual Perceptions

In Chapter 13 of this text, we discuss the topographic diagnosis of disorders of visual processing distal to the primary visual cortex. Because many of these disorders result from lesions in the extrastriate cortex of the oc-

cipital lobes, it is worth mentioning a few of the more prominent syndromes here.

The human visual cortex is specialized with respect to specific functions. For example, an area in the lingual and fusiform gyri of the prestriate cortex corresponds to area V4 in the monkey and subserves the perception of color. Lesions in this region may spare the visual field but produce acquired dyschromatopsia in the contralateral hemifield. The area of functional specialization for visual motion is localized to the temporoparieto-occipital junction, a region corresponding to area V5 in the monkey. Lesions in this region, especially when bilateral, may cause a selective deficit in the perception of visual movement without

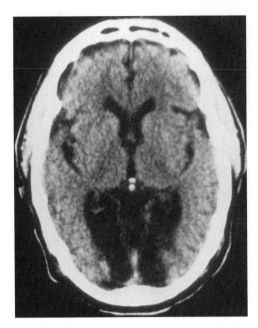

Figure 12.36. Bilateral simultaneous posterior cerebral artery occlusion secondary to embolic infarction from a cardiac arrhythmia. The patient was initially cortically blind with no light perception vision. Over the course of a few weeks, his vision improved to 20/30 vision in each eye because of 5 degrees of macular sparing.

Table 12.1. *Circumstances of Cerebral Blindness*

Acute intermittent porphyria
Bacterial endocarditis
Blood transfusions
Cardiac arrest
Cerebral angiography
Correction of hyponatremia
Creutzfeldt-Jakob disease
Diseases of white matter
   Adrenoleukodystrophy
   Metachromatic leukodystrophy
   Pelizaeus-Merzbacher disease
   Progressive multifocal leukoencephalopathy
   Schilder's disease
Electroshock
Epilepsy
Exposure to or ingestion of toxins
   Carbon monoxide
   Cisplatin
   Cyclosporin
   Ethanol
   Interferon
   Lead
   Mercury
   Methamphetamine
   Methotrexate
   Nitrous oxide
   Tacrolimus (FK506)
   Vincristine
   Vindesine
Hypoglycemia
Infarction
Infectious and neoplastic meningitis
Mitochondrial encephalopathy, lactic acidosis, and
   stroke-like episodes (MELAS)
Neoplasm
Malignant hypertension
Subacute sclerosing panencephalitis
Sudden elevation or reduction in intracranial pressure
Syphilis
Toxemia of pregnancy
Trauma
Uremia
Ventriculography

a visual field defect and without impairment of nonvisual movement perception (i.e., movement perceived by acoustic or tactile stimulation).

In some patients, damage to an occipital lobe can cause a complete homonymous hemianopia to non-moving objects with retention of the ability to detect moving objects within the blind hemifield—this is static-kinetic dissociation, also called the **Riddoch phenomenon.** Such dissociation may have prognostic significance, because it usually means that some degree of recovery can be expected to occur. Static-kinetic dissociation is not a pathologic phenomenon that is purely limited to the occipital lobe. In fact, even normal individuals perceive moving objects better than static objects of the same size, shape, and luminance. The Riddoch phenomenon may occur in patients with lesions of the optic nerves and chiasm, as well as in patients with retrochiasmal visual pathway damage that spares the occipital lobes.

The Riddoch phenomenon is one form of a general category of visual phenomena designated as "blindsight." Some patients with extensive damage to the occipital lobes appear to retain a rudimentary form of vision involving the perception of visual stimuli other than just moving objects. Most patients are not consciously aware of this ability to look, point, detect, and discriminate without truly "seeing." In many cases, blindsight is most likely a result of islands of preserved area 17. However, in some cases, blindsight is a genuine phenomenon that reflects nonstriate visual pathways, such as a direct geniculoextrastriate cortical projection and a retinocollicular projection that reaches extrastriate cortical visual areas via the pulvinar nucleus.

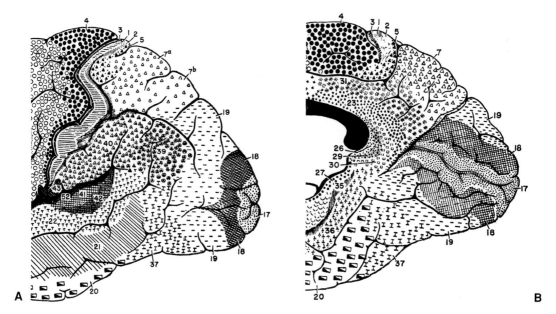

Figure 12.37. The areas occupied by the primary visual cortex and the extrastriate areas, according to Brodmann's classification. **A:** Mesial surface. **B:** Lateral surface. (Reprinted from: R. Lindenberg, FB Walsh, JG Sacks. *Neuropathology of Vision: An Atlas.* Philadelphia: Lea & Febiger; 1973, with permission.)

Another way in which visual perceptions may be dissociated is in the syndrome of unilateral inattention or neglect. Patients with this defect may appear to have normal visual function if tested in routine fashion, because they are able to correctly perceive objects in each hemifield with either eye. However, when two test objects are presented in the right and left hemifields of each eye simultaneously, the patient perceives only the test object in the hemifield ipsilateral to the lesion. This phenomenon, called **visual extinction**, can occur following damage to the parietal or occipitoparietal cortex as well as to several different regions of the brain, reflecting the complex integrated network that exists for the modulation of directed attention within extrapersonal space.

Nonvisual Symptoms and Signs of Occipital Lobe Disease

Except with regard to the visual system, lesions of the occipital lobe are usually asymptomatic. However, many patients with occipital infarctions experience acute pain of the head, brow, or eye ipsilateral to the lesion. This presumably reflects the dual trigeminal innervation of the posterior dural structures and the periorbital region. Patients with homonymous hemianopia may also complain of disturbances of equilibrium, a sense that their body is swaying toward the side

of the hemianopia. This so-called "visual ataxia" may reflect unopposed tonic input of vision from the intact hemifield rather than any true vestibular impairment or neglect.

If the posterior cerebral artery is occluded proximally, patients with an infarct in the occipital lobe may also have hemiplegia from damage to the posterior internal capsule or cerebral peduncle, language dysfunction from damage to posterior parietal and temporal structures, and symptoms indicating damage to the ipsilateral thalamus. In addition, because the condition is ordinarily seen in patients with severe atherosclerosis, there may be other evidence of vertebrobasilar insufficiency, including ocular motor abnormalities referable to the rostral brainstem. Patients who develop a bilateral homonymous hemianopia in this setting may be more severely impaired than patients with blindness from bilateral retinal or optic nerve disease. Such patients present major problems as regards rehabilitation.

Tumors of the occipital lobe may cause nonvisual manifestations by virtue of their mass effect. Headache is the most common symptom, occurring in up to 90% of the patients. Other symptoms and signs include nausea and vomiting, ataxia, hallucinations that are usually unformed (e.g., flashing lights, geometric shapes), seizures, and mental status changes. Many of these symptoms are nonlocalizing and related to increased intracranial pressure.

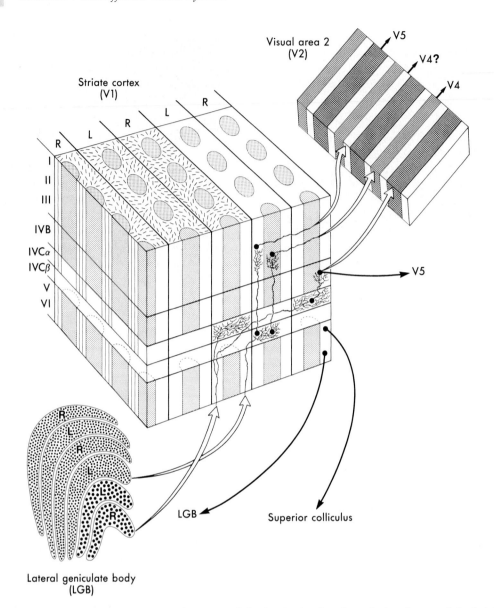

Figure 12.38. Schematic diagram showing the magnocellular (originating from large dots) and parvocellular (originating from small dots) pathways from the lateral geniculate body through areas V1 and V2 to areas V4 and V5. Each module of striate cortex contains a few complete sets of ocular dominance columns (R and L), orientation columns, and about a dozen cytochrome oxidase-positive blobs (stippled cylinders). The orientation columns, depicted with hash marks on the cortical surface, extend through all layers except IVC_α. Their borders are not discrete. The magnocellular stream courses through layer IVC_α to layer 4B and then to dark thick stripes in area V2 and to area V5. The parvocellular stream courses through layer IVC_β to layers 2 and 3. Cells within the cytochrome oxidase blobs project to dark thin stripes in area V2, whereas cells within interblob regions project to pale thin stripes in V2. Both dark and pale thin stripes in area V2 probably project to area V4 and other regions. Note that layers 5 and 6 in area V1 send projections to the superior colliculus and the lateral geniculate body, respectively. (Reprinted from: Horton JC. The central visual pathways. In: Hart WM Jr, ed. *Adler's Physiology of the Eye*. 9th ed. St Louis: CV Mosby; 1992:751.)

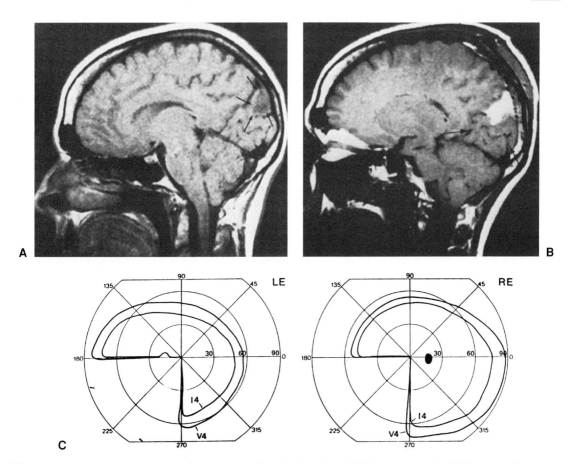

Figure 12.39. A 39-year-old woman had experienced multicolored visual hallucinations in her left lower quadrant since childhood. **A:** T1-weighted sagittal MRI reveals a lesion within the cuneus of the right occipital lobe which on en bloc resection was found to be a grade I astrocytoma. **B:** Postoperative T1-weighted sagittal MRI reveals the area of resection. **C:** Postoperative visual fields demonstrate a left inferior homonymous quadrantanopia with precise respect of the horizontal and vertical meridia. The patient could detect gross hand motion within the quadrantic defect. (Reprinted from: Horton JC, Hoyt WF. Quadrantic visual field defects: a hallmark of lesions in extrastriate (V2/V3) cortex. *Brain.* 1991;114:1703–1718, with permission.)

Treatment and Rehabilitation for Homonymous Hemianopia

Some spontaneous recovery of homonymous visual field defects occurs in no more than 20% of the patients, typically within the first several months after brain injury. Despite a certain amount of plasticity even in the adult cerebral cortex, patients with visual field defects have a consistently poor rehabilitation outcome. The exact anatomic location of the lesion causing the homonymous hemianopia does not appear to affect the functional outcome; however, the greater the number of associated neurologic deficits, the more difficult the rehabilitation and the poorer the functional performance. Contributing further to poor functional improvement is the advanced age of most of these patients, a factor associated even in normal individuals with progressive cognitive, sensory, and motor deficits. Finally, the presence of neglect, especially in patients with nondominant hemisphere lesions, also interferes with the rehabilitation process.

Several techniques may assist in the treatment and rehabilitation of patients with homonymous hemianopia. A mirror attachment can be used to project the mirror image of the blind field into the seeing half-field. The mirror is attached to the nasal side of the spectacle frame behind the lens. For many patients, however, such mirrors do not prove satisfactory; the patient has to turn the head toward the mirror, the mirror produces a scotoma that blocks a portion of the seeing field, and spatial disorientation is common (images seen in the mirror are reversed and projected to the opposite side of the midline).

Fresnel prisms can be placed on glasses for use in the rehabilitation of patients with homonymous hemi-anopias. One option is to place the prism on the outside half of the spectacle lens ipsilateral to the hemianopia with the base oriented toward that side. For example, for a patient with a left homonymous hemianopia, a 30-prism diopter prism is placed base-out on the left half of the left lens, thus displacing the image of an object in the patient's left hemifield 15 degrees to the right. Alternatively, 20-prism diopter Fresnel prisms can be placed on both spectacle lenses, allowing for a 5-degree movement of the eyes before they encounter the prism edge. The power and placement of the prisms can then be modified, depending on patient adaptation. The goal is to increase the patient's scanning skills over time, although the effects on activities of daily living are likely minimal.

Patients with hemianopia commonly experience reading difficulties. Patients with right hemianopias cannot see which letters or words follow those that they have already deciphered. Patients with left hemi-anopias may read without difficulty until they come to the end of the line, but in attempting to return to the beginning of the next line, they move into their blind hemifield and lose their place, often beginning again on an unrelated line. Simple maneuvers to help improve reading include the use of a ruler placed under the line of text, maintaining the left index finger or thumb at the beginning of each line, or even turning the material 90 degrees and reading vertically within the intact hemifield.

Another strategy that may help rehabilitate patients with homonymous hemianopia who have difficulty reading is assessment of the saccadic strategy that the patient uses during attempted reading, followed by systematic retraining of saccadic eye movements and ocular scanning techniques. Many hemianopic patients exhibit a restricted field of ocular motor visual exploration, so practice with spatially organized visual searching can improve functional outcome for these patients.

Another proposed approach to patients with neurogenic visual field loss, including those with homonymous hemianopia, is to use training techniques which purportedly achieve actual restoration of visual field, presumably on the basis of neuroplasticity. Expansion of the visual field on average of 5 degrees has been reported in up to two thirds of the patients with subjective improvement in activities of daily living reported by more than 80% of patients. The mechanisms underlying these improvements, however, are controversial and the subject of much ongoing debate.

FOR FURTHER INFORMATION

See *Walsh & Hoyt's Clinical Neuro-Ophthalmology*, 6th edition, Volume 1, Chapter 12, pages 503–573; and Volume 2, Chapter 28, pages 1348–1371.

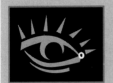

CHAPTER 13

Central Disorders of Visual Function *

This chapter addresses aspects of behavior disorders caused by damage to the visual cortex and white matter connections. These conditions are often referred to as "central disorders of vision," "cerebral disorders of vision," or "higher disorders of vision." The understanding of these disorders continues to improve with the development of new techniques for measuring visual dysfunction, imaging the behaving brain, rehabilitating visual dysfunction in patients with brain damage, and even creating visual sensations in the blind with prostheses to stimulate visual cortex.

Vision was once thought to be primarily a serial (or hierarchic) process in which visual signals were altered or enhanced at successive way stations from retina to brain until an image of the physical world somehow emerged at the level of conscious experience. It has subsequently become clear that serial processing is only one of several mechanisms used by the brain to process visual signals. The primate visual system also uses parallel processing, beginning in the retina. Different types of retinal ganglion cells are specialized to transduce different types of physical signals and give rise to different channels. There is cross-talk between these channels at several levels from the retina to the cortex, and there also are feed-forward and feed-back connections between early and late stages of the visual sensory system. Instead of just serial processing, visual functions are explained in terms of multiple interactions among specialized brain regions in the same hemisphere and across the corpus callosum. Central disorders of vision thus can be interpreted as a conse-

quence of disturbing the processing in different sectors or pathways in a complex interconnecting network.

SEGREGATION OF VISUAL INPUTS

The functional segregation of visual inputs in the primate visual system is well documented (Figs. 12.38 and 13.1). Retinal information is communicated to cortical neurons through a set of pathways that appear specialized to convey a particular class of visual information. For example, the **parvocellular** or P-pathway, named for its connections to simian striate cortex (area V1) via parvocellular layers 3 to 6 of the lateral geniculate body (LGB), is characterized by color opponency and slow-conducting axons that convey sustained signals. This pathway has strong projections to secondary areas such as V4 and inferior temporal (IT) cortex, located in the inferior occipital lobe and adjacent temporo-occipital regions. These regions, along the ventral or temporal cortical pathway (the "what" pathway), are presumed to play a role in the perception of color, luminance, stereopsis, and pattern recognition. In contrast, the **magnocellular** or M-pathway is characterized by large, fast-conducting axons that convey information about more transient visual signals. This pathway connects to areas in visual association cortex, including the middle temporal (MT) and medial superior temporal (MST) areas. These regions, located along the dorsal or parietal cortical pathway (the "where" pathway), are thought to analyze the spatial location and movement of objects in the panorama (Fig. 13.1).

Analyses of data from a large number of patients with focal lesions of the visual cortex and its connections support the general concept of separate dorsal and ventral processing pathways as a framework for interpreting human clinical disorders. For example, damage to the inferior visual cortex and adjoining temporal regions impairs pattern recognition and learning,

*Adapted from: Rizzo M, Barton JJS. Central disorders of visual function. In: Miller NR, Newman NJ, Biousse V, Kerrison JB, eds. *Walsh & Hoyt's Clinical Neuro-Ophthalmology*. 6th ed. Vol. I. Philadelphia: Lippincott Williams & Wilkins; 2005:575–645.

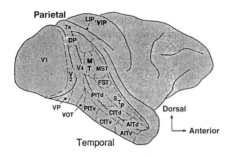

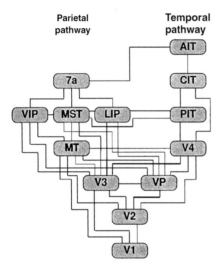

Figure 13.1. Parallel pathways for visual function in the cerebral cortex of the nonhuman primate. Borders between visual areas are indicated by fine dashed lines. The superior temporal sulcus has been opened to show areas that are normally out of sight. The medial hemisphere is not shown. The lower panel shows a flow diagram from area V1 (primary visual cortex) to the parietal pathway that includes area MT and the temporal pathway that includes area V4. The visual information encoded by neurons varies greatly among these different areas. The human brain is likely to respect a similar organization. 7*a*, Brodmann's area 7a. *AIT*, anterior inferotemporal area (*d*, dorsal subdivision; *v*, ventral subdivision). *CIT*, central inferotemporal area (*d*, dorsal subdivision; *v*, ventral subdivision). *DP*, dorsal parietal area. *FST*, fundus of the superior temporal area. *LIP*, lateral intraparietal area. *MST*, medial superior temporal area. *MT*, middle temporal area. *PIT*, posterior inferotemporal area (*d*, dorsal subdivision; *v*, ventral subdivision). *STP*, superior temporal polysensory area. *V*1, visual area 1 (striate cortex). *V*2, visual area 2. *V*4, visual area 4. *VIP*, ventral intraparietal area. *VOT*, ventral occipitotemporal area. *VP*, ventral posterior area. (Reprinted from: Maunsell JHR. The brain's visual world: representation of visual targets in cerebral cortex. *Science.* 1995;270:765–769, with permission.)

producing agnosia for objects and faces (prosopagnosia) or inability to read despite previous literacy (alexia). It can also reduce color perception in the contralateral field—cerebral achromatopsia. By contrast, damage to the superior visual cortex and the adjacent parietal cortex produces disorders of spatial-temporal analysis—inability to judge location, distance, orientation, size, or motion of objects, as well as marked disturbances of visually guided eye and hand control. Balint's syndrome is a striking example.

Each of these major divisions probably has functional subdivisions. Furthermore, although the dorsal and ventral visual cortex are associated with different, behaviorally separable functions, there is growing evidence that these two major divisions also have overlapping functions.

BLINDSIGHT AND RESIDUAL VISION

Some patients with lesions of area V1 causing an homonymous field defect perform better than chance on simple forced-choice detection tasks or on localization tasks measuring the accuracy of finger pointing or eye movements toward targets presented in the defective field of vision. Some of these patients deny any conscious experience of the objects they reportedly localize or detect and are thus said to have **blindsight.**

Precise anatomic analyses are critical to the interpretation of cases of presumed blindsight. For example, it would be highly undesirable to mistake residual vision from sparing of the cortical representation of the monocular temporal crescent with blindsight. In addition, a distinction should be made between blindsight and residual vision. Some studies describing patients with blindsight indicate that the patients are aware of visual stimuli within an homonymous scotoma from damage to the striate cortex. This "residual vision" differs from the nonconscious visual abilities in patients with true blindsight.

The dominant hypothesis in blindsight research is that the phenomenon represents residual function in a visual pathway parallel to the retino-geniculo-calcarine system. The initial candidate was an alternative pathway involving the superior colliculus, and indeed this remains so for investigators who report blindsight in hemidecorticate patients. However, remnant perception of pattern and motion are not easily explained on the basis of known tectal response properties, and these findings led to suggestions that tectal projections to the pulvinar may provide an indirect visual input to extrastriate cortex. This would require a pathologic adaptation of pulvinar function, because the visual responses in this thalamic nucleus normally derive solely from visual cortex. Moreover, the retino-tecto-pulvino-cortical relay can also be challenged because some patients with blindsight demonstrate perception of color in their blind hemifields, and tectal neurons lack color opponency. Another theory is that blindsight results from a projection to extrastriate cortex from a few remnant lateral geniculate neurons that survive the retrograde degeneration after a striate lesion.

There are also explanations of blindsight that do not invoke parallel pathways. Remnant striate cortex is one possibility, especially given the difficulty of proving complete destruction without an autopsy. Of course, blindsight may simply reflect a testing phenomenon known as **criterion shift,** in which patients tend to use fairly conservative criteria when asked to respond Yes or No during a detection task but use more relaxed criteria when forced to choose an alternative (i.e., guess) in a discriminatory paradigm. Furthermore, studies that attempt to determine if hemianopic patients have blindsight must eliminate all potential testing artifacts, including inadequate fixation, light scatter, nonvisual cues, and nonrandom presentation of targets.

Even if blindsight does exist, it is clear that visual discriminations in blind hemifields are less accurate and more variable than those in normal hemifields. However, the range of visual function demonstrated in patients with either blindsight or residual vision is impressive, including perception of spatial location and discrimination of form, orientation, color, and motion. No clear pattern of visual abilities that are preserved or destroyed has emerged in such patients. The variability in blindsight profiles may have an anatomic basis in the inevitable variability of naturally occurring human lesions. Most lesions of striate cortex also involve some extrastriate regions, but the degree and the areas affected differ from one patient to the next. The fact is, not all patients with cortical field defects have blindsight. Why some patients have blindsight and others do not is unclear. Its presence or absence may reflect differences in lesion anatomy, but this is not proven. Some studies have found that blindsight was present only in patients with hemianopia occurring in childhood, a period of presumably greater neural plasticity, but other studies have not confirmed this impression. A requirement for childhood onset is inconsistent with reports that training in older patients can lead to blindsight. If blindsight truly exists, it is uncommon.

CEREBRAL ACHROMATOPSIA

Cerebral achromatopsia, also called central achromatopsia, is an uncommon defect of color perception caused by damage to the visual cortex. Some patients with this condition complain that colors look dull, wrong, or less bright, whereas others report that their world is completely colorless and that objects appear only in shades of gray, like in old black and white movies. Although the term *cerebral achromatopsia* is sometimes used to include all degrees of cerebral color deficits, we believe that this term is best reserved for the most severe cases and that the term **cerebral dyschromatopsia** should be used in cases where there is residual color sensation.

Either cerebral achromatopsia or cerebral dyschromatopsia may be a presenting symptom or may evolve during recovery from cortical blindness. The most common setting is vertebrobasilar ischemia affecting the posterior cerebral arterial blood supply to the occipital lobes. Other causes of achromatopsia include herpes simplex encephalitis, cerebral metastases, recurrent focal seizures, and dementia with visual cortical involvement. Transient achromatopsia may also occur as part of the aura of migraine.

Anatomic and functional imaging studies indicate that color is processed by a large network of structures, including V1, V2, V3, V4 (the most emphasized), and IT. Nevertheless, the lesions causing cerebral achromatopsia are rather restricted and usually affect the ventromedial sectors of the occipital lobe in the lingual and fusiform gyri (Fig. 13.2). Lesions of the middle third of the lingual gyrus or the white matter immediately behind the posterior tip of the lateral ventricle are said to be critical. Bilateral lesions are necessary for complete achromatopsia; unilateral right or left occipital lesions may produce a hemiachromatopsia.

Common accompaniments of cerebral achromatopsia include superior homonymous quadrantanopia, visual agnosia, and acquired alexia. The **quadrantanopia** may be complete or incomplete; but in either case, the achromatopsia affects the remaining inferior quadrants of the visual fields on the side opposite the lesion (i.e., on the same side as the visual field defect). **Visual agnosia**—the inability to recognize previously familiar objects or to learn the identity of new objects by sight alone despite adequate visual sensory abilities—is also seen in patients with cerebral achromatopsia, particularly in patients with bilateral lesions. The syndrome in such patients includes **prosopagnosia,** in which the agnosic defect is most striking for faces and **topographagnosia** or topographic disorientation, in which patients tend to get lost in familiar visual surroundings, partly because of an inability to recognize previously familiar local landmarks. Some patients have **pure alexia,** also known as alexia without agraphia, the acquired inability to read in previously literate individuals (see below). Defects of visual memory and even generalized amnesia can accompany cerebral achromatopsia, depending on the extent of the lesion into more anterior and mesial structures in the temporal lobes.

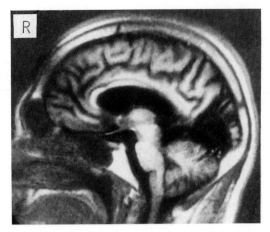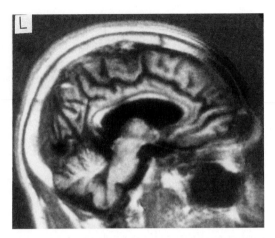

Figure 13.2. Magnetic resonance imaging in a patient with cerebral dyschromatopsia. Nonenhanced sagittal T1-weighted images show bilateral lesions in the visual cortices. The lesion of the right hemisphere (**R**) is responsible for the left homonymous hemianopia. The lesion of the left hemisphere (**L**) is located below the calcarine fissure in the inferior visual association cortex in regions thought to process color. (Reprinted from: Rizzo M, Nawrot M, Blake R, et al. A human visual disorder resembling area V4 dysfunction in the monkey. *Neurology.* 1992;42:1175–1180, with permission.)

One should be cautious in interpreting the verbal report of a patient with cerebral achromatopsia. Assessment of color naming and associations should be conducted independently of color perception testing. This allows the best opportunity to distinguish cerebral achromatopsia and dyschromatopsia from color anomia, agnosia, and related defects of language and memory. Using matching tasks in addition to naming tasks is crucial.

Color anomia is often part of a more general anomia in aphasic patients, but there are instances in which color naming is disproportionately affected. These cases tend to occur with left occipital lesions and are associated with a complete right homonymous hemianopia, rather than just the upper quadrantanopia seen with cerebral achromatopsia. One possible mechanism in such cases is an interhemispheric disconnection syndrome associated with right homonymous hemianopia and pure alexia. Because of the complete right homonymous hemianopia, visual input to language areas in the left hemisphere must arise from the right visual cortex. However, a concurrent lesion of the splenium of the corpus callosum interrupts this process. Affected patients can perceive colors yet not name them (color anomia) and may also see letters but not be able to read them (pure alexia). Preserved tactile naming in such patients suggests preservation of callosal fibers anterior to those required for reading and color naming. Color anomia, together with pure alexia, can also occur without a callosal lesion when there is damage near the posterior aspect of the occipital horn on the left, interrupting connections from both visual fields to language areas.

PROSOPAGNOSIA AND RELATED DISTURBANCES OF OBJECT RECOGNITION

Visual agnosia is an inability to recognize familiar objects, despite adequate visual perception attention, intellect and language. Prosopagnosia is a restricted form of visual agnosia characterized by the impaired ability to recognize familiar faces or to learn to recognize new faces. It is a specific functional disorder with a specific neuroanatomic basis. Prosopagnosia may actually cover a spectrum of deficits, with individual patients varying in the degree of perceptual versus memory dysfunction or even having disconnections between the two processes. Furthermore, abnormal face recognition may be part of more generalized perceptual, cognitive, or memory problems. We will reserve the term *prosopagnosia* for cases in which the facial recognition deficit is disproportionately more severe than other associated deficits (Fig. 13.3).

Patients with prosopagnosia are usually aware of their difficulty and complain of the social embarrassment of not recognizing acquaintances. When they do recognize others, it is often by reliance on specific facial features or paraphernalia (e.g., a hairstyle, glasses, beards and mustaches, a missing tooth, or a particular scar) that bypass the need for an overall analysis of the shape of the face. They may also use nonfacial visual cues, such as gait and posture, or nonvisual cues, such as voice. The context of the encounter is also important. For example, patients with prosopagnosia may be able to recognize hospital staff but are unable to recognize

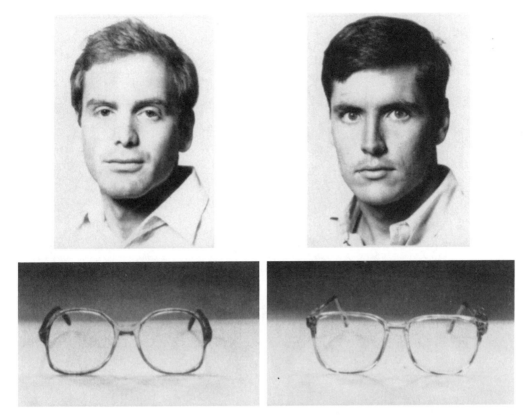

Figure 13.3. Matching the complexity of face and object recognition. Most tests of object recognition use stimuli that are much easier to distinguish from each other than are faces. To increase the level of difficulty in object recognition, one study asked patients to match pairs of glasses that differed in subtle individual details. Patients with prosopagnosia still had more trouble matching faces **(top)** than matching glasses **(bottom)**, suggesting that the recognition defect is specific for faces. (Reprinted from: Farah MJ, Levinson KL, Klein KL. Face perception and within-category discrimination in prosopagnosia. *Neuropsychologia.* 1995;33:661–674, with permission.)

the same persons when they meet them later on the street. Persons with childhood onset of prosopagnosia and, occasionally, persons with onset in adulthood may be ignorant of their deficit.

Despite abnormal recognition of familiar faces, many patients with prosopagnosia can accurately discriminate among unfamiliar faces, even with varying lighting conditions or facial views (i.e., Benton Facial Recognition Test). However, patients with prosopagnosia may require much more time than normal to arrive at correct judgments, suggesting that they use an inefficient and abnormal route for processing face information.

Some individuals with prosopagnosia can judge the age, gender, and emotional expression of faces they cannot recognize, and some even lip-read. Again, prosopagnostics may use different perceptual processes from those used by normal individuals to make such judgments. For example, a patient with prosopagnosia might rely on wrinkles to tell age, whereas normal in-

dividuals can still make age judgments in the absence of such local features. Other prosopagnostic patients, usually those with more pervasive perceptual dysfunction, are impaired with respect to judgments about facial age, sex, emotional expression, and the direction of the person's gaze, the last item being an important social signal.

An important theoretical issue is whether the prosopagnostic defect is specific for faces or also affects perception of other objects. Some patients have difficulty distinguishing types of objects, such as makes of cars, flowers, food, and coins. They also have trouble identifying previously familiar items, such as buildings, handwriting, and personal belongings or clothing. These cases imply that in prosopagnosia, impaired facial recognition may simply be the most prominent manifestation of a more general recognition or perceptual problem. On the other hand, some patients can distinguish nonface objects relatively well despite severe prosopagnosia. Specific tests of face versus

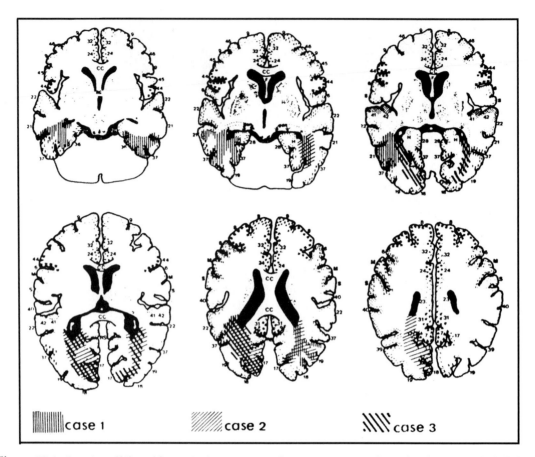

Figure 13.4. Location of bilateral lesions in three patients with prosopagnosia. Axial template drawings with shaded areas representing the lesions of three patients with prosopagnosia. Bilateral damage, greater on the left than the right, is present in all three cases. (Reprinted from: Damasio AR, Damasio H, van Hoesen GW. Prosopagnosia: anatomic basis and behavioral mechanisms. *Neurology.* 1982;32:331–341, with permission.)

object recognition appear to confirm this dissociation (Fig. 13.3).

Although patients with prosopagnosia deny familiarity with and cannot identify known faces, some patients retain covert (i.e., nonconscious) recognition of these faces at a variety of levels. Investigators have shown two main phenomena: **covert familiarity,** in which the patient is able to distinguish previously familiar but unrecognized faces from completely unknown faces, and **covert semantic knowledge,** in which the patient retains information about name, occupation, and other facts associated with a face.

Patients with prosopagnosia usually have difficulty recognizing faces of people with whom they were familiar before the start of the illness (retrograde prosopagnosia) as well as people whom they meet after the onset of the condition (anterograde prosopagnosia). Some patients have slightly better recognition of people long known to them, whereas others have only anterograde prosopagnosia. Prosopagnosia his-

torically has been segregated into two main forms: **apperceptive prosopagnosia,** in which there is a failure to form a sufficiently accurate facial percept; and **associative prosopagnosia,** in which there is an inability to match an accurate percept to facial memories.

In most cases of prosopagnosia, the lesion is in the inferior temporo-occipital cortex, usually in the lingual and fusiform gyri (Fig. 13.4). In occasional cases, the lesion appears to be located in the more anterior temporal cortex. All autopsied cases of prosopagnosia have **bilateral** lesions, often symmetric, presumably affecting homologous regions of both hemispheres. However, the position of the left-sided lesion can be more variable. A left-sided hemisphere lesion or a lesion of the splenium of the corpus callosum might disconnect a right hemispheric locus for facial recognition from visual input of the right hemifield, with critical effects in cases with left homonymous hemianopia. Furthermore, reports of neuroimaging showing apparently unilateral right temporo-occipital lesions have accumulated. The type of face perception deficits caused by unilateral as opposed to bilateral cerebral lesions may differ. It has been suggested that apperceptive types of prosopagnosia occur with damage to right ventral and dorsal temporo-occipital areas, whereas bilateral ventral temporo-occipital lesions result in an associative or dysmnesic form.

Almost all patients with prosopagnosia have other visual deficits. Visual field defects are frequent, the most common being left homonymous hemianopia, left superior homonymous quadrantanopia, bilateral superior quadrantanopia, or combinations of these. The visual field defect, achromatopsia or hemiachromatopsia, and topographagnosia often form a common tetrad with prosopagnosia. Nevertheless, cases of prosopagnosia associated with normal color vision exist, showing that prosopagnosia and achromatopsia are dissociable. Visual object agnosia is said to be absent in some patients with prosopagnosia and present, though proportionately milder, in others.

A frequent finding in patients with prosopagnosia is impaired visual memory. In some of these patients, the memory deficit also affects verbal material. Other patients with prosopagnosia also have simultanagnosia, palinopsia, visual hallucinations, constructional difficulties, and left hemineglect. Hemisensory deficits or hemiparesis occur in some patients with unilateral right-sided lesions, although in some of these cases, the motor and sensory findings are related to other lesions. Pure alexia (see below) can occur in some patients with prosopagnosia.

The most common lesions causing prosopagnosia are posterior cerebral artery infarctions and, less often, viral encephalitis. The predominance of these conditions may be related to their potential to inflict bilateral damage, although the neuroimaging in some cases shows only a unilateral lesion. Other unilateral lesions, such as tumors, hematomas, abscesses, and surgical resections, are less frequently reported.

Impaired facial recognition can occur as part of the generalized dementia in Alzheimer's disease, in Parkinson's disease, and rarely in elderly patients with bilateral or unilateral right temporal lobar degeneration. The last disorder is one of the focal progressive atrophies, others of which affect the frontal, parietal, or left temporal lobes possibly related to Alzheimer's or Pick's disease.

Developmental prosopagnosia also has been described. Patients with this condition usually are not aware that they have problems with face recognition until they experience social difficulties related to the impairment. In addition to problems with facial recognition, these patients have difficulty judging facial age, sex, and expressions. They also perform facial matching tasks very slowly, suggesting a perceptual process differing from normal. In some cases, developmental prosopagnosia is present in other family members, possibly as an autosomal-dominant trait, and coexists with the Asperger syndrome of autism. The prevalence of prosopagnosia among all autistic individuals is unknown, as are the effects of the face perception disorder on other aspects of psychosocial development.

ACQUIRED ALEXIA

Acquired alexia is the loss of efficient reading for comprehension, despite adequate visual acuity. Reading is a complex behavior involving perception of form, spatial attention, ocular fixation, scanning saccadic eye movements, and linguistic processing. Not surprisingly, many types of cerebral or visual dysfunction can disrupt the reading process. Although other clinical signs may overshadow the difficulty, impaired reading is sometimes the chief complaint. The severity of reading difficulty can range from a mild defect with slow reading and occasional errors, which may only be identified by comparison with normal controls matched for educational level, to a complete inability to read even numbers and letters. Analysis of not only the severity but also the type of reading errors can help differentiate among the various forms of reading impairment and their causes.

Note that the term *alexia* implies a complete inability to read. The term *dyslexia* is more appropriate in persons who have preservation of aspects of reading. Unfortunately, dyslexia is also used to describe developmental reading impairments, creating potential confusion. In this chapter, we use the term *dyslexia* only when describing *acquired* reading impairments of cerebral origin.

Most syndromes of alexia can be explained by the disconnectionist theories. The left angular gyrus stores the visual representation of words necessary for reading and writing. Therefore, disconnecting the visual inputs of both hemispheres from the left angular gyrus could disrupt reading but leave writing intact—that is, pure alexia.

The key feature of **pure alexia (alexia without agraphia, or word blindness),** is a dramatic dissociation between the ability to read and the ability to write. Patients with this condition can write fluently and spontaneously, but having done so are unable to read what they have just written. The severity varies from a slow, laborious reading of words one letter at a time (letter-by-letter reading; spelling alexia) to complete inability to read words or letters (global alexia) and sometimes even numbers or other symbols. Covert reading ability can be detected in at least some patients with pure alexia. These patients have aspects of preserved reading ability of which they are not aware.

Lesions causing pure alexia are almost always located in the left hemisphere, most commonly in the

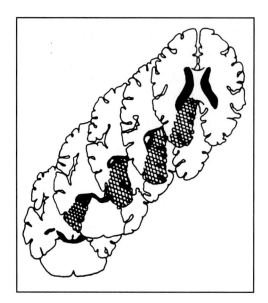

Figure 13.5. Location of lesions causing pure alexia, right homonymous hemianopia, and color dysnomia. Template drawings of axial CT images, combined from five patients, show lesions affecting the left medial and lateral occipital lobes, medial temporo-occipital lobe and paraventricular white matter, and forceps major, sometimes extending into the splenium proper. (Reprinted from: Damasio AR, Damasio H. The anatomic basis of pure alexia. *Neurology.* 1983;33:1573–1583, with permission.)

medial and inferior temporo-occipital region (Fig. 13.5). Most are caused by infarction within the vascular territory of the left posterior cerebral artery, but other causes include primary and metastatic tumors, arteriovenous malformations, hemorrhage, herpes simplex, encephalitis, and a rare focal posterior cortical dementia.

One popular explanation of pure alexia is that it is a disconnection of visual information from linguistic processing centers. Visual information from the right hemifield is either absent in cases with right hemianopia, or it is interrupted in its course through left extrastriate centers to the reading center in the left angular gyrus. Callosal pathways transmitting visual information from visual association cortex of the right hemisphere to homologous regions in the left hemisphere are interrupted by a lesion in the splenium, forceps major, or periventricular white matter surrounding the occipital horn of the lateral ventricle. Thus, words in the left hemifield also cannot access the left angular gyrus. Similarly, other visual information is isolated, causing an associated anomia for colors and objects.

Associated signs with pure alexia are common. There is often a right homonymous field defect, usually a complete homonymous hemianopia but sometimes only a superior quadrantanopia, in which case there may also be a right hemiachromatopsia. Pure alexia cannot be attributed to the field defect, however, because pure alexia can occur without a field defect, and many patients with a right homonymous hemianopia that splits (i.e., does not spare) the macula do not have pure alexia. Although associated dyschromatopsia is generally restricted to the right homonymous hemifield, naming of colors in the whole field may be abnormal. Anomia is not necessarily restricted to the visual modality but can include objects perceived by touch, implying some nonvisual language disturbance from extension of the lesion outside the visual association cortex. Verbal memory deficits and visual agnosia can occur. Some authors describe a form of optic ataxia (see the subsequent text) in which the dominant right hand has difficulty with purposeful movements to objects in the nondominant left visual field.

Pure alexia without an homonymous hemianopia occurs in some patients with lesions of the white matter underlying the angular gyrus. Such "subangular" lesions presumably disconnect the input from both hemispheres to the angular gyrus very distally. This phenomenon suggests to some authors that the right hemispheric callosal fibers travel in the white matter ventral to the occipital horn. Others speculate that some callosal fibers travel dorsal to the occipital horn, and that these are preserved in letter-by-letter or spelling alexia, which they consider a partial form of pure alexia, but are destroyed in global alexia, which they consider the complete form.

Although some cases of pure alexia may be a visual agnosia from left extrastriate damage, at least some cases do represent a true visual-verbal disconnection. For example, pure alexia can occur with the combination of a splenial lesion and a left geniculate nuclear lesion causing a right homonymous hemianopia; there is no damage to striate or extrastriate cortex in such patients. These cases demonstrate that disconnection is sufficient to cause pure alexia.

The disconnection hypothesis involves two deafferentations of the left angular gyrus: the disconnection of right-hemisphere vision and the disconnection or destruction of left-hemisphere vision. Each of these can occur independently and is called a **hemi-alexia.** In left hemi-alexia, reading is impaired in the left hemifield only, because of isolated damage to the posterior corpus callosum or callosal fibers elsewhere. Right hemi-alexia occurs when a lesion of the left medial and ventral occipital lobe spares other visual functions in the right field.

Left **hemiparalexia** is a rare syndrome attributed to damage to the splenium of the corpus callosum. The reading pattern in patients with this condition is similar to that in patients with left hemineglect, in that

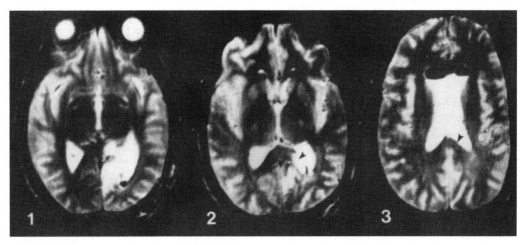

Figure 13.6. Neuroimaging in a patient with left hemiparalexia. **1–3,** Axial T2-weighted MRI at three successive levels from a 40-year-old woman who underwent embolization of a left medial parieto-occipital arteriovenous malformation. After the procedure, she had a right homonymous hemianopia, left unilateral tactile dysnomia, and alien hand syndrome on the left. During reading, she missed the letters on the left side of words, even though she had an intact left homonymous hemifield and no left hemineglect. The images show changes consistent with infarction in the left ventral-caudal splenium (*arrowhead*, level 2) and medial occipital lobe (levels 1 and 2), with sparing of the rostral splenium (*arrowhead*, level 3). (Reprinted from: Binder JR, Lazar RM, Tatemichi TK, et al. Left hemiparalexia. *Neurology.* 1992;42:562–569, with permission.)

substitution and omission errors occur for the first letter of words. However, these patients do not have evidence of hemineglect, and although patients with left hemineglect usually have a right hemispheric lesion and an associated left homonymous hemianopia, some of the patients with left hemiparalexia have left occipital lesions and a right homonymous hemianopia (Fig. 13.6). Patients with left hemiparalexia may have other signs of callosal disconnection, such as inability to name objects felt by the nondominant (left) hand, left-hand agraphia, and inability to duplicate the unseen movements of one hand by the other.

A combination of impaired reading and writing constitutes **alexia with agraphia.** This syndrome usually is associated with lesions of the left angular gyrus, although lesions of the adjacent temporoparietal junction have also been implicated. In patients with left parietal lesions, alexia with agraphia may be accompanied by acalculia, right-left disorientation, and finger agnosia, the other elements of **Gerstmann's syndrome.** In some rare cases, there is relative preservation of oral and auditory language functions, although more often there are other elements of aphasia.

Another form of alexia and agraphia is described as an accompaniment of Broca's aphasia (nonfluent aphasia), which is caused by lesions of the dominant (left) inferior frontal lobe. These patients have difficulty reading aloud and writing, attributable to their problems with all forms of expressive language output. However,

comprehension of text is also often impaired in such patients, despite relatively preserved comprehension of auditory language. In contrast with the letter-by-letter reading in pure alexia, these patients are better at occasionally grasping a whole word, even though they are unable to name the letters of the word. Thus, this type of alexia with agraphia sometimes is called **literal alexia** or "letter blindness." These patients also have impaired comprehension of syntactic structure, just as their speech output often demonstrates a significant impairment of syntax called **agrammatism.** The underlying mechanism is unknown. Gaze paresis and difficulty in maintaining verbal sequences have been proposed but not proven. It may be that this frontal alexia is a variant of deep dyslexia, a type of central dyslexia (see below).

Some patients with visual field defects have reading problems despite normal or near normal visual acuity. In particular, patients with complete homonymous hemianopia may have significant difficulty reading. Such patients are said to have **hemianopic dyslexia.** This condition mainly occurs when the field defect affects parafoveal vision and is more often evident in the acute aftermath of the hemianopia. With languages written from left to right, patients with a left homonymous hemianopia may encounter trouble when they reach the end of one line and try to find the beginning of the next line, because the left margin disappears into the scotoma as they scan rightward. A right homonymous hemianopia prolongs reading times, causing prolonged fixation and reduced amplitude of reading saccades to the right

Disturbances of attention can also cause a number of so-called peripheral dyslexias. Simultanagnosia, in which perception of single items is adequate but perception of several objects simultaneously is impaired, has been implicated in **attentional dyslexia.** Patients with this condition read single words normally but not several words together. They also identify single letters but not the letters in a word. Attentional dyslexia occurs from lesions in the left temporo-occipital junction and the left parietal lobe. Its diagnosis rests upon the difference between reading of single versus multiple words and the presence of simultanagnosia for other visual items besides words.

Left hemineglect is an attentional deficit that causes **neglect dyslexia,** a condition characterized by left-sided reading errors. This can occur for a whole text, so that the reader misses the left side of an entire line or page, or with individual words, so that the reader makes omissions, additions, or substitutions at the beginning. These defects are specific for left hemispace rather than word beginnings; such errors do not occur for vertically printed words. Many patients with left hemineglect also have a left homonymous hemianopia. The underlying lesion is often in the right parietal lobe, although right frontal and subcortical lesions can also cause hemineglect.

Subtle acquired dyslexic deficits occur in addition to the more overt disturbances described previously. Many of these deficits occur in association with other aphasic features and thus could be classified as aphasic alexias; however, they can occasionally occur as isolated deficits. These reading defects are sometimes labeled **central dyslexias,** because they reflect dysfunction of central reading processes rather than "peripheral" attention or visual deficits.

DISORDERS OF MOTION PERCEPTION (CEREBRAL AKINETOPSIA)

Akinetopsia (cerebral akinetopsia) is the term used to describe complete loss of movement perception from an acquired cerebral lesion. Although akinetopsia requires bilateral cerebral lesions, subtle and generally asymptomatic disturbances of motion perception can occur with unilateral cerebral lesions.

Motion perception plays many roles in vision. One is the perception of moving objects in the environment. Because objects usually occupy only a small part of the visual field, their perception is facilitated by comparing their motion with that of the background. Object motion guides limb-reaching movements and smooth-pursuit eye movements, and it influences saccadic accuracy. In addition to object motion, information about self-motion can be obtained from motion perception. As the observer moves or turns the head or eyes, the image of the entire visual environment moves in the opposite direction. Thus, motion of large portions of the visual field usually implies self-motion rather than motion of an external object. This large-field motion generates optokinetic responses that complement the vestibulo-ocular reflex in stabilizing sight during head- or self-motion. Information about object identity is also available from visual motion.

PET scanning studies performed in normal humans during motion perception show activation in the lateral occipital gyri at the junction of Brodmann areas 19 and 37. This motion-selective area is most consistently related to the conjunction of the anterior limb of the inferior temporal sulcus with the lateral occipital sulcus. Other areas activated during motion perception include V1, V2, and the dorsal cuneus, which may correspond to V3 in nonhuman primates (Fig. 13.7). Similarly, studies with functional MRI show motion-selective responses in the lateral temporo-occipital cortex as well as in V2 and the superior and inferior parietal lobules. Signal changes in lateral temporo-occipital cortex also correlate with motion after-effects. Both motion perception and pursuit-related signals are present in lateral temporo-occipital cortex. Magnetic stimulation can be used to create temporary dysfunction within specific cortical areas. Stimulation over lateral temporo-occipital cortex impairs motion direction discrimination but not form discrimination in the contralateral hemifield and, to a lesser degree, in the ipsilateral hemifield.

There are few clinical tests of motion perception. Smooth pursuit and optokinetic nystagmus can be observed and measured, but only indirect conclusions about the underlying state of motion perception can be made from these. More definitive tests of motion perception—such as animated displays of moving dots (random-dot kinematograms) or moving gratings—can be designed to probe discrimination of motion direction, motion speed, the presence of a motion boundary, and forms defined by motion, but these are experimental tools, not widely used in the clinical setting.

Cerebral akinetopsia appears to require bilateral lesions affecting the lateral temporo-occipital cortex. The cause in one well-described case was sagittal sinus thrombosis with bilateral infarctions involving the lateral aspects of Brodmann areas 18, 19, and 39 (lateral occipital, middle temporal, and angular gyri) (Fig. 13.8). In another well-studied case, acute hypertensive hemorrhage resulted in bilateral lesions in the lateral temporo-occipital regions.

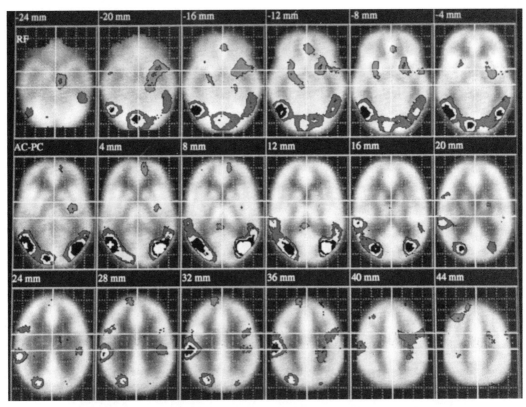

Figure 13.7. Positron emission tomographic (PET) study of motion perception. Areas with changing regional cerebral blood flow during motion perception, averaged over all normal subjects. Results are shown in axial section, with numbers indicating distance from a line joining the anterior and posterior commissures (negative values are inferior). Pixels indicate changes in blood flow, with black and white pixels indicating areas with highly significant increases in blood flow. Several areas of activation are seen, including the lateral temporo-occipital cortex. (Reprinted from: Dupont P, Orban GA, de Bruyn B, et al. Many areas in the human brain respond to visual motion. *J Neurophysiol.* 1994;72:1420–1424, with permission.)

Unilateral lesions of extrastriate cortex in the lateral temporo-occipital or inferior parietal lobule regions can cause more subtle abnormalities of motion perception (Fig. 13.9). There are reports of contralateral hemifield defects for speed discrimination, for detection of boundaries between regions with different motion, and for discrimination of direction from backgrounds of motion noise. Most of the patients with unilateral lesions have predominantly vascular lesions in the right more than left temporo-occipital or parieto-occipital regions. There is also some evidence that lesions of the cerebellum adversely affect the perception of motion.

Patients with motion perception deficits may have other abnormalities caused by lesions of the lateral temporo-occipital area. Perception of form may be abnormal, as may be object recognition, spatial vision and stereopsis. Hemianopias of various degrees are more often left-sided, reflecting the right brain predominance of the causative lesions.

BALINT'S SYNDROME AND RELATED VISUOSPATIAL DISORDERS

In 1909, Balint described a triad of visual defects in a man with bilateral parieto-occipital lesions (Fig. 13.10). The most significant deficit was an inability to perceive together at any one time the several items of a visual scene, which Balint interpreted as a "spatial disorder of attention." Other terms used to describe this deficit subsequently included *visual disorientation* and *simultanagnosia* (an inability to interpret the totality of a picture scene despite preservation of ability to apprehend individual portions of the whole). The patient described by Balint also had an inability to move the eyes voluntarily to objects of interest despite unrestricted eye rotations, so-called "psychic paralysis of gaze," "spasm of fixation," or "acquired ocular apraxia." The third deficit present in the patient described by Balint was a defect of hand movements under visual

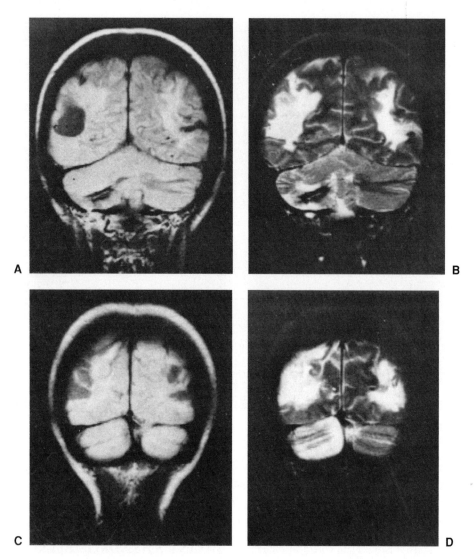

Figure 13.8. Conventional coronal MRI through the occipital lobes in same patient whose three-dimensional MRI is seen in Figure 13.11. **A:** T1-weighted image through midoccipital region shows hypointense areas, right greater than left, consistent with infarcts, surrounded by mild hyperintense areas consistent with edema. **B:** T2-weighted image at same location, showing large hyperintense areas with minimal mass effect on both sides. Note similar areas in cerebellum, primarily in right hemisphere and in the midline. **C:** T1-weighted image through posterior occipital lobes shows persistent bilateral hypointense areas with surrounding minimal hyperintensity. **D:** T2-weighted image at same location shows large areas of hyperintensity in both occipital lobes. (Reprinted from: Zihl J, von Cramon D, Mai N, et al. Disturbance of movement vision after bilateral posterior brain damage: further evidence and follow-up observations. *Brain.* 1991;114:2235–2252, with permission.)

guidance despite normal limb strength and position sense, termed *optic ataxia*.

Among the many reported causes of so-called **Balint's syndrome** are cerebrovascular disease (especially watershed infarctions as in Balint's original case), tumor, trauma, Creutzfeldt-Jakob disease, and degenerative conditions such as Alzheimer's disease.

The definition of simultanagnosia can be operationalized as an inability to report all the items and

relationships in a complex visual display despite unrestricted head and eye movements. A suitable screening tool is the Cookie Theft Picture from the Boston Diagnostic Aphasia Examination or any similar picture containing a balance of information among the four quadrants (Fig 13.11). The patient's report can be correlated with a checklist of the items in the picture. Exclusion criteria should include aphasia severe enough to impair the verbal descriptions of a display, so as to

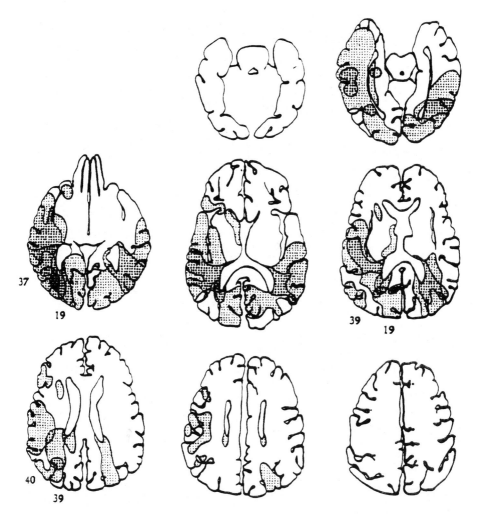

Figure 13.9. Abnormal central motion direction discrimination. Axial template drawings from CT or MRI scans, showing lesions (stippled areas) of six patients with abnormal signal-to-noise thresholds for the discrimination of motion direction in foveally presented displays. In most, the defect affected motion primarily toward the side of the lesion. Numbers indicate Brodmann areas. Areas of denser stippling indicate greater overlap, with the highest density at the junction of Brodmann areas 19 and 37. (Reprinted from: Barton JJS, Raymond J, Sharpe JA. Retinotopic and directional defects in motion direction discrimination after human cerebral lesions. *Ann Neurol.* 1995;37:665–675, with permission.)

avoid confusing a defect of language with one of visual perception. It is also crucial to exclude or at least be aware of defective visual acuity or visual fields. For example, objects may seem to vanish into a central scotoma, paracentral scotoma, or a hemianopia, causing symptoms that mimic simultanagnosia.

Balint's syndrome may not exist as a sufficiently autonomous complex. Affected patients often have a number of other devastating defects in behavior, and the classic three components originally described by Balint are not as closely bound as is often assumed. Moreover, individual components of the syndrome appear to represent relatively broad categories comprising other more specific defects. Furthermore,

Balint's syndrome does not appear to have a specific neuroanatomic significance, because bilateral damage to the parieto-occipital regions can cause other defects, and damage elsewhere in the brain can cause similar clinical disorders. It is probably best to consider Balint's syndrome a variety of combined deficits from lesions of the dorsolateral visual association cortices, which include the putative human area MT complex and its projections to the parieto-occipital cortex. Damage to these areas and to the cortices surrounding the angular gyrus and parietal insular cortex can disturb multiple aspects of spatial and temporal processing, including the perception of visual motion, perceptions of structure from motion and

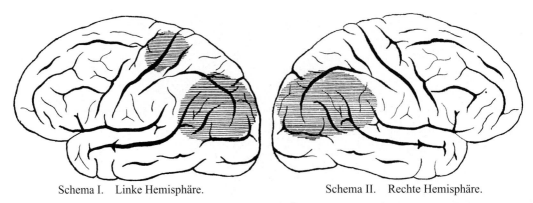

Schema I. Linke Hemisphäre.   Schema II. Rechte Hemisphäre.

Figure 13.10. Drawing of the locations of the major lesions in the case described by Balint in 1909, as pictured on lateral views of the hemispheres. The views are idealized and do not convey the full extent of the pathology. The surface of the brain was actually atrophic. Not seen in this view are several lesions of potential importance to the patient's behavior presentation. These included lesions of the posterior white matter in which optic radiations travel on both sides, and of the pulvinar, a critical structure for visuospatial integration in primates. (Reprinted from Balint R. Seelenlahmung des "Schauens," optische Ataxie, räumliche Störung der Aufmerksamkeit. *Monatschr Psychiatr Neurol.* 1909;25:51–181, with permission.)

dynamic stereopsis, the perception of egomotion, and coordination of visual (eye-centered) and vestibular (gravity-centered) coordinate systems that orient us in the physical world. Bilateral lower quadrantanopsias may also occur from damage to the primary visual cortex lining the dorsal banks of the calcarine fissure (human area V1), thus adding to a patient's overall problem.

The observations of Balint on what he called "optic ataxia" sparked interest in the neural basis of visually guided **reaching and grasping.** Reaching and grasping external objects is a fundamental activity that demands the coordination of several different nervous system functions. To accomplish this task, the brain transforms a target's visual coordinates to body-centered space, plans a hand path and trajectory (the

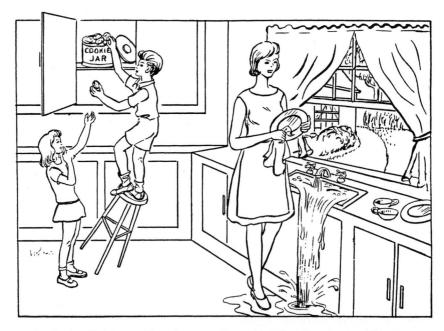

Figure 13.11. The "Cookie Theft Picture" from the Boston Diagnostic Aphasia Examination. This picture contains a balance of information among the four quadrants. The patient is asked to describe the events depicted in the picture.

sequence of hand position and velocity to target), and computes multiple joint torques, especially about the shoulder and elbow. It also specifies the necessary limb segment orientations from among many possibilities, activates appropriate muscle groups, and inhibits others to meet those specifications.

Reaching can be separated into two different phases. In the transport phase of reaching, the hand is moved toward an object whose position is determined by vision or memory. In the acquisition phase, grasp formation depends on somatosensory and visual information on the limb and target, familiarity with the target, and perhaps on predetermined motor programs. These two phases mature at different rates, may be controlled independently before becoming coordinated, and can be dissociated by focal brain lesions. Posterior parietal damage may affect neurons coding eye position in the head and stimulus location on the retina that, together with neurons in motor and premotor cortex, permit hand movements to visual targets in a body-centered coordinate system.

In "optic ataxia" as described by Balint, patients reportedly reach as if blind toward targets they nevertheless can see and describe. Limb strength and position sense are normal; however, there is severe visual sensory loss and poor visuospatial perception, and patients may even appear demented because of their extensive bilateral lesions. Inability to reach and grasp targets in these cases is often multifactorial, including V1-type visual field defects, defective visual attention, and inability to locate targets with the eyes. Indeed, in screening for optic ataxia, the examiner should verify that the patient has foveated the target for a reach before making any observations on limb movement control. Another possible cause of defective reaching is abnormal sensorimotor transformation, an inability to transform the visual coordinates of external objects to appropriate limb coordinates for generating accurate reaches.

Lesions in the right inferior and superior parietal lobules, as in Balint's original case, are likely to produce visuomotor difficulty in reaches conducted with the left hand to both visual fields (hand effects) and with both hands to the left visual fields (field effects). Subsequent studies of patients with defective reaching have demonstrated lesions in the inferior parietal lobule, the occipitotemporal region, or both. Distance and direction errors may be dissociable, especially with lesions of the inferior posterior parietal cortex, suggesting that localization of a target with reaching movements depends on a network of structures in the visual association cortex.

POSITIVE VISUAL PHENOMENA

Cerebral lesions that affect vision usually create deficits in the visual fields—that is, **negative phenomena.**

On occasion, however, they create **positive phenomena,** in which false visual images are seen by the patient. These false visual images can be classified as visual perseverations, hallucinations, and distortions (dysmetropsia).

VISUAL PERSEVERATION

Visual perseveration is the persistence, recurrence, or duplication of a visual image. It is a rare complaint in patients with cerebral lesions. Several varieties exist: palinopsia (or paliopsia)—the perseveration of a visual image in time; cerebral diplopia or polyopia—the perseveration of a visual image in space; and illusory visual spread—the contents or surface appearance of an object spread beyond the spatial boundaries of the object.

The content of visual hallucinations is often imagery created de novo, or sometimes from the distant past (experiential hallucinations), but the palinopsic illusion contains elements of a more recently viewed scene or even one that is still being viewed. There are at least two forms of **palinopsia,** an immediate and a delayed type. With the *immediate type* of palinopsia, an image persists after the disappearance of the actual scene, usually fading after a period of several minutes. This type of palinopsia bears some similarity to the normal phenomenon of an afterimage experienced after prolonged viewing of a bright object. With the *delayed type* of palinopsia, an image of a previously seen object reappears after an interval of minutes to hours, sometimes repeatedly for days or even weeks. Some patients have both immediate and delayed types of palinopsia.

A perseverated image can assume almost any location in the visual field. It may persist in the same retinal location as the original image, which is usually at the fovea, and thus move as the eyes move, much as a normal afterimage does. Sometimes, the image is translocated into a coexistent visual field defect and indeed can be a transient feature in the evolution of cerebral homonymous field defects. In other cases, the image is multiplied across otherwise intact visual fields. On rare occasions, the location of palinopsic images is contextually specific, as when patients report that after viewing a face on television, everyone else in the room has the same face as the person on television, or that the sign over one shop reappears on the boarding over other shops. Although some of these cases may represent a complex form of palinopsic polyopia, others may also be consistent with a constant foveal or perifoveal perseverative image that repeatedly manifests itself when the context is appropriate.

A wide range of other symptoms can accompany palinopsia. An associated homonymous visual field defect is almost always present and may be a complete hemianopia, incomplete hemianopia, superior quadrantanopia, or inferior quadrantanopia. There may be other spatial illusions, such as metamorphopsia, macropsia, and micropsia. Less frequently, ventral stream deficits occur, such as topographagnosia, prosopagnosia, and achromatopsia.

The natural history of palinopsia is variable. In some patients, palinopsia is a transient phase in either the resolution or progression of a visual field defect and lasts from days to months, eventually resolving. Other cases of palinopsia persist for months or even years. Anticonvulsant medication may prove helpful in prolonged cases.

The pathophysiologic mechanisms of palinopsia are unclear. The main hypotheses include: 1) a pathologic exaggeration of the normal afterimage; 2) a seizure disorder; 3) hallucinations; and 4) psychogenic. It is likely that different mechanisms account for similar palinoptic phenomena in different patients.

In etiologic investigations, drug-induced palinopsia must first be considered. Intoxication with hallucinogens such as mescaline, lysergic acid diethylamide (LSD), and 3,4-methylenedioxymethamphetamine (Ecstasy) can cause palinopsia, sometimes permanently. Isolated reports assert that palinopsia and other visual illusions may occur with prescribed medication, such as clomiphene, interleukin 2, and trazodone, or with abnormal metabolic states such as nonketotic hyperglycemia. Palinopsia can also occur in psychiatric conditions, such as schizophrenia and psychotic depression, but it is always accompanied by other signs of mental illness. Once intoxication and psychiatric conditions are excluded, visual perseveration almost always indicates a cerebral lesion.

The localizing value of palinopsia is not clear. Most studies find a predominance of right parieto-occipital lesions in patients with palinopsia, although left hemispheric lesions may be under-represented because of aphasia. There are also reports of medial occipital and temporo-occipital lesions verified by neuroimaging and autopsy results.

Patients with **cerebral polyopia** see two or more copies of a single object simultaneously. This form of visual perseveration is described much less frequently than is palinopsia. It occurs with monocular viewing, which distinguishes it from the binocular diplopia caused by misalignment of the eyes. Cerebral polyopia can generally be differentiated from monocular polyopia caused by ocular abnormalities, such as uncorrected or miscorrected refractive errors, corneal opacities, and cataract, because the images of cerebral polyopia are all seen with equal clarity, do not resolve during viewing with a pinhole, and are unchanged in appearance whether the patient is viewing binocularly or monocularly with either eye. Some patients experience cerebral polyopia only in certain positions of gaze, causing confusion with tropic diplopia until the monocular nature of the polyopia is recognized. Some patients see only two images; others see dozens.

Cerebral polyopia is most commonly encountered after parietal lobe or parito-occipital region strokes. It can occur as a transient phase in the recovery from cortical blindness secondary to strokes or traumatic injury. Other reported causes of cerebral polyopia include encephalitis, multiple sclerosis, and tumors. Associated clinical manifestations are usually present in patients with cerebral polyopia. These include homonymous visual field defects, difficulties with visually guided reaching, cerebral achromatopsia or dyschromatopsia, object agnosia, fluctuations in the visual image, and abnormal visual afterimages.

Patients with **illusory visual spread** see the contents or surface appearance of an object spread beyond the spatial boundaries of the object. Thus, wallpaper patterns spread beyond the surface of the wall, and cloth patterns spread from a shirt to the wearer's face. Illusory visual spread may occur in isolation or may be a feature of palinopsic images.

VISUAL HALLUCINATIONS

Hallucinations are perceptions without external stimulation of the relevant sensory organ. They are common in patients with dementia or confusional states secondary to metabolic insults, including alcohol withdrawal, where they form the predominant type of hallucination. Drugs reported to cause hallucinations include digoxin, bupropion, ganciclovir, vincristine, cyclosporine, lithium, lidocaine, itraconazole, dopaminergic agonists, and baclofen withdrawal. Visual hallucinations can occur in patients with a variety of psychiatric disorders. In such cases, they are usually accompanied by hallucinations in other sensory modalities (especially auditory) and by other signs of mental illness.

Isolated visual hallucinations in persons with intact cognition and mental function are often a sign of underlying neurologic or ophthalmologic disease. Isolated visual hallucinations can be separated into three main pathophysiologic groups: (a) release hallucinations, (b) visual seizures, and (c) migraine.

Release Hallucinations (Charles Bonnet Syndrome)

Bilateral simultaneous or sequential visual loss from any cause can result in visual hallucinations. These are often called **release hallucinations,** because it is thought that they arise from, or are "released" in, visual cortex that is no longer receiving the incoming visual sensory impulses that usually filter out nonvisual stimuli. Release visual hallucinations usually occur in patients with visual acuity in the better eye of 20/60 or worse. Any type of visual loss, whether ocular or cerebral in origin, can lead to release hallucinations. When the disease causing visual loss is ocular and occurs first in one eye and then in the other, hallucinations usually do not develop until the second eye loses vision.

Some series report that up to 57% of patients with a variety of causes of visual loss have release hallucinations. In fact, the true incidence of release hallucinations may be much higher because of a reluctance on the part of affected patients to tell their physicians that they are experiencing hallucinations, for fear of being labeled "crazy." Patients with release hallucinations are mentally lucid; the majority are aware that the visions are not real; and, in general, they are not distressed by them. Notable is the absence of other sensory hallucinations.

Release hallucinations can be classified as simple (unformed) or complex (formed) (Fig. 13.12). Simple hallucinations consist of brief flashes or points of light, colored lines, shapes, or patterns (phosphenes). Complex hallucinations contain recognizable objects and figures, such as flowers, animals, and humans, with a potential for bizarre, dreamlike imagery of considerable detail and clarity, including dragons and angels. Sometimes the vision is a recognizable image from the patient's past, such as a deceased friend or relative. Simple hallucinations are at least twice as common as complex ones. In most series, complex hallucinations account for 10% to 30% of release hallucinations.

Some authors reserve the term *Charles Bonnet syndrome* for the association of visual loss with complex formed hallucinations. However, some patients have simple hallucinations initially and later experience complex ones. A similar progression in visual hallucinatory content is reported in normal people subjected to sensory deprivation. Also, because the type of release hallucination does not correlate with the site of visual loss, the distinction between complex and simple release hallucinations lacks diagnostic value.

There must be other contributing factors besides visual loss in the development of release hallucinations, because they do not develop in all patients with visual loss. Older age may be one risk factor, but even patients as young as 10 years can have release hallucinations. Social isolation is another potential factor, thought to act by accentuating the sensory deprivation of visual loss.

In the brain, visual experience is represented by patterns of coordinated impulses within the visual cortex. These patterns are generated by sensory stimuli and represent the current experience of the individual; however, the brain can generate these neural patterns spontaneously and, in fact, does so during sensory deprivation from either imposed isolation or pathologic denervation. These spontaneous neural patterns could correspond to hallucinations. A similar explanation has been invoked for the phantom-limb phenomenon after amputation and presumably also underlies other release phenomena, such as musical hallucinations in cases of deafness. Supporting evidence for the analogy with sensory deprivation includes the fact that these hallucinations tend to occur when patients are alone or inactive, and in the evening or night when the lighting is poor.

Release hallucinations may be brief, with each episode lasting a few seconds or minutes, or nearly continuous. Hallucinations most often follow the onset of visual loss by several days or weeks, but the delay can be longer. That loss of vision triggers the hallucinations is supported by the observation that release hallucinations disappear in patients whose vision subsequently improves. In many patients, release hallucinations last for a few days to a few months and then spontaneously disappear even though visual function remains stable. In others, however, the hallucinations persist for years or even decades.

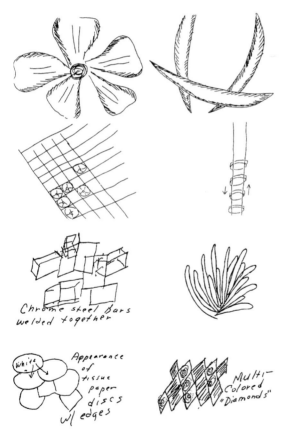

Figure 13.12. Appearance of both simple and complex hallucinations. Drawing by a patient with occipital lobe damage showing his most frequent hallucinations. Note that some are complex (**above**), whereas others are simple (**middle** and **below**). (Reprinted from: Anderson SW, Rizzo M. Hallucinations following occipital lobe damage: the pathological activation of visual representations. *J Clin Exp Neurol.* 1994;16:651–663, with permission.)

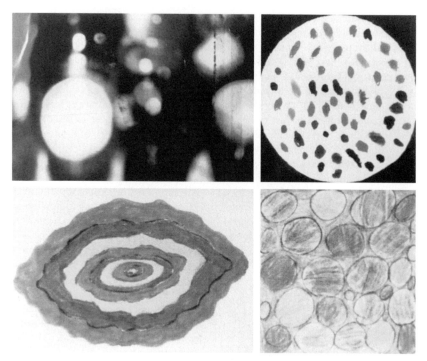

Figure 13.13. Visual illusions of occipital lobe epilepsy as perceived by four different patients. (Reprinted from: Panayiotopoulos CP. Elementary visual hallucinations in migraine and epilepsy. *J Neurol Neurosurg Psychiatry.* 1994;57:1371–1374, with permission.)

Release hallucinations do not bother most patients, and some persons even enjoy them. Treatment of the visual disturbance in such patients, other than reassurance concerning the significance of the hallucinations, is usually not indicated. However, some patients find the hallucinations annoying, upsetting, or distracting. Unfortunately, there is no proven effective treatment for such patients. Moving socially isolated patients into a more stimulating environment may lessen the hallucinations, and anticonvulsant drugs may improve the hallucinations but not consistently.

Visual Seizures

Visual seizures are not common in patients with epilepsy. When they do occur, they can be confused with migraine and release hallucinations. Much of the confusion related to the localizing value of the visual content of hallucinations stems from failure to distinguish between release hallucinations and true visual seizures. The content of release hallucinations is highly variable and independent of the site of pathology, whereas the content of visual seizures may have more localizing value. Older human stimulation experiments found that simple flashes of light and colors resulted from electric activity in striate cortex, whereas stimulation of visual association cortex in areas 19 and temporal regions resulted in complex formed images. A sim-

ilar distinction probably holds for epileptic visual hallucinations (Fig. 13.13). Nevertheless, temporal lobe lesions can occasionally produce simple unformed hallucinations, and occipital lesions can produce complex hallucinations. In the latter setting, spread of ictal activity into extrastriate cortex probably is responsible for the complex character of the hallucinations. Hence, the content at the onset of a visual seizure has the most localizing value.

The association with other ictal phenomena or an homonymous visual field defect may be helpful in identifying visual seizures from a cerebral lesion. Accompanying head or eye deviation (usually but not always contralateral) and rapid blinking are common accompaniments of occipital seizures. Other features that also strongly support ictal origin are signs of more distant spread of seizure activity, such as confusion, dysphasia, tonic-clonic limb movements, and the automatisms of complex partial seizures. Because routine scalp electroencephalographic leads often do not localize an occipital focus accurately, suspicion of such a focus usually requires intracranial electrodes for confirmation.

Although a variety of pathologies in the visual cortex may be associated with visual seizures, one syndrome requiring emphasis is **benign childhood epilepsy with occipital spike-waves.** This idiopathic epilepsy syndrome begins between 5 and 9 years of age and ceases spontaneously in the teenage years. Seizures are characterized by blindness and/or hallucinations of both simple and complex types, and it may progress to motor or partial complex seizures. Some children develop nausea and headache following the visual seizure, leading to an erroneous diagnosis of migraine. The diagnosis is established by occipital spike-waves occurring during eye closure on electroencephalography.

Migrainous Hallucinations

A variety of visual phenomena can occur in migraine. In migraine with visual aura (classic migraine), the visual phenomena generally precede the headache, whereas in migraine aura without headache (acephalgic migraine), visual phenomena occur alone. Photopic images are most common in both settings and are described as spots, wavy lines, or shimmering of the environment similar to heat waves over a road on a hot day. The scintillating scotoma is a blind region surrounded by a margin of sparkling lights, which often slowly enlarges over time and which may move across the visual field or expand concentrically from a small point to distort some or all of the field of vision of both eyes. In some patients, the sparkling margin can be discerned as a zig-zag pattern of lines oriented at 60 degrees to each other, usually in one hemifield and on the leading edge of a C-shaped scotoma (Fig. 13.14). This is the fortification spectrum or teichopsia (from the Greek word *teichos*, meaning "town wall"), which is so-named because of the resemblance of the zig-zag margin to the ground plan of town fortifications in Europe. There may be several sets of zig-zag lines in parallel, often shimmering or oscillating in brightness. They may be black and white or vividly colored. These zig-zag lines begin near the center of the field and expand toward the periphery with increasing speed over a period of about 20 minutes, with both the speed and the size of the lines increasing with retinal eccentricity. The relation of speed and size to eccentricity is predicted by the cortical magnification factor, which is a measure of the area of visual field represented in a given amount of striate cortex as a function of retinal eccentricity. This suggests that migrainous hallucinations are generated by a wave of neuronal excitation spreading from posterior to anterior striate cortex at a constant speed, leaving a transient neuronal depression that causes the temporary scotoma in its wake. It is also hypothesized that the zig-zag nature of the lines reflects the sensitivity to line orientation of striate cortex and the pattern of inhibitory interconnections within and among striate columns.

Although both migraine and visual seizures can feature abnormal hallucinations followed by headache and vomiting, the two disorders can sometimes be distinguished by their visual imagery, with black and white

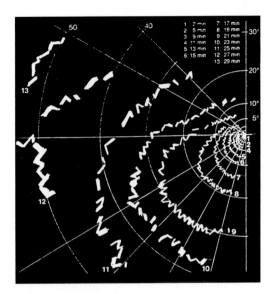

Figure 13.14. Photographic negative of a migraine phosphene protocol. The scintillating phosphene was progressing through the lower quadrant and part of the upper quadrant of the left visual hemifield. Thirteen drawings were made between 2 and 29 minutes after the phosphene first appeared near the center of the visual field. To evaluate the distance between the phosphene and the center of the visual field, several radii were drawn across the protocol. The angular distance from the fovea center, computed in degrees of visual angle, is indicated by circles. Circles and radii were added to the sheet after the observations were made. Observation distance = 34 cm. (Reprinted from: Grüsser O-J. Migraine phosphenes and the retino-cortical magnification factor. *Vision Res.* 1995;35:1125–1134, with permission.)

zig-zag lines being more suggestive of migrainous hallucinations and colored circular patterns being more common in ictal hallucinations. Seizures are briefer, usually lasting a few seconds or minutes, spread more rapidly, and always occur in the same hemifield.

Other Types of Hallucinations

Hallucinations associated with lesions of the mesencephalon, so-called **peduncular hallucinations** (or peduncular hallucinosis), are rare. They have many similarities to the complex release hallucinations associated with visual loss. They can be continuous or episodic, with detailed formed imagery, such as flying birds, dogs, roaring lions, crawling snakes, gangsters with knife wounds, and men herding cattle. These hallucinations are not stereotyped and vary from one episode to the next. In some cases with thalamic rather than midbrain infarcts, the hallucinations are from events in the patient's past. Many patients with peduncular hallucinations realize that the hallucinations are not real. Similar hallucinations occur for sounds, and some patients have multimodality hallucinations, involving vision, touch, sound, and even the sense of body posture.

The most frequently described etiology of peduncular hallucinations is infarction involving the substantia nigra pars reticulata and its connections to the pedunculo-pontine nucleus, and/or the reticular formation and the ascending reticular activating system. Peduncular hallucinations are almost invariably associated with inversion of the sleep-wake cycle—that is, diurnal somnolence and nocturnal insomnia. Other associated signs from damage to adjacent structures in the midbrain include unilateral or bilateral oculomotor nerve palsy, hemiparkinsonism, hemiparesis, and gait ataxia. In cases caused by infarction, the hallucinations can resolve, but they usually persist indefinitely, although the episodes may become shorter.

Rare patients experience **hallucinations with eye closure.** Causative settings include drug toxicity from atropine and probably lidocaine, infection with high fever, and after major surgery. It has been proposed that they are similar to hypnagogic hallucinations, suggesting a disturbance in sleep-wake cycle mechanisms.

VISUAL DISTORTIONS (DYSMETROPSIA)

Illusions about the spatial aspect of visual stimuli can be separated into three main categories: (a) micropsia—the illusion that objects are smaller than in reality; (b) macropsia—the illusion that objects are larger than in reality; and (c) metamorphopsia—the illusion that objects are distorted.

Micropsia is the most common of the visual distortions and has the largest variety of possible etiologies. Convergence-accommodative micropsia is a normal and physiologic phenomenon in which an object at a set distance appears smaller when the observer focuses at near rather than far, even though there is no change in the retinal angle covered by the object and no change in its spatial relations to the surround. It is unusual for accommodative micropsia to be a source of complaints.

Psychogenic micropsia occurs in psychiatric patients. It is the subject of extensive psychoanalytic interpretations, with the most prevailing theory being that it occurs in patients who are literally trying to "distance" themselves from environments fraught with conflict.

Retinal micropsia occurs when the distance between photoreceptors is increased. The micropsia usually occurs in foveal vision and is caused by macular edema. There may be associated metamorphopsia if the receptor separation is irregular. Visual acuity is also reduced in such cases. Causes of macular edema and micropsia include central serous chorioretinopathy, diabetic retinopathy, severe papilledema, and reti-

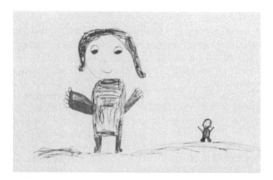

Figure 13.15. Drawing of cerebral micropsia by a child with migraine. The child stated that during some of her attacks, other children **(right)** appeared unusually small to her **(left)**. (Reprinted from: Hachinski VC, Porchawka J, Steele JC. Visual symptoms in the migraine syndrome. *Neurology.* 1973;23:570–579, with permission.)

nal detachment. The condition may resolve or persist for years.

Cerebral micropsia, in contrast to retinal micropsia, is always binocular. Unusual variants include hemimicropsia, which occurs in the hemifield contralateral to the cerebral lesion. Given the small number of cases, the localization value of cerebral micropsia is uncertain. Temporo-occipital lesions are present in some cases, with either medial or lateral involvement. One survey of over 3,000 adolescent students revealed that complaints of episodic micropsia or macropsia were not rare, occurring in 9%. Some occurred in the hypnagogic state or during fever, and there was a correlation with a history of migraine. Indeed, micropsia occurs not infrequently in migraine, particularly in childhood, and migraine is probably the most common setting in which cerebral micropsia is encountered (Fig. 13.15).

Macropsia is much less frequently described than micropsia. Retinal macropsia can occur in the late scarring stage of macular edema, and it can be a side effect of the drug zolpidem. Cerebral macropsia can rarely occur during seizures. Cerebral hemimicropsia was reported in a patient with a left occipital tumor and also in a patient with a right occipital infarct. As noted previously, both micropsia and macropsia occur episodically in children and seem to correlate with childhood migraine.

Ocular causes of **metamorphopsia** are far more common than cerebral causes. Most often, the metamorphopsia occurs from retinal pathology, such as macular edema, and in such cases, it often coexists with micropsia. Disorders that cause traction and distortion of the macula, such as an epiretinal membrane, may also cause metamorphopsia. As with retinal micropsia, metamorphopsia from ocular disease is usually monocular. In those rare cases in which it is binocular, the distortions are almost never identical in the two eyes. Metamorphopsia is most often tested using an Amsler grid.

Cerebral metamorphopsia occurs in some patients during seizures. Other reported causes include right parietal glioma, right parietal arteriovenous malformation, medial posterior cerebral artery infarction, a transient stage in the development of cortical blindness, and even brainstem lesions.

TESTS OF HIGHER VISUAL FUNCTION

Chapter 1 of this text contains detailed descriptions of the standard vision tests used to measure the visual abilities in patients. However, standard vision and screening tools generally do not provide a measure of higher order visual functions, nor are they meant to do so. Basic categories of higher visual function tests include tests of

1. *Reading,* such as the reading subtest of the Wide Range Achievement Test and Chapman-Cook Speed of Reading Test.
2. *Visual recognition,* such as the recognition of famous faces, the Boston Naming Test, and the Visual Naming Test from the Multilingual Aphasia Examination.
3. *Mental imagery,* such as the Hooper Visual Organization Test (Fig. 13.16).

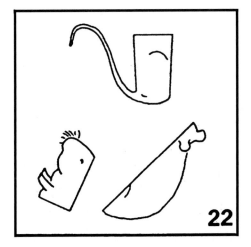

Figure 13.16. Tests of higher visual function. A plate (number 22/30) from the Hooper Visual Organization Test (HVOT). The patient is required to identify each of the 30 items on the plate from their cut-up rearranged line drawings. This test is memory dependent, in that it depends on the history of exposure of the patient to the items on the plate.

Rey-O Complex Figure Test

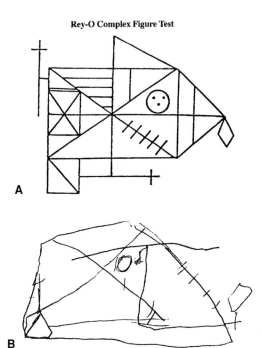

Figure 13.17. Tests of higher visual function. **A:** The Rey-Osterreith Complex Figure. **B:** Defective copy of this figure by a 74-year-old woman with Alzheimer's disease.

4. *Visual perception,* such as the Facial Recognition Test and Judgment of Line Orientation.
5. *Visual attention,* such as the Cookie Theft Picture (see Fig. 13.11), and the line bisection task.
6. *Visuoconstruction,* such as drawing to dictation and copy (Fig. 13.17), writing to dictation copy and spontaneously, and the 3-D Block Construction Test.
7. *Visual memory,* such as the Benton Visual Retention Test, BVRT (Fig. 13.18).

GLOSSARY OF CEREBRAL VISUAL DEFICITS

Agnosia (also known as associative agnosia). The inability to recognize previously familiar objects despite adequate perception. Objects are effectively stripped of their meanings.

Alexia without agraphia (also known as pure alexia or acquired dyslexia). The acquired inability to read in previously literate individuals. Should not be confused with developmental dyslexia.

Anosognosia. Failure to recognize one's own impairment (see Anton's syndrome).

Anton's Syndrome. The denial of cerebral blindness.

Benton Visual Retention Test
Form C, Design 5

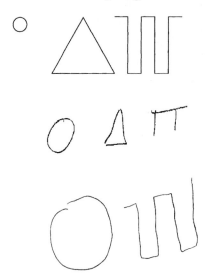

Figure 13.18. Tests of higher visual function. **A:** Plate (design 5) from the Benton Visual Retention Test (BVRT). **B:** Defective reproduction by a patient with Alzheimer's disease. **C:** Omission of the one of the left figures in a patient with a right hemisphere lesion causing left hemineglect.

Apperceptive agnosia. Failure to identify previously familiar objects due to impaired perception.

Balint's syndrome. Simultanagnosia, ocular apraxia, and optic ataxia.

Blindsight. Residual vision in the fields of a putative striate scotoma; redefined more broadly as a "visual capacity in a field defect in the absence of acknowledged awareness."

Central (paracentral) scotoma. A visual field defect at (or near) the fixation point.

Cerebral achromatopsia (also known as central achromatopsia). An uncommon defect of color perception caused by damage to the visual cortex and connections. The term *achromatopsia* implies complete color loss. The term *dyschromatopsia* should be used when there is some sparing of color sensation.

Cerebral akinetopsia. Defective processing of visual motion cues due to cerebral lesions. The ability to perceive motion direction, shape from motion, and other "higher order" motion processes may be impaired.

Cerebral blindness. Bilateral loss of vision from bilateral damage to the optic radiations or striate cortex. Cortical blindness (see below) is a form of cerebral blindness.

Color agnosia. Inability to identify colors despite preserved ability to discriminate among colors.

Color anomia. Inability to name colors despite adequate color perception and recognition.

Cortical blindness. Inability to see following bilateral damage to the visual cortex. Affected patients generally have considerable damage that extends well beyond V1. Cortical blindness is a specific form of cerebral blindness (see above).

Foveal (macular) sparing. An homonymous hemianopia in which 2° to 10° of the central vision are preserved on the affected side.

Foveal (macular) splitting. An homonymous hemianopia that includes the entire foveal representation on the affected side.

Keyhole vision (cerebral tunnel vision). Homonymous hemianopias may be bilateral (double homonymous hemianopia) leading to a severe loss of peripheral vision; if there is bilateral foveal sparing, a tunnel or keyhole of vision remains around fixation.

Macropsia. The illusion that objects are larger than in reality.

Metamorphopsia. The illusion that objects are distorted.

Micropsia. The illusion that objects are smaller than in reality.

Ocular apraxia (also called psychic paralysis of gaze or spasm of fixation). An inability to move the eyes to objects of interest despite unrestricted ocular rotations.

Optic ataxia. A defect of hand movements under visual guidance despite adequate limb strength, position sense, and coordination.

Palinopsia. Persistence of visual after-images of an object despite looking away.

Prosopagnosia. Inability to recognize previously familiar faces or to learn new faces despite adequate perception. This is a restricted form of (associative) agnosia.

Scotoma. An area of blindness surrounded by intact vision. The physiologic blind spot is a scotoma.

Simultanagnosia (simultagnosia). This is often equated with Balint's "spatial disorder of attention." An inability to interpret the totality of a picture scene despite preservation of ability to apprehend individual portions of the whole.

FOR FURTHER INFORMATION

See *Walsh & Hoyt's Clinical Neuro-Ophthalmology*, 6th edition, Volume 1, Chapter 13, pages 575–645.

THE PUPIL

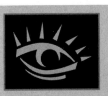

ASSESSMENT OF PUPILLARY SIZE, SHAPE, AND FUNCTION

Assessment of the pupils requires a precise history and careful examination. Often, it is followed by pharmacologic testing.

HISTORY

Patients are often not aware of any abnormality of pupil size. A spouse, friend, or physician may bring the abnormality to attention. The pupil abnormality may be intermittent or episodic. Dating the onset of the pupillary abnormality is aided by reviewing readily available photographs with the aid of a magnifying lens.

Symptoms associated with abnormalities of pupillary size and shape include: light sensitivity, difficulty focusing while adjusting to changing lighting conditions, or blurring vision. Complaints of blurry vision are typically nonspecific.

Important past medical history includes a history of previous infections, trauma, operations (particularly on the neck), or migraine. Occupational history may be important. Farmers or gardeners may be exposed to

plants or pesticides that produce pupillary dilation or constriction. Physicians, nurses, or other health professionals may work with or have access to topical dilating or constricting substances. Medication history may be important as opiates may cause pupil constriction and anticholinergics used in inhalers for asthmatics may cause pupillary dilation.

EXAMINATION

Slit lamp examination of the anterior segment is essential in patients with a pupillary abnormality. It may reveal a corneal injury that could affect pupillary size or anterior chamber inflammation, which may be associated with ciliary spasm and miosis. Examination of the iris should include assessment of the iris sphincter for small traumatic tears and transillumination of the iris for defects. In addition, by placing a wide beam at an angle to the iris and turning the light off and on, the light reflex can be assessed for segmental defects, such as occur in eyes with tonic pupils or aberrant regeneration of the oculomotor nerve.

Pupil measurements may be performed using a handheld pupil gauge, handheld pupil camera, or infrared video pupillometry. The handheld pupil gauge is held next to the eye to determine pupil size in both light and darkness. Pupil gauges consist of a series of solid or open circles or half-circles with diameters that increase by 0.2 mm in steps (Fig. 14.1). A handheld pupil camera is a more accurate method for measuring pupillary size and comparing pupils before and after

---

*Adapted from: Digre KB. Principles and techniques of examination of the pupils, accommodation, and lacrimation. In: Miller NR, Newman NJ, Biousse V, Kerrison JB, eds. *Walsh & Hoyt's Clinical Neuro-Ophthalmology*. 6th ed. Vol. I. Philadelphia: Lippincott Williams & Wilkins; 2005: 715–737, with permission.

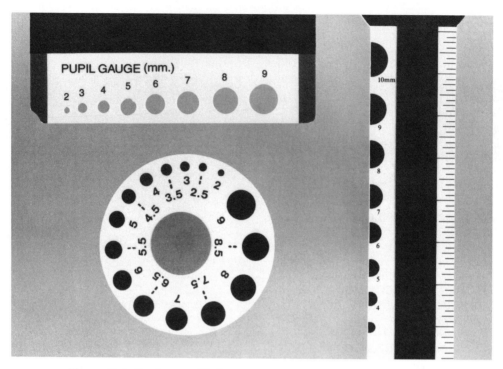

Figure 14.1. Pupil gauges. The best gauges measure in 0.5 millimeter steps.

pharmacologic testing and in various illuminations, although not in darkness. Infrared video pupillometry is perhaps the most accurate method of assessing the size of the pupil. An infrared video pupillometer permits observation of pupils not only in lighted conditions but also in total darkness.

During clinical evaluation, the examiner should first assess the size of the pupils. The examiner should determine if the pupils are equal. If they are not equal, the examiner should determine whether the difference in size is greater in light or darkness. Other questions that should be answered pertain to whether the pupils constrict with the same velocity, whether they redilate equally with the same velocity, and how the pupillary reaction to light compares to the pupillary reaction to near. Finally, the examiner must assess whether a relative afferent pupillary defect is present.

Assessing Pupillary Size

The diameter of both pupils should be estimated or measured in light, using either normal room light or a handheld light source. The diameter of the pupils should then be assessed in darkness, using the dimmest room light in which the examiner can still see the edge of the pupil. Finally, the pupillary size should be assessed during near stimulation using an accommodative target to achieve maximum constriction of the pupils.

Measurements of the pupil in light and dark should determine if **anisocoria,** a difference in the pupils of 0.4 mm or more, is present. A substantial percentage (20%) of the normal population has clinically detectable anisocoria, referred to as "physiologic anisocoria." Anisocoria may be produced by damage to the iris sphincter or dilator muscles or to their nerve supply. The amount of anisocoria may be affected by illumination. For example, a greater degree of anisocoria is present in darkness than in light in patients with physiologic anisocoria or Horner's syndrome. Anisocoria can also be affected by the degree of accommodation, by fatigue, and by sympathetic drive.

Testing the Pupillary Reaction to Light

When testing the reaction of a pupil to light shined in the eye—the **direct pupillary light reaction**—it is important to have a quiet and dimly lit room. The patient must be fixating on a distance target to eliminate any effect of accommodation on pupillary size.

The light source used to illuminate the pupils should be bright enough to produce a maximum rate of constriction and redilation. If the light source is too bright, a prolonged contraction lasting several seconds will occur, making determination of the normal light reflex difficult. It may be helpful to use a dim secondary light source to provide oblique illumination

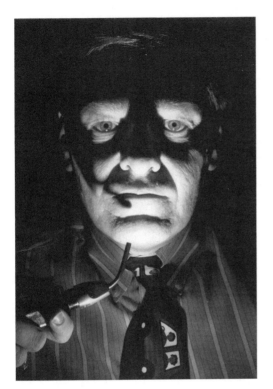

Figure 14.2. Use of indirect lighting to view pupils in darkness.

of the pupil in some cases as this technique increases visualization of darkly pigmented irides (Fig. 14.2).

The light source should be directed straight into the eye for a few seconds and then moved downward away from the eye to eliminate the stimulation. The pupil response should be assessed during this maneuver, which should be repeated several times. The normal response to a bright light is a contraction called "pupillary capture." "Pupillary escape," on the other hand, is a phenomenon in which the pupil initially constricts and then slowly redilates and returns to its original size. Pupillary escape most often occurs on the side of a diseased optic nerve or retina and in normal persons tested with a low-intensity light source. The initial size of the pupil is important in assessing both pupillary capture and pupillary escape. A larger pupil is more likely to show pupillary escape, whereas a smaller pupil is more likely to show pupillary capture.

The latency and speed with which a pupil constricts to light and redilates after light stimulation can be assessed using pupillography. The use of pupillography to record waveforms of pupillary constriction and dilation is generally limited to research.

When light is shined in one eye, the contralateral pupil constricts as well in a **consensual light response**. The consensual light response to light is assessed using a light source for illumination of the pupil of one eye and a dimmer light source that is held obliquely to the side of the contralateral eye being observed. The consensual pupillary response should be approximately equal in both velocity and extent to the direct response, because the pupillary decussation in the midbrain is about 50% to each eye.

Testing the Pupillary Near Response

The near response, a co-movement of the near triad that also includes accommodation and convergence, should be tested in a room with light that is adequate for the patient to fixate an accommodative target. A nonaccommodative target, such as a pencil, may not be a sufficient stimulus to produce a normal near response even in a normal person. The near response should not be induced by having the patient look at a bright light stimulus, because the light itself may produce pupillary constriction. One can document the light and near response with photographs or pupillometry (Fig. 14.3).

Assessment of Pupillary Dilation

Dilation of the pupils occurs in a variety of settings. Most often, the pupils dilate after they have constricted to light or near stimulation. In patients with certain retinal and, less often, optic nerve disease, they may actually dilate when light is shined in one eye (paradoxical pupillary response). Reflex pupillary dilation can also be elicited by sudden noise or by pinching the back of the neck.

When assessing pupillary dilation, the examiner should look specifically for dilation lag. This phenomenon is present when there is more anisocoria 4 to 5 seconds after pupillary constriction to light than there is 15 seconds after pupillary constriction. Dilation lag typically occurs in patients with a defect in the sympathetic innervation of the pupil (i.e., Horner's pupil), although it also occurs in some normal subjects.

Dilation lag may be tested by observing both pupils simultaneously in a very dim light after a bright light has been turned off. Normal pupils return to their widest size within 12 to 15 seconds, with most of their dilation occurring in the first 5 seconds. Pupils that show dilation lag may take up to 25 seconds to return to maximum size in darkness with most of the dilation occurring about 10 to 12 seconds after the light goes out. Dilation lag may also be tested by taking flash photographs at 5 and 15 seconds after the lights are turned off.

Testing for Light-Near Dissociation

A dissociation between the pupillary response to light stimulation and the pupillary response to near stimulation (light-near dissociation) occurs in patients with a variety of disorders (see Chapter 15). In almost

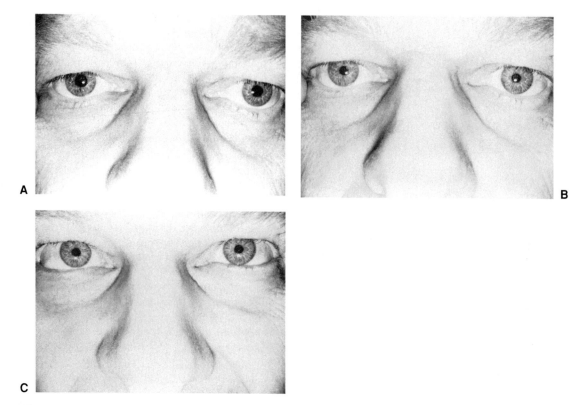

Figure 14.3. Use of a handheld camera to document size of the pupils in light and darkness in a normal subject. **A:** In room light without any other stimulation. **B:** In room light during stimulation with a bright light. **C:** In room light during stimulation with an accommodative target. Note associated convergence.

all cases, the pupillary reaction to light is impaired, whereas the pupillary response to near is normal or near normal. Thus, light-near dissociation should be considered in any patient with an impaired pupillary light reaction. Essentially all cases of light-near dissociation in which there is a normal pupillary reaction to light and a poor pupillary response to near are caused by lack of effort on the part of the patient during attempted near viewing.

Testing for a Relative Afferent Pupillary Defect

When a patient has an optic neuropathy in one eye or an asymmetric bilateral optic neuropathy, covering one eye and then the other reveals that the pupil of the normal eye constricts when it is uncovered and the abnormal eye is covered, whereas the pupil of the abnormal eye dilates when it is uncovered and the pupil of the normal eye is covered (Fig. 14.4). The abnormal pupil is often called a *Marcus Gunn pupil*. The term *relative afferent pupillary defect* is preferred because it describes the nature of the pupillary abnormality.

The **swinging flashlight test** (Fig. 14.5), which accentuates differences in the pupillary response to light,

is probably the most valuable clinical test of optic nerve dysfunction available to the general physician. The patient focuses on a distant target in a darkened room, and a light is swung back and forth multiple times to bring out the best response.

The swinging flashlight test should be performed with a bright hand light in a darkened room in order to maximize the amplitude of the pupillary movement and make it easier to see a small RAPD. Using too bright a light will produce an afterimage that may keep the pupils small for several seconds, obscuring the pupillary dilation in the abnormal eye. The patients must fixate on a distant target during testing in order to prevent miosis that occurs in the near response. In patients with ocular misalignment (i.e., strabismus or displacement of the globe by an orbital or intracranial process), care must be taken to shine the light along the visual axis. The light should cross from one eye to the other fairly rapidly but should remain on each eye for 3 to 5 seconds to allow pupillary stabilization. Thus, there are really two parts of the pupillary response that must be observed during the swinging flashlight test: (a) the initial pupillary constriction response and (b) the pupillary escape that is observed for 2 to 5 seconds after the

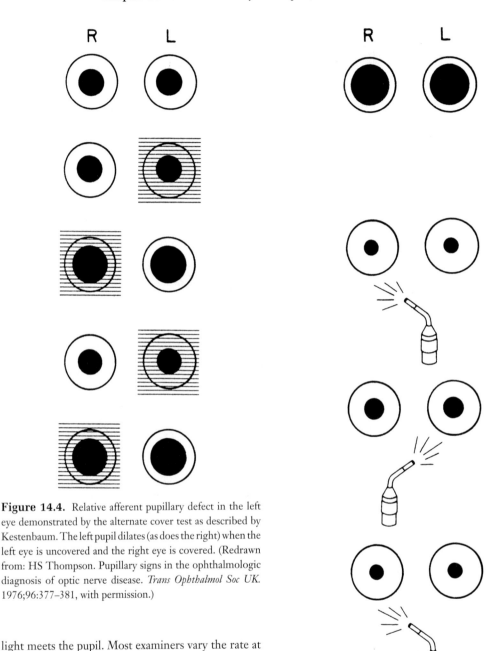

Figure 14.4. Relative afferent pupillary defect in the left eye demonstrated by the alternate cover test as described by Kestenbaum. The left pupil dilates (as does the right) when the left eye is uncovered and the right eye is covered. (Redrawn from: HS Thompson. Pupillary signs in the ophthalmologic diagnosis of optic nerve disease. *Trans Ophthalmol Soc UK.* 1976;96:377–381, with permission.)

Figure 14.5. Relative afferent pupillary defect in the left eye demonstrated using the swinging flashlight test. The pupils constrict when the light is shined directly into the right eye; however, when the flashlight is swung back to the left eye, both pupils dilate. (Redrawn from: HS Thompson. Pupillary signs in the ophthalmologic diagnosis of optic nerve disease. *Trans Ophthalmol Soc UK.* 1976;96:377–381, with permission.)

light meets the pupil. Most examiners vary the rate at which they move the light from eye to eye. There is often an optimum swing rate that brings out an RAPD and that varies among patients.

Some authors recommend moving the light from one pupil to the other before the latter can escape from the consensual response to bring out an afferent defect. However, **the light should never be left longer on one eye than on the other.** This might create a RAPD in the eye with the longer light exposure, because the longer the light is kept on the eye, the more pupillary dilation occurs as the eye adapts to the light.

In addition, if the retina becomes bleached in one eye and not in the other, a small RAPD will be

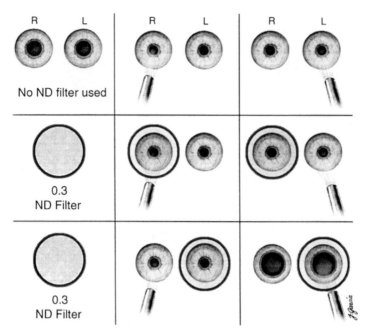

Figure 14.6. The use of neutral density filters to bring out a relative afferent pupillary defect (RAPD). A previous swinging flashlight test has failed to demonstrate a convincing RAPD. A 0.3 log unit neutral density filter is placed over the right eye and a swinging flashlight test is performed. The filter is then placed over the left eye, and the test is repeated. If there is a subtle optic neuropathy in the left eye, placing the filter in front of that eye will reduce the light stimulation even further, and there will now be a RAPD during the swinging flashlight test. When the filter is placed in front of the right eye, however, the reduced brightness in the right eye will tend to balance the reduced brightness in the left eye (from the optic neuropathy), and no RAPD will be seen.

produced. Special care must be taken to keep retina bleach equal, especially when measuring with neutral density filters greater than 1.2 log units in density (see subsequent text).

Finally, the swinging flashlight test can be performed as long as there are two pupils, even when one pupil is nonreactive and dilated or constricted from neurologic disease, iris trauma, or topical drugs. Recall that as the light is shifted from the normal to the abnormal eye, the total pupillomotor input is reduced. Thus, the efferent stimulus for pupillary constriction is reduced in *both* eyes so that both pupils dilate. In performing the swinging flashlight test, one tends to observe only the pupil that is being illuminated; however, the opposite pupil is responding *in an identical fashion.* Thus, if one pupil is mechanically or pharmacologically nonreactive, one can simply perform a swinging flashlight test observing only the reactive pupil. If the abnormal eye is the eye with a fixed pupil, the pupil of the normal eye will constrict briskly when light is shined directly in it and will dilate when the light is shined in the opposite eye. If the abnormal eye is the eye with the reactive pupil, the pupil will constrict when light is shined in the opposite eye and dilate when the light is shined directly in it. This is extremely helpful in at-

tempting to determine if a patient with an oculomotor nerve paresis or traumatic iridoplegia also has an optic neuropathy or retinal dysfunction.

The swinging flashlight test can be further refined in patients in whom a unilateral optic neuropathy is suspected but who do not seem to have a RAPD when a standard swinging flashlight test is performed. In such patients, the use of a neutral density filter with a transmission of 0.3 logarithmic units often permits the detection of the defect (Fig. 14.6). The test is performed as follows. The filter is first placed over one eye, and the swinging flashlight test is performed. The filter is then placed over the opposite eye, and the swinging flashlight test is repeated. If there is truly no defect in the afferent system in either eye, placing the filter over either eye will simply induce a slight but symmetric RAPD in the eye covered by the filter, from reduction in the amount of light entering the system through that eye. On the other hand, if one eye already has a mild RAPD, placement of the filter over that eye will further reduce the amount of light entering the system through that eye, thus increasing the previously inapparent defect and causing it to become recognizable; placement of the filter over the opposite (normal) eye will simply balance the afferent defect in the opposite

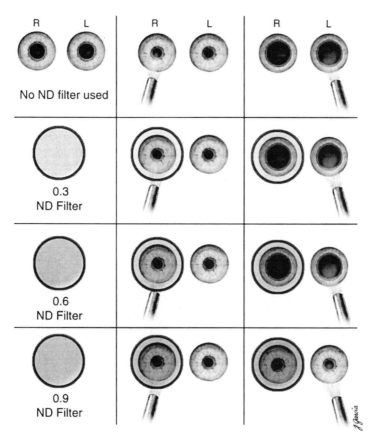

Figure 14.7. Quantification of the relative afferent pupillary defect (RAPD) using neutral density filters and the swinging flashlight test. Neutral density filters of increasing density are placed in front of the normal eye in a patient with a contralateral RAPD, and a swinging flashlight test is performed until the RAPD disappears. In this case, the RAPD is balanced with a 0.9 log unit filter.

eye, and there will be no significant asymmetry in pupillary responses to light.

One can quantify the RAPD using graded neutral density filters that are calibrated in percent transmittance. After determining that a RAPD is present, the examiner balances the defect by adding successive neutral density filters in 0.3 logarithmic steps over the **normal** eye while performing the swinging flashlight test until the defect disappears (Fig. 14.7). The most useful neutral density filters are those ranging in transmission from 80% (0.1 log unit) to 1% (2.0 log units) (Fig. 14.8).

To reach the endpoint of the test, the examiner should "overshoot the endpoint"—that is, produce a RAPD in the normal (covered) eye. The examiner should then rebleach the retina of that eye and perform the swinging flashlight test with another filter at the next lower amount. Several "rules of thumb" in measuring the RAPD for various conditions are found in Table 14.1.

There is some correlation between the severity of a RAPD and the size of the peripheral field defects detected with kinetic perimetry using a Goldmann perimeter. There is less convincing evidence of a correlation between the pupillary response and field defects in the central field detected using static perimetry.

Tests used to detect a RAPD, particularly the swinging flashlight test, are sensitive tests for optic nerve dysfunction; however, they represent only one type of test used to determine whether a patient has an optic neuropathy, and, if so, what the degree of severity of the optic nerve dysfunction is.

PHARMACOLOGIC TESTING (TABLE 14.2)

If a judgment is to be made about the dilation or constriction of the pupil in response to a drop of some drug in the conjunctival sac, then whenever possible one pupil should be used as an internal control. Thus, if the condition is unilateral, the drug should be placed in both eyes so that the responses of the two eyes can

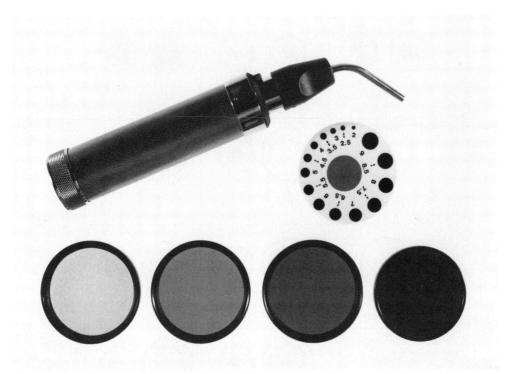

Figure 14.8. The equipment needed to quantify or bring out a relative afferent pupillary defect includes a bright handheld light source, a pupil gauge, and a set of photographic neutral density filters in 0.3, 0.6, 0.9, and 1.2 steps.

Table 14.1. *Expected RAPD in Various Situations—Rules to Follow*

Condition	Expected Rapd in Log Units	Comment
Optic neuritis	0.3 to over 3 log units	If no RAPD, suspect bilateral disease
Optic tract	0.4–0.6 contralateral eye	Look for temporal visual field defect
Pretectal lesion	Contralateral RAPD without VF loss	
Visual field defect	Correlates with Goldmann/Humphrey	
Amblyopia	Less than 0.5 log units	If greater than 1.0 log unit, look for other disease
Anisocoria	0.1 log unit for every 1 mm	Test in light
Macular disease	Better than 20/200, no more than 0.5	Worst macular disease less than 1.0 log unit
Central serous	Less than 0.3 log units	
Central retinal vein occlusion	Ischemic 0.9–1.2 log units	
Central retinal vein occlusion	Nonischemic <0.6 log units	
Retinal detachment	1 Quad 0.3; 2 Quad 0.6; macular 0.9; complete 2.0	
Retinitis pigmentosa	0.3 log units or less	
Cataract	None	If dense, expect RAPD in opposite eye
Patching; dark adaptation	Up to 1.5 log units in unoccluded eye	Maximum RAPD in 30 min; reverses in 10 min
Glaucoma	Varies	Corresponds with retinal rim
Nonorganic visual loss	None	

Table 14.2. *Pharmacologic Testing in Diagnosing Common Pupil Conditions*

Agent	Purpose	Dose	Time	Lighting	Measure
Dilute Pilocarpine	Supersensitivity testing	0.625%	30 min	Dim light or darkness	Change in pupil diameter
Pilocarpine 2%	Pharmacologic pupil blockade	2%	40 min	Darkness	Change in pupil diameter
Cocaine	To demonstrate sympathetic defect	10%	60 min	Light	Postcocaine anisocoria
Hydroxyamphetamine	To detect postganglionic sympathetic defect		50–60 min	Light	Absolute dil. OU or anis. >1 mm or change in anis. >1 mm

be compared. When the condition is bilateral, no such comparison is possible, but an attempt should be made to make certain that the observed response is indeed caused by the instilled drug. In such cases, the drug may be placed in one eye only so that the responses of the medicated and unmedicated eyes can be compared.

Other problems can occur when performing pharmacologic testing of the pupil using topical drugs. The drug may be outdated and thus more or less potent; the patient may develop sufficient tearing that the strength of the drug is altered by dilution or washed out of the inferior conjunctival sac before it can be absorbed; the patient may squeeze the eyes tightly during instillation of the drug, thus preventing a sufficient amount of drug from being placed in the inferior conjunctival sac. One must also consider individual variations in the action of the drug on patients of different ages or with different-colored irides. Determining the results of pupillary testing can also be difficult depending on the initial size of the pupil.

ASSESSMENT OF ACCOMMODATION, CONVERGENCE, AND THE NEAR RESPONSE

Accommodation may be too great, too little, or too slow. Disturbances of the other two components of the near response—convergence and pupillary miosis—may manifest themselves as overactive or impaired.

HISTORY

While the symptoms of patients with disturbances of accommodation tend to be nonspecific, some aspects of the history may be important. Patients with accommodative insufficiency, for instance, usually complain of blurred vision at near and not in the distance. Patients with the most common problem with accommo-

dation, presbyopia, may report that the farther away they hold an object, the better they can see it. Frequently, presbyopia and other accommodative insufficient states can be precipitated with medications having anticholinergic effects.

Accommodative excess or spasm is typically associated with clear vision at near but poor distance vision. In addition, these patients often complain of brow ache. When convergence is affected in addition to accommodation, other symptoms may be present. Convergence excess is often associated with diplopia in the distance, blurring of vision, oscillopsia, or pain. On the other hand, convergence insufficiency is associated with trouble reading, diplopia at near, blurred vision that clears when either eye is covered, and pain or discomfort during near tasks.

In patients with spasm of the near reflex, symptoms are related to dysfunction of all three components. Such patients have accommodative spasm (up to 8 to 10 diopters), extreme miosis, and strabismus caused by convergence.

EXAMINATION
General Principles

Accommodation is the ability of the lens to change its refractive power in order to keep the image of an object clear on the retina. The primary stimulus for accommodation is blur, and most tests of accommodation depend on producing or eliminating blur. Stimuli for accommodation besides blur, including chromatic aberration and perceived nearness, may also be used to test accommodation.

Accommodation is part of a complex triad that maintains clear near vision: the **near response** (also called the *near reflex*). Even though the components of the near response—accommodation, convergence, and pupillary miosis—normally work in concert during near viewing, each component can be tested separately.

For example, one can weaken the stimulus to accommodation with plus lenses or strengthen the stimulus to accommodation with weak minus lenses without stimulating convergence or miosis. One can use weak base-out prisms to stimulate convergence without changing accommodation. Under certain conditions, one can test accommodation without inducing pupillary constriction. Even in presbyopia, in which accommodation fails, convergence and miosis continue. Furthermore, if one paralyzes accommodation with drugs, convergence remains intact.

The **near point of accommodation** (NPA) is the point closest to the eye at which a target is sharply focused on the retina. Accommodation is measured by the **accommodative amplitude**—the power that the lens can vary from the nonaccommodative state to full accommodation. This power is measured in units called **diopters**. A diopter (D) is the reciprocal of the fixation distance. For example, 1 meter is 1 D; 0.5 m is 2 D; 0.33 m is 3 D; etc. The **range of accommodation** is the distance between the farthest point an object is in clear sight and the nearest point at which the eye can maintain clear vision.

Convergence is a vergence adduction movement that increases the visual angle to permit single binocular vision during near viewing. Convergence can be voluntary but need not be; that is, no stimulus needs to be present to elicit it. It is also reflexive and a comovement in the near response. Accommodation and convergence are related; a unit change in one normally causes a unit change in the other. Convergence may be separated into four subtypes: tonic convergence, accommodative convergence, fusional convergence, and voluntary convergence.

The eyes normally tend to diverge. Keeping the eyes straight thus requires increased tone in the medial rectus muscles. This tone is **tonic convergence.**

Accommodative convergence is the amount of convergence elicited for a given amount of accommodation. The relationship between accommodation and convergence is usually expressed as the ratio of accommodative convergence in prism diopters to accommodation in diopters: the AC/A ratio. Because accommodation decreases with age, the AC/A ratio increases with age.

Fusional convergence is convergence that is stimulated not by changes in accommodation but by disparate retinal images. It is thought to "fine tune" normal convergence.

Voluntary convergence is measured by determining the near point of convergence (NPC)—the nearest point to which the eye can converge. It is closer to the eyes than the near point of accommodation and, in general, does not deteriorate with age as the NPA does. The NPC is usually 10 cm or less.

The pupil constricts when changing fixation from distance to near—this is **miosis.** This movement can occur in darkness, is slower than the light reflex, and is maintained as long as the near reaction is maintained. Miosis improves the range through which an object is seen clearly without any change in accommodation, called the **depth of field.** In patients with presbyopia, pupil size continues to decrease even when accommodation has reached its maximum.

In testing accommodation and the near vision response, the previously mentioned relationships must be remembered. Furthermore, one must remember that accommodation is never measured or tested in an absolute sense, but rather in response to how it changes under certain testing conditions.

Accommodation

The principal handicaps in the clinical application of adequate tests of accommodation are the subjective nature of the end points and the number of variables that must be controlled. The first step in any testing of components of accommodation or the near response is to perform an adequate refraction in the distance and at near. In children and some adults, a cycloplegic refraction with an agent like cyclopentolate (Cyclogyl) is mandatory. This accurately determines the far point. Pseudomyopia may be the first clue to accommodative spasm. Excellent distance vision and poor near vision may indicate accommodative insufficiency or presbyopia.

The NPA is the most frequent measure of accommodation. It is best measured using a scale device such as the Prince, Krimsky, or Behrens Rules—rulers with markings in both centimeters and diopters on which there is a small sliding chart containing Snellen letters (Fig. 14.9). The technique of testing accommodation is called the *push-up method*. One eye is tested at a time. Wearing an optimum distance refraction and with the opposite eye occluded, the patient fixes on small (usually 5-point) type on a card that is attached to the rule and that can be slid forward and backward. The zero point of the rule should be 11 to 14 mm in front of the cornea. This corresponds to the approximate position of the spectacle correction. The card is moved from a distance to the closest point at which the patient can see the print before it starts to blur. This is the NPA. The maneuver should be repeated several times until the test gives reproducible results.

Once the measurement is made in centimeters, the accommodative amplitude can be calculated by dividing 100 by the NPA in centimeters. For example, in a person with an NPA of 10 cm, the accommodative amplitude is 10 D; if the NPA is 25 cm, the amplitude is 4 D. This means that the accommodative power of

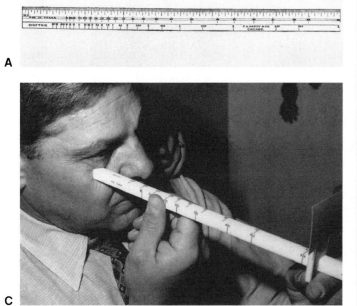

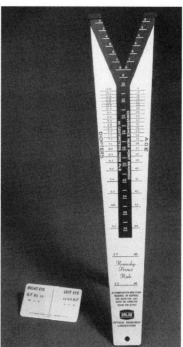

Figure 14.9. Photographs of accommodative rules. **A:** The Prince Rule. (Reprinted from: CA Wood. *The American Encyclopedia and Dictionary of Ophthalmology*. Chicago: Cleveland Press, 1919:10961, with permission.) **B:** The Krimsky-Prince rule. (Photo courtesy of Paul Montague, CRP.) **C:** The Behrens rule.

the eyes in these two examples corresponds to a lens with a focal distance of 10 or 4 diopters, respectively.

Using the push-up method, age-related normative data for accommodation have been developed (Fig. 14.10). If, on repeated testing, the NPA or range of accommodation is consistently out of the range considered to be normal for age, the results should be considered truly abnormal. Illumination is a critical factor in performing the test. By increasing illumination from 1 to 25 foot candles, the accommodative range can be increased by 28% in nonpresbyopes and by 73% in presbyopes.

The range of accommodation can be tested in a fashion similar to that used to test the accommodative amplitude. The patient should be instructed to indicate when the object blurs at near (the near point) and when it blurs in the distance (the far point). The range of accommodation is then calculated by determining the far point and near point in diopters and by subtracting the far point from the near point. For an emmetrope, the near point is the range of accommodation, because the far point is at infinity. For a myope whose far point is 50 cm or 2 diopter in front of the eye and whose near point is 10 cm or 10 D, the range of accommodation is $10 - 2 = 8D$. For a hyperopic eye with a far point of 25 cm or 4 diopters *behind* the eye and a near

point of 10 cm or 10 D, the range of accommodation is $10 - (-4) = 14$ D.

If the patient is too presbyopic or myopic to do the test, corrective lenses should be used. One must then adjust the results to reflect the correction. If a minus lens has been used, the diopteric power of the lens is added to the result; if a plus lens has been used, the diopteric power of the lens is subtracted.

A second method of measuring accommodative amplitude is the *method of the spheres*. The patient fixates on a reading target at 40 cm, and accommodation is stimulated by adding minus (concave) lenses until the print blurs. Accommodation is subsequently relaxed by adding stronger plus (convex) lenses until the print blurs. The sum of the lenses is the measure of the accommodative amplitude.

Convergence

Total convergence is usually measured by testing the NPC. This is usually done by asking the patient to fixate on an accommodative target held 33 cm from the eyes. The target is then moved toward the nose, with the patient being instructed to try to keep the target in focus. The end point of the test is when the patient reports horizontal diplopia or one of the inward turning

Numerical Values of Limits for Each Age

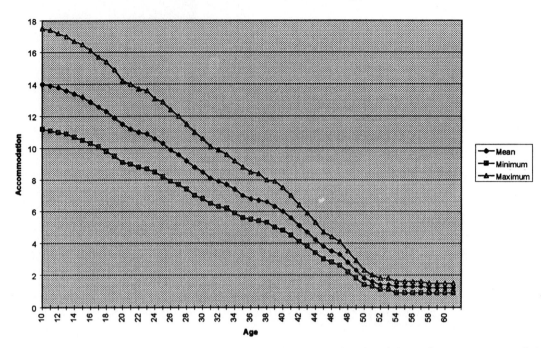

Figure 14.10. The relationship between accommodation and age. Note the relatively linear decrease in accommodation with age until about age 52, when almost all accommodation has been lost. (Graph obtained using data from: A. Duane. The accommodation and Donders curve and the need of revising our ideas regarding them. *J Am Med Assoc.* 1909;52:1992–1996, with permission.)

eyes is observed to turn suddenly outward. The distance at which this occurs can be determined with a millimeter ruler placed alongside the patient's nose. In normal persons, the NPC is usually between 5 and 10 cm. An NPC greater than 30 cm indicates convergence insufficiency.

Another way to determine whether or not convergence is normal is to perform a cover-uncover test while the patient is reading. This is helpful only if the patient has full versions and no previous strabismus.

A way of determining if convergence is sufficient for the amount of accommodation is measuring the AC/A ratio. There are two different methods for measuring the AC/A ratio. The **gradient method** determines the AC/A ratio by the change in deviation in prism diopters that occurs when a lens of varied power is placed over both eyes to stimulate or relax accommodation. An accommodative target must be used, and the working distance is held constant. Plus or minus lenses (+1, +2, –1, –2, etc.) are used to vary the accommodative requirement. The difference between the ocular alignment with and without the lens, divided by the power of the lens, is the AC/A ratio. The **heterophoria method** uses the distance-near relationship to determine the AC/A ratio. A similar ocular alignment

should be present for both distance and near viewing. If a patient is more exotropic or less esotropic at near, this indicates less convergence—that is, a low AC/A ratio; if more esotropic or less exotropic at near, this indicates a high AC/A ratio.

The normal AC/A ratio is between 3 and 6, regardless of the method of testing that is used. Values above 6 indicate an excess of convergence per unit of accommodation, whereas values below 3 suggest convergence insufficiency.

Testing convergence accommodation—that is, the CA/A ratio—requires that the patient experience no blur during the test. This can be accomplished by the use of a pin-hole device, dim illumination, or a Gaussian target. Measurements of accommodation are made as convergence is produced using base-out prisms. The CA/C ratio decreases with decreasing accommodation amplitude and therefore with age, and, of course, with cycloplegics.

ASSESSMENT OF LACRIMATION

The tear film is a trilaminar structure having a superficial oil layer, an aqueous middle component, and a mucin component. In order to discern a problem of the tear secretion, one should attempt to determine if only one layer is affected or all the layers are affected.

The main function of the **oil layer** is to retard evaporation of the tear film. Removal of the oil layer causes a 19-fold increase in evaporation, and abnormalities in the oil layer are often present with blepharitis and ocular rosacea.

The **aqueous layer** is the thickest component of the tears. It contributes the most to the volume of the tear film, and most of the tests that measure the quantity of the tear film test the aqueous layer. This layer is produced by the primary lacrimal gland and also by the accessory lacrimal glands of Krause and Wolfring. The glands of Krause are located in the upper fornix, whereas the glands of Wolfring are situated farther down on the eyelid, above the tarsus. It is generally accepted that the main lacrimal gland, having an efferent parasympathetic innervation, functions primarily during reflex tear secretion, whereas the accessory lacrimal glands provide nonreflex basal tear secretion.

The **mucin layer** is a biphasic layer that allows the aqueous component to adhere to the hydrophobic cornea epithelium. This layer thus helps to maintain the integrity of the aqueous component of tears and the quality of the tear film. Abnormalities in this layer (and also in the oil layer) can create tear film disturbances despite good aqueous tear production. The mucin layer is produced by goblet cells located in the conjunctiva.

The normal basal tear volume is 5 to 9 microliters, and the normal flow rate averages 0.5 to 2.2 microliters per minute. In general, neither basal tear volume nor flow changes with increasing age, but reflex tearing does decrease with age.

The main disturbances of lacrimation relate to excess or insufficient tear production and to obstruction of the normal passage of tears through the lacrimal drainage apparatus. Thus, the assessment of patients with difficulties should be oriented to an evaluation of tear production and drainage.

HISTORY

Excessive drying of the eyes occurs in several settings. It may result from reduced production, increased evaporation, or excessive drainage of tears. **Epiphora**—excessive tearing—also occurs under several different circumstances. An increased production of tears may be present; the lacrimal drainage system may be obstructed; or the excess tearing may actually be reflexive in nature and related to a *deficiency* of normal basal tearing.

Patients with dry eyes often complain of a scratchy sensation in or around the eyes, as if there is a foreign body present. The patient may also complain of blurred vision that seems to improve with blinking or prolonged closure of the eyes.

Episodic epiphora may, in fact, be a symptom of dryness of the eyes. Patients with dry eyes from a variety of causes related to dysfunction of the glands of Krause and Wolfring may nevertheless have a functioning lacrimal gland. Irritation from a dry cornea may stimulate excess tearing from the lacrimal gland, thus creating the paradoxical situation of a patient with dry eyes who complains of excess tearing.

EXAMINATION

The examination of a patient with a disturbance of lacrimation is directed toward the three potential abnormalities described earlier: decreased tear production, increased tear production, and partial or complete obstruction of the lacrimal drainage apparatus.

Lid function is critical to spreading the tear film and should be assessed in any patient suspected of having an abnormality of tear function. Disturbances of eyelid structure and function can be detected both by simple external examination and by slit lamp biomicroscopy. Slit lamp examination can also detect punctate staining of the inferior cornea related to dry eyes, exposure (lagophthalmos), or a lid abnormality.

Specific tests of the mucin layer of the tears include a conjunctival biopsy to determine the number of goblet cells. A qualitative test for mucin can also be performed. In this test, a cotton strip which has been placed in the inferior cul de sac of an unanesthetized eye for 5 minutes is stained with periodic acid-Schiff (PAS) stain and microscopically examined for the presence of mucin. Impression cytology can also be used to determine if goblet cells are present and in what numbers. In this simple technique, cellulose acetate filter strips are placed on the conjunctival epithelium and then stained with hematoxylin and PAS. This procedure can be used to diagnose not only dry eye conditions but also vitamin A deficiency.

Examination of the aqueous layer should begin with an assessment of the tear meniscus. The eyelids and lashes should be observed for evidence of entropion, ectropion, and stray lashes and for the position and integrity of the lower lacrimal punctum. Such abnormalities may cause disturbances that simulate those caused by abnormal tear production.

Nonspecific tests of tear secretion are usually performed in patients with symptoms that suggest insufficient tear production. The sensitivity and specificity of these tests vary greatly, depending on the specific test used and the reference criteria for normal values. Judging the height of the tear meniscus is a common method used to predict the amount of tear production.

The "noninvasive tear film break-up time" is perhaps the simplest test used to determine the adequacy of the tear film. The examiner applies fluorescein, which stains the mucin layer of the tear film, to an unanesthetized eye. The patient is asked to look straight ahead without blinking. A normal test is characterized by the persistence of the fluorescein over the cornea for 10 seconds or longer. A break up and disappearance of the fluorescein in less than 10 seconds is abnormal and indicates an abnormality in one of the layers of the tear film. The test has relatively good sensitivity (82%) and specificity (86%).

Another test of tear function is the "rose bengal test." The examiner applies a drop of 1% rose bengal solution, which stains dead and degenerating cells, to an anesthetized eye. Normal patients have little if any staining, whereas patients with a dry eye or a poor mucin layer will have mild to severe staining.

As noted above, tear secretion may be classified as basal, reflex, or total. Tests of tear secretion can thus be separated into those that test basal tear production (from the glands of Krause and Wolfring) and those that test reflex tear production (from the primary lacrimal gland). The Schirmer test is a simple and practical clinical way of measuring both reflex secretion and basal secretion. Total tear secretion is usually tested first, because no anesthetic drop is applied to the eye in this test (often called the Schirmer 1 test). After drying the inferior conjunctival fornices on both sides with soft cotton, the examiner places a strip of special absorbent filter paper in the lower conjunctival sac. After 5 minutes, the strip is removed, and the amount of wetting is measured from the folded end. This wetting is the result of both basal tear secretion and reflex secretion.

A variant of the Schirmer 1 test can be performed by anesthetizing the eyes with a topical proparacaine 0.5%. After the eye has been anesthetized, the paper strips are placed as indicated above, and the nasal mucosa is stimulated using a cotton-tipped applicator that has been soaked with benzene or a similar trigeminal stimulant. Regardless of the technique used, normal persons wet 10 to 30 mm in 5 minutes. By multiplying the millimeters of wetting in 1 minute by a factor of three, the standard 5-minute Schirmer 1 test could be shortened by 4 minutes.

Basal tear secretion is determined using the Schirmer 2 test. A topical anesthetic is placed in the lower fornix of both eyes. After a minute or so, the examiner uses a small piece of cotton or filter paper to dry the inferior fornices. The paper strips are then placed in the manner of the Schirmer 1 test. After 5 minutes, the strips are removed, and the amount of wetting is measured. The wetting in this test should represent only the basal tear secretion, as the topical anesthetic should prevent stimulation of the main lacrimal gland. In addition, by subtracting the amount of basal tear secretion obtained from the Schirmer 2 test from the total secretion measured in the Schirmer 1 test, one should obtain the amount of reflex tearing.

All of the previously mentioned tests can be criticized for providing inexact and highly variable results; The best balance between specificity and sensitivity was may be achieved by performing both a rose bengal test and a Schirmer 1 test.

Patients who have epiphora should be evaluated not only for excess tear production but also for possible blockage of the tear drainage system. The punctae should be examined to see if they are patent, and the examiner should gently press on the lacrimal sac to see if there is regurgitation of contents through the punctae, indicating a block at the nasolacrimal duct.

The patency of the drainage system can next be tested by instillation of one drop of 2% fluorescein dye into the inferior conjunctival sac of both eyes, followed by observation of the difference at the end of 5 minutes between the two eyes in the residual fluorescein in the conjunctival sac and on the sclera, graded in terms of color intensity. A slightly more quantitative version of this test is to instill the dye in both inferior conjunctival sacs and to place a small cotton pledget or cotton-tipped applicator in the nose just below both inferior turbinates within 1 to 5 minutes. The pledgets or applicators are then examined to see if they are stained with dye that should have passed through the lacrimal punctae into the lacrimal canaliculi and then to the lacrimal sac, eventually exiting the lacrimal duct just below the inferior turbinate. If no dye is present, a secondary dye test is performed. The lacrimal system is flushed with clear saline, and the fluid emanating from the nose is checked for fluorescein staining. If there is still no dye, the nasolacrimal apparatus can be probed. If, after probing, dye is present at the inferior turbinate, then incomplete blockage exists and the lacrimal pump is functioning. If, however, there is clear fluid at the inferior turbinate, then a nonfunctioning pump exists and a complete block is present.

Dacryocystography is a radiologic evaluation of the lacrimal drainage system in which contrast is placed into the lower fornix on the side of the presumed obstruction, and radiographs, computed tomographic (CT) scans, magnetic resonance images (MRI), or angiographic images are obtained to determine if and where the contrast material stops, thus localizing the obstruction.

FOR FURTHER INFORMATION

See *Walsh & Hoyt's Clinical Neuro-Ophthalmology*, 6th edition, Volume 1, Chapter 15, pages 715–737.

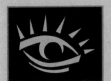

CHAPTER 15

Disorders of Pupillary Function, Accommodation, and Lacrimation*

DISORDERS OF PUPILLARY FUNCTION

The value of observation of pupillary size and motility in the evaluation of patients with neurologic disease cannot be overemphasized. In many patients with visual loss, an abnormal pupillary response is the only objective sign of organic visual dysfunction.

EFFERENT ABNORMALITIES: ANISOCORIA

Efferent disturbances of the pupil are usually unilateral and thus produce a difference in the size of the pupils called **anisocoria.** When assessing the pupils, one should always attempt to determine if anisocoria is present. If anisocoria is present, there is often something wrong with one or both irises or with the innervation of the iris muscles.

Once it is determined that anisocoria is present, the physician should determine if the degree of anisocoria is greater in light or darkness. This is best tested by illuminating the eyes from below with a hand light and turning the room lights off and on. If there is more anisocoria in darkness, the anisocoria may be caused by weakness of the dilator muscle in the eye with the smaller pupil (as in Horner's syndrome), or it may be a physiologic (simple) anisocoria. If there is more anisocoria in light (assuming that the condition is recent), the iris sphincter can be presumed to be weak in the

eye with the bigger pupil. This could be due to anticholinergic medication, a tonic pupil, an oculomotor nerve palsy, or spasm of the dilator muscle. Causes of anisocoria are described subsequently and are outlined in Table 15.1.

More Anisocoria in Darkness

Physiologic Anisocoria (Simple Anisocoria, Central Anisocoria, Benign Anisocoria)   In dim light, almost 20% of the normal population has an anisocoria of 0.4 mm or more at the moment of the examination. In room light, this number drops to about 10%. This form of anisocoria, called **physiologic anisocoria,** is rarely more than 0.6 mm, but it may be as much as 1.0 mm (Fig. 15.1) The anisocoria is almost the same in light and in dark, but there is a tendency for it to decrease in light, perhaps because the smaller pupil reaches the zone of mechanical resistance first, giving the larger pupil a chance to catch up. Other terms for physiologic anisocoria are *simple anisocoria, central anisocoria,* and *benign anisocoria.*

In a patient with physiologic anisocoria, the amount of pupillary inequality may vary. Physiologic anisocoria may be observed in prior pictures, even back to infancy or early childhood. The anisocoria seldom reverses.

Horner's Syndrome   When the sympathetic innervation to the eye is interrupted, the retractor muscles in the eyelids are weakened, allowing the upper lid to droop and the lower lid to rise. The dilator muscle of the iris is weakened, allowing the pupil to become smaller. Vasomotor and sudomotor control of parts of the face may be lost. This combination of ptosis, miosis, and anhidrosis is called **Horner's syndrome** (Fig. 15.2).

*Adapted from: Kawasaki A: Disorders of pupillary function, accommodation, and lacrimation. In: Miller NR, Newman NJ, Biousse V, Kerrison JB, eds. *Walsh & Hoyt's Clinical Neuro-Ophthalmology.* 6th ed. Vol. I. Philadelphia: Lippincott Williams & Wilkins; 2005:739–805.

Table 15.1. *Causes of Anisocoria*

More Anisocoria in Darkness

Simple (physiologic) anisocoria
Inhibition of the sympathetic pathway
 • Horner's syndrome
 • Pharmacologic (dapiprazole, thymoxamine)
Stimulation of the sympathetic pathway
 • Tadpole pupils
 • Intermittent dilation of one pupil caused by
  sympathetic hyperactivity
 • Pharmacologic (cocaine, eye-whitening drops,
  adrenergic drugs)
Pharmacologic stimulation of the parasympathetic
 pathway (eserine, organophosphate esters,
 pilocarpine, methacholine, arecoline)

More Anisocoria in Light

Damage to the parasympathetic outflow to the iris
 sphincter muscle
 • Oculomotor nerve paresis
 • Tonic pupil syndromes (including Adie's)
 • Intermittent dilation of one pupil caused by
  inhibition of the parasympathetic pathway
Trauma to the iris sphincter
Acute glaucoma
Siderosis
Pharmacologic inhibition of the parasympathetic
 pathway (atropine, scopolamine)

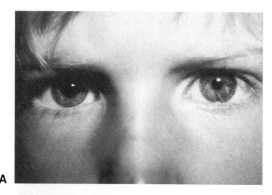

A

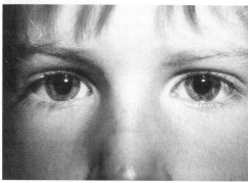

B

Figure 15.1. Physiologic (simple) anisocoria. The patient was a 5-year-old boy whose parents noted that the right pupil was larger than the other. The anisocoria was more obvious in dark than in light, and both pupils reacted normally to light stimulation. **A:** Appearance of the patient. Note anisocoria, with right pupil larger than left. **B:** Both pupils are dilated 45 minutes after instillation of a 10% solution of cocaine into both inferior conjunctival sacs, indicating that anisocoria is not caused by sympathetic denervation.

CLINICAL FEATURES   The affected eye often looks small or sunken in patients with Horner's syndrome. The upper eyelid is slightly drooped because of paralysis of the sympathetically innervated smooth muscle (Müller's muscle) that contributes to the position of the opened upper eyelid. This **ptosis** is sometimes so slight or so variable that it escapes attention. Similar smooth muscle fibers in the lower eyelid also lose their nerve supply in Horner's syndrome. Thus, the lower lid is usually slightly elevated, producing an "upside-down ptosis," further narrowing of the palpebral fissure, and an **apparent enophthalmos.**

The palsy of the iris dilator muscle in Horner's syndrome allows the iris sphincter to constrict, producing **miosis.** If the dilator muscle is stimulated (e.g., after an adrenergic eye drop is used), the pupil will dilate widely. Endogenous catecholamines can produce a similar phenomenon if the iris dilator muscle is supersensitive because of denervation. This "paradoxical pupillary dilation" is caused by denervation supersensitivity of the dilator muscle to circulating adrenergic substances.

In Horner's syndrome, the weakness of the dilator muscle is most apparent in darkness. The anisocoria is greater in the dark and almost disappears in light.

The anisocoria of Horner's syndrome is diminished in bright light because the normal action of both sphincters tends to make the two pupils more nearly equal.

Paresis of the dilator muscle in Horner's syndrome can be detected in several ways. When the lights are turned out, the Horner's pupil dilates more slowly than the normal pupil **(dilation lag)** (Fig. 15.3). A sudden noise will produce an increased sympathetic discharge to the dilator muscle resulting in a transient increase in anisocoria. When looking for dilation lag in a patient with anisocoria that may be caused by Horner's syndrome, it is helpful to interject a sudden noise just after the lights go out.

Depigmentation of the ipsilateral iris is not usually seen in patients with an acquired Horner's syndrome, but it is a typical feature of congenital Horner's syndrome. Nevertheless, it rarely can occur after injury to the sympathetic nervous system in adults.

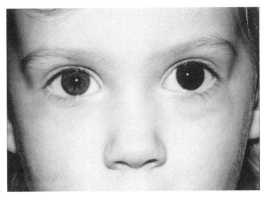 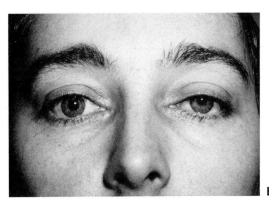

Figure 15.2. Horner's syndrome in two patients. **A:** Congenital right Horner's syndrome. Note associated heterochromia iridis and minimal ptosis. **B:** Left Horner's syndrome after neck trauma.

Characteristic vasomotor and sudomotor changes of the facial skin occur on the affected side in some patients with Horner's syndrome. The best known of these is loss of sweating **(anhidrosis)**. In a warm environment, the skin on the affected side will feel dry whereas the skin on the normal side will be damp. The postganglionic sympathetic sudomotor fibers for the face, after synapsing at the superior cervical ganglion, follow the external carotid artery to the face, whereas the sympathetic fibers to the eye travel via the carotid plexus of the internal carotid artery, carrying only a few sweat fibers for the skin of the forehead. Thus, anhidrosis occurs only in patients with a central or preganglionic Horner's syndrome, never with a postganglionic Horner's syndrome.

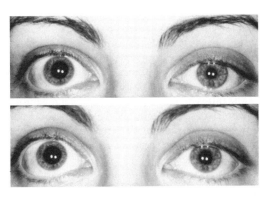

Figure 15.3. Dilation lag in a patient with a left Horner's syndrome, observed using infrared pupillary videography. Photo taken 5 seconds after room lights turned off **(top).** Photo taken after 15 seconds of darkness **(bottom).** Note that the right pupil is already maximally dilated within 5 seconds of turning the room lights off; however, the left pupil still has not dilated maximally after 15 seconds of darkness.

After acute, preganglionic sympathetic denervation, the temperature of the skin rises on the side of the lesion because of loss of vasomotor control and consequent dilation of blood vessels. Acutely, there may be some flushing and some conjunctival hyperemia, epiphora, and nasal stuffiness.

DIAGNOSIS   It is important to differentiate a Horner's syndrome from physiologic anisocoria. The diagnosis of Horner's syndrome can be made by pharmacologic testing. The **cocaine test** is most commonly used and is based on the failure of cocaine to dilate a sympathetically denervated eye. Cocaine blocks the re-uptake of norepinephrine into the sympathetic nerve endings. In a normal eye, a 10% solution of cocaine causes dilation of the pupil, often to 8 mm or more, within about 45 minutes. However, a sufficient quantity of norepinephrine does not accumulate at the receptors of effector cells unless norepinephrine is continually being released by action potentials within the sympathetic nerves to those cells, which does not occur when there is sympathetic denervation of the pupillary dilator muscle (Fig. 15.4).

The first drop of topical cocaine stings briefly until the anesthetic effect occurs. Peak effect is attained in 40 to 60 minutes. There are no apparent psychoactive effects from a 10% solution of cocaine, but metabolites of the drug can be found in the urine in 100% of patients after 24 hours and in 50% at 36 hours.

Cocaine affects only the sympathetic system, not the parasympathetic system. If the patient is observed while seated in a lighted room, the pupils may appear not to have responded to the cocaine because the light tends to produce pupillary constriction. The patient must be brought into the examination room and the lights dimmed, at which time the pharmacologic dilation of one or both pupils can easily be appreciated.

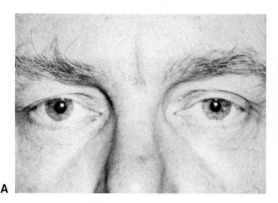
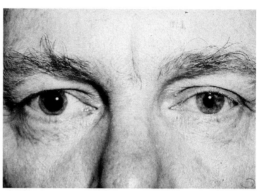

A   B

Figure 15.4. Response of Horner's pupils to cocaine. **A:** Left Horner's syndrome associated with Raeder's paratrigeminal neuralgia in a 55-year-old man. **B:** Photo taken 45 minutes after conjunctival instillation of 2 drops of a 10% cocaine solution in each eye. The right pupil is dilated, whereas the left pupil remains unchanged.

The odds of an anisocoria being caused by an oculosympathetic palsy increase with the amount of anisocoria measured 45 minutes after the instillation of 10% cocaine into both eyes. It is not necessary to compare the before and after measurements; a postcocaine anisocoria of 0.8 mm is sufficient to diagnose a Horner's syndrome.

LOCALIZATION   Regardless of the site of the lesion in the long sympathetic pathway, all patients with Horner's syndrome have a similar ptosis and miosis. It is, however, clinically important to separate the pathway into three major divisions: the central (first-order), the preganglionic (second-order), and the postganglionic (third-order) neurons.

Central Horner's Syndromes. The **central** (first-order) neuron begins in the ipsilateral hypothalamus and extends to the ciliospinal center of Budge and Waller in the intermediolateral gray column of the spinal cord at C8–T1 (Fig. 15.5). The path may actually be polysynaptic, but it seems to stay lateral in the brainstem and cervical cord. Thus, Horner's syndrome caused by damage to the central neuron is almost always unilateral. There is no pharmacologic test that identifies a central-neuron Horner's syndrome, so the clinician must put localizing weight on the associated clinical signs. For example, lesions of the hypothalamus that cause an ipsilateral Horner's syndrome are often associated with a contralateral hemiparesis, and some of these patients also have a contralateral hypesthesia.

Another neurologic syndrome characterized in part by a central Horner's syndrome is **Wallenberg's syndrome.** This condition, which is caused by damage to the lateral medulla, is also characterized by ipsilateral impairment of pain and temperature sensation over the face, limb ataxia, and a bulbar disturbance causing dysarthria and dysphagia. Contralaterally, pain and temperature sensation are impaired over the trunk and limbs. Lateropulsion, a compelling sensation of being pulled toward the side of the lesion, is often a prominent complaint of patients with Wallenberg's syndrome and is also evident in the ocular motor findings.

The occurrence of a unilateral Horner's syndrome and a contralateral trochlear nerve paresis indicates involvement either of the trochlear nucleus on the side of the Horner's syndrome or of the ipsilateral fascicle before its decussation. However, not all patients with a first-order neuron Horner's syndrome have other neurologic manifestations. Patients with cervical spondylosis, for example, may have no symptoms or signs of spinal cord disease. Such patients may present only with a Horner's syndrome and perhaps some neck pain.

Preganglionic Horner's Syndromes. The **preganglionic** (second-order) neuron exits from the ciliospinal center of Budge and passes across the pulmonary apex (Fig. 15.5). It then turns upward, passes through the stellate ganglion, and goes up the carotid sheath to the superior cervical ganglion, near the bifurcation of the common carotid artery.

The ptosis and miosis of a preganglionic Horner's syndrome are nonspecific, but the distribution of anhidrosis is characteristic. The entire side of the head, the face, and the neck down to the clavicle are usually involved.

Malignancy is a common cause of a preganglionic Horner's syndrome. The most common tumors, not surprisingly, are lung and breast cancer, but Horner's syndrome is usually not an early sign of these tumors. Tumors that spread behind the carotid sheath at the C6 level may produce a preganglionic Horner's syndrome associated with paralysis of the phrenic, vagus, and recurrent laryngeal nerves: the "Rowland Payne syndrome." Benign tumors in this region, such as a

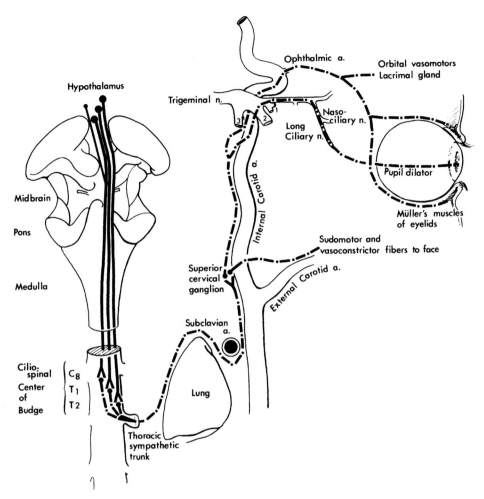

Figure 15.5. The oculosympathetic pathway. Note location of central (first-order), preganglionic (second-order), and post-ganglionic (third-order) neurons. (Reprinted from: Glaser JS. *Neuro-Ophthalmology*. 1st ed. Hagerstown, MD: Harper & Row; 1978:173, with permission.)

schwannoma of the sympathetic chain, can also produce a preganglionic Horner's syndrome.

A preganglionic Horner's syndrome can be caused by accidental or surgical injury (e.g., disc herniation at C8 or T1, trauma to the brachial plexus, pneumothorax, coronary artery bypass surgery, or insertion of a pacemaker). The preganglionic neuron can also be transiently blocked by an epidural anesthetic that flows the wrong way or by an interpleural anesthetic that soaks through the pleura at the pulmonary apex to reach the stellate ganglion. Chest tubes, vascular catheters, and stray bullets can directly injure the preganglionic sympathetic nerves.

Postganglionic Horner's Syndromes. The **postganglionic** (third-order) neuron of the sympathetic pathway to the iris dilator muscle extends from the superior cervical ganglion behind the angle of the mandible and up along the internal carotid artery, where it is called the "carotid plexus" or the "carotid nerve." Within the cavernous sinus, the sympathetic fibers leave the internal carotid artery, join briefly with the abducens nerve, and then leave it to join the ophthalmic division of the trigeminal nerve, entering the orbit with its nasociliary branch. The sympathetic fibers in the nasociliary nerve divide into the two long ciliary nerves that travel with the lateral and medial suprachoroidal vascular bundles to reach the anterior segment of the eye and innervate the iris dilator muscle.

Lesions that affect the postganglionic third-order sympathetic neuron may be extracranial or intracranial. Extracranial lesions damage the cervical sympathetics in the neck, whereas intracranial lesions damage the sympathetic chain at the base of the skull, in the carotid canal and middle ear, or in the region of the cavernous sinus. It is very unusual for an orbital lesion to produce an isolated Horner's syndrome.

Lesions of or along the internal carotid artery are a common cause of a postganglionic Horner's syndrome. Both traumatic and spontaneous **dissections of the internal carotid artery** can produce sudden ipsilateral face and neck pain associated with a postganglionic Horner's syndrome. Raeder's paratrigeminal neuralgia, the name given to a headache syndrome characterized by persistent trigeminal pain associated with a postganglionic Horner's syndrome, likely represents unrecognized carotid dissection in many patients.

A postganglionic Horner's syndrome may be caused by tumors, inflammatory lesions, and other masses in the neck. Any neoplasm that extends or metastasizes to the cervical lymph nodes may also damage the cervical sympathetic chain. A postganglionic Horner's syndrome, paralysis of the tongue, anesthesia of the pharynx, and dysphagia, all on the same side, may indicate a tumor of the nasopharynx or jugular foramen.

Tumors, aneurysms, infections, and other lesions in the cavernous sinus may produce a postganglionic Horner's syndrome. In many of these cases, there is associated ipsilateral ophthalmoplegia as well as pain or dysesthesia of the ipsilateral side of the face caused by involvement of one or more ocular motor nerves and the trigeminal nerve within the sinus. Because the abducens nerve and oculosympathetic nerves are briefly joined in the cavernous sinus, an abducens palsy and a postganglionic Horner's syndrome occurring together without other neurologic signs should immediately suggest a cavernous sinus lesion.

Cluster headaches often occur at night and usually last 30 to 120 minutes. The patient is completely preoccupied with a very severe lancinating or dysesthetic pain. In addition, the eye is red and half closed from an associated sympathetic palsy, and there is ipsilateral nasal stuffiness. Typically, the Horner's syndrome persists after the headache resolves. Other ischemic conditions, such as giant cell arteritis, can cause a postganglionic Horner's syndrome.

A middle fossa mass encroaching on Meckel's cave and on the internal carotid artery at the foramen lacerum can also produce a postganglionic Horner's syndrome associated with pain. Other lesions at the base of the skull, including a basal skull fracture, can produce a similar clinical picture.

Differentiating Localizations. The **hydroxyamphetamine test** can be used to differentiate between a postganglionic and a preganglionic or central Horner's syndrome (Fig. 15.6). This test should be performed only after a cocaine test has established the diagnosis of a Horner's syndrome or in a setting in which the diagnosis of Horner's syndrome is clear cut. If a cocaine test has been performed, the hydroxyamphetamine test should not be performed for 24 to 48 hours, to allow the corneas and pupils to recover from the effects of the cocaine. The hydroxyamphetamine test is performed as follows. Two drops of hydroxyamphetamine hydrobromide 1% (Paredrine) are placed in the lower cul-de-sac of each eye, and the pupils are assessed in a dim light about 45 minutes later. Hydroxyamphetamine releases norepinephrine from the stores in the adrenergic nerve ending, producing variable but usually significant mydriasis in normal subjects. When the lesion causing a Horner's syndrome is in the *postganglionic neuron*, the nerve endings themselves are destroyed, there are no stores of norepinephrine to release, and hydroxyamphetamine thus has no mydriatic effect. If the lesion is in the *preganglionic or central neuron*, the pupil will dilate fully and may even become larger than the opposite pupil, presumably because of up-regulation of the postsynaptic receptors on the dilator muscle. Although there are occasional false-negative responses to the hydroxyamphetamine test, such responses usually occur only in patients who are tested within the first week after the Horner's syndrome has developed, presumably before the stores of norepinephrine at the presynaptic terminals have been depleted.

A smaller pupil that fails to dilate to cocaine and subsequently does not dilate after topical administration of hydroxyamphetamine or a similar substance is likely to be caused by a lesion of the postganglionic sympathetic neuron. Such a pupil should show evidence of denervation supersensitivity to adrenergic substances and should dilate to a weak, direct-acting topical adrenergic drug. Indeed, such a pupil not only will dilate but will become larger than the opposite pupil. Denervation supersensitivity of the iris to adrenergic drugs may take as long as 17 days to develop.

ACQUIRED HORNER'S SYNDROME IN CHILDREN While an acquired Horner's syndrome in childhood is sometimes associated with neoplasia, including spinal cord tumors, embryonal cell carcinoma, neuroblastoma, and rhabdomyosarcoma, this association is quite rare. A Horner's syndrome in childhood is usually *not* associated with a tumor and is often an isolated finding of no significance. Other causes of an acquired Horner's syndrome in childhood include traumatic brachial plexus palsy, intrathoracic aneurysm, and thrombosis of the internal carotid artery. If old photographs clearly indicate that a Horner's syndrome in a child is acquired, it is recommended to begin further evaluation with CT scanning or MRI of the chest.

CONGENITAL HORNER'S SYNDROME Congenital Horner's syndrome is an uncommon disorder. In its fully developed form, the syndrome consists of ptosis, miosis, facial anhidrosis, and hypochromia of the affected iris. Injury to the brachial plexus at birth is responsible for

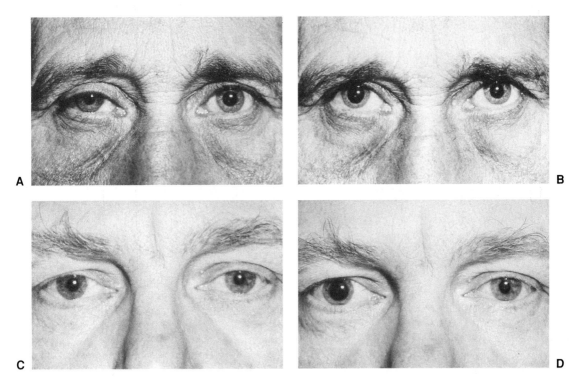

Figure 15.6. Response of Horner's pupils to hydroxyamphetamine. **A:** Right Horner's syndrome in a 45-year-old man with an apical lung tumor. **B:** At 45 minutes after conjunctival instillation of 2 drops of 1% hydroxyamphetamine solution (Paredrine) in each eye, both pupils are dilated, indicating an intact postganglionic neuron (i.e., a preganglionic Horner's syndrome). **C:** Left Horner's syndrome associated with cluster headaches in a 55-year-old man. **D:** At 45 minutes after conjunctival instillation of 2 drops of 1% hydroxyamphetamine solution in each eye, only the right (normal) pupil is dilated. The left pupil is unchanged, indicating damage to the postganglionic neuron (i.e., a postganglionic Horner's syndrome).

many of these cases (Fig. 15.7), but some cases occur in association with congenital tumors, and others occur after viral infections.

Most patients with congenital Horner's syndrome can be separated into one of three groups: patients with evidence of obstetric trauma to the internal carotid artery sympathetic plexus, patients without a history of birth trauma but with a lesion that is clinically and pharmacologically localized to the superior cervical ganglion, and those with evidence of surgical or obstetric injury to the preganglionic sympathetic pathway.

The first group of patients tends to have had substantial perinatal head trauma as a result of difficult forceps deliveries. Clinically, such patients have obvious ptosis and miosis with generally intact facial sweating. Pharmacologic testing is consistent with a postganglionic lesion.

In the second group of patients, pharmacologic testing also is consistent with a postganglionic lesion but such patients have facial anhidrosis, indicating a lesion proximal to the separation of the sudomotor fibers with

the external carotid artery. The causes of such a lesion could include an embryopathy directly involving the superior cervical ganglion, damage to the vascular supply of the superior cervical ganglion, or transsynaptic dysgenesis of the superior cervical ganglion following a defect located more proximally in the sympathetic pathway.

The third group of patients has suffered trauma to the preganglionic oculosympathetic pathway. Injuries include trauma to the brachial plexus and surgery in the thoracic region. Although patients in this group should have a preganglionic Horner's syndrome, some have pharmacologic testing consistent with a postganglionic lesion, presumably indicating transsynaptic degeneration occurring in the postganglionic neuron following preganglionic injury.

Parents of infants with congenital Horner's syndrome sometimes report that the baby develops a hemifacial flush when it is nursing or crying. It is likely that the hemifacial flushing seen in infants is on the side opposite the Horner's syndrome and is simply the normal response, which appears more obvious because

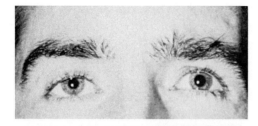

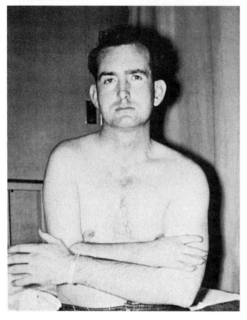

Figure 15.7. Horner's syndrome **(top)** associated with injury of the right brachial plexus at birth. Note the underdeveloped right arm and forearm **(bottom).**

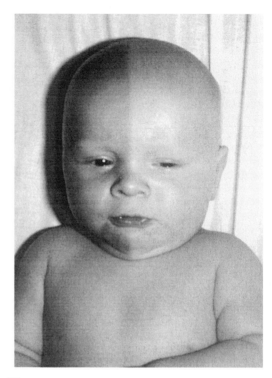

Figure 15.8. Lack of atropinic flushing in a child with a congenital left Horner's syndrome. Note that the atropinic flush is present only on the side of the face opposite the Horner's syndrome.

of the impaired facial vasodilation on the side of a congenital Horner's syndrome.

When a child has unilateral ptosis and ipsilateral miosis, and there is doubt as to whether or not a sympathetic defect is present, a cycloplegic refraction can sometimes unexpectedly solve the problem by producing an atropinic flush. This reaction only occurs when there is an intact sympathetic innervation to the skin and thus is absent on the side of the Horner's syndrome (Fig. 15.8).

A child with Horner's syndrome and very blue eyes will not develop visible iris heterochromia, but most children with Horner's syndrome have the more pale iris on the affected side. This occurs whether the lesion is preganglionic or postganglionic because of anterograde transsynaptic dysgenesis. When the sympathetic pathway is interrupted in the preganglionic neuron, the next distal ganglion—the superior cervical ganglion—does not develop normally. There are fewer cells in the ganglion and less norepinephrine stores to release with

hydroxyamphetamine. This results in impaired development of iris melanophores, causing hypochromia of the iris stroma.

Sympathetic Hyperactivity   Sympathetic hyperactivity occurs in a number of settings in which the pupils are affected. In such cases, there may be anisocoria that is more obvious in darkness than in light.

A **tadpole pupil** is an intermittent and benign phenomenon in which the pupil of one eye becomes becomes distorted for a minute or two. The pupil is pulled in one direction like the tail of a tadpole. It is thought to be caused by repeated bursts of sympathetic innervation, an irritation that eventually causes loss of fibers and a Horner's syndrome. This condition is different from the **episodic unilateral mydriasis** that occurs in some young patients during a typical migraine attack, although there is some similarity.

Some patients who sustain trauma (e.g., whiplash injury) to the low cervical or high thoracic spinal cord experience episodes of unilateral pupillary dilation associated with unilateral sweating. Pharmacologic testing in such patients suggests that the mydriasis is caused by episodic sympathetic irritation.

Pharmacologic Stimulation of the Iris Sphincter
Almost all cases of acute anisocoria in which one pupil is nonreactive are caused by pharmacologic blockade of the iris sphincter muscle. In such cases, the anisocoria is worse in light than in darkness because the affected pupil cannot constrict. In rare instances, however, a pharmacologic agent, such as an organophosphate used in pesticides, may produce anisocoria by stimulating rather than blocking the parasympathetic system, thus producing a nonreactive, **miotic** pupil. In such cases and in other cases of pharmacologic stimulation of the ocular parasympathetic pathway, a 1% solution of tropicamide will dilate the larger, reactive pupil but will fail to dilate the small, nonreactive pupil.

Pharmacologic Stimulation of the Iris Dilator
Topical cocaine placed in the nose for medical or for other reasons can back up the lacrimal duct into the conjunctival sac. Most eye-whitening drops that contain sympathomimetic components are too weak to dilate the pupil, but if the cornea is abraded (e.g., by a contact lens), enough of the oxymetazoline or the phenylephrine may get into the aqueous humor to dilate the pupil. Other adrenergic drugs given in a mist for pulmonary therapy may escape around the edge of the face mask and condense in the conjunctival sac, causing pupillary dilation that is more evident in darkness than in light.

More Anisocoria in Light

Damage to the Parasympathetic Outflow to the Iris Sphincter Muscle   The final common pathway for pupillary reactivity to light and near stimulation begins in the mesencephalon with the visceral oculomotor nuclei, continues via the oculomotor nerve to the ciliary ganglion, and reaches the iris sphincter through the short ciliary nerves. Lesions that affect this parasympathetic pathway can produce absolute paralysis of pupillary constriction. The pupil is then dilated and nonreactive, and all constrictor reflexes are absent. In many cases, all parasympathetic input to the eye is damaged simultaneously so that accommodation is also lost. This combination of iridoplegia and cycloplegia is often called **internal ophthalmoplegia** to distinguish it from the external ophthalmoplegia that occurs when the extraocular muscles are paralyzed in the setting of normal pupillary responses.

Topical diagnosis of paralysis of the iris sphincter is simplified when signs of an oculomotor nerve palsy are present. In the setting of ptosis and paralysis of the superior, inferior, and medial rectus muscles, as well as the inferior oblique muscle, a nonreactive, dilated pupil is but a part of the classic picture of a lesion of the oculomotor nerve. However, isolated iris paralysis can be a difficult diagnostic problem. One must consider lesions of the mesencephalon, the oculomotor nerve, the ciliary ganglion, the short ciliary nerves, and the eye itself.

Damage to the Edinger-Westphal Nuclei   Lesions of the rostral mesencephalon almost never produce an isolated unilateral, nonreactive, dilated pupil. When there is isolated damage to the Edinger-Westphal nuclei, bilateral pupillary abnormalities are the rule. In addition, most lesions in this region that produce pupillary abnormalities also affect other parts of the oculomotor nucleus, causing ptosis, ophthalmoparesis, or both.

Damage to Pupillomotor Fibers in the Oculomotor Nerve Fascicle   The fascicle of the oculomotor nerve can be damaged within the mesencephalon by a variety of processes, including ischemia, inflammation, and infiltration. Such processes can produce a complete or incomplete isolated oculomotor nerve paresis or a syndrome in which an oculomotor nerve paresis is associated with other neurologic signs, such as contralateral hemiparesis or tremor. Because the fibers emerging from the Edinger-Westphal nucleus are among the most rostral in the oculomotor group (Fig. 15.9), it is possible for a lesion to damage just the fibers serving pupillary function, thus producing a unilateral, dilated, nonreactive pupil. In other patients, a lesion affecting the oculomotor fascicle may damage only the fibers destined for the extraocular muscles, levator palpebrae superioris, or both, sparing the bundle headed for the iris sphincter and thus producing a pupil-sparing complete or incomplete oculomotor nerve palsy.

Damage to Pupillomotor Fibers in the Subarachnoid Portion of the Oculomotor Nerve   The separate bundles of the oculomotor nerve that leave the mesencephalon merge to form the oculomotor nerve in the subarachnoid space. The nerve takes a short course between the posterior cerebral and superior cerebellar arteries and then enters the cavernous sinus. In this part of the preganglionic path, the pupillary fibers are superficial and migrate from a superior medial position to the inferior part of the nerve (Fig. 15.10).

Noxious influences carried by the cerebrospinal fluid (CSF) are a hazard to the oculomotor nerve within the subarachnoid space. In basal meningitis, for example, the nerve is surrounded by pus, and the superficially located pupillary fibers are particularly at risk. Basal meningitis from a variety of organisms, including bacteria, viruses, and spirochetes, can produce unilateral or bilateral poorly reactive pupils.

Although intracranial aneurysms, particularly those at the junction of the internal carotid artery and the posterior communicating artery, may produce a dilated, nonreactive pupil, this is nearly always associated with other evidence of oculomotor nerve dysfunction.

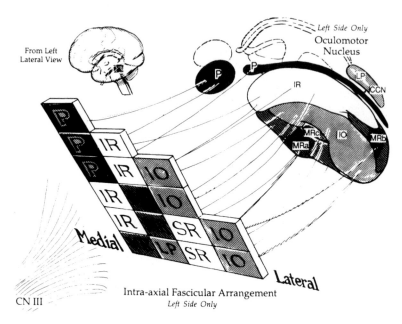

Figure 15.9. Position of the pupillomotor fibers in the fascicle of the human oculomotor nerve. Note that the fibers destined to innervate the iris sphincter muscle (*P*) are located rostral and medial to the fibers that innervate the extraocular muscles and the levator palpebrae superioris (*LP*). *IO*, inferior oblique. *IR*, inferior rectus. *MR*, medial rectus. *SR*, superior rectus. *MRa*, *MRb*, and *MRc*, subnuclei serving medial rectus function in the oculomotor nuclear complex. *CCN*, central caudal nucleus. (Reprinted from: Ksiazek SM, Slamovits TL, Rosen CE, et al. Fascicular arrangement in partial oculomotor paresis. *Am J Ophthalmol.* 1994;118:97–103, with permission.)

Cases of aneurysmal oculomotor nerve palsies characterized *only* by a dilated, nonreactive pupil are extremely unusual. Nevertheless, such cases do occur. Aneurysms of the tip of the basilar artery are more likely to produce isolated pupillary dilation than are aneurysms of the internal carotid artery.

Intrinsic lesions of the oculomotor nerve in the subarachnoid space can produce an oculomotor nerve paresis that begins with a dilated pupil. Such lesions include schwannomas and angiomas.

Damage to the Cavernous Portion of the Oculomotor Nerve   The pupillomotor fibers are located inferiorly and superficially in the portion of the oculomotor nerve located within the cavernous sinus. Damage to the intrinsic aspect of the nerve, particularly ischemia in the setting of diabetes mellitus, not uncommonly produces a pupil-sparing oculomotor nerve palsy; however, it is exceptionally rare to observe an isolated, dilated, nonreactive pupil from damage to the pupillomotor fibers in this region.

Damage to the Ciliary Ganglion and its Roots in the Orbit: Tonic Pupil   Damage to the postganglionic parasympathetic innervation of the intraocular muscles produces a characteristic syndrome. Initially, there may

be an isolated internal ophthalmoplegia. Later, one or more of the following abnormalities may be observed: a poor pupillary reaction to light that can be seen to be a regional palsy of the iris sphincter by slit lamp biomicroscopy, paresis of accommodation, cholinergic supersensitivity of the denervated muscles, a pupillary response to near stimuli that is unusually strong and tonic, and a slow and tonic redilation after constriction to near stimuli.

Pupils that react in this manner are called **tonic pupils** (Fig. 15.11). The lesions that produce them damage the ciliary ganglion or the short ciliary nerves in the retrobulbar space or in the intraocular, suprachoroidal space (Figs. 15.12). The slowness and tonicity of the pupillary movement is caused by aberrant regeneration of ciliary nerves into the iris sphincter. Tonic pupils can be separated into three categories: local, neuropathic, and the Holmes-Adie (Adie's) syndrome.

Local Tonic Pupil. Acute internal ophthalmoplegia followed by the development of a tonic pupil occurs from a variety of inflammations, infections, and infiltrative processes that affect the ciliary ganglion in isolation or as part of a systemic process. Disorders that can cause a **local** tonic pupil include herpes zoster, chickenpox, measles, diphtheria, syphilis (both congenital and

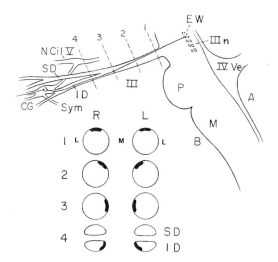

Figure 15.10. Course of preganglionic autonomic nerve fibers from the brainstem to the ciliary ganglion in humans. A sagittal reconstruction of the brainstem with the course of the oculomotor nerve is shown at top. The corresponding locations of the preganglionic autonomic fibers for pupillo-constriction and accommodation within the right (**R**) and left (**L**) oculomotor nerves are shown in black in coronal sections through slices at 1 (emergence from the brainstem), 2 (midpoint in the subarachnoid space), 3 (at the point where the third nerve enters the dura), and 4 (in the anterior cavernous sinus where the fibers have entered the anatomical inferior division of the third nerve). The autonomic fibers are located superiorly as the oculomotor nerve exits the brainstem and then come to lie more medially as the oculomotor nerve passes toward the orbit. *A*, dorsal, and *B*, ventral side of brainstem; *P*, pons; *M*, medulla; *EW*, Edinger-Westphal nucleus; *IIIn*, somatic portion of 3rd nerve nucleus; *III*, 3rd nerve; *ID*, inferior division of 3rd nerve; *SD*, superior division of 3rd nerve; *NCilV*, nasociliary branch of the 5th nerve; *CG*, ciliary ganglion; *Sym*, sympathetic route; *m*, medial; *l*, lateral. (Reprinted from: Kerr FWL, Hallowell OW. Location of pupillomotor and accommodation fibers in the oculomotor nerve: experimental observations on paralytic mydriasis. *J Neurol Neurosurg Psychiatry.* 1964;27:473–481, with permission.)

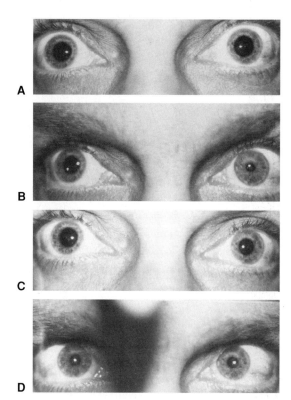

Figure 15.11. Tonic pupil syndrome. About 4 months earlier, this 38-year-old man noted that his right pupil was larger than this left pupil. **A:** In the dark looking in the distance, both pupils are dilated and relatively equal in size. **B:** In bright light, the right pupil does not constrict, whereas the left pupil constricts normally, producing a marked anisocoria. **C:** In room light looking in the distance, there is a moderate anisocoria. **D:** During near viewing, however, both pupils constrict. The right pupil constricted much slower than the left and redilated slowly.

acquired), sarcoidosis, scarlet fever, pertussis, smallpox, influenza, sinusitis, Vogt-Koyanagi-Harada syndrome, rheumatoid arthritis, viral hepatitis, choroiditis, primary and metastatic choroidal and orbital tumors, blunt injury to the globe, and penetrating orbital injury. Siderosis from an intraocular iron foreign body apparently damages the nerves more than the sphincter muscle and may produce an iron mydriasis. Various ocular or orbital surgical procedures, including retinal reattachment surgery, inferior oblique muscle surgery, orbital surgery, optic nerve sheath fenestration, photo-

coagulation, transconjunctival cryotherapy, transscleral diathermy, and retrobulbar injections of alcohol can cause a local tonic pupil, as can inferior dental blocks with local anesthesia. Ischemia of the ciliary ganglion or short ciliary nerves from migraine, giant cell arteritis, and other vasculitides also can cause a tonic pupil.

Neuropathic Tonic Pupil. **Neuropathic tonic pupils** occur in patients in whom a tonic pupil is part of a generalized, widespread, peripheral or autonomic neuropathy that also involves the ciliary ganglion, the short ciliary nerves, or both. In some cases, there is evidence of both a sympathetic and a parasympathetic disturbance. Diseases that produce this syndrome include syphilis, chronic alcoholism, diabetes mellitus, some of the spinocerebellar ataxias, Guillain-Barré syndrome (GBS), and the Miller Fisher variant of GBS. Other systemic diseases involving autonomic nervous system

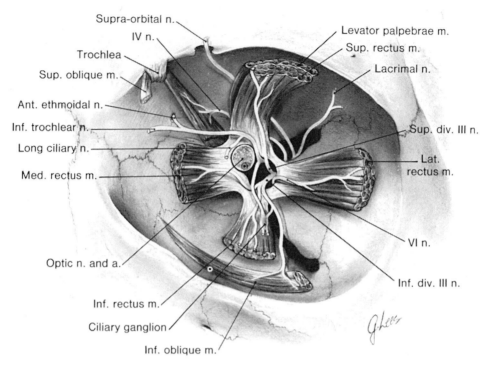

Figure 15.12. View of the posterior orbit showing the relationship of the optic nerve to the ocular motor nerves and extraocular muscles. Note the location of the ciliary ganglion. (Redrawn from: Wolff E. *Anatomy of the Eye and Orbit.* 6th ed. Philadelphia: WB Saunders; 1968.)

dysfunction that may be associated with a tonic pupil are acute pandysautonomia, Shy-Drager syndrome, and Ross syndrome (hyporeflexia, progressive segmental hypohidrosis, and tonic pupil). Patients with systemic lupus erythematosus may develop tonic pupils in association with a more generalized autonomic neuropathy, as may patients with Sjögren's syndrome, in whom the pupillary disturbance may even be the first sign of the disorder. Tonic pupils can also develop in patients with systemic amyloidosis, hereditary sensory neuropathy, a paraneoplastic syndrome, and hereditary motor-sensory neuropathy (Charcot-Marie-Tooth disease).

Holmes–Adie Tonic Pupil Syndrome. The **Holmes-Adie tonic pupil syndrome** (also called Adie's syndrome) consists of unilateral or bilateral tonically reacting pupils developing in otherwise healthy persons and in patients with unrelated conditions. Most of these patients also have a disturbance in deep-tendon reflexes, but they have no evidence of local ocular or orbital disease or of generalized peripheral or autonomic nervous system dysfunction.

Adie's syndrome is not common. It nearly always occurs as a sporadic entity, although it can be familial. Most patients are between 20 and 50 years of age when the condition is noticed. Seventy percent of cases occur in women and 30% in men. Adie's syndrome is unilateral in about 80% of cases. When the condition is bilateral, the onset is occasionally simultaneous but usually occurs in separate episodes months or even years apart.

Most patients with Adie's syndrome have visual complaints including photophobia, blurred near vision, an enlarged pupil, and headaches. Over time, the dilated pupil becomes smaller, and accommodation improves; however, many patients continue to have difficulty focusing. If, some years later, the other eye is similarly affected, as occurs in about 4% of cases per year, it seems to produce far fewer symptoms, and may in fact pass unnoticed.

It may also be confused with a pharmacologically induced mydriasis and cycloplegia until a slit lamp examination is performed, at which time segmental contractions of the iris sphincter are observed (Fig. 15.13). These segmental contractions or "vermiform movements" are observed in all forms of tonic pupil, including Adie's syndrome, whereas a pharmacologic anticholinergic blockade always paralyzes the *entire* sphincter. Segmental palsy of the iris sphincter is a critical diagnostic observation. Almost every Adie's pupil that has any reaction to light (about 90%) has such a segmental palsy of the sphincter.

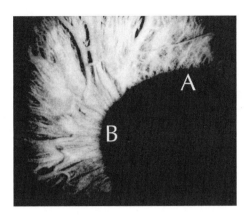

Figure 15.13. Segmental palsy of the iris sphincter in Adie's tonic pupil syndrome. **A:** This part of the iris sphincter is denervated and does not react to light. **B:** This sphincter segment constricts to light.

In most patients with Adie's syndrome, the accommodative paresis resolves over several months. In some patients, however, aberrant regeneration within the ciliary muscle produces an accommodative paresis that may persist until presbyopia develops and diminishes the symptoms.

Hyporeflexia or areflexia is present in a substantial number of patients with Adie's syndrome. The most likely explanation is that the responsible lesion is located centrally within the spinal cord. Indeed, pathologic studies in a few patients with Adie's syndrome report atrophic changes in the dorsal columns. It thus seems most likely that degeneration of cell bodies in the dorsal columns similar to that which occurs in the ciliary ganglion is responsible for the loss of deep-tendon reflexes that occur in the majority of patients with Adie's syndrome.

The tonic pupil of patients with Adie's syndrome is supersensitive to acetylcholine and similar substances, including pilocarpine. For example, conjunctival administration of 2 drops of a 0.1% solution of pilocarpine causes intense miosis in most tonic pupils (Fig. 15.14), whereas such solutions do not generally cause any change in the size of normal pupils. Unfortunately, the clinical usefulness of the **denervation supersensitivity test** for a tonic pupil is limited because the pupils of many patients with oculomotor nerve palsies constrict about as much as Adie's pupils to weak solutions of pilocarpine.

Denervation supersensitivity is caused by an effector cell becoming more sensitive to a transmitter substance or its analogs after the nerves have been severed. This increased sensitivity occurs whether the preganglionic or the postganglionic neuron is damaged, although the degree of supersensitivity is generally somewhat greater after a postganglionic denervation than after a preganglionic denervation. If the diagnosis of a tonic pupil is uncertain, it is certainly appropriate to test for cholinergic supersensitivity. We use a 0.1% pilocarpine solution, prepared in a syringe from 1 part commercially available 1% pilocarpine and 9 parts normal saline. The sphincter should not be considered supersensitive unless it becomes the smaller of the two medicated pupils.

Five features of Adie's syndrome change over time: the accommodation paresis seems to recover; the pupillary light reaction does not recover and may become even weaker, deep-tendon reflexes tend to become increasingly hyporeflexic, the affected pupil gradually becomes smaller, and there is a tendency for patients with unilateral Adie's syndrome to develop a tonic pupil in the opposite eye with time.

The etiology of Adie's syndrome remains obscure. Both pharmacologic studies and pathologic studies

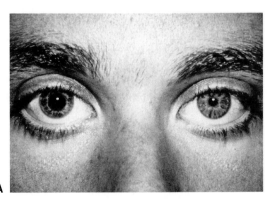
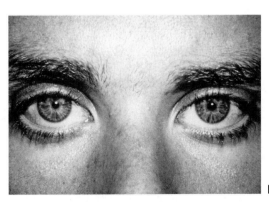

Figure 15.14. Postganglionic supersensitivity in the tonic pupil syndrome. **A:** A right tonic pupil in a 36-year-old woman. **B:** At 45 minutes after conjunctival instillation of 2 drops of 0.1% pilocarpine solution in each eye, the right pupil is constricted and nonreactive. The left pupil remains unchanged and normally reactive.

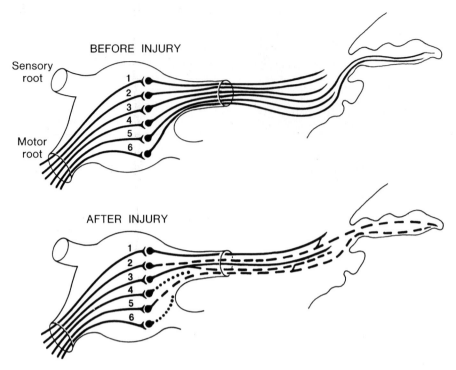

Figure 15.15. Misregeneration theory as it pertains to the findings in the tonic pupil syndrome. Before injury, most of the fibers in the ciliary ganglion are destined for the ciliary muscle to produce accommodation **(Above).** Following injury, it is more likely that a regenerating postganglionic fiber will be one for accommodation; however, many of these fibers send branches or collaterals to the iris, producing pupillary constriction during attempted accommodation-convergence **(Below).** In this drawing, postganglionic fiber 1, for accommodation, has not been injured; fibers 2 and 5, also accommodative, have regenerated, sending sprouts to both the ciliary muscle and the iris sphincter; fiber 3, for pupillary constriction, has sent a sprout to the ciliary muscle via the remaining nerve sheath of fiber 4, which has been damaged; fiber 6, for pupillary constriction, has been destroyed and has not regenerated. Thus, accommodation and pupillary constriction will occur primarily on attempted accommodation-convergence.

indicate that the ciliary ganglion, short ciliary nerves, or both are the location of the lesion that produces Adie's syndrome.

The explanation for why the light reflex is so much more severely impaired than the near vision constriction is that the near vision reaction is not so much **spared** as it is **restored.** Fibers originally destined for the ciliary muscle resprout randomly, with some of the fibers reaching the iris sphincter and causing a miosis every time the ciliary muscle is stimulated. In addition, pupillomotor fibers to the iris sphincter muscle constitute only about 3% of the total number of postganglionic neurons that leave the ciliary ganglion; the remainder innervate the ciliary muscle. Thus, when the ciliary ganglion is injured, there is a greater chance of survival for cells or fibers that serve accommodation than for those that innervate the iris. When the new collateral fibers sprout, the probability is much greater that these new fibers arise from accommodative elements than from those that originally innervated the

iris. These new fibers now innervate both the ciliary muscle and the iris, and the pupil once again constricts when the patient looks at a near object (Fig 15.15).

Damage to the Iris Sphincter   Tears in the iris sphincter or in the iris base may occur from blunt trauma to the eye. Such damage may produce a nonreactive or poorly reactive irregularly dilated pupil that may be mistaken for the dilated pupil of an oculomotor nerve palsy. In most cases, iris tears or dialysis are easily observed using a standard or portable slit lamp. Other signs suggesting damage to the eye, which may be present in a patient with iris sphincter damage, include scattered pigment on the anterior iris stroma, pigment on the anterior lens capsule (Vossius' ring), focal cataract, choroidal rupture, commotio retinae, and retinal hemorrhages.

Pharmacologic Blockade with Parasympatholytic Agents   A dilated, nonreactive pupil can be caused

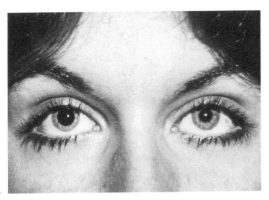
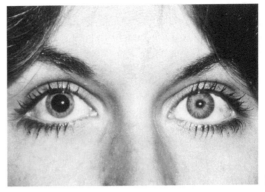

A

B

Figure 15.16. Pharmacologically dilated pupil. **A:** Nonreactive, dilated right pupil in an 18-year-old woman complaining of headache and blurred vision. **B:** At 45 minutes after conjunctival instillation of 2 drops of 1% pilocarpine in each eye, the right pupil is unchanged, whereas the left pupil is markedly constricted. The patient subsequently admitted having placed topical scopolamine in the right eye.

by topical administration of one of several parasympatholytic agents, many of which are described later in the section on drug effects. It should be emphasized that pharmacologic mydriasis is extreme, usually more than 8 mm. Because an acute tonic pupil may have a somewhat similar appearance, it is necessary to be able to distinguish between these two entities. In addition, although a dilated pupil from oculomotor nerve involvement is rarely widely dilated and is nearly always associated with other signs of oculomotor nerve dysfunction, clinicians occasionally become concerned that a dilated, nonreactive pupil may be the earliest sign of an acute oculomotor nerve palsy. A 1% solution of pilocarpine can be used to differentiate a pupil that is dilated from pharmacologic blockade of the iris sphincter cells from a pupil that is dilated from neurologic damage to the parasympathetic pathway from the brainstem to the iris sphincter. A pupil that is dilated from pharmacologic blockade will be unchanged

or poorly constricted by a topical solution of pilocarpine strong enough to maximally constrict the opposite pupil (Fig. 15.16), and a tonic pupil will constrict to even weaker solutions of pilocarpine because of denervation supersensitivity (see previous text) and should certainly constrict to 1% pilocarpine. A pupil that is dilated from oculomotor nerve dysfunction will also constrict maximally after instillation of pilocarpine.

Anisocoria That May Be More Obvious in Darkness or in Light When some normal persons look in extreme lateral gaze, the pupil on that side becomes larger than the pupil on the opposite side, which becomes smaller. This phenomenon is called **Tournay's phenomenon.** It is of no clinical significance.

Transient unilateral dilation of the pupil occurs in otherwise healthy young adults in association with blurred vision and headaches (Fig. 15.17). No other signs of oculomotor nerve palsy are present in these

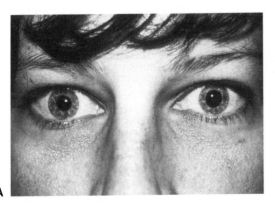
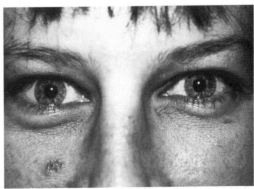

A

B

Figure 15.17. Intermittent unilateral pupillary dilation in a young woman during a severe migraine headache. **A:** During the migraine attack, the left pupil is dilated and poorly reactive. Accommodation is normal, however, suggesting that the dilation is caused by sympathetic hyperactivity rather than parasympathetic hypoactivity. **B:** Between attacks, the pupils are isocoric.

patients, and neuroimaging studies, including cerebral arteriography, show no intracranial abnormalities. Such patients were once thought to have a variant of ophthalmoplegic migraine, and it was believed that damage to efferent pupillomotor fibers along the oculomotor nerve or in the orbit were responsible; however, some patients demonstrate sympathetic hyperactivity of the iris rather than parasympathetic weakness.

Thus, the first step in determining the management of a patient with a headache and a unilateral dilated pupil is to determine, by assessing the reactivity of the pupils to light and the amount of accommodative amplitude if the anisocoria is caused by parasympathetic or sympathetic dysfunction. If sympathetic hyperactivity is present, no further assessment is necessary. Although some patients with parasympathetic insufficiency may require angiography to exclude an aneurysm, the availability of increasingly sensitive neuroimaging tests, such as standard MRI, MR angiography, and CT angiography, allows such patients to be evaluated in a noninvasive manner, and, if the studies are negative, to be followed for either resolution of pupillary dilation or development of other signs of oculomotor nerve dysfunction.

Transient unilateral pupillary dilation occurs in some healthy persons unassociated with headache, and this phenomenon may also be caused by parasympathetic interruption or sympathetic irritation. Such episodes may last minutes, hours, or even weeks, and they may recur for several years. In some patients, the pupillary dilation is associated with evidence of loss of accommodation in the affected eye, thus implicating a parasympathetic process; however, in others, there is other evidence of autonomic dysfunction, including labile blood pressure and erythromelalgia of the neck and thorax. These features, along with normal accommodation, suggest hyperactivity of the sympathetic system. Thus, episodic unilateral pupillary mydriasis, whether or not it is associated with headache, may be caused by parasympathetic hypofunction or sympathetic hyperfunction.

Differentiation of Anisocoria   From a practical standpoint, anisocoria that is more evident in darkness than in light indicates that the iris sphincter muscles and the parasympathetic pathway that constricts them are intact. There is more dilation in darkness of one pupil than the other, because both pupils constrict to light stimulation, but one pupil dilates more in darkness than the other. Anisocoria that is more evident in light than in darkness indicates a defect of the ocular parasympathetic pathway, the iris sphincter muscles, or both. This permits a relatively straightforward approach to the patient with anisocoria, using the reaction of the pupils to light stimulation as the initial differentiating feature (Fig. 15.18).

If there is a good light reaction in both eyes, the patient almost always has either physiologic anisocoria or a Horner's syndrome. These two entities are then differentiated using the cocaine test. If the cocaine test indicates that the patient has a Horner's syndrome, the hydroxyamphetamine test is performed on another occasion at least 24 hours later to differentiate a central or preganglionic Horner's syndrome from a postganglionic Horner's syndrome. We do not routinely test for sympathetic denervation sensitivity; however, this can be done using a 1% solution of phenylephrine or a similarly weak solution of epinephrine.

If there is a poor light reaction in one or both eyes, the patient has a defect of the parasympathetic system or the iris sphincter muscle. The iris should be examined using a slit lamp biomicroscope to determine if there is a sphincter tear or other iris damage and to see if there is any evidence of a segmental palsy of the iris sphincter or vermiform movements. If there is no evidence of iris damage, a 1% solution of pilocarpine can be used to distinguish between a pharmacologically blockaded pupil and a neurogenic cause. If the results of the test indicate neurogenic anisocoria, but there is no other evidence of an oculomotor nerve paresis, a 0.1% solution of pilocarpine can be used at another time to detect denervation supersensitivity of the parasympathetic system that most often occurs in association with a tonic pupil syndrome. Alternatively, one can begin with a 0.1% solution of pilocarpine to test for denervation supersensitivity. If neither pupil constricts, a 1% solution of pilocarpine can then be used at the same sitting.

AFFERENT ABNORMALITIES
The Relative Afferent Pupillary Defect

The relative afferent pupil defect (RAPD) is one of the most important objective signs in ophthalmology. It may be the only evidence of organic afferent visual sensory system dysfunction in a patient who complains of visual loss in one or both eyes but who has a normal ocular fundus.

Most patients with a unilateral or pathologically asymmetric bilateral **optic neuropathy,** regardless of the cause, have a RAPD (Fig. 15.19). Patients with **glaucoma** have a RAPD only if the glaucoma is unilateral or asymmetric, and patients with **optic disc drusen** have a RAPD only when there is associated visual field loss in one eye only or asymmetrically in both eyes. If visual acuity is 20/200 or better and is caused by **macular disease,** such as macular degeneration, any RAPD will usually be 0.5 log units or less. Indeed, it is difficult to produce a RAPD greater than 1.0 log units with a lesion confined to the macula. Central serous maculopathy, which can occasionally mimic an optic neuropathy, produces a minimal RAPD, usually 0.3

ANISOCORIA

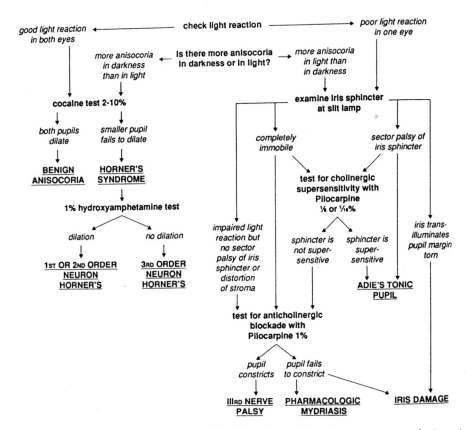

Figure 15.18. Flow chart indicating steps that should be taken to differentiate among causes of anisocoria.

log units or less. A RAPD can occur in a patient with a **retinal detachment.** Each quadrant of a fresh, bullous retinal detachment produces about 0.3 log of RAPD, and when the macula detaches, the RAPD increases by about another 0.7 log units. A RAPD can be produced by a **central retinal vein occlusion** (CRVO), particularly when the occlusion is of the ischemic variety. About 90% of nonischemic CRVOs are associated with a RAPD that is 0.3 log units or less, and none have a RAPD larger than 0.9 log units. In contrast, over 90% of ischemic CRVOs are associated with a RAPD of 1.2 log units or more, and none have a RAPD smaller than 0.6 log units.

In **anisocoria,** the eye with the smaller pupil has a relatively shaded retina, and when less light strikes one retina during the swinging flashlight test it can look like a RAPD. This asymmetry only becomes clinically significant when one pupil is very small or when the anisocoria is large (2 mm or more). In suppression **amblyopia,** a small RAPD can often be seen in an am-

blyopic eye. It is generally less than 0.5 log units, and the number does not correlate well with the visual acuity. An eye that is **occluded** becomes increasingly dark-adapted and light-sensitive during the first 30 minutes of occlusion. This can temporarily produce up to 1.5 log units of a false RAPD in the unpatched eye.

A unilateral **cataract,** even one that is very dense and brunescent, produces little or no RAPD. This may be partly because of the dark-adapted retina behind the cataract and partly because the beam of light coming through the pupil is caught by the cataract and lights up the crystalline lens like an intraocular Chinese lantern. The light then shines in all directions, causing excess retinal stimulation. Indeed, a unilateral, white, opaque cataract routinely seems to produce a small RAPD in the opposite eye.

A complete or nearly complete lesion of the **optic tract** not only produces a contralateral homonymous hemianopia, it also produces a definite RAPD (0.3 to 1.8 log units) in the contralateral eye—the eye with

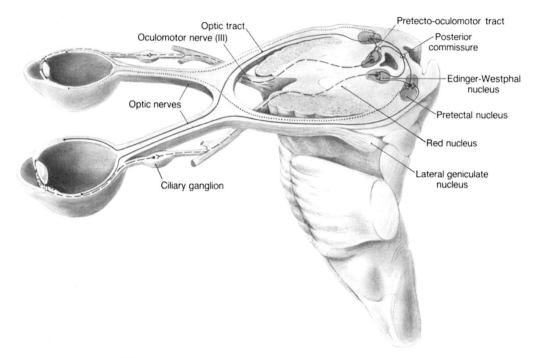

Figure 15.19. Diagram of the path of the pupillary light reflex.

the temporal field loss. This is partly because there are more crossed than uncrossed fibers in the chiasm and also because there are more crossed than uncrossed fibers in the midbrain hemidecussation of the pupillary pathways.

Most patients with homonymous hemianopias do not have a RAPD unless the lesion affects the contralateral optic tract. An exception is the patient with a **postgeniculate congenital homonymous hemianopia.** In such cases, the RAPD is on the side opposite the lesion (on the side of the hemianopia) and results from transsynaptic degeneration of the optic tract ipsilateral to the lesion. Such patients also have bilateral, hemianopic retinal and optic nerve atrophy.

A unilateral lesion in the **pretectal nucleus or in the brachium of the superior colliculus** will damage the pupillary fibers coming from the ipsilateral optic tract. This can produce a contralateral RAPD without any loss of visual acuity or color vision and without any visual field defect, although the RAPD may occasionally be associated with an ipsilateral or contralateral trochlear nerve paresis. In addition, lesions that involve the lateral geniculate body or the proximal portion of the retrogeniculate pathway may be associated with a contralateral RAPD not from involvement of that pathway but from involvement of the adjacent intercalated neurons between the visual pathway and the pupillomotor centers in the pretectum.

Neither nonorganic loss of visual acuity nor nonorganic constriction of the visual field in one eye ever produces a RAPD. In contrast, the vast majority of patients with monocular neurogenic loss of the visual field do have a RAPD. Thus, the absence of this sign in a patient with monocular loss of vision and no evidence of a refractive error, opacified media, or small macular lesion should suggest a nonorganic process. If a patient with a suspected unilateral optic neuropathy, regardless of the cause, has no RAPD, either the patient does not have an optic neuropathy or the patient has a bilateral optic neuropathy.

Some normal subjects show a persistent but small RAPD in the absence of any detectable pathologic disease. The RAPD in such cases is quite small, usually 0.3 log units or less, and variable in degree.

Wernicke's Pupil

When the optic chiasm is bisected sagittally, the nasal halves of each retina become insensitive to light so that there is not only a bitemporal hemianopia but also a bitemporal pupillary hemiakinesia. Light falling on the nasal retina of either eye will fail to produce pupillary constriction.

Poorly Reacting Pupils from Midbrain Disease

Dilated, nonreactive pupils and pupils that react poorly to both light and near stimuli may be produced by damage to the afferent input to the visceral oculomotor nuclei or by damage to the nuclei and their efferent fiber tracts. The precise location of such lesions is almost impossible to determine unless there is associated evidence of ocular motor nerve dysfunction. A variety of pupillary abnormalities can be detected in patients with tumors in the pineal region. Some patients have markedly impaired light reactions but relatively intact responses to near stimuli (classic light-near dissociation), whereas others have impairment of both light and near reactions, and rare patients have relatively intact light reactions but impaired responses to near stimuli (inverse Argyll Robertson pupils).

Dilated, nonreactive or poorly reactive pupils that occur in patients with pinealomas and other tumors that damage the dorsal mesencephalon are usually bilateral and may precede the development of supranuclear paralysis of conjugate upward gaze. In some cases, there may initially be light-near dissociation.

Bilateral, dilated, nonreactive pupils rarely occur in isolation when caused by damage to the rostral oculomotor nuclear complex. Lesions that produce these changes must be located in the periaqueductal gray matter near the rostral end of the aqueduct. Vascular, inflammatory, neoplastic, and demyelinating diseases that affect this area almost always produce associated signs, including nuclear ophthalmoplegia, paralysis of vertical gaze, loss of convergence, exotropia, ptosis, and other defects of ocular movement.

Paradoxical Reaction of the Pupils to Light and Darkness

Patients with congenital stationary night blindness, congenital achromatopsia, blue-cone monochromatism, and Leber's congenital amaurosis often exhibit a "paradoxical" pupillary response characterized by constriction in darkness. In a lighted room, such patients often have moderately dilated pupils; however, when the room lights are extinguished, the patients' pupils briskly constrict and then slowly redilate. Such responses occasionally occur in patients with optic disc hypoplasia, autosomal-dominant optic atrophy, and bilateral optic neuritis. These pupillary responses probably occur not from abnormalities in the CNS but from selective delays in afferent signals from the retinal photoreceptors to the pupillomotor center.

LIGHT-NEAR DISSOCIATION

Normal pupils constrict not only from light stimulation but also during near viewing as part of the **near response** of convergence, accommodation, and miosis. A constriction of the pupils during near viewing that is stronger than the light response—**light-near dissociation**—may be caused by a defect in the afferent or the

efferent system subserving pupillary function. For example, this is the primary feature of the Argyll Robertson pupils that occur from efferent dysfunction, but it is also seen in patients with pregeniculate blindness, compressive and infiltrative mesencephalic lesions, and damage to the parasympathetic innervation of the iris sphincter.

Argyll Robertson Pupils

The characteristic features of this syndrome as first described are (a) retinas sensitive to light, (b) pupils unresponsive to light, (c) normal pupillary constriction during accommodation and convergence for near objects, and (d) very small pupils (Fig. 15.20). The Argyll Robertson pupil is widely accepted as being almost pathognomonic of neurosyphilis.

Argyll Robertson pupils are typically small and dilate poorly in darkness. An additional important feature is irregularity of the pupil. In the fully developed Argyll Robertson pupil, there is complete loss of pupillary constriction. Although constriction of the pupils to near stimulation often appears normal, the reaction usually is slightly impaired. Argyll Robertson pupils are usually bilateral and symmetric.

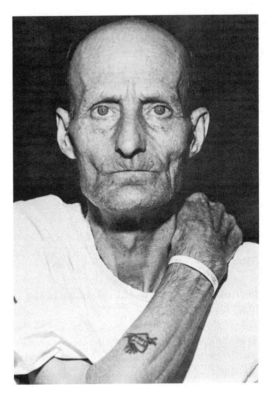

Figure 15.20. Argyll Robertson pupils in a tabetic merchant seaman. Even in the semidarkness that preceded the photographer's flash, the pupils are so small as to be hidden behind the corneal reflection.

The site of the lesion responsible for the production of Argyll Robertson pupils is the region of the sylvian aqueduct in the rostral midbrain. In this location, the damage interferes with the light reflex fibers and the supranuclear inhibitory fibers as they approach the visceral oculomotor nuclei, but it spares the fibers subserving pupillary constriction for near viewing.

The "complete" Argyll Robertson syndrome may be observed in patients with diabetes mellitus, chronic alcoholism, encephalitis, multiple sclerosis, age-related and degenerative diseases of the CNS, some rare midbrain tumors, and, rarely, in systemic inflammatory diseases, including sarcoidosis and neuroborreliosis. However, a patient with Argyll Robertson pupils should still be assumed to have neurosyphilis until proven otherwise.

Mesencephalic Lesions

Pressure on the dorsal mesencephalon may produce Parinaud's syndrome (also called the sylvian aqueduct syndrome or dorsal midbrain syndrome). This syndrome of the rostral midbrain in the region of the posterior commissure consists of supranuclear paralysis of upward gaze (often worse for saccades than pursuit), lid retraction, accommodation difficulties, convergence-retraction nystagmus on attempted upward gaze, and disturbances of pupillary function. The pupils in such patients are typically large, fail to constrict to light or do so very poorly, and yet react well to near stimuli (Fig. 15.21). Such pupils may be the first sign of a pineal or other tumor that compresses or infiltrates the dorsal midbrain or of hydrocephalus, particularly that caused by aqueductal stenosis or a blocked shunt.

Lesions of the Afferent Pathway

Lesions of the visual sensory pathway from the retina to the point at which the pupillomotor fibers exit impair the light reaction but spare the near response. If the patient is blind from optic nerve disease, for example, there will be no reaction of the pupil in the blind eye to direct light stimulation, but the near reaction may be well preserved when tested using proprioception as a stimulus.

Aberrant Regeneration after Damage to the Innervation of the Iris Sphincter

In some patients who have damage to the innervation of the iris sphincter, the light reaction is not truly "spared," rather it is restored by aberrant regeneration of damaged fibers. This phenomenon occurs in the setting of aberrant regeneration after structural damage to the **preganglionic** oculomotor nerve. Fibers headed for extraocular muscles or the ciliary muscle may be diverted into the iris sphincter, which is such a small muscle that only a few of these fibers are sufficient to

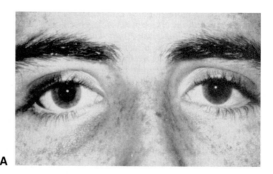

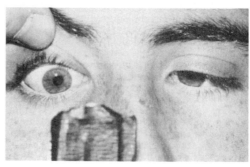

A

B

Figure 15.21. Pupillary light-near dissociation in a patient with a dysgerminoma producing a dorsal midbrain syndrome. In a dimly lighted room, both pupils were large and slightly anisocoric. **A:** When a bright light is shined in either eye, both pupils constrict sluggishly and incompletely. **B:** When the patient is asked to look at an accommodative target, both pupils constrict briskly and extensively. The patient also had difficulty with upward gaze.

make the iris sphincter contract. Although such pupils are often called "tonic" pupils, two cardinal features of the tonic pupil—a slow sustained contraction to near effort and a slow redilation after constriction—are absent.

DISTURBANCES DURING SEIZURES

Some patients, most of them children, experience unilateral, transient pupillary mydriasis during and after seizures. In most instances, the seizures are of the petit mal type. The mechanism of the pupillary dilation that occurs during and following seizure activity appears to be a combination of interruption of parasympathetic impulses and irritation of the sympathetic system.

Not all patients with pupillary disturbances during a seizure have dilation of the pupils. Some experience ictal unilateral or bilateral pupillary constriction, with and without ptosis.

DISTURBANCES IN COMA

Coma is a state of unarousable psychologic unresponsiveness in which the patient lies with eyes closed.

Patients in coma show no psychologically understandable response to external stimuli or inner needs. Causes of coma include supratentorial lesions, infratentorial lesions, and diffuse brain dysfunction from a variety of inflammatory, infectious, degenerative, and metabolic processes. The prevalence of pupillary abnormalities in comatose patients is high and may, in some instances, help in the initial understanding and localization of the process.

Cerebral lesions that cause coma may produce primary abnormalities of pupillary size and reactivity. For example, damage to the **hypothalamus,** especially in the posterior and ventrolateral regions, may produce an ipsilateral central Horner's syndrome. Downward displacement of the hypothalamus with unilateral Horner's syndrome is often the first clear sign of incipient transtentorial herniation. Damage to the **diencephalon,** particularly during rostral-caudal brainstem deterioration caused by supratentorial lesions, produces symmetrically small but briskly reactive pupils.

Lesions of the dorsal tectal or pretectal regions of the **mesencephalon** interrupt the pupillary light reflex but may spare the response to near stimuli (light-near dissociation). The pupils are either in midposition or slightly dilated and are round. Mesencephalic lesions in the region of the oculomotor nerve nucleus nearly always damage both sympathetic and parasympathetic pathways to the eye. The resulting pupils are usually slightly irregular and unequal. They are midposition and nonreactive to light stimuli.

Lesions of the tegmental portion of the **pons** may interrupt descending sympathetic pathways and produce bilaterally small pupils. In many cases, especially those with pontine hemorrhage, the pupils are pinpoint, presumably from a combination of sympathetic interruption and parasympathetic disinhibition.

The pupillary fibers within the **peripheral oculomotor nerve** are particularly susceptible when uncal herniation compresses the nerve against the posterior cerebral artery or the edge of the cerebellar tentorium. In these instances, pupillary dilation may precede other signs of ocular motor nerve paralysis, and such patients may present with nonreactive, dilated, or oval pupils.

Supratentorial lesions produce neurologic dysfunction by two mechanisms: primary cerebral damage and secondary brainstem dysfunction from displacement, tissue compression, swelling, and vascular stasis. Of the two processes, secondary brainstem dysfunction is the more threatening to life. It usually presents as one of two main patterns. Most patients develop signs of bilateral diencephalic impairment: **the central syndrome.** In this syndrome, pupillary, ocular motor, and respiratory signs develop that indicate that diencephalic, mesencephalic, pontine, and, finally, medullary function are being lost in an orderly rostral-caudal fashion. Other patients develop signs of uncal herniation with oculomotor nerve and lateral mesencephalic compression, either ipsilaterally or contralaterally: **the uncal syndrome.**

In patients in deep coma, the state of the pupils may become the single most important criterion that clinically distinguishes between metabolic and structural disease. Pupillary pathways are relatively resistant to metabolic insults. Thus, the presence of preserved pupillary light reflexes despite concomitant respiratory depression, caloric unresponsiveness, decerebrate rigidity, or motor flaccidity suggests **metabolic coma.** Conversely, if asphyxia, drug ingestion, or preexisting pupillary disease can be eliminated as a cause of coma, the absence of pupillary light reflexes in a comatose patient strongly implicates a structural lesion rather than a metabolic process.

DISTURBANCES IN DISORDERS OF THE NEUROMUSCULAR JUNCTION

Despite being of neuroectodermal origin, the iris musculature may be affected by systemic myopathies and by generalized disorders of the neuromuscular junction. Although most investigators describe no pupillary abnormalities in patients with **myasthenia gravis,** rare patients with ocular myasthenia gravis have anisocoria, sluggishly reactive pupils, or both that show fatigue on prolonged light stimulation. This dysfunction **is not clinically significant** and should not confuse the diagnosis.

Botulism is a life-threatening disease that occurs from the effects of the toxin produced by one of several strains of the organism, *Clostridium botulinum.* In most instances, the source of the botulism is oral ingestion of the toxin in spoiled foods. Nearly all patients who develop botulism have multiple symptoms and signs of cholinergic dysfunction, including dilated, poorly reactive or nonreactive pupils, paresis of accommodation, ptosis, and ophthalmoplegia.

DRUG EFFECTS
Drugs That Dilate the Pupils

Parasympatholytic (Anticholinergic) Drugs   The pharmacology of the parasympathetic innervation of the iris is illustrated in Figure 15.22.

Sympathomimetic (Adrenergic) Drugs   The pharmacology of the sympathetic innervation of the iris is illustrated in Figure 15.23.

Drugs That Constrict the Pupils

Parasympathomimetic (Cholinergic) Drugs   The pharmacology of the parasympathetic innervation of the iris is illustrated in Figure 15.22.

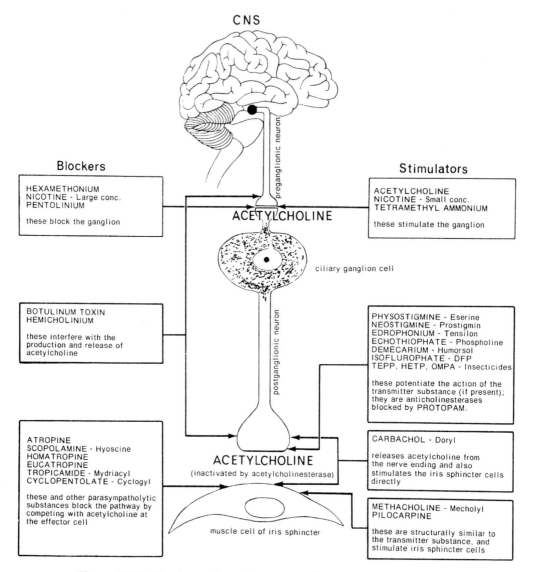

Figure 15.22. The pharmacology of the parasympathetic innervation of the iris.

Sympatholytic (Antiadrenergic) Drugs   The pharmacology of the sympathetic innervation of the iris is illustrated in Figure 15.23.

STRUCTURAL DEFECTS OF THE IRIS
Congenital

Aniridia is a congenital abnormality in which the iris appears clinically to be absent (Fig. 15.24A). In almost all cases, histologic or gonioscopic examination reveals small remnants of iris tissue. The condition is usually bilateral and may occur as a hereditary condition or as a sporadic phenomenon. When the condition is hereditary, it is usually transmitted in an autosomal-dominant

fashion; however, rare cases of recessive transmission occur. Patients with aniridia usually have poor visual acuity and other ocular abnormalities, including nystagmus, glaucoma, cataracts, ectopia lentis, corneal degeneration, and optic nerve or macular hypoplasia or aplasia. Systemic abnormalities found in patients with aniridia include polydactyly, oligophrenia, cranial dysostosis, malformations of the extremities and external ears, hydrocephalus, cerebellar ataxia, and mental retardation. The most important association, however, is with the childhood cancer Wilms' tumor.

A **coloboma** is a full-thickness defect that may be limited to the iris tissue or may be part of a larger defect involving the ciliary body, choroid, and optic disc

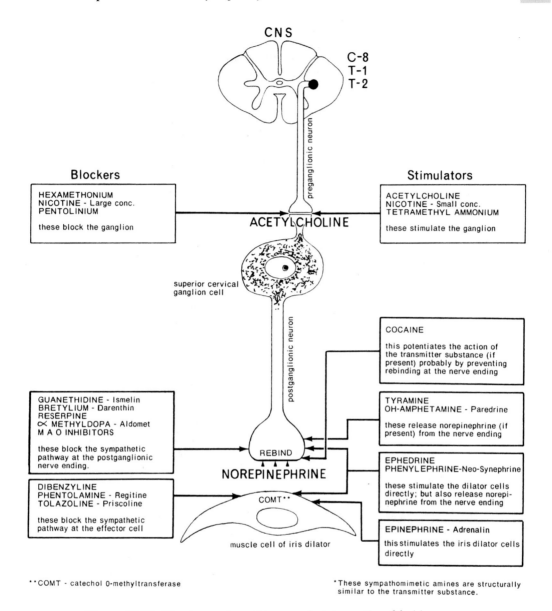

CNS

C-8
T-1
T-2

preganglionic neuron

Blockers

HEXAMETHONIUM
NICOTINE - Large conc.
PENTOLINIUM

these block the ganglion

ACETYLCHOLINE

Stimulators

ACETYLCHOLINE
NICOTINE - Small conc.
TETRAMETHYL AMMONIUM

these stimulate the ganglion

superior cervical
ganglion cell

postganglionic neuron

COCAINE

this potentiates the action of
the transmitter substance (if
present) probably by preventing
rebinding at the nerve ending

GUANETHIDINE - Ismelin
BRETYLIUM - Darenthin
RESERPINE
∝ METHYLDOPA - Aldomet
M A O INHIBITORS

these block the sympathetic
pathway at the postganglionic
nerve ending.

TYRAMINE
OH-AMPHETAMINE - Paredrine

these release norepinephrine (if
present) from the nerve ending

REBIND

NOREPINEPHRINE

DIBENZYLINE
PHENTOLAMINE - Regitine
TOLAZOLINE - Priscoline

these block the sympathetic
pathway at the effector cell

COMT**

muscle cell of iris dilator

EPHEDRINE
PHENYLEPHRINE-Neo-Synephrine

these stimulate the dilator cells
directly; but also release norepinephrine from the nerve ending

EPINEPHRINE - Adrenalin

this stimulates the iris dilator cells
directly

**COMT - catechol 0-methyltransferase

*These sympathomimetic amines are structurally
similar to the transmitter substance.

Figure 15.23. The pharmacology of the sympathetic innervation of the iris.

(Fig. 15.24B). Coloboma of the iris may be transmitted either as a dominant or a recessive trait.

Misplaced or **ectopic pupils** (corectopia, ectopia pupillae) are usually bilateral and symmetric. They are typically displaced up and out from the center of the cornea. Such displacement of the pupils may be isolated but is frequently associated with ectopia lentis, congenital glaucoma, microcornea, ocular coloboma, albinism, external ophthalmoplegia, and high myopia (Fig. 15.24C).

Persistent pupillary membrane remnants are vestiges of the embryonic pupillary membrane that can be seen as thread-like bands running across the pupillary space and attaching to the lesser circle of the iris (Fig. 15.24D). These remnants do not interfere with pupillary movements, and they rarely have clinical significance.

In true **polycoria,** the extra pupil(s) has a sphincter muscle that contracts on exposure to light. In fact, most additional pupils are actually just holes in the iris without a separate sphincter muscle. This **pseudopolycoria** may be a congenital disorder, such as an iris coloboma or persistent pupillary membrane, or it may be part of one of several syndromes

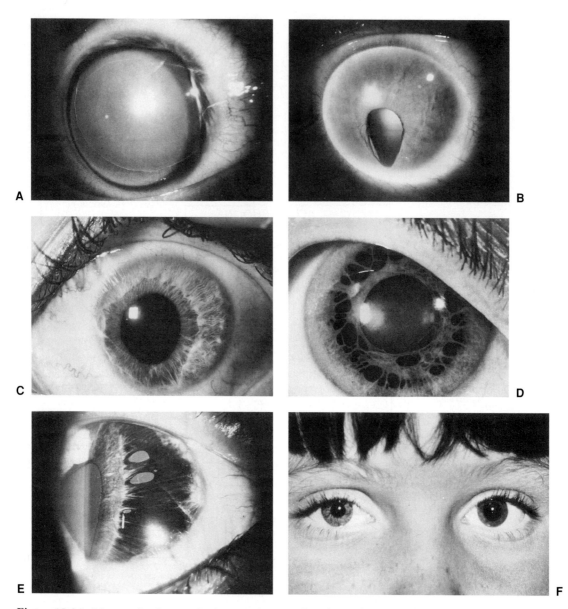

Figure 15.24. Iris anomalies that may simulate neurologic pupillary abnormalities. **A:** Aniridia. Note associated upward lens dislocation. (Courtesy of Dr. Irene H. Maumenee.) **B:** Typical iris coloboma. (Courtesy of Dr. Irene H. Maumenee.) **C:** Acquired corectopia in iridocorneal-endothelial adhesion syndrome. (Courtesy of Dr. Harry A: Quigley.) **D:** Persistent pupillary membrane. (Reprinted from: Gutman ED, Goldberg MF. Persistent pupillary membrane and other ocular abnormalities. *Arch Ophthalmol.* 1976;94:156–157, with permission.) **E:** Pseudopolycoria from iridocorneal-endothelial adhesion syndrome. (Courtesy of Dr. Harry A. Quigley.) **F:** Heterochromia iridis in a patient with congenital Horner's syndrome. Note that the lighter iris is the abnormal iris.

characterized by mesodermal dysgenesis. More commonly, pseudopolycoria occurs as an acquired disorder from direct iris trauma, including surgery, photocoagulation, ischemia, and glaucoma, or as part of a degenerative process such as the ICE syndrome (Fig. 15.24E).

Congenital miosis, which is usually bilateral, is characterized by extremely small pupils that react slightly to light stimuli and dilate poorly after instillation of sympathomimetic agents. The anomaly appears to result from congenital absence of the iris dilator muscle. Congenital miosis may be an isolated phenomenon, or it may be associated with other ocular abnormalities, including microcornea, iris atrophy, myopia, heterochromia iridis, and anterior chamber angle deformities.

Congenital mydriasis is a unilateral or bilateral disorder that may be difficult to distinguish from aniridia unless a careful ocular examination is performed. There appear to be numerous causes of congenital mydriasis. It may occur as an isolated phenomenon or in association with developmental delay and has been reported in a patient with Waardenburg syndrome.

The color of the iris depends upon the pigment in the iris stroma. In albinism, there is failure of mesodermal and ectodermal pigmentation. Consequently, the iris has a transparent, grayish-red color and transilluminates readily. In a number of congenital and acquired conditions, the iris of one eye differs in color from the iris of the other eye. In other instances, one iris is entirely normal, and a part of the iris in the opposite eye has a different color than the rest of the iris surrounding it ("iris bicolor"). These abnormalities, collectively called **heterochromia iridis,** may occur as: (a) an isolated congenital anomaly; (b) in association with other ocular abnormalities, such as iris or optic disc coloboma; (c) in association with systemic congenital abnormalities, as in patients with Waardenburg's syndrome, congenital Horner's syndrome, or incontinentia pigmenti; or (d) from an acquired ocular condition (Fig. 15.24F).

Acquired

Iritis or **iridocyclitis** in its acute stages produces swelling of the iris, miosis, and slight reddening of the circumcorneal tissues. The miosis of iritis results from the release of a neurohumor, substance P, that produces miosis through interaction with a specific receptor in the iris sphincter muscle. In patients with intraocular inflammation, dilation of the pupil with mydriatics may be difficult because of adhesions between the iris and the lens (posterior synechiae). These adhesions in chronic iritis may distort the shape of the pupil. They may also fix the pupil in a dilated position.

Ischemia of the anterior segment of the globe can produce iridoplegia. Transient dilation of the pupil may occur during an episode of monocular amaurosis associated with carotid occlusive disease, migraine, giant cell arteritis, or Raynaud's disease. This unilateral pupillary change is *not* caused by the blindness but by the hypoxic process that affects the entire eye, including the iris sphincter. If the whole globe is ischemic (as in angle-closure glaucoma), iris ischemia will relax the iris sphincter and dilate the pupil. Chronic ischemia of the anterior segment of the globe results in neovascularization of the chamber angle and the surface of the iris (rubeosis iridis), producing iris atrophy, ectropion

of the pigment layer at the pupillary margin (ectropion uveae), glaucoma, and immobility of the iris.

Very few **tumors** affect the iris, but those that do can cause irregularity of the iris border, anisocoria, and an abnormally reactive pupil. Leiomyoma, malignant melanoma, and lymphoma can all present in this fashion.

Spastic miosis is a constant and immediate result of **trauma** to the globe and occurs immediately after blunt trauma to the cornea or perforating injury to the eye. The constriction of the pupil is profound but usually transient and often followed by iridoplegia. Dilation of the pupil frequently occurs after concussion of the globe and is often followed by paralysis of accommodation after the initial intense miosis has resolved. The frequent absence of detectable pathologic change suggests that the effect may occur from injury of the fine nerves of the ciliary plexus. In other cases, tears in the iris or rupture of the iris sphincter may be identified using slit lamp biomicroscopy with transillumination, and a traumatic, peripheral iridodialysis may be present, with resultant distortion of the normally round pupil.

An acute attack of **angle-closure glaucoma** usually presents no problem in diagnosis, but, occasionally, the pain is minimal or nonexistent. Redness of the eye is common. The pupil is usually mid-dilated and nonreactive (Fig. 15.25), but it may be oval. If the acute rise in intraocular pressure abates in an hour or two, the patient may never complain about the pain but instead may seek medical attention for the subsequent iridoplegia.

Iris **atrophy** may be caused by inflammation, ischemia, or trauma. It may be circumscribed or diffuse and may involve the anterior border layer, the stroma and sphincter muscle, the anterior epithelium and dilator muscle, the posterior pigmented epithelium, or a combination of these structures.

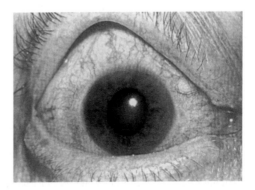

Figure 15.25. Appearance of the eye during an attack of acute angle closure glaucoma. The pupil is dilated and nonreactive. Note the slightly opaque cornea and dilation of the conjunctival vessels.

Some patients experience an irreversible mydriasis and pupillary immobility after an otherwise uncomplicated keratoplasty or uneventful cataract extraction. This **postoperative mydriasis** or "atonic pupil" probably results from direct damage to the iris sphincter muscle during surgery.

DISORDERS OF ACCOMMODATION

Abnormalities of accommodation are usually acquired, although congenital anomalies do occur. Acquired disturbances of accommodation occur most frequently as part of the normal aging process (presbyopia); however, disturbances of accommodation may also occur in otherwise healthy persons, in persons with generalized systemic and neurologic disorders, and in persons with lesions that produce a focal interruption of the parasympathetic (and, rarely, the sympathetic) innervation of the ciliary body. Finally, accommodation may be voluntarily disrupted.

ACCOMMODATION INSUFFICIENCY AND PARALYSIS

Congenital and Hereditary Accommodation Insufficiency and Paralysis

Congenital defects are a rare cause of isolated lack of accommodation. The ciliary body is, however, defective in a number of congenital ocular anomalies. In most cases, vision is so defective that the inability to accommodate is never noted by either the patient or the physician. Aniridia and choroidal coloboma cause obvious defects of the ciliary body, but ciliary aplasia also occurs in well-formed eyes in which the iris is intact and reacts normally to light.

Acquired Accommodation Paresis

Isolated Accommodation Insufficiency   Accommodation insufficiency may be separated into two groups: static insufficiency and dynamic insufficiency.

Patients with **static insufficiency** of accommodation have normal ciliary body innervation and normal innervational impulses, but there is an inadequate response of either the lens or the ciliary muscle. A majority of patients in this group suffer from presbyopia. Static accommodation insufficiency usually occurs gradually as changes occur in either the lens or the ciliary body. In some cases, however, there is sudden loss of accommodation that does not recover. Patients with static accommodation insufficiency require appropriate spectacle correction.

Patients with **dynamic insufficiency** have inadequate parasympathetic impulses required to stimulate the ciliary musculature. Patients with isolated dynamic accommodation insufficiency have normal pupillary size and reactivity. The diagnosis of dynamic accommodation insufficiency is made by measurements of accommodation that are found to be below the minimum for the age of the patient. Such patients often have associated convergence insufficiency. The symptoms of dynamic accommodation insufficiency are asthenopia, tiring of the eyes sometimes associated with brow ache, irritation and burning of the eyes, blurred vision particularly for near work, inability to concentrate, and photophobia. Dynamic insufficiency of accommodation usually occurs in asthenopic persons who become ill with some unrelated condition, although it may also occur suddenly in otherwise healthy individuals. As a general rule, accommodation recovers once the patient's illness is successfully treated.

The management of dynamic accommodation insufficiency is treatment of the underlying illness, after which the patient's symptoms often disappear. If accommodation insufficiency remains, the prescription of convex (plus) lenses is indicated, regardless of the patient's age. In patients with an associated convergence insufficiency, convergence exercises or base-out prisms added to the patient's near correction may be of benefit.

Accommodation Insufficiency Associated with Primary Ocular Disease   **Iridocyclitis** may cause profound dysfunction of the ciliary body. In the acute stage, there may be ciliary spasm and loss of accommodation. In the chronic stage, atrophy of the ciliary body results in accommodation insufficiency.

Glaucoma in children or young adults causes accommodation insufficiency from secondary atrophy of the ciliary body. The drugs used in the management of glaucoma affect the ciliary body as well as the iris. In patients who are still able to accommodate, miotic drugs frequently produce ciliary spasm with symptoms of blurred vision.

Choroidal metastases to the suprachoroidal space may produce cycloplegia and pupillary dilation from damage to the ciliary neural plexus.

Internal ophthalmoplegia is associated with **contusion of the globe.** When accommodation is paralyzed, the pupil is dilated and nonreactive. Recovery of accommodation is common. Following trauma to the globe, rupture of zonular fibers with partial subluxation of the lens may also produce loss of accommodation.

Iatrogenic trauma to the eye, such as that which occurs during retinal reattachment surgery, cryotherapy, or panretinal photocoagulation may injure the ciliary nerves, producing accommodation paresis and mydriasis. Sector palsy of the iris sphincter can also occur after argon laser trabeculoplasty.

Accommodation Insufficiency Associated with Neuromuscular Disorders   Some diseases produce myopathic changes in the smooth muscle fibers of the ciliary body. Isolated ocular involvement of this type is rare, however.

Myotonic dystrophy frequently produces degenerative changes in the lens, the region of the ora serrata, and the anterior chamber angle. Because other smooth muscle dysfunction occurs in such patients, the ciliary muscle also may be affected.

Myasthenia gravis may cause defective accommodation, and this may be the first symptom of the disorder.

Accommodation paralysis is a common and early sign of **botulism.** In some cases, it is the initial sign of nervous system involvement, usually heralding the onset of complete internal and external ophthalmoplegia and various bulbar palsies. It persists for as long as a year, if the patient survives.

Tetanus can produce accommodation paralysis. In most cases, the accommodation paralysis occurs in the setting of generalized ophthalmoparesis.

Accommodation Insufficiency Associated with Focal or Generalized Neurologic Disease Accommodation paresis may be caused by both focal and generalized neurologic disorders that interrupt the innervation of the ciliary body. In some cases, focal lesions of the oculoparasympathetic pathway produce characteristic abnormalities of accommodation combined with disturbances of pupillary function, ocular motility, or both. In other instances, the parasympathetic innervation to the ciliary body is interrupted as part of the overall involvement of the nervous system.

Accommodation may become paretic in both eyes from lesions of the parasympathetic nuclei in the midbrain (e.g., following encephalitis). The pupils may or may not be affected. Vague visual complaints resulting from an abnormality of accommodation can be one of the earliest symptoms of pressure on the **dorsal mesencephalon,** either from hydrocephalus or from an extrinsic mass lesion such as a pineal tumor. Multiple sclerosis, Guillain-Barré syndrome, and ischemia can all cause accommodation paralysis through their effects on the mesencephalon. In most patients, there are other signs of mesencephalic dysfunction.

Acute neurologic dysfunction of the hemispheres may cause accommodation insufficiency. The lesions that can produce this phenomenon include acute ischemic **stroke** and **hematoma**; thus far, reported cases are confined to the left cerebral hemisphere.

Wilson's disease is a hereditary disorder of copper metabolism that is characterized by a progressive degeneration of the CNS associated with hepatic cirrhosis. Ocular findings in patients with Wilson's disease include a peripheral corneal ring of copper deposition involving Descemet's membrane (Kayser-Fleischer ring), copper pigment under the lens cap-

sule, and various ocular motor disturbances. Paresis of accommodation is common in such patients.

Most patients with **tonic pupil syndromes** initially have an accommodative paresis. In most cases of tonic pupil syndrome, particularly in Adie's syndrome, the accommodation insufficiency shows marked improvement over several months; however, because of denervation supersensitivity of the ciliary body, some patients have persistent tonic accommodation, and others have persistent fluctuations in accommodation.

Accommodation Insufficiency Associated with Systemic Disease Children and adults may develop transient accommodation paresis following various systemic illnesses. In such cases, the accommodation paresis often appears to occur as an indirect complication of the systemic disorder rather than from direct damage to the ciliary body or its innervation. There are, however, certain systemic diseases that produce accommodation insufficiency through direct effects on the ciliary body and lens or on their innervation.

In patients who develop **diphtheria,** accommodative paralysis is usually bilateral and often occurs during or after the third week following the onset of infection. Patients typically have normal pupillary responses to light but almost no movement of the pupil during attempted near viewing.

Transient loss of accommodation may occur in patients with **diabetes mellitus,** particularly in the young. It develops in 14% to 19% of new diabetics in all age groups, but in 77% of patients under 30 years of age who also have refractive changes. Although the accommodation paresis may develop in patients with uncontrolled diabetes, it usually occurs after treatment has begun. Hyperopia and accommodation weakness develop concurrently within a few days after the patient's blood glucose has been lowered and then gradually return to normal over 2 to 6 weeks. Either metabolic or neurologic mechanisms can be responsible for accommodation paresis in a patient with this disease.

Accommodation Insufficiency Associated with Trauma to the Head and Neck Symptoms of difficulty with focusing at near and at far, commonly associated with headache and pains about the eyes, are common complaints in patients who have experienced cerebral concussion or craniocervical extension injuries. These vague and ill-defined complaints are most prominent during the first weeks or months after injury. The persistence of such complaints for many months or even years is most common in patients who are seeking compensation for their injury through litigation. An organic basis for these complaints is difficult, if not impossible, to establish. Theoretically, any cerebral injury could impair the highly complex neurophysiologic system involved in the coordination of the near response.

Accommodation Insufficiency and Paralysis from Pharmacologic Agents   Some pharmacologic agents that produce pupillary mydriasis after ocular instillation also produce cycloplegia, including atropine, scopolamine, homatropine, eucatropine, tropicamide, cyclopentolate, and oxyphenonium. None of these agents ever causes persistent paralysis of accommodation after discontinuation.

When cycloplegic agents or related substances are incorporated in medications that are taken internally or applied to the skin, there may be sufficient absorption to produce paresis of accommodation. In such cases, there is never complete paralysis of accommodation, and recovery begins shortly after the medication is discontinued.

Accommodation Paralysis for Distance: Sympathetic Paralysis   Lesions of the cervical sympathetic outflow may produce a defect that prevents the patient from accommodating fully from near to far, but most reports describe an *increase* in accommodative amplitude on the side of the Horner's syndrome. Accommodation paresis for distance may also occur periodically in patients with Raeder's paratrigeminal neuralgia.

ACCOMMODATION SPASM AND SPASM OF THE NEAR REFLEX

Accommodation Spasm Associated with Organic Disease

Accommodation crises or spasms produce an increase in myopia or pseudomyopia. This increase in myopia is often associated with convergence and miosis—that is, a **spasm of the near reflex.** In rare instances, these spasms are caused by or associated with a variety of diverse organic ocular motor and neurologic diseases, such as hepatic encephalopathy, neurosyphilis, ocular inflammation, Raeder's paratrigeminal syndrome, cyclic oculomotor palsy, coma, and myasthenia gravis.

Patients with both primary and secondary **aberrant reinnervation of the oculomotor nerve** have pupillary disturbances, and such patients may also have aberrant reinnervation of the ciliary body. Accommodation in these patients may thus be increased, compared with a normal age-matched population.

Accommodation Spasm Unassociated with Organic Disease

Many young persons, when undergoing a noncycloplegic refraction, consistently accept overcorrecting concave (minus) lenses. When the same patients undergo a cycloplegic refraction, they are found to be emmetropic or at least significantly less myopic than they appeared to be when not cycloplegic. Such persons are exhibiting an increase or "spasm" of accommodation. In some patients, the accommodation spasm may be significant, as much as 10 diopters, and may persist for several years. Accommodation spasm of such magnitude is often associated with excessive convergence that produces a variable esotropia with miosis.

Spasm of accommodation occurs most often in patients who are malingering or who have conversion hysteria. In these patients, it usually occurs as intermittent attacks of accommodative spasm, convergence, and miosis—spasm of the near reflex. The degree of accommodation and convergence spasm in such patients is variable; however, miosis is always present and impressive (Fig. 15.26).

Spasm of the near reflex may be associated with headache, photophobia, defective vision for near and distance, inability to concentrate, and diplopia with bilateral or unilateral limitation of horizontal eye movements. The observation of **miosis** in a patient with apparent unilateral or bilateral limitation of abduction and severe myopia (8 to 10 diopters) is crucial in arriving at the correct diagnosis. This miosis generally resolves as soon as either eye is occluded with a hand-held occluder or patch. In addition, despite apparent bilateral abduction weakness with both eyes open, such patients usually show full abduction in each eye when the opposite eye is patched and ductions are tested directly. Refraction with and without cycloplegia will establish the presence of pseudomyopia.

The management of patients with spasm of the near reflex depends on the setting in which it occurs. Some patients require only simple reassurance that they have no irreversible visual or neurologic disorder. For others, psychiatric counseling is appropriate. In some patients, symptomatic relief may be achieved with a cycloplegic agent and bifocal spectacles or reading glasses. Glasses with an opaque inner third of the lens can be used to treat some patients with spasm of the near reflex. These glasses are designed to occlude vision when the eyes are esotropic, thus interrupting the convergence spasm.

Accommodation Spasm from Pharmacologic Agents

Most of the cholinergic agents that are mentioned in the earlier section of this chapter concerning pharmacologically induced miosis also produce an increase in accommodation and, occasionally, accommodation spasm. Pilocarpine, physostigmine, and the

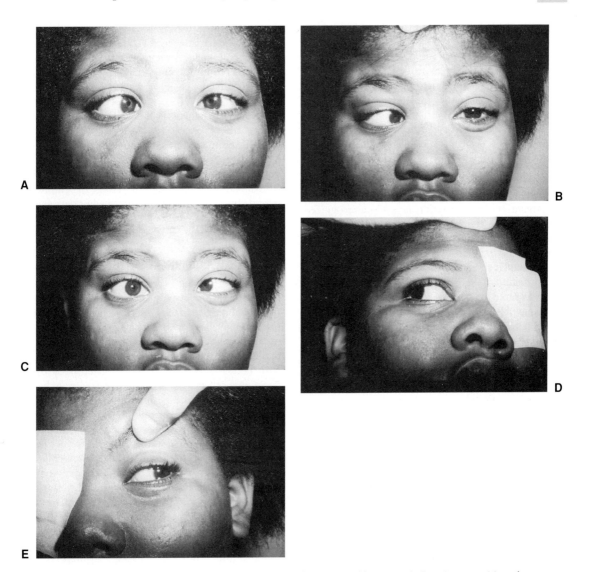

Figure 15.26. Spasm of the near reflex in an otherwise healthy 15-year-old woman. **A:** In primary position, the eyes are esotropic, and the pupils are constricted. **B:** On attempted left gaze, the left eye does not abduct, and both pupils become even smaller. **C:** On attempted right gaze, the right eye does not abduct, and both pupils become smaller. **D:** With the left eye patched, the right eye abducts fully on oculocephalic testing, and the pupil dilates. **E:** With the right eye patched, the left eye abducts fully on oculocephalic testing, and the pupil dilates.

organophosphate esters produce the most accommodation, whereas the effect of aceclidine on accommodation is minimal.

DISORDERS OF LACRIMATION

Tear secretion may be altered by supranuclear lesions as well as by lesions along the pathway from the brainstem to the lacrimal gland. In most cases, there are other

neurologic abnormalities, particularly those that relate to facial or trigeminal nerve function.

TOPICAL DIAGNOSIS

Supranuclear Lesions

A few cerebral diseases produce distinct abnormalities of tear secretion. The most common abnormality is associated with signs of pseudobulbar palsy. The patient experiences inappropriate and unexpected spells of crying accompanied by profuse weeping. During the episodes, he or she shows all the outward expressions of grief without an inward emotional counterpart. These signs suggest hypothalamic involvement, usually in its posterior ventral region. This type of spontaneous crying can occur in patients with signs of pseudobulbar palsy from parkinsonism, various senile dementias, giant cell arteritis, hypothalamic tumors, encephalitis, meningitis, and even mass lesions such as recurrent craniopharyngioma with hypothalamic compression.

Brainstem Lesions

Abnormalities of tear secretion are seldom recognized in patients with lesions of the brainstem. The **congenital paradoxic gustolacrimal reflex** is a rare phenomenon that may be associated with congenital absence of ocular abduction or Duane's syndrome on the involved side.

An acquired brainstem syndrome may produce unilateral involvement of the superior salivary nucleus when one of the small vessels supplying the area near the 4th ventricle at the level of the superior salivary nucleus becomes thrombosed. The vascular accident that develops when this vessel becomes occluded is characterized by a peripheral type of facial paralysis from inclusion of motor fibers in the lesion and an associated dry eye from involvement of the lacrimal nucleus. Salivary flow from the submaxillary gland is also decreased or absent. The rostral end of the vestibular nucleus lies in the immediate vicinity, and these patients usually have vertical or torsional nystagmus. The pathways and neurons concerned with lateral gaze may also be affected, causing an ipsilateral palsy of horizontal gaze.

It might be assumed that any lesion of the brainstem that involves the facial motor nucleus might automatically produce decreased tearing and loss of taste because of the proximity of the structures conveying these modalities. In fact, lesions in this area that produce facial weakness may spare both taste and tearing, because the motor fibers to the facial muscles are anatomically separate from the nerve's sensory-parasympathetic components.

Lesions Affecting the Nervus Intermedius, Facial Nerve Trunk, and Geniculate Ganglion

The secretory fibers to the lacrimal gland pass peripherally from the brainstem in the **nervus intermedius.** This nerve is adjacent to the facial nerve trunk and the vestibulocochlear nerve in the cerebellopontine angle and the internal auditory meatus, after which it joins the facial nerve before it reaches the geniculate ganglion (Fig. 15.27). Lesions in this area, usually tumors, can produce ipsilateral loss of hearing, vestibular palsy, facial palsy, loss of taste, hyperacusis, and a dry eye. Peripheral facial palsy associated with ipsilateral reduction of reflex tearing usually suggests a lesion in the petrous bone, the cerebellopontine angle, or both. For example, many patients with vestibular schwannomas (acoustic neuromas) have a demonstrable but asymptomatic deficiency of tearing on the side of the lesion.

Occasional patients with small vestibular schwannomas report **excessive lacrimation** on the side of their deafness. This symptom may only be apparent during meals. The explanation for this rare gustolacrimal reflex is thought to be compression, demyelination, and short-circuiting of autonomic neural impulses in the nervus intermedius between the afferent fibers for taste and the secretomotor fibers for lacrimation.

Lesions Affecting the Greater Superficial Petrosal Nerve

Any lesion that involves the floor of the middle fossa in the neighborhood of the gasserian ganglion may injure the lacrimal fibers in the greater superficial petrosal nerve (Figs. 15.27 and 15.28). The resulting deficiency of tears on the affected side is rarely noted by the patient unless he or she has an associated palsy of the trigeminal or facial nerve and develops signs of keratitis from drying and exposure of the cornea. Acquired lesions that may damage the greater superficial petrosal nerve include nasopharyngeal tumors, meningeal sarcomas, schwannomas, inflammations of the gasserian ganglion (e.g., herpes zoster), petrositis, sphenoid sinus disease, aneurysms of the petrous portion of the carotid artery, fractures through the middle fossa, alcohol injections, and extradural operations for trigeminal neuralgia.

The finding of impaired tear secretion on the side of an acquired palsy of the abducens nerve is of great value because it indicates a lesion (usually extradural) in the middle fossa. Thus, patients with "isolated" abducens nerve palsies should also have careful testing of tear function in addition to other tests of facial and trigeminal nerve function.

Lesions Affecting the Sphenopalatine Ganglion

Lesions of the sphenopalatine ganglion produce unilateral diminution of reflex tearing, dryness of the nasal mucosa, and frequently paresthesia or hypesthesia in the area supplied by the maxillary division of the trigeminal nerve. The finding of diminished tearing in a patient with ipsilateral pain and hypesthesia in the cheek indicates a lesion, usually a malignant tumor, in the pterygopalatine fossa. Unilateral reduction of tear secretion in a patient with a known tumor or infection of the maxillary (or sphenoid) sinus indicates extension of the disease beyond the confines of the sinus.

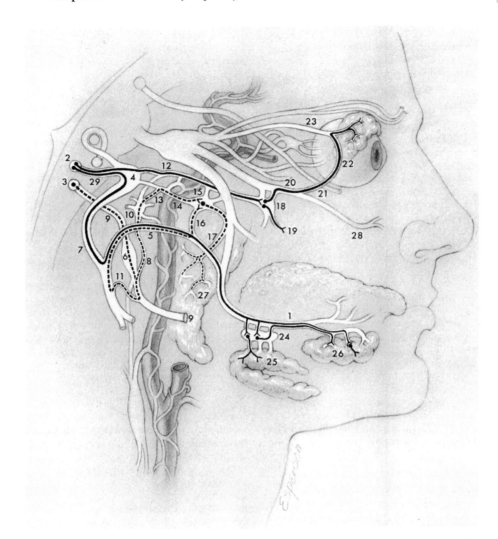

Figure 15.27. Secretomotor pathways for lacrimation and salivation: the efferent visceromotor (parasympathetic) outflow. *1*, lingual nerve; *2*, superior salivatory and lacrimal nucleus; *3*, inferior salivatory nucleus; *4*, geniculate ganglion of the seventh nerve; *5*, chorda tympani; *6*, petrosal ganglion; *7*, facial nerve; *8*, tympanic nerve; *9*, glossopharyngeal nerve; *10*, tympanic plexus; *11*, anastomotic branch (cranial nerves 9 to 7); *12*, greater superficial petrosal nerve; *13*, deep petrosal nerve; *14*, lesser superficial petrosal nerve; *15*, otic ganglion; *16*, anastomotic branch; *17*, auriculotemporal nerve; *18*, sphenopalatine ganglion; *19*, branches to nasal mucosa and palatine glands; *20*, maxillary division of trigeminal nerve; *21*, zygomatic nerve; *22*, zygomaticolacrimal anastomosis; *23*, lacrimal nerve; *24*, submaxillary ganglion; *25*, submaxillary gland; *26*, sublingual gland; *27*, parotid gland; *28*, infraorbital nerve; *29*, nervus intermedius.

Some patients with an abducens nerve palsy have associated maxillary pain. Such patients usually have a lesion in the pterygopalatine fossa, most often a malignant nasopharyngeal tumor, and it is likely that the abducens nerve in some of these cases is affected in its extradural course posterior to the cavernous sinus. Transient abducens nerve palsy and decreased tearing may occur following a dental injection into the sphenopalatine area. This syndrome usually results from an inadvertent injection of anesthetic into the maxillary artery, a branch of which may supply the lateral rectus muscle via a meningeal-lacrimal anastomosis.

Lesions of the Zygomaticotemporal Nerve

Damage to the zygomaticotemporal nerve produces postganglionic denervation of the lacrimal gland. Such damage usually occurs from trauma involving the posterior lateral orbital wall. Occasionally, tumors in this area, particularly metastatic carcinoma, will damage these fibers, resulting in a reduction of reflex tearing.

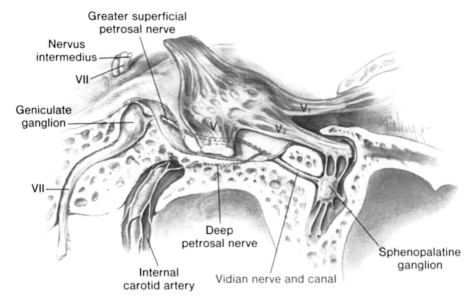

Figure 15.28. Vertical section through the axis of the petrous pyramid of the temporal bone showing the location of the geniculate ganglion and the course of the greater superficial petrosal nerve from the geniculate ganglion to the sphenopalatine ganglion. Note that some sympathetic fibers leave the internal carotid artery at the foramen lacerum to form the deep petrosal nerve. This nerve joins with the greater superficial petrosal nerve to form the vidian nerve. Also note the connections between the sphenopalatine ganglion and the maxillary nerve trunk (V_2). V_1, ophthalmic nerve; V_3, mandibular nerve.

GENERALIZED DISTURBANCES OF AUTONOMIC FUNCTION

Pupillary and accommodation abnormalities may occur as part of generalized dysfunction of various portions of the autonomic nervous system. These disorders include, but are not restricted to, familial dysautonomia (Riley-Day syndrome); congenital familial sensory neuropathy with anhidrosis; hereditary anhidrotic ectodermal dysplasia; neural crest syndrome; congenital cholinergic nervous system dysfunction;

tonic pupils, areflexia, and progressive segmental hypohidrosis (Ross syndrome); primary acquired autonomic dysfunction (Shy-Drager syndrome); acute pandysautonomia; autonomic hyperreflexia; and the Miller Fisher variant of Guillain-Barré syndrome (ophthalmoplegia, ataxia, and areflexia).

FOR FURTHER INFORMATION

See *Walsh & Hoyt's Clinical Neuro-Ophthalmology*, 6th edition, Volume 1, Chapter 16, pages 739–805.

THE EFFERENT SYSTEM

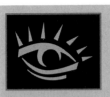

CHAPTER **1 6**

Examination of Ocular Motility and Alignment*

HISTORY
  Diplopia
  Visual Confusion
  Blurred Vision
  Vestibular Symptoms: Vertigo, Oscillopsia,
    and Tilt

EXAMINATION
  Fixation and Gaze-Holding Ability
  Range of Eye Movements
  Ocular Alignment
  Performance of Versions
  Quantitative Analysis of Eye Movements

HISTORY

A careful history should always precede a complete examination of the ocular motor system. Patients with ocular motor disorders may complain of a number of visual difficulties, including diplopia, visual confusion, blurred vision, and the vestibular symptoms of vertigo, oscillopsia, or tilt.

DIPLOPIA

Because misalignment of the visual axes causes the image of an object of interest to fall on noncorresponding parts of the two retinas, usually the fovea of one eye and extrafoveal retina of the other eye, a sensory phenomenon occurs that is usually interpreted as **diplopia**, the visualization of an object in two different spatial locations. Diplopia may be horizontal, vertical, torsional, or a combination of these.

Diplopia that results from ocular misalignment disappears with either eye closed—it is a **binocular** phenomenon. Binocular diplopia is almost never caused by intraocular disease, although it may occur in rare patients in the setting of a monocular macular lesion, such as a subretinal neovascular membrane. The pathophysiology of binocular diplopia with uniocular disease may

represent the establishment of rivalry between central and peripheral fusion mechanisms.

Diplopia that persists with one eye closed, **monocular diplopia**, is rarely caused by neurologic disease. In almost all cases, it is produced by local ocular phenomena, including uncorrected astigmatism or other refractive errors, corneal and iris abnormalities, cataract, and macular disease. Most patients with this type of monocular diplopia recognize a difference in the intensity of the two images that they see and may be describe as a "ghost image" that overlaps the clear image.

Cases of monocular diplopia and polyopia are occasionally reported in patients with central nervous system (CNS) disease. Patients with "cerebral polyopia" generally see each image with equal clarity. In addition, the monocular diplopia in these patients is always seen with either eye covered. Such patients usually have lesions in the parieto-occipital region. The mechanism of cerebral diplopia-polyopia is unknown.

In any patient complaining of "double vision," one must first determine if the double vision is binocular or monocular. If it is monocular, and the patient is otherwise healthy, the examiner may concentrate on ocular disorders, rather than on neurologic or myopathic disorders that affect ocular alignment. In patients with binocular diplopia, the eyes are presumably misaligned, and the examiner should ascertain if the diplopia is horizontal, vertical, or oblique; better or worse in any particular direction of gaze; different when viewing at distance or near; or affected by head posture.

*Adapted from: Borchert MS. Principles and techniques of the examination ocular motility and alignment. In: Miller NR, Newman NJ, Biousse V, Kerrison JB, eds. *Walsh & Hoyt's Clinical Neuro-Ophthalmology*. 6th ed. Vol. I. Philadelphia: Lippincott Williams & Wilkins; 2005:887–905.

VISUAL CONFUSION

In patients with misalignment of the visual axes, the maculae of the two eyes are simultaneously viewing two different objects or areas, interpreted as existing at the same point in space. This sensory phenomenon is called **visual confusion.** Patients with visual confusion complain that the images of objects of interest are superimposed on inappropriate backgrounds.

BLURRED VISION

Misalignment of the visual axes does not always produce diplopia or visual confusion. In some patients, the images of an object seen by noncorresponding parts of the retina are so close together that the patient does not recognize diplopia but instead complains that the vision is blurred when both eyes are open. In such patients, the blurred vision clears completely if **either eye** is closed.

Blurred vision that resolves with one but not either eye closed usually suggests a primary visual sensory disturbance. Blurred vision that does not resolve with either eye closed also usually occurs from visual sensory disease but may also occur in some patients with disorders of saccades (e.g., saccadic oscillations such as ocular flutter) and in patients with impaired pursuit leading to disordered tracking.

VESTIBULAR SYMPTOMS: VERTIGO, OSCILLOPSIA, AND TILT

Patients with disorders that affect the vestibular system may complain of disequilibrium or unsteadiness, symptoms that reflect imbalance of vestibular tone. A common complaint of patients with vestibular imbalance is **vertigo,** the illusory sensation of motion of self or of the environment. Vertigo usually reflects a mismatch among vestibular, visual, and somatosensory inputs concerning the position or motion of one's body in space. It is best to evaluate the vestibular sense alone by asking the patient about the perceived direction of self-rotation with the **eyes closed,** thus eliminating conflicting visual stimuli.

Oscillopsia is an illusory to-and-fro movement of the environment that may be horizontal, vertical, torsional, or a combination of these directions. It is usually caused by an instability of fixation from mechanical or neurologic disorders. When oscillopsia is produced or accentuated by head movement, it is usually of vestibular origin. Oscillopsia is rarely present when ocular motor dysfunction is congenital.

A third group of vestibular symptoms include the perception of **tilts,** static rotations of the perceived world or the body. These complaints usually reflect a disturbance of the otolith organs from either peripheral or central causes. When dealing with such patients, as with patients who complain of vertigo, the examiner should ask about the perception of the positions of the body with the eyes closed, to eliminate conflicting visual stimuli.

EXAMINATION

The examination of the ocular motor system generally consists of the assessment of (a) fixation and gaze-holding ability, (b) range of monocular and binocular eye movements, (c) ocular alignment, and (d) performance of versions (saccades, pursuit). In addition, depending on the findings of the basic examination, it may be appropriate to test the vestibulo-ocular and optokinetic reflexes and to attempt to mechanically move the eyes using forced duction testing.

FIXATION AND GAZE-HOLDING ABILITY
Principles

In a normal, awake person, the eyes are never absolutely still. Fixation is interrupted by three distinctive types of miniature eye movements including microsaccades, continuous microdrift, and microtremor. Square-wave jerks—spontaneous, horizontal saccades of about 0.5°, followed about 200 msec later by a corrective saccade and occurring at a rate of less than 9 per minute—can also be observed during fixation in most normal individuals.

When no efforts are being made toward ocular fixation or accommodation, the eyes are said to be in a "physiologic" position of rest. With total ophthalmoplegia, there is usually a slight divergence of the visual axes, and this position usually also occurs during sleep, deep anesthesia, and death.

Technique

In patients complaining of intermittent diplopia, visual confusion, or strabismus, tests of sensory fusion (e.g., stereoacuity) and fixation should be performed before the eyes are dissociated by tests of monocular visual function (e.g., visual acuity, color vision, visual fields).

The initial part of the ocular motor examination consists of a study of fixation. The patient should be instructed to focus on a distant target, and the eyes should be observed carefully. If strabismus is present, any preference for fixation with one eye should be noted. Constant or intermittent monocular and binocular eye movements, whether conjugate or dissociated, should be noted. Subtle degrees of abnormal fixation can often be easily detected during the ophthalmoscopic examination.

RANGE OF EYE MOVEMENTS
Principles

To discuss eye movements, it is necessary to have a frame of reference against which any movement may

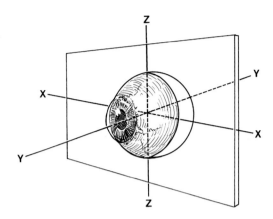

Figure 16.1. The axes of rotation of the eye. The Y axis corresponds to the line of sight when the eye is in the primary position, looking straight ahead.

be quantified. Accordingly, the **primary** position of the eyes is arbitrarily designated as that position from which all other ocular movements are initiated or measured.

All movements of the globe around the hypothetical center of rotation can be analyzed in terms of a coordinate system with three axes perpendicular to each other and intersecting at the center of rotation (Fig. 16.1). The Y axis is equivalent to the visual axis; the Z axis is vertical (around which the eye rotates horizontally); and the X axis is horizontal (around which the eye rotates vertically).

Rotations of either eye alone without attention to the movements of the other eye are called **ductions.** Horizontal rotation is termed **adduction** if the anterior pole of the eye is rotated nasally and **abduction** if the anterior pole of the eye is rotated temporally. Vertical rotation is called **elevation** if the anterior pole of the eye rotates upward and **depression** if it rotates downward.

Rotation around either the horizontal or vertical axis places the eye in a **secondary** position of gaze. In achieving this position, there is no rotation of the globe around the Y axis (i.e., there is no torsion). The oblique positions of gaze are called **tertiary** positions. They are achieved by a simultaneous rotation around the horizontal and vertical axes. When an eye moves obliquely out of primary position, the vertical axis of the globe tilts with respect to the X and Z axes.

True ocular torsion is defined by the direction of the rotation around the Y axis (i.e., the visual axis) relative to the nose. If the 12 o'clock region of the limbus rotates toward the nose, the movement is called **intorsion** (incycloduction; incyclotorsion). If the same area rotates away from the nose, the movement is called **extorsion** (excycloduction; excyclotorsion).

Torsion occurs mainly as part of the involuntary compensatory eye movements that take place during head tilt. In this setting, the torsion movements are called **countertorsion** or **counter rolling. Dynamic countertorsion** occurs during head tilt and reflects the semicircular canal-induced torsional vestibulo-ocular reflex (VOR). **Static countertorsion** persists at a given angle of any head tilt, but the amount of rotation is minor compared with that which occurs from dynamic countertorsion. Static countertorsion reflects a tonic otolith-ocular reflex. Each utricle influences both eyes in both directions but primarily controls tilt to the contralateral side.

The actions of the extraocular muscles are typically discussed in terms of individual antagonist pairs. The two horizontal rectus muscles have only the primary action of either adduction (for the medial rectus) or abduction (for the lateral rectus). The primary action of the two vertical rectus muscles is vertical eye movement (elevation for the superior rectus; depression for the inferior rectus), with both muscles additionally having secondary actions of adduction and torsion (intorsion for the superior rectus; extorsion for the inferior rectus). Torsion is the primary action of the two oblique muscles, with the superior oblique producing intorsion and the inferior oblique producing extorsion. The secondary actions of these muscles are abduction and vertical movement (depression for the superior oblique; elevation for the inferior oblique).

Normal eye movements are binocular. Such movements are called **versions** if the movements of the two eyes are in the same direction and **vergence** movements if they are in opposite directions (i.e., divergence or convergence). For practical purposes, the extraocular muscles of each eye work in pairs during both versions and vergence movements, with one muscle of each eye contracting (the **agonist**) while its opposing muscle relaxes (the **antagonist**). The three agonist-antagonist muscle pairs for each eye are the medial and lateral rectus muscles, the superior and inferior rectus muscles, and the superior and inferior oblique muscles. Whenever an agonist muscle receives a neural impulse to contract, an equivalent inhibitory impulse is sent to the motor neurons supplying the antagonist muscle so that it will relax. This is called **Sherrington's law of reciprocal innervation.**

For the eyes to move together to produce a horizontal version, the lateral rectus of one eye and the medial rectus of the opposite eye must contract together. These muscles constitute a **yoke pair.** The other two yoke pairs are the superior rectus muscle of one eye and the inferior oblique muscle of the other eye, and the superior oblique muscle of one eye and the inferior rectus muscle of the other eye. Implicit in the concept of a yoke pair is that such muscles receive equal innervation so that the eyes move together. This is the simplest statement of **Hering's law of motor correspondence.**

Techniques

When testing the range of ocular movement, the examiner should ask the patient to follow a target through the full range of movement, including the cardinal (or diagnostic) positions of gaze. The eyes are tested individually with one eye covered and together with both eyes open. The normal range of movements is fairly stable throughout life for all directions except upgaze. Normal abduction is usually 50 degrees; adduction, 50 degrees; and depression, 45 degrees. Limitation of upward gaze in an older individual may simply be age-related and not necessarily a new, pathologic process.

When the range of motion is limited, it is necessary to determine if the limitation is mechanical, and if not, whether the disturbance is supranuclear or peripheral.

Several tests may be used to determine if a mechanical restriction of ocular motion is present. Mechanical limitation of motion (such as that seen in patients with thyroid ophthalmopathy or orbital floor fracture with entrapment) can be inferred if intraocular pressure increases substantially when the patient attempts to look in the direction of gaze limitation.

Mechanical limitation of motion can more reliably be detected with **forced duction** testing. In such tests, an attempt is made to move the eye forcibly in the direction(s) of gaze limitation while the patient is attempting to look in that direction (Fig. 16.2). After adequate topical anesthesia, the conjunctiva is grasped with a fine-toothed forceps near the limbus on the side opposite the direction in which the eye is to be moved. The patient is instructed to try to look in the direction of limitation, and an attempt is made to move the eye in that direction. If no resistance is encountered, the motility defect is not restrictive; however, if resistance is encountered, then mechanical restriction exists. In children or when testing restriction of the oblique muscles, forced duction test can be performed only under general anesthesia.

Nonrestrictive limitation of eye movements may occur from disease of supranuclear or infranuclear structures. Because the workup and management of the patient will vary considerably depending on the location of the lesion, it is imperative that supranuclear disorders be distinguished from infranuclear disorders. From a practical standpoint, supranuclear disorders that cause abnormalities in the range of eye movements usually result from lesions of the cerebral hemispheres or the brainstem premotor structures, whereas infranuclear disorders may be caused by lesions of the brainstem, ocular motor nerves, or the extraocular muscles

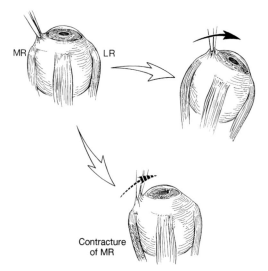

Figure 16.2. Forced duction testing. After the eye has been anesthetized with topical proparacaine and cocaine, the conjunctiva just posterior to the limbus is grasped with a fine-toothed forceps at a point opposite the direction of limitation. An attempt is then made to rotate the eye in the direction of limitation. If no mechanical limitation is present, the eye can be moved fully into the direction of limitation (*solid black arrow*). If mechanical limitation is present, the eye will resist attempts to rotate it into the field of limitation (*dashed black arrow*).

themselves. In all cases, stimulation of the vestibular apparatus can be used to assess the integrity of the peripheral ocular motor pathways either by **oculocephalic testing (the doll's head maneuver)** or by **caloric testing.**

In the oculocephalic test, the awake patient is asked to fixate on a target straight ahead while the head (or the entire body) is rotated from side to side and up and down. A normal response consists of a conjugate eye deviation in the direction away from head or body rotation such that the eyes remain stable with respect to space despite the head movement. Normal responses during oculocephalic testing indicate that the nuclear and infranuclear ocular motor structures are intact and capable of being stimulated by an intact vestibular system. This test can also be used in unconscious patients and with nonorganic limitation of gaze to show that a full range of eye movement can be elicited.

The vestibular system may also be stimulated by caloric irrigation. In this test, performed in the light with the patient in a supine position with the head is flexed 30 degrees. This places the lateral (horizontal) semicircular canals in a nearly vertical position allowing the thermal stimulus to induce maximal convection currents in the endolymph. Up to 200 mL of warm

(44°C) or cold (30°C) water is infused into the external canal using a small tube fitted onto a syringe. In the awake patient, a normal response consists of conjugate nystagmus, with the slow phase toward the side of cold water irrigation (or away from the side of warm water irrigation) and the fast phase away from the side of cold water irrigation (or toward the side of warm water irrigation). The nystagmus occurs because an initial slow-phase movement of the eyes produced by stimulation of the vestibular system is followed by a refixation movement (quick phase or saccade). If the induced nystagmus is consistently less when one ear is irrigated, regardless of the stimulus temperature, a peripheral vestibular disturbance is present on that side. If the nystagmus is consistently greater in one direction, regardless of which ear is stimulated, the patient has a directional preponderance of the vestibular system that may occur with central or peripheral vestibular lesions and is otherwise nonlocalizing.

The eye movements that occur during caloric irrigation can best be observed by placing Frenzel's spectacles on the patient. These spectacles eliminate patient fixation and provide magnification for the examiner.

In comatose patients with intact nuclear and infranuclear ocular motor structures and an intact vestibular system, a normal response is simply a tonic, conjugate ocular deviation toward the side of cold water irrigation and away from the side of warm water irrigation. There are no significant refixation movements, because all horizontal quick phases are generated by the paramedian pontine reticular formation (PPRF), which is not functioning in such patients. Absence of the VOR by either oculocephalic or caloric stimulation in comatose patients is consistently associated with poor outcome.

In some patients with paresis of upward gaze, **Bell's phenomenon** may be helpful in differentiating an infranuclear from a supranuclear lesion. Bell's phenomenon consists of outward and upward rolling of the eyes when forcible efforts are made to close the eyelids against resistance. The presence of this movement in persons who cannot voluntarily elevate their eyes usually indicates that brainstem pathways between the facial nerve nucleus and that portion of the oculomotor nucleus responsible for ocular elevation are intact and, thus, that an upward gaze paresis is supranuclear in origin. Absence of a Bell's phenomenon has less diagnostic usefulness because about 10% of normal subjects do not have this facio-ocular movement.

OCULAR ALIGNMENT
Principles

When the eyes are not aligned on the same object, **strabismus** is present. The strabismus may be congenital or acquired and may be caused by central or peripheral dysfunction. In some persons, particularly those with isolated congenital strabismus, the amount of ocular misalignment is unchanged regardless of the direction of gaze or of which eye is fixating the target. This type of strabismus is termed **comitant** or **concomitant.** When the amount of an ocular deviation changes in various directions of gaze, with either eye fixing or both, the strabismus is said to be **incomitant** or **noncomitant.** Congenital comitant strabismus is occasionally associated with other neurologic dysfunction, and acquired comitant strabismus may be a sign of intracranial disease. In addition, comitant strabismus may appear in otherwise normal children and adults, as well as in persons with neurologic or systemic disease, from **decompensation** of a preexisting phoria. Nevertheless, most instances of neuropathic or myopathic strabismus are of the incomitant variety.

Primary and Secondary Deviations

Any patient with a manifest deviation of one eye (heterotropia) will fixate a target with only one eye at a time. During viewing with that eye, the visual axis of the opposite (nonfixing) eye will be deviated a certain amount away from the target. Patients with a comitant strabismus have the same amount of deviation of the nonfixing eye regardless of the eye that is fixing or the field of gaze. Most patients with incomitant (and especially paralytic) strabismus tend to fix with the nonparetic eye if visual acuity is equal in the two eyes. In these patients, the deviation of the nonfixing eye is called the **primary** deviation. When such patients are forced to fix the same target with the paretic eye, the deviation that results, the **secondary** deviation, is always greater than the primary deviation (Fig. 16.3).

When the paretic eye is fixating a target, it is held in an orbital position farther in the direction of action of the paretic muscle than when the nonparetic eye is fixating the same target. This results in a secondary deviation that is greater than the primary deviation simply because of the change in eye position toward the direction of action of the paretic muscle when the paretic eye is forced to take up fixation. The innervation to both muscles in the yoke pair is increased in that direction as predicted by Hering's law, and this increased innervation is more effective in the nonparetic muscle. However, the innervation is not increased any more than if the nonparetic eye is forced to take up fixation in eccentric gaze to achieve the same final orbital position.

Past-Pointing and Disturbances of Egocentric Localization

Patients with paralytic strabismus often have anomalies of spatial localization called **past-pointing** or **false**

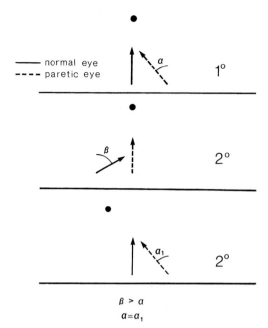

normal eye
paretic eye

$1°$

$2°$

$2°$

$\beta > \alpha$
$\alpha = \alpha_1$

Figure 16.3. The principle of primary and secondary deviations. When the normal eye fixes on a target directly ahead, the paretic eye deviates from the primary position by a certain amount (α) **(top)**. This is called the primary deviation. When the paretic eye fixes on a target in primary position, the normal eye also deviates from primary position by a certain amount (β), but this secondary deviation of the normal eye when the paretic eye is fixing is greater than the amount of deviation of the paretic eye when the normal eye is fixing ($\beta > \alpha$) **(middle)**. Although the common explanation of primary and secondary deviation is based on Hering's law of equal innervation to yoke muscles, some authors believe that the secondary deviation is greater than the primary deviation in paretic strabismus, because when the paretic eye is fixing in primary position it is forced farther into its field of limitation **(bottom)**. If the paretic eye were fixing on an object in the opposite direction, the deviation of the eye from primary position (α_1) would be the same as if the normal eye were fixing on an object straight ahead ($\alpha = \alpha_1$). Thus, although Hering's law is maintained, the explanation for primary and secondary deviations is based upon the position of the eyes within the orbit and not upon which eye is fixing.

orientation. If a patient is asked to point at an object in the field of action of a paretic muscle while the paretic eye is fixating, the patient's finger will point beyond the object *toward* the field of action of the paretic muscle. During this test, it is important that the hand be covered or that the patient point rapidly toward the object so as to avoid visual correction of the error of localization while the hand is still moving toward the object.

Head Turns and Tilts

Patients with strabismus commonly turn or tilt the head to minimize diplopia. Head turns are frequently associated with paresis of the horizontal extraocular muscles, with the turn being toward the side of the weakness. Similarly, patients with vertical extraocular muscle paresis may carry their head flexed or extended. Some patients adopt a head posture that actually increases the distance between the two images, allowing one of the images to be more easily ignored.

Head tilts are most commonly observed in patients with paresis of the oblique muscles, particularly the superior oblique. With an acquired superior oblique palsy, for example, the face is usually turned away from the paretic eye, the chin is down slightly, and the head is tilted toward the side opposite the paretic muscle. This permits fusion of images.

Techniques

Ocular alignment may be tested subjectively or objectively, depending on the circumstances under which the examination is performed and the physical and mental state of the patient.

Subjective Testing When a patient is cooperative, subjective testing of diplopia reliably indicates the disparity between retinal images. The simplest subjective tests of ocular alignment use colored filters to dissociate the deviation and to emphasize and differentiate the images so that the patient and the observer can interpret them. A fixation light is used to provide the image. A red filter held over one eye suffices in most cases; however, the addition of a green filter over the opposite eye gives better results. The use of complementary colored filters, one over each eye, produces maximum dissociation of images because there is no part of the visible spectrum common to both eyes.

The red filter is always placed over the patient's right eye, and all questions posed to the patient relate to the relationship of the red image with respect to the white (or green) image. The patient is first asked if he or she sees one or two lights. If the patient sees two lights, he or she is then asked what color they are. After the appropriate answer, the patient is asked if the red light is to the right or left of the other light and if it is above or below the other light.

It should be remembered that the image of an object is always displaced in the *opposite* direction to the position of the eye (Fig. 16.4). Thus, if an eye is exotropic, the patient will have **crossed** diplopia, and (with a red filter over the right eye) the patient will see the red image to the *left* of the other image. Similarly, if the patient has an esotropia, the red image will be seen to

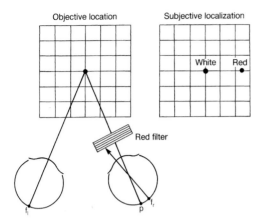

Figure 16.4. The principle of diplopia tests. A red filter is placed in front of the right eye, and the patient fixes a single light in the distance. If the eyes are misaligned, the light is imaged on the fovea of one eye (f_l) and the nonfoveal retina (p) of the opposite eye. The patient thus sees two images, white and red, in different locations in space.

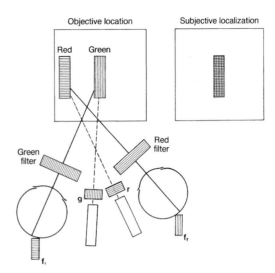

Figure 16.5. The principle of haploscopic tests. Red and green test objects are used, and the patient has a red filter placed in front of one eye and a green filter in front of the other eye.

the *right* of the other image (**uncrossed** diplopia). If the patient has a vertical deviation of the eyes, the eye that is higher will see the image of an object *below* that of the opposite eye.

Once a patient indicates that there is a clear separation of images when he or she is fixing on a light held straight ahead, the examiner can determine the area of maximum vertical separation, horizontal separation, or both, by having the patient look at a light held in the eight other cardinal positions of gaze.

In addition to the use of filters placed over one or both eyes, one can place a red Maddox rod over one eye and have the patient fixate on a white light. The "rod" is, in fact, a set of small half-cylinders aligned side by side in a frame in such a way that when the eye views a light through the cylinders, the image seen is that of a line perpendicular to the cylinder axis. Thus, if one views a white light with one eye covered by a red Maddox rod, the images will be those of a red line and a white light. The Maddox rod can be placed in such a manner as to produce a vertical, horizontal, or oblique line. Persons who are orthophoric see the line pass through the light. When the rod is oriented to produce the image of a vertical line, patients with a horizontal strabismus will see the line to the left or right of the light. When the rod is oriented so that a horizontal line image is produced, patients with a vertical strabismus will see the line above or below the light.

Torsional misalignment of the eyes (e.g., superior oblique palsy) can be tested with two Maddox rods, one over each eye. This is best performed using a trial lens frame. If both rods are oriented so as to produce a horizontal line image, an eye with torsional dysfunction will see the line as oblique, rather than horizontal. The patient is then asked to rotate the rod until the line is perceived as horizontal. By this method, the amount of torsion can be measured and followed.

Other subjective techniques to assess ocular misalignment may be used in which two test objects rather than one are presented to the patient in such a way that each object is viewed with only one eye (Fig. 16.5). The patient is then required to place the two objects in such a fashion that they appear to be superimposed. The objects only appear superimposed when their images fall on the fovea of each eye. Misalignment of the foveas results in the patient placing the objects in different locations in space. The eyes are differentiated and dissociated in various ways. Each eye may be presented with a different target, or complementary colors may be placed into the visual field, either directly or by projection, with each eye being provided with a corresponding colored filter. These **haploscopic** tests include the use of a major amblyoscope, and the Hess screen and Lancaster red-green tests.

Objective Testing

CORNEAL LIGHT REFLEX   The simplest objective method of determining ocular alignment is the use of a hand light to cast a reflection on the corneal surfaces of both eyes in the cardinal positions of gaze. If the images from the two corneas appear centered, then

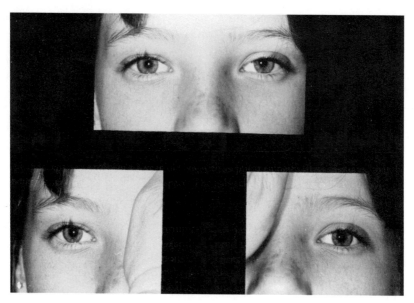

Figure 16.6. Positive angle kappa with the corneal light reflex test. With both eyes open **(top)** the eyes appear exotropic because the light reflection is decentered nasally in the left eye. The reflex remains centered in the right eye when the left eye is covered **(bottom left)**. When the right eye is covered **(bottom right)**, there is no shift of fixation, and the light reflection remains nasally displaced.

the visual axes are usually correctly aligned. If the light reflexes are not centered, one can estimate the amount of misalignment based on the apparent amount of decentration of the light reflex (the **Hirschberg test**). With the fixation light held 33 cm from the patient, 1 mm of decentration equals 7 degrees of ocular deviation.

Alternately, prisms can be placed over either of the eyes until the light reflexes appear centered (the **Krimsky test**). In general, prisms are always placed over the fixing eye; however, in circumstances where the non-fixing eye is so eccentric and limited in its excursion that centration of the light reflex is impossible or requires excessive prism over the fixing eye, holding the prism over the fixing eye results in a measurement of the deviation only in eccentric gaze. This is essentially the same as measuring the secondary, rather than the primary, deviation.

A number of conditions other than a heterotropia may cause decentration of the corneal light reflex and must be considered in order to interpret correctly tests based on centration of the light reflex. The **angle kappa** is defined as the angle between the visual line (the line connecting the point of fixation with the fovea) and the pupillary axis (the line through the center of the pupil perpendicular to the cornea). The angle is measured at the center of the pupil. It is considered positive when the light reflex is displaced nasally, and negative when the light reflex is displaced temporally. A positive angle kappa may simulate an exodeviation

(Fig. 16.6), and a negative angle kappa may simulate an esodeviation.

Other ocular abnormalities that produce decentration of the corneal light reflex include eccentric fixation and ectopic macula.

COVER TESTS   The most precise, objective methods of measuring ocular alignment are the **cover tests.** Although these tests require that the patient be able to fixate a target with either eye, they generally require less cooperation than do the subjective tests described above. The three types of cover tests used by most clinicians are the single-cover test, the cover-uncover test, and the alternate-cover (cross-cover) test.

In the **single-cover test,** the patient fixates an accommodative target at 33 cm (near target) or 6 meters (distant target). An opaque occluder is placed in front of one eye, and the examiner observes the opposite eye to see if it moves to take up fixation of the target (Fig. 16.7). If the patient has a manifest ocular deviation **(heterotropia)**, the previously nonfixing eye will be observed to change position in order to take up fixation when the fixing eye is covered. On the other hand, when the nonfixing eye is covered, no movement of the fixing eye will be observed (because it is already fixing on the target).

In the **cover-uncover test**, the patient fixates on an accommodative target, and one eye is occluded. The behavior of that eye is then observed as the cover is removed (Fig. 16.7). The direction of any deviation

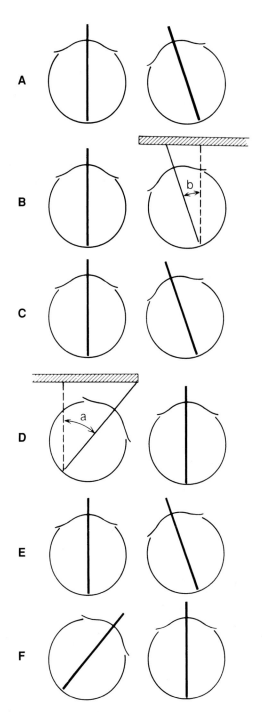

and the speed and rate of recovery to binocular fixation are noted.

If no movement of the uncovered eye is observed when the cover-uncover test is performed, an **alternate-cover test** may be used to detect a latent deviation of the eyes **(heterophoria)**. Instead of occluding one eye and then taking the occluder away, first one eye and then the other is alternately occluded. The cover should remain in front of each eye long enough to allow the patient to take up fixation with the uncovered eye. This test prevents fusion and dissociates the visual axes. Any movement of either uncovered eye suggests that although the eyes are straight during binocular viewing, loss of fusion (i.e., by the alternate occlusion of the two eyes) results in a deviation of whichever eye is covered (Fig. 16.8).

The importance of distinguishing between heterophorias and heterotropias cannot be overemphasized, because patients with heterophorias have binocular central fusion, whereas patients with heterotropias do not.

If either the cover-uncover or alternate-cover tests detect evidence of ocular misalignment, prisms can be used to neutralize the movement and thereby measure the deviation, whether it is a heterotropia or heterophoria. Prisms are placed in front of either eye such that the apex of the prism is oriented in the direction of the deviation, and the prism strength is altered until the deviation is no longer observed.

HEAD TILT TEST   When there is a vertical ocular deviation, it is often helpful to perform cover tests with the head tilted first toward one side and then toward the other. This test is useful primarily in the diagnosis of superior oblique palsy, because patients with this disorder consistently show a hypertropia of the involved eye when the head is tilted toward the involved side.

When a patient with a trochlear nerve palsy tilts the head toward the affected side, intorsion of that eye should occur to keep the vertical meridian perpendicular to the horizon. This intorsion is usually about 10 degrees and is produced by the otolith-ocular reflex,

Figure 16.7. The single-cover and cover-uncover tests. In both tests, one eye is covered at a time; however, in the single-cover test, one eye is covered, and the opposite eye is observed. In the cover-uncover test, one eye is covered, and the behavior of that eye is observed when the cover is removed. **A:** Initially, with both eyes viewing, the left eye is fixating the target, and the right eye is esotropic. **B:** When the right eye is covered, no movement of the left (uncovered) eye is observed.

Figure 16.7. (*Continued*) **C:** Nor is any movement of the right eye observed when the cover is removed (**C**). **D:** When the left eye is covered, the right eye moves outward to take up fixation. Note that the deviation of the normal eye under cover (the secondary deviation, **A**) is greater than that of the paretic eye under cover (primary deviation, **B**). When the cover is removed, either (**E**) the left eye again takes up fixation, or (**F**) the paretic right eye continues to fixate.

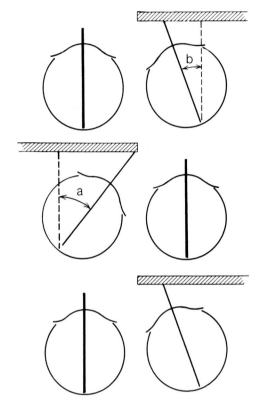

Figure 16.8. The alternate-cover test. This test prevents fusional vergence and thus tests both phorias and tropias but does not differentiate between them. In this test, the cover is quickly moved from one eye to the other, and any movement of either eye is noted. In this example, there is an esodeviation.

resulting in synergistic contractions of the superior rectus and superior oblique muscles. If the superior oblique muscle is paretic, its secondary actions, one of which is depression, is also impaired. The superior rectus muscle is therefore the only means by which the eye is intorted, and its main action, elevation of the eye, is unopposed, resulting in hypertropia with head tilt toward the involved eye.

THREE-STEP DIAGNOSTIC TEST   The head tilt test is best used as part of a "three-step" diagnostic test. This test is used to isolate the involved paretic muscle in concomitant or incomitant vertical deviations. It is only useful if the paresis is of a single cycloverted muscle. The steps are as follows:

1. The presence of a vertical heterotropia is determined in primary position. Depending on the eye that is hypertropic, one of four muscles may be paretic: the ipsilateral inferior rectus, the ipsilateral superior oblique, the contralateral superior rectus, or the contralateral inferior oblique. Thus, if the patient has a right hypertropia, the muscles that may be paretic are the right superior oblique, the right inferior rectus, the left superior rectus, or the left inferior oblique.

2. Whether the hypertropia increases in right or left horizontal gaze is determined. This reduces the potential paretic muscles to two. Thus, in a patient with a right hypertropia, if the deviation increases in right gaze, the affected muscles can only be the right inferior rectus (which has its maximum vertical action when the eye is in an abducted position) or the left inferior oblique (which has its maximum vertical action when the eye is in an adducted position). If the deviation increases in left gaze, the affected muscles could be either the right superior oblique or the left superior rectus.

3. The differential diagnosis between the two muscles, one in each eye, that are potentially responsible for the vertical heterotropia, is now made using the head tilt test as described above. Thus, if the patient has a right hypertropia that increases in left gaze, an increase in the hypertropia when the head is tilted to the right side indicates a paretic superior oblique muscle.

Although the three-step test is extremely useful in patients with presumed trochlear nerve palsies, its reliability in the diagnosis of pareses of other vertical muscles is questionable. Furthermore, restrictive ophthalmoplegia, myasthenia gravis, and skew deviation can mimic superior oblique palsy using the three-step test.

DIRECT OBSERVATION OF THE FUNDUS   A final objective method of determining ocular torsion is direct observation of the ocular fundus. The normal fovea is generally located about 7 degrees below the center of the optic disc (range, 0° to 16°) or along a horizontal line originating from a point between the middle and lower thirds of the optic disc. When an eye is extorted, the foveal reflex rotates below this plane, whereas intorsion results in upward rotation of the reflex (Fig. 16.9). The amount of torsion can be determined using a variety of ophthalmoscopic and photographic methods.

PERFORMANCE OF VERSIONS

Versions may be tested by examining the saccadic, pursuit, vestibular, and optokinetic systems.

Clinical Examination of Saccades

Saccadic eye movements are examined clinically by instructing the patient to alternately fixate upon two targets—usually the examiner's finger and nose. Saccades in each direction can be examined in each field of

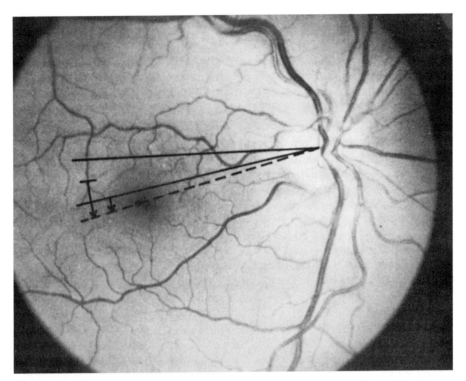

Figure 16.9. Torsion of the ocular fundus. Photograph of an extorted right fundus, direct view, with a dashed line drawn from the center of the optic disc through the fovea. The normal angular range of the fovea from the center of the disc is shown by the two solid lines. The amount of extorsion can be measured in degrees from the center of the normal range (*long arrow*) or from the limit of the normal range (*short arrow*). (Courtesy of Dr. David L Guyton.)

gaze in both the horizontal and vertical planes. The examiner must determine if the saccades are (a) promptly initiated, (b) of normal velocity, and (c) accurate.

Saccadic latencies can be appreciated by noting the time it takes the patient to initiate the saccade. Abnormal voluntary saccadic velocities may be accentuated by using a handheld drum or tape with repetitive patterns.

Disorders of saccadic accuracy—such as **saccadic dysmetria**—can be inferred from the direction and size of corrective saccades that the patient must make to ultimately acquire the fixation target. Because saccades as small as 0.5° can be easily identified during clinical observation, minimal degrees of saccadic dysmetria can be easily appreciated during the clinical examination. Normal persons may undershoot a target by a few degrees when refixations are large. Similarly, such individuals may overshoot a target during centripetal, and especially downward, saccades. This dysmetria is transient, however, gradually disappearing during repetitive refixations between the same targets.

When a saccadic abnormality is detected during the clinical examination, the examiner must attempt to lo-

calize the disturbance within the hierarchic organization of the saccadic eye-movement system. The first step in localization is to establish whether or not reflex types of saccades are affected by the disease process. Quick phases can be examined by spinning the patient in a swivel chair to elicit vestibular and optokinetic nystagmus. Next, an attempt should be made to determine if saccades can be performed without visual targets or in response to auditory targets. This is achieved by asking the patient to refixate under closed lids. The eye movements thus generated can be observed, palpated, and even heard (with a stethoscope applied to the lids).

Clinical Examination of Pursuit

Patients with isolated deficiency of smooth pursuit do not usually complain of visual symptoms, because they can track moving objects with a series of saccades. Only very demanding tracking tasks (e.g., playing tennis, handball, or baseball) may cause patients with impaired pursuit to report difficulties. The vision of normal subjects deteriorates during tracking of targets moving at high frequencies, however, so that even complaints of inability to track fast-moving objects may not signify a disorder of smooth pursuit.

To test the pursuit system, the examiner should ask the patient to track a small target, such as a pencil tip held a meter or more from the eyes, with the head held still. The target should initially be moved at a low, uniform velocity. Pursuit movements that do not match the target velocity result in corrective saccades. If these are "catch-up" saccades, then the pursuit gain is low. If pursuit gain is too high, then "back-up" saccades are observed. Small children, uncooperative patients, or persons thought to have nonorganic blindness may be tested with a slowly rotating large mirror held before their eyes.

Although handheld drums or tapes with repetitive targets do not truly test the optokinetic system, they do stimulate pursuit and may be useful in the detection of pursuit asymmetries and other abnormalities of the pursuit system.

The smooth-pursuit system can also be assessed using the VOR. The VOR normally generates eye movements that compensate for angular displacement of the head and maintain the visual axes "on target." If one observes a slowly moving target by moving the head, so that the target remains stationary relative to the head, the eye movements generated by the VOR are inappropriate and must be suppressed. The ability of a patient to suppress (or cancel) the VOR can be evaluated by using a central fixation target that moves in the same direction and at the same velocity as the head. Patients often do this best by fixating their thumbnail with their arm outstretched while being rotated in the examination chair. When suppression of the VOR and pursuit are compared in normal human subjects, similar frequency response curves are obtained, leading to the hypothesis that suppression of the VOR depends directly on information derived from the smooth-pursuit system. This hypothesis is supported by the clinical observation that patients with impaired smooth pursuit also have abnormal suppression of the VOR. The evaluation of VOR suppression is thus another way to test the integrity of the pursuit system. Deficits in VOR suppression, however, are nonlocalizing, because they may occur with either cerebral or cerebellar disease.

Clinical Examination of the Vestibular and Optokinetic Systems

The clinical methods used to test the vestibular system (oculocephalic and caloric testing) are described above. Although the optokinetic system can be tested in the laboratory (see below), the system cannot be tested as part of a routine clinical examination. As noted above, so-called "optokinetic" handheld drums and tapes ac-

tually assess the smooth-pursuit system, not the optokinetic system.

QUANTITATIVE ANALYSIS OF EYE MOVEMENTS
Voluntary Eye Movements

Most disturbances of ocular motility and alignment can be detected during a standard clinical examination; however, some subtle abnormalities of the pursuit, saccadic, optokinetic, and vestibulo-ocular systems may be more easily and accurately assessed by performing a quantitative analysis of eye movements. The most common methods used to record eye movements are electro-oculography and infrared oculography. These techniques may be used to distinguish myopathic (restrictive) from neuropathic conditions that affect ocular motility and to determine the presence or absence of improvement of ocular motor function during therapy.

Although electro-oculography can yield reasonable recordings of horizontal eye movements, vertical measurements with this technique are affected by eyelid artifacts and nonlinearities. Infrared oculography provides higher resolution measurements of both horizontal and vertical eye movements, but over a limited range, especially vertically. In addition, the signal is lost when the eyes are closed. Finally, neither electro-oculography nor infrared oculography measures ocular torsion.

The magnetic field-search coil method, which uses coils embedded in a silicone rubber ring that adheres to the sclera by suction, overcomes most of the problems that limit both electro-oculography and infrared oculography and enable this technique to be used with great accuracy to measure almost all types of normal and abnormal eye movements.

The Vestibulo-Ocular Reflex

The oculocephalic and caloric tests that are performed in patients with apparent limitation of eye movement primarily test the function of the semicircular canals of the vestibular system. More extensive testing is usually directed toward determining gain, phase, and balance. Rotation tests give more accurate and reproducible results than do caloric tests. The gain of the VOR may be obtained by measuring the peak eye velocity in response to a velocity step (e.g., sudden sustained rotation at 60°/second) in darkness. This is usually done in vestibular laboratories equipped with servo-controlled chairs and eye-monitoring equipment, although portable systems for this purpose are available.

The Optokinetic System

The handheld "optokinetic" drums or tapes that are used to elicit smooth movements primarily test the pursuit system. True optokinetic testing requires a stimulus that fills the field of vision. A common technique is to have the patient sit inside a large, patterned optokinetic drum that is rotated around the patient. A true optokinetic stimulus induces a sensation of self-rotation. Another method of eliciting a true optokinetic response is rotation of an individual at a constant velocity in the light for over 1 minute. The sustained nystagmus that results is caused by purely visual stimuli (the vestibular response having died away); however, it is still difficult to separate its pursuit and optokinetic components.

FOR FURTHER INFORMATION

See *Walsh & Hoyt's Clinical Neuro-Ophthalmology*, 6th edition, Volume 1, Chapter 18, pages 887–905.

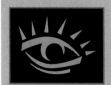

CHAPTER 17

Supranuclear and Internuclear Ocular Motor Disorders*

Supranuclear ocular motor disorders can be caused by lesions in the brainstem, cerebellum, or cerebral hemispheres. Internuclear ocular motor disorders, by definition, are caused by damage to brainstem pathways that coordinate the movements of the two eyes. In this chapter, we discuss the features and causes of supranuclear and internuclear ocular motor disorders.

OCULAR MOTOR SYNDROMES CAUSED BY LESIONS OF THE MEDULLA

The medulla contains a number of structures that are important in the control of eye movements: vestibular

nuclei, perihypoglossal nuclei, medullary reticular formation, inferior olive, and restiform body (Fig. 17.1). The perihypoglossal nuclei consist of the nucleus prepositus hypoglossi (NPH), which lies in the floor of the 4th ventricle, the intercalatus nucleus, and ventrally the nucleus of Roller. These nuclei have rich connections with other ocular motor structures. The NPH and the adjacent medial vestibular nucleus (MVN) are of critical importance for holding horizontal positions of gaze (the neural integrator). These structures also participate in vertical gaze-holding, although more rostral structures, especially the interstitial nucleus of Cajal (INC), also contribute. When lesions are present in the paramedian structures of the medulla, nystagmus—commonly upbeat, but sometimes horizontal with a gaze-evoked component—is the most common finding.

Lesions of the **inferior olivary nucleus** or its connections may produce the **oculopalatal myoclonus syndrome.** This condition usually develops weeks to

---

*Adapted from: Zee DS, Newman-Toker D. Supranuclear and internuclear ocular motility disorders. In: Miller NR, Newman NJ, Biousse V, Kerrison JB, eds. *Walsh & Hoyt's Clinical Neuro-Ophthalmology.* 6th ed. Vol. I. Philadelphia: Lippincott Williams & Wilkins; 2005:907–967.

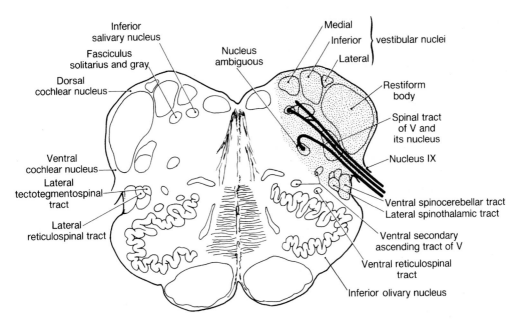

Figure 17.1. Schematic drawing of the medulla oblongata. The specific neural structures that are commonly damaged in Wallenberg's syndrome are shaded.

months after a brainstem or cerebellar infarction, although it may also occur with degenerative conditions. The term *myoclonus* is misleading, because the movements of affected muscles are to-and-fro and are approximately synchronized, typically at a rate of 2 to 4 cycles/second.

The ocular movements present in a majority of cases consist of pendular oscillations that are often vertical but may have a horizontal or torsional component. These oscillations are associated with unilateral or asymmetric palatal myoclonus. Occasionally, the oscillations resolve spontaneously. Gabapentin and ceruletide may partially ameliorate the eye oscillations. The main pathologic finding with palatal myoclonus is hypertrophy of the inferior olivary nucleus, which may be identified by magnetic resonance imaging (MRI).

Occasionally, acute disease processes are restricted to the **vestibular nuclei.** For example, vertigo may be the sole symptom of an exacerbation of multiple sclerosis (MS) and of brainstem ischemia. Nystagmus caused by disease of the vestibular nuclei may be purely horizontal, vertical, or torsional. Mixed patterns also may occur. Moreover, nystagmus from a central vestibular lesion can mimic that caused by peripheral vestibular disease. Dolichoectasia of the basilar artery may produce a variety of combinations of central and peripheral vestibular syndromes. Microvascular compression of the vestibulocochlear nerve may also give rise to paroxysmal vertigo.

WALLENBERG'S SYNDROME (LATERAL MEDULLARY INFARCTION)

Typically, lesions of the vestibular nuclei also affect neighboring structures, especially the cerebellar peduncles and perihypoglossal nuclei. The best recognized syndrome involving the vestibular nuclei is caused by a lateral medullary infarction (Wallenberg's syndrome) (Fig. 17.1). The typical findings of Wallenberg's syndrome are **ipsilateral** impairment of pain and temperature sensation over the face, central Horner's syndrome, limb ataxia, and a bulbar disturbance causing dysarthria and dysphagia. **Contralaterally,** pain and temperature sensation are impaired over the trunk and limbs. The facial nerve may also be affected if the infarct extends more rostrally. The disorder is most commonly caused by occlusion of the ipsilateral vertebral artery; occasionally, the posterior inferior cerebellar artery (PICA) is selectively involved (Fig. 17.2). Dissection of the vertebral artery (either spontaneous or traumatic, such as following chiropractic manipulation) is occasionally the cause. Rarely, demyelinating disease produces this syndrome.

Lateropulsion, a compelling sensation of being pulled toward the side of the lesion, is often a prominent complaint of patients with Wallenberg's syndrome and is also evident in the ocular motor findings. If the patient is asked to fixate straight ahead and then gently close the lids, the eyes deviate conjugately toward the side of the lesion. This is reflected

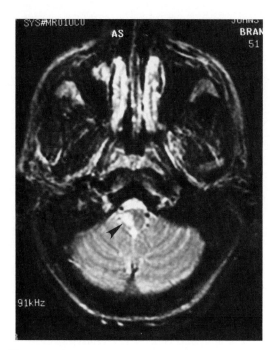

Figure 17.2. Neuroimaging of Wallenberg's syndrome. The T2-weighted magnetic resonance image (MRI), axial view, in a 51-year-old man with Wallenberg's syndrome—characterized in part by lateropulsion of saccades toward the right side, a skew deviation with the right eye being hypotropic, and the ocular tilt reaction—shows a hyperintense area (*arrowhead*) consistent with an infarct on the right side of the medulla.

by the corrective saccades that the patient must make on eye opening to reacquire the target. Lateropulsion may even appear with a blink.

Saccadic eye movements are also affected by lateropulsion (Fig. 17.3). Horizontally, saccades directed toward the side of the lesion usually overshoot the target, and saccades directed away from the side of the lesion undershoot the target; this is referred to as **ipsipulsion** of saccades and should be differentiated from the **contrapulsion** of saccades that occurs with infarcts from occlusion of the superior cerebellar artery (SCA). Quick phases of nystagmus are similarly affected in Wallenberg's syndrome, so saccades directed away from the side of the lesion are smaller than those directed toward the lesion. On attempting a purely vertical refixation, the patient produces an oblique saccade directed toward the side of the lesion. Corrective saccades then bring the eyes back to the target.

When present, spontaneous **nystagmus** in Wallenberg's syndrome is usually horizontal or mixed horizontal-torsional with a small vertical component. In primary position, the slow phase is directed toward the side of the lesion, although it may reverse direction in eccentric positions, suggesting co-existent abnormalities of the gaze-holding mechanism. Lid nystagmus (synkinetic lid twitches with horizontal quick phases) can also occur. The **ocular tilt reaction** (OTR) commonly occurs in Wallenberg's syndrome, as does a **skew deviation** with an ipsilateral hypotropia. The eyes counter-roll toward the side of the lesion, but unequally, so that there is a cyclodeviation. The lower eye is usually more extorted. Some patients show ipsilateral head tilt. The skew deviation and head tilt arise from imbalance in pathways mediating otolith responses (Fig. 17.4). The subjective sensations of tilt or inversion of the world probably also reflect involvement of central projections from the gravireceptors, the utricle and saccule.

Many of the findings in Wallenberg's syndrome, including the bizarre visual disturbances and the skew deviation, may reflect imbalance of otolith influences caused by direct damage to the caudal aspects of the vestibular nuclei. Damage to the restiform body, which carries olivocerebellar projections, may also account for some of the ocular motor findings.

SYNDROME OF THE ANTERIOR INFERIOR CEREBELLAR ARTERY

The anterior inferior cerebellar artery (AICA) supplies portions of the vestibular nuclei, adjacent dorsolateral brainstem, and inferior lateral cerebellum. In addition, the AICA is the origin of the labyrinthine artery in most persons and also sends a twig to the cerebellar flocculus in the cerebellopontine angle. Consequently, ischemia in the distribution of the AICA may cause vertigo, vomiting, hearing loss, facial palsy, and ipsilateral limb ataxia, along with gaze-holding and pursuit deficits as well as vestibular nystagmus (Fig. 17.5). The ocular motor signs reflect a combination of involvement of the labyrinth, vestibular nuclei, and the flocculus.

SKEW DEVIATION AND THE OCULAR TILT REACTION

Skew deviation is a vertical misalignment of the visual axes caused by a disturbance of prenuclear inputs. Torsional and horizontal deviations may be associated findings. The hypertropia may be the same in all positions of gaze (comitant) or it may vary and may even alternate (e.g., right hypertropia on right gaze, left hypertropia on left gaze) (incomitant or noncomitant). When skew deviation is incomitant—and especially in the pattern of an individual muscle palsy—it can only be differentiated from a vertical extraocular muscle palsy by the co-existence of signs of central neurologic dysfunction. Rarely, patients show a slowly **alternating skew deviation** with each eye being hypertropic for about 30 seconds to a minute.

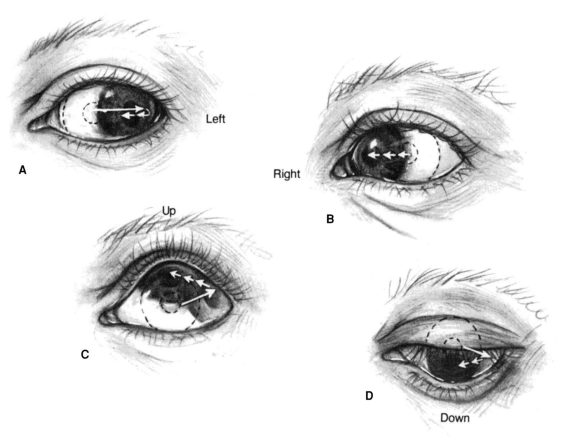

Figure 17.3. Lateropulsion of saccades in a patient with a left Wallenberg's syndrome. **A:** On attempted leftward gaze, the patient overshoots the target and must make a corrective saccade. **B:** On attempted rightward gaze, the patient makes a series of hypometric saccades. **C and D:** On attempted upward and downward gaze, the eyes move obliquely to the left and must make several refixation movements back to center. (Redrawn from: Kommerell G, Hoyt WF. Lateropulsion of saccadic eye movements: electro-oculographic studies in a patient with Wallenberg's syndrome. *Arch Neurol.* 1973;28:313–318.)

In some patients, skew deviation is associated with ocular torsion and head tilt, the **ocular tilt reaction,** which may be tonic (sustained) or paroxysmal (Fig. 17.4). Such patients also show a deviation of the subjective vertical. The ocular torsion may be dissociated, producing a cyclodeviation. The OTR is usually attributed to an imbalance in otolith-ocular and otolith-collic reflexes that are part of a phylogenetically old righting response to a lateral tilt of the head. In patients with more rostral lesions, interruption of descending pathways involved with controlling head posture may also contribute to the head tilt of the OTR.

Skew deviation occurs with a variety of abnormalities in the vestibular periphery, brainstem, or cerebellum and as a reversible finding with raised intracranial pressure (ICP) from supratentorial tumors or pseudotumor cerebri. In infants, a skew deviation may be the harbinger of a subsequent horizontal strabismus.

Why does skew deviation occur with lesions at a variety of sites throughout the posterior fossa? Current evidence suggests that skew deviation occurs whenever peripheral or central lesions cause an **imbalance of otolithic inputs** (Fig. 17.4). An imbalance of posterior semicircular canal inputs may also play a role, although in this setting, nystagmus should also be present.

Lesions of the **vestibular organ or its nerve** can cause both skew deviation and the OTR by producing an imbalance in utricle inputs. The utricle projects predominantly to the ipsilateral lateral vestibular nucleus, whereas the saccule projects to the y-group of vestibular nuclei. Thus, disease of the **vestibular nuclei** may also cause skew deviation with hypotropia on the side of the lesion. In addition, some patients show an ipsilateral head tilt and disconjugate ocular torsion. The latter is an excyclotropia with excyclodeviation of the ipsilateral, lower eye, but small or absent incyclodeviation of the contralateral, higher eye. It is the absence

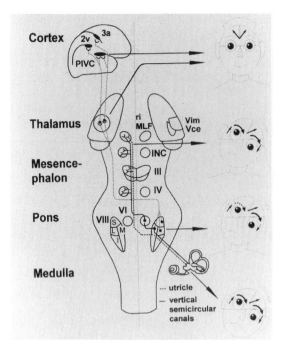

Figure 17.4. Graviceptive pathways from the otoliths and vertical semicircular canals mediating the vestibular reactions in the roll plane. The projections from the otoliths and the vertical semicircular canals to the ocular motor nuclei (trochlear nucleus *IV*, oculomotor nucleus *III*, abducens nucleus *VI*) and the supranuclear centers of the interstitial nucleus of Cajal *(INC)*, and the rostral interstitial nucleus of the medial longitudinal fasciculus *(riMLF)* are shown. They subserve vestibuloocular reflex (VOR) in three planes. The VOR is part of a more complex vestibular reaction that also involves vestibulospinal connections via the medial and lateral vestibulospinal tracts for head and body posture control. Furthermore, connections to the assumed vestibular cortex (areas *2v* and *3a* and the parietoinsular vestibular cortex, *PIVC*) via the vestibular nuclei of the thalamus (*Vim, Vce*) are depicted. Graviceptive vestibular pathways for the roll plane cross at the pontine level. Ocular tilt reaction (OTR) is depicted schematically on the right in relation to the level of the lesion—ipsiversive OTR with peripheral and pontomedullary lesions, contraversive OTR with pontomesencephalic lesions. In vestibular thalamus lesions, the tilts of the subjective visual vertical may be contraversive or ipsiversive; in vestibular cortex lesions, they are preferably contraversive. OTR is not induced by supratentorial lesions above the level of INC. (Reprinted from: Brandt T, Dieterich M. Vestibular syndromes in the roll plane: topographic diagnosis from brainstem to cortex. *Ann Neurol.* 1994;36:337–347, with permission.)

of excyclotorsion in the hypertropic eye that allows a skew deviation to be differentiated from a trochlear nerve palsy.

Utricular projections from the vestibular nuclei probably cross the midline and ascend in the medial longitudinal fasciculus (MLF). Therefore, unilateral **internuclear ophthalmoplegia** (INO) is often associated with a skew deviation. The INO usually is on the side of the hypertropic eye, possibly because lesions of one MLF cause an imbalance of ascending otolithic inputs.

In the **midbrain,** otolith projections contact the oculomotor and trochlear nerve nuclei, as well as the INC. Mesencephalic lesions in or around the INC thus may cause skew deviation and the OTR (Fig. 17.4). When the head tilt is sustained (tonic), it is contralateral to the side of the lesion; in addition, there is usually a hypertropia that is ipsilateral to the lesion and a conjugate cyclotorsion that is characterized by intorsion of the ipsilateral eye. Associated defects of vertical eye movements and oculomotor or trochlear nerve function are common, including seesaw nystagmus. Combined prenuclear and fascicular or nuclear lesions in the midbrain may create torsion of one eye and the OTR.

Rarely, skew deviation slowly alternates or varies in magnitude over the course of a few minutes. The periodicity of the phenomenon is reminiscent of periodic alternating nystagmus, and the two phenomena can, in fact, co-exist. Patients with this condition usually have midbrain lesions.

OCULAR MOTOR SYNDROMES CAUSED BY LESIONS OF THE CEREBELLUM

Clinicians are appropriately cautious in attributing eye movement abnormalities specifically to cerebellar dysfunction, because the brainstem is so frequently damaged in patients with lesions of the cerebellum. Nevertheless, most clinical and experimental studies provide convincing evidence that cerebellar lesions alone can cause specific ocular motor abnormalities (Figs. 17.6 and 17.7). In essence, three principal syndromes can be identified: the syndrome of the dorsal vermis and underlying posterior fastigial nuclei; the syndrome of the flocculus and paraflocculus; and the syndrome of the nodulus and ventral uvula. The main features of each of these syndromes are summarized in Table 17.1.

LOCATION OF LESIONS AND THEIR MANIFESTATIONS

Experimental lesions of the **dorsal vermis** (lobules VI and VII) and of the underlying fastigial nuclei (called the fastigial oculomotor region or FOR) cause saccadic dysmetria, typically hypometria, when the vermis alone

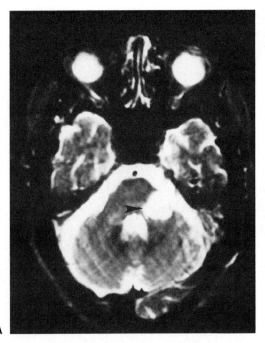
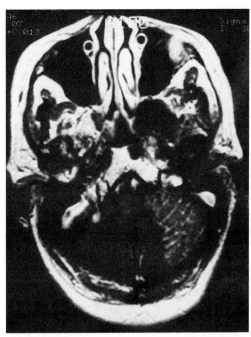

A

B

Figure 17.5. Neuroimaging of an infarct in the territory of the left anterior inferior cerebellar artery (AICA). **A:** T2-weighted axial MRI scan shows hyperintense area in the region of the left middle cerebellar peduncle (*arrowhead*). **B:** T1-weighted axial MRI scan after intravenous injection of paramagnetic contrast material shows diffuse enhancement in the distal distribution of the AICA involving the left cerebellar hemisphere. The 69-year-old patient had, among other manifestations, left-beating gaze-evoked nystagmus.

is involved, and hypermetria when the deep nuclei are affected (Fig. 17.7). Lesions of the deep nuclei may sometimes lead to macrosaccadic oscillations, an extreme degree of hypermetria.

Experimental lesions of the **flocculus and paraflocculus** cause gaze-evoked nystagmus, rebound nystagmus, and downbeat nystagmus (Fig. 17.6). Such lesions also cause impaired smooth tracking, either with eyes alone (smooth pursuit) or with eyes and head; postsaccadic drift; and loss of some adaptive capabilities, such as the ability to adjust the gain and direction of the vestibulo-ocular reflex (VOR) or the pulse-step match for saccades. Unilateral lesions produce ipsilateral deficits in pursuit and gaze holding.

Experimental lesions of the **nodulus** lead to an increase in the duration of vestibular responses that predisposes the animal to the development of periodic alternating nystagmus. Such lesions also produce other abnormalities of the "velocity-storage mechanism," including a failure of tilt suppression of postrotatory nystagmus and loss of habituation. Positional nystagmus usually occurs with lesions of the nodulus.

Another ocular motor sign attributable to a focal cerebellar lesion is torsional nystagmus during vertical pursuit. Patients with lesions in the middle cerebellar peduncle show this phenomenon. The direction of the

torsional nystagmus changes with the direction of the pursuit, with the eye velocity of the slow phase of the torsional nystagmus being directly proportional to the eye velocity of the slow phase of pursuit.

The cerebellum is also important in long-term **adaptive functions** that keep eye movements appropriate to the visual stimulus. For example, adaptation of the gain of the VOR is impaired in patients with cerebellar lesions. This adaptive or "repair shop" function of the cerebellum probably accounts for both the enduring nature of the ocular motor deficits that accompany diffuse cerebellar lesions and, perhaps, the somewhat variable effects of cerebellar lesions. Thus, inherent, idiosyncratic abnormalities in brainstem or peripheral ocular motor mechanisms that are normally "repaired" by the cerebellum may reappear after cerebellar lesions.

ETIOLOGIES
Developmental Anomalies

The **Arnold-Chiari malformation** is an anomaly of the hindbrain involving the caudal cerebellum (including the vestibulocerebellum, flocculus, paraflocculus (tonsils), uvula, and nodulus) and the caudal medulla. In the type 1 malformation, the cerebellar tonsils are

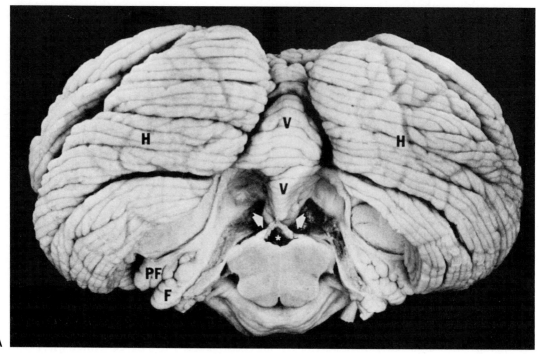

A

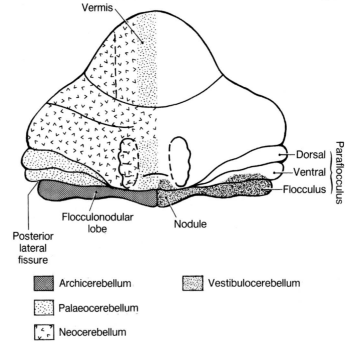

B

Figure 17.6. The human cerebellum. **A:** Anterior inferior view shows the cerebellar hemispheres (*H*), vermis (*V*), flocculus (*F*), and paraflocculus (*PF*). *White arrowheads,* nodulus; *asterisk,* 4th ventricle. (Reprinted from: Ghuhbegovic N, Williams TH. *The Human Brain: A Photographic Guide.* Hagerstown, MD: Harper & Row; 1980, with permission.) **B:** Schematic drawing of the subdivisions of the human cerebellum. The left half of the drawing shows the three main subdivisions: the archicerebellum—the flocculonodular lobe; the paleocerebellum—the anterior vermis, the pyramis, the uvula, and the paraflocculus; and the neocerebellum. The right half of the diagram shows the structures of the vestibulocerebellum—the flocculonodular lobe and the dorsal and ventral parafloculi. (After Brodal A. *Neurological Anatomy in Relation to Clinical Medicine.* 3rd ed. New York: Oxford University Press; 1981.)

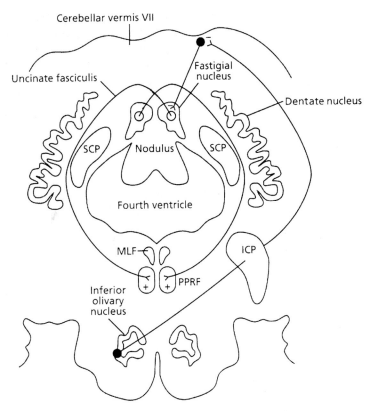

Figure 17.7. Schema of projections from the inferior olivary nuclei through the inferior cerebellar peduncle *(ICP)* to lobule VII of cerebellar cortex, where Purkinje cells inhibit the fastigial nucleus *(FN)*. The caudal part of the fastigial nucleus probably excites the contralateral paramedian pontine reticular formation *(PPRF)* via its projections in the uncinate fasciculus. A lesion in the left inferior cerebellar peduncle increases Purkinje cell activity, leading to decreased firing of the ipsilateral fastigial nucleus and decreased activation of the contralateral (right) paramedian pontine reticular formation. This causes ipsipulsion of saccades. A lesion of the left uncinate fasciculus (from the right fastigial nucleus) decreases activity in the ipsilateral paramedian pontine reticular formation, causing contrapulsion of saccades. *MLF*, medial longitudinal fasciculus; *SCP*, superior cerebellar peduncle. (Reprinted from: Sharpe JA, Morrow MJ, Newman NJ, et al. *Continuum, Neuro-Ophthalmology*. American Academy of Neurology, 1995, with permission.)

Table 17.1. *Localization of Cerebellar Eye Movement Abnormalities*

Structure	Function	Disorder
Dorsal vermis and posterior fastigial nucleus	Saccade accuracy, smooth pursuit	Saccadic dysmetria, impaired pursuit
Flocculus and paraflocculus	Retinal-image stabilization (smooth tracking with head still or free suppression of inappropriate vestibular nystagmus, holding positions of gaze, adaptive control of the VOR and pulse-step match)	Impaired smooth pursuit, VOR cancellation and fixation suppression of caloric nystagmus; gaze-evoked, rebound, centripetal and downbeat nystagmus; postsaccadic drift; inappropriate amplitude or direction of the VOR
Nodulus and ventral uvula	Control of low-frequency response of the VOR	Periodic alternating nystagmus, impaired tilt suppression of postrotatory nystagmus, positional nystagmus, impaired habituation of the VOR, increased duration of vestibular responses.

displaced caudally into the foramen magnum, and the medulla is elongated. A meningomyelocele usually is not present. Such patients often present with symptoms in adult life. In the type 2 malformation, both the 4th ventricle and the inferior vermis extend below the foramen magnum, the brainstem and spinal cord are thin, and a lumbar meningomyelocele is usually present. Patients with a type 2 malformation usually present in childhood, but in milder cases, the onset of symptoms is delayed until adulthood. Presenting symptoms include oscillopsia that is brought on or exacerbated by head movements, and Valsalva-induced dizziness, vertigo, cervical pain, and headaches. A variety of ocular motor abnormalities, especially downbeat nystagmus (both spontaneous and positional), occur in patients with the Chiari malformation (Table 17.2). Diagnosis is by MRI with sagittal views of the craniocervical junction being most useful (Fig. 17.8). Patients often improve after suboccipital decompression, although it may take months for the eye movement abnormalities to diminish. A similar ocular motor syndrome may be observed in patients with other lesions located at the craniocervical junction.

The **Dandy-Walker syndrome** consists of a malformation of the cerebellar vermis, a membranous cyst of the 4th ventricle, and malformations of the cerebellar cortex and deep cerebellar nuclei. Patients with this condition often show a mild saccadic dysmetria, although some patients have normal eye movements. Ocular motor abnormalities, including nystagmus and

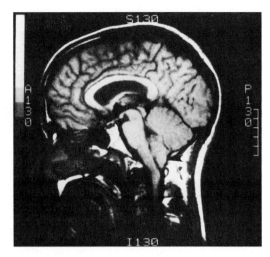

Figure 17.8. Neuroimaging of an Arnold-Chiari malformation. T1-weighted sagittal MRI shows herniation of cerebellar tonsils below the foramen magnum (*arrowhead*). Note flattening of the brainstem in this region.

strabismus, also occur in patients with agenesis of the vermis or hypoplasia of the entire cerebellum.

Degenerative Diseases

Many degenerative processes can affect the cerebellum or its connections and produce cerebellar eye signs. These disorders include the cerebellar cortical degenerations, ataxia telangiectasia, and various spinocerebellar and olivopontocerebellar degenerations (OPCDs). Moreover, many of these conditions also affect brainstem structures. Thus, other, presumably noncerebellar, ocular motor signs may be present (e.g., slow saccades, prolonged saccadic latencies, decreased or absent vestibulo-ocular responses, and ophthalmoplegia).

Paraneoplastic cerebellar degeneration is a rare remote effect of cancer, usually occurring with breast, ovarian, or small-cell lung cancer, and typically associated with serum and cerebrospinal fluid anti-Yo antibodies. The onset of symptoms is usually acute or subacute, with the development of severe midline and appendicular ataxia, dysarthria, and downbeat nystagmus. Pathologic studies indicate total loss of Purkinje cells in patients with this condition. Such patients have lost all output from the cerebellar cortex, and the common finding of primary-position downbeat nystagmus thus tends to confirm that asymmetric, inhibitory projections of the cerebellum to the central connections of the semicircular canals can be the cause of this nystagmus. A cerebellar syndrome may also complicate treatment of cancer or leukemia with cytosine arabinoside.

Table 17.2. *Eye Signs in the Chiari Malformation*

1. Downbeat nystagmus (occasionally with a torsional component), worse on lateral gaze
2. Sidebeat nystagmus (primary position, unidirectional, horizontal nystagmus)
3. Periodic alternating nystagmus
4. Divergent nystagmus
5. Esotropia
6. Gaze-evoked nystagmus
7. Rebound nystagmus including torsional rebound
8. Impaired pursuit (and VOR cancellation)
9. Impaired OKN with slow build-up of eye velocity in response to a constant-velocity stimulus
10. Convergence nystagmus
11. Divergence paralysis
12. Skew deviation accentuated or alternating on lateral gaze
13. Saccadic dysmetria
14. Internuclear ophthalmoplegia
15. Increased VOR gain
16. Shortened VOR time constant
17. Positional nystagmus

Vascular Diseases

The cerebellum is supplied by three branches of the vertebrobasilar circulation: the PICA, the AICA, and the SCA. Occlusion of one or more of these vessels often produces concurrent brainstem infarction, making precise clinicopathologic correlation difficult. Infarction in the distribution of the distal PICA may cause a syndrome of acute vertigo and nystagmus that often simulates an acute peripheral vestibular lesion. These symptoms probably reflect a central vestibular imbalance created by asymmetric infarction of the vestibulocerebellum. The vestibulocerebellum normally has a tonic inhibitory effect upon the vestibular nuclei, and patients with lesions in this region may have prominent gaze-evoked nystagmus that helps differentiate this cerebellar lesion from an acute peripheral vestibulopathy.

Infarction in the territory of the AICA, the branches of which often supply the flocculus, may cause vertigo, vomiting, hearing loss, facial palsy, and ipsilateral limb ataxia, along with gaze-holding and pursuit deficits as well as vestibular nystagmus (Fig. 17.5). The ocular motor signs reflect a combination of involvement of the labyrinth, vestibular nuclei, and the flocculus.

Infarction in the territory of the SCA causes ataxia of gait and limbs and vertigo (Fig. 17.9). A characteristic abnormality is **saccadic contrapulsion.** This consists of an overshooting of contralateral saccades and an undershooting of ipsilateral saccades. Attempted vertical saccades are oblique, with a horizontal component away from the side of the lesion. Thus, this saccadic disorder is the opposite of the saccadic ipsipulsion seen in Wallenberg's syndrome and probably reflects interruption of outputs from the fastigial nucleus running in the uncinate fasciculus next to the superior cerebellar peduncle. Infarction restricted to the posterior-inferior vermis can selectively impair pursuit and optokinetic eye movements.

Mass Lesions

Cerebellar hemorrhage, tumors, infarcts, abscesses, cysts, and extra-axial hematomas may all cause cerebellar eye signs by direct damage to the cerebellar parenchyma. Cerebellar lesions, however, may also compress the brainstem and produce additional signs. Vertical or horizontal gaze disorders can occur, depending on whether the direction of compression is rostral or forward, respectively. The oculomotor, trochlear, and abducens nerves may also be affected. Ocular motor dysfunction may also be caused by secondary obstructive hydrocephalus and increased ICP.

Medulloblastomas arising in the posterior medullary velum frequently produce or are associated with positional nystagmus. Involvement of the nodulus and uvula are presumably responsible for this finding.

Vestibular schwannomas (acoustic neuromas) may compress the cerebellar flocculus (which lies in the cerebellopontine angle) and produce eye signs of vestibulocerebellar lesions, including Brun's nystagmus in which there is a coarse nystagmus beating to the side of the lesion (reflecting a gaze-holding deficit) and a fine nystagmus beating away from the side of the lesion (reflecting a vestibular imbalance). Acute cerebellar hemorrhage frequently causes nystagmus, gaze palsy (usually toward the side of the lesion), abducens nerve palsy, and skew deviation. These signs are, caused, in part, by compression of the brainstem.

OCULAR MOTOR SYNDROMES CAUSED BY LESIONS OF THE PONS

LESIONS OF THE INTERNUCLEAR SYSTEM: INTERNUCLEAR OPHTHALMOPLEGIA

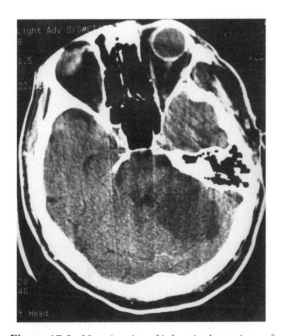

Figure 17.9. Neuroimaging of infarct in the territory of the superior cerebellar artery (SCA) in a 69-year-old man with hypertension. Computed tomographic scan shows a large hypodense area in the left cerebellar hemisphere corresponding to the distribution of the left SCA. The patient had a left horizontal gaze palsy from compression of the left side of the brainstem.

Among the fibers that comprise the MLF, many carry a conjugate horizontal eye movement command from abducens internuclear neurons in the pons to the medial rectus subdivision of the **contralateral** oculomotor nuclear complex in the midbrain. Other fibers in the MLF carry signals for holding vertical eye position, for vertical smooth pursuit, and for the vertical VOR.

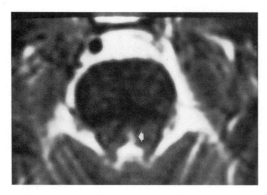

Figure 17.10. Neuroimaging in a patient with a left internuclear ophthalmoplegia. T2-weighted MRI, axial view, shows a tiny area of hyperintensity consistent with an infarct in the region corresponding to the location of the left medial longitudinal fasciculus (*arrowhead*). The patient also had a skew deviation.

Manifestations

Lesions of the MLF produce **internuclear ophthalmoplegia** (Fig. 17.10). When the lesion is unilateral, the INO is characterized by weakness of adduction ipsilateral to the side of the lesion (Fig. 17.11). This weakness can vary from a complete loss of adduction beyond the midline to a mild decrease in the velocity of adduction without any limitation in range of motion. The fibers subserving horizontal gaze in the MLF each carry commands for all types of conjugate eye movements. Thus, vestibular slow phases, pursuit and optokinetic following movements, and saccades and quick phases of nystagmus are all affected by the MLF lesion.

When patients with INO are able to converge, despite absence of voluntary adduction, a caudal lesion with preservation of the medial rectus subdivision of the oculomotor nuclear complex can be assumed. Patients with INO and intact convergence were said to have a **posterior internuclear ophthalmoplegia** by Cogan. Although the presence of intact convergence is important in such cases, the absence of convergence in the setting of an INO (the "anterior" internuclear ophthalmoplegia of Cogan) does not necessarily imply a rostral lesion involving the medial rectus nuclear subdivision. Some patients simply are not able to produce a strong convergence effort, and the vertical disparity that occurs when a unilateral INO is associated with a skew deviation (see below) also may interfere with convergence effort.

The second cardinal sign of an INO is **nystagmus on abduction in the contralateral eye.** This nystagmus consists of a centripetal (inward) drift, followed by a corrective saccade that may be hypermetric, hypometric, or orthometric. It is present in nearly all patients with INO. The cause of abduction nystagmus must relate either to lesions outside the MLF or to an adaptive response to the initial adduction weakness.

Skew deviation (Fig. 17.12) commonly occurs with unilateral INO but is rarely seen with bilateral INO. When skew deviation is associated with an INO, the higher eye is usually on the side of the lesion. **Dissociated vertical nystagmus** (downbeat in the ipsilateral eye, torsional in the contralateral eye) may occur with an INO. This pattern of dissociated nystagmus reflects the finding that posterior semicircular canal pathways mediating excitation pass through the MLF, but some anterior semicircular canal pathways do not.

Lesions that damage the MLF may also damage the abducens nucleus, fascicle, or both on either side of the brainstem. Lesions that damage the MLF on one side and the ipsilateral abducens nucleus produce the one-and-a-half syndrome (see below), whereas lesions that damage the ipsilateral abducens fascicle produce horizontal ophthalmoplegia in the ipsilateral eye from the combination of an INO and an abducens nerve palsy. Lesions that damage the MLF on one side and the paramedian pontine reticular formation (PPRF) or abducens nucleus on the opposite side produce a horizontal gaze palsy toward the side of the damaged PPRF

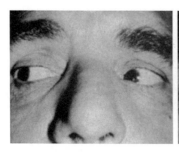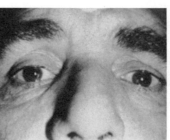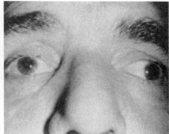

Figure 17.11. Unilateral, right internuclear ophthalmoplegia in a 32-year-old man with multiple sclerosis. Note complete lack of adduction in the right eye on attempted left horizontal gaze.

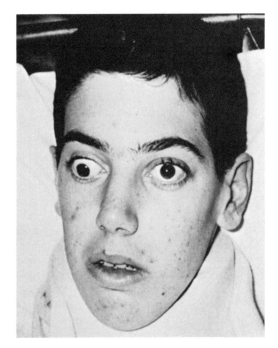

Figure 17.12. Skew deviation in a patient following an operation on the posterior fossa for a superiorly placed vermis tumor. The deviation persisted for 3 weeks. The patient also had a left internuclear ophthalmoplepia.

Table 17.3. *Etiology of Internuclear Ophthalmoplegia*

1. Multiple sclerosis (commonly bilateral); postirradiation demyelination
2. Brainstem infarction (commonly unilateral), including complication of arteriography; hemorrhage
3. Brainstem and 4th ventricular tumors and mesencephalic clefts
4. Chiari malformation, and associated hydrocephalus and syringobulbia
5. Infection: bacterial, viral and other forms of meningoencephalitis; in association with AIDS
6. Hydrocephalus; subdural hematoma; supratentorial arteriovenous malformation
7. Nutritional disorders: Wernicke's encephalopathy and pernicious anemia
8. Metabolic disorders: hepatic encephalopathy, maple syrup urine disease, abetalipoproteinemia, Fabry's disease
9. Drug intoxications: phenothiazines, tricyclic antidepressants, narcotics, propranolol, lithium, barbiturates, D-penicillamine, toluene
10. Cancer: either due to carcinomatous infiltration or remote effect
11. Head trauma, including cervical hyperextension or manipulation
12. Degenerative conditions: progressive supranuclear palsy
13. Syphilis
14. Pseudo-internuclear ophthalmoplegia of myasthenia gravis and Fisher's syndrome

or abducens nucleus. In such cases, the INO cannot be diagnosed because of the overriding horizontal gaze palsy. Damage to the MLF on one side and to the contralateral abducens nerve fascicle will produce abduction weakness of the contralateral eye combined with adduction weakness of the ipsilateral eye. In this setting, there will be a "pseudo-horizontal gaze palsy" on attempted horizontal gaze away from the side of the MLF lesion. The diagnosis may be suspected in a patient who appears to have a horizontal gaze palsy that is asymmetric, with one eye (usually the adducting eye) being much more limited than the other.

Etiologies

Table 17.3 summarizes some etiologies of INO. In general, a unilateral INO is most commonly caused by ischemia, although even in these cases there is often subtle involvement of the other side. Bilateral INO is commonly caused by demyelination. Although MRI frequently shows a lesion in the MLF in patients with INO (Fig. 17.10), there are many exceptions.

LESIONS OF THE ABDUCENS NUCLEUS

Lesions of the abducens nucleus cause an ipsilateral palsy of horizontal conjugate gaze because the abducens nucleus contains two groups of neurons: abducens motoneurons that innervate the ipsilateral lateral rectus muscle and abducens internuclear neurons that innervate the contralateral medial rectus motor neurons via the MLF (Fig. 17.13). Vergence movements of the eyes are spared however, so adduction is possible with a near stimulus. Most often, the abducens nucleus is affected in association with adjacent tegmental structures, particularly the genu of the facial nerve, the MLF, and the PPRF (Fig. 17.14). Lesions restricted to the abducens nucleus can often be distinguished from those in the adjacent caudal PPRF, because only in the latter may pursuit and vestibular movements be spared, and only in the former may ipsilateral saccades in the contralateral field be spared by virtue of intact inhibition upon the contralateral abducens nucleus. Gaze-evoked nystagmus on contralateral gaze also occurs in patients with presumed abducens nucleus lesions. Possible mechanisms for the gaze-evoked nystagmus include damage to adjacent vestibular or NPH

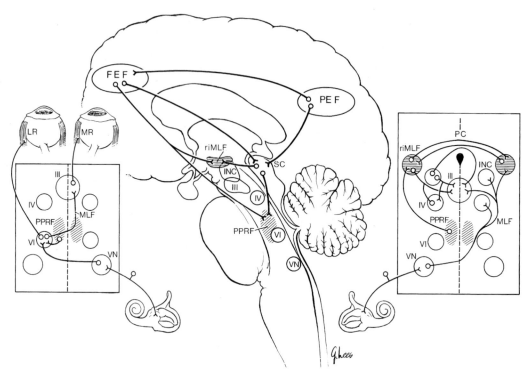

Figure 17.13. Summary of saccadic and vestibular eye movement control. The center figure shows the supranuclear connections from the frontal eye fields *(FEF)* and the parietal eye field *(PEF)* to the superior colliculus *(SC)*, rostral interstitial nucleus of the medial longitudinal fasciculus *(riMLF)*, and the paramedian pontine reticular formation *(PPRF)*. The FEF, PEF, and SC are involved in the production of saccades. The schematic drawing on the left shows the brainstem pathways for horizontal gaze. Axons from the cell bodies located in the PPRF travel to the ipsilateral abducens nucleus *(VI)*, where they synapse with abducens motoneurons whose axons travel to the ipsilateral lateral rectus muscle *(LR)* and with abducens internuclear neurons whose axons cross the midline and travel in the medial longitudinal fasciculus *(MLF)* to the portions of the oculomotor nucleus *(III)* concerned with medial rectus *(MR)* function (in the contralateral eye). The schematic drawing on the right shows the brainstem pathways for vertical gaze. Important structures include the riMLF, PPRF, the interstitial nucleus of Cajal *(INC)*, and the posterior commissure *(PC)*. Note that axons from cell bodies located in the vestibular nuclei *(VN)* travel directly to the abducens nuclei and, most via the MLF, to the oculomotor nuclei. *IV*, trochlear nucleus.

pathways that are involved in neural integration for gaze holding, or damage to the paramedian cells and tracts that lie in part in the rostral abducens nucleus and have reciprocal connections with the cerebellar flocculus, a structure also involved in gaze holding.

LESIONS OF THE PARAMEDIAN PONTINE RETICULAR FORMATION

The PPRF, which corresponds principally to medial portions of the nucleus pontis centralis caudalis, contains burst neurons that are important in the generation of saccades, and the paramedian nucleus raphe interpositus contains pause neurons that inhibit burst neurons at all times except during saccades.

Destructive lesions of the PPRF, such as infarction and hemorrhage, tend to affect all cell groups, along with fibers of passage that convey pursuit and vestibular signals to the ipsilateral abducens nucleus. **Unilateral** destructive lesions cause an ipsilateral, conjugate, horizontal gaze palsy. With acute lesions, the eyes may be deviated contralaterally. Nystagmus occurs when gaze is directed into the intact contralateral field of movement with quick phases directed away from the lesioned side; this is usually accentuated in darkness. Ipsilaterally directed saccades and quick phases are small and slow and do not carry the eye past the midline. Vertical saccades may be slightly slow, and an inappropriate horizontal component, directed away from the side of the lesion, may occur during attempted vertical saccades.

Bilateral pontine lesions may impair vertical eye movements. It is well established that signals for vertical vestibular and smooth-pursuit eye movements ascend in the MLF and other pathways through the pons,

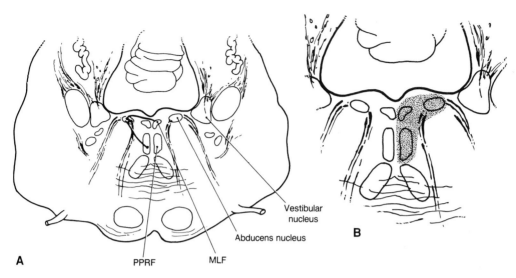

Figure 17.14. Drawing of the pons at the level of the abducens nuclei. **A:** Drawing illustrates the important structures involved in the production of horizontal gaze. *MLF*, medial longitudinal fasciculus; *PPRF*, paramedian pontine reticular formation. Note that neurons project from the PPRF to the abducens nucleus and that neurons in the abducens nucleus are both motoneurons whose axons represent the abducens nerve and internuclear neurons whose axons ascend in the *contralateral* MLF. **B:** The areas that may be involved when a one-and-a-half syndrome is present. Note that involvement of either the abducens nucleus or the PPRF can cause the horizontal gaze palsy. Damage to the ipsilateral medial longitudinal fasciculus produces the internuclear ophthalmoplegia. (Modified from: Sharpe JA, Rosenberg MA, Hoyt WF, et al. Paralytic pontine exotropia: a sign of acute unilateral pontine gaze palsy and internuclear ophthalmoplegia. *Neurology.* 1974;24:1076–1081.)

and it also seems likely that pontine lesions can cause impairment of vertical saccades.

COMBINED UNILATERAL CONJUGATE GAZE PALSY AND INTERNUCLEAR OPHTHALMOPLEGIA (ONE-AND-A-HALF SYNDROME)

Combined lesions of the abducens nucleus or PPRF and adjacent MLF on one side of the brainstem cause an ipsilateral horizontal gaze palsy and an INO. The only preserved horizontal eye movement is abduction of the contralateral eye, hence the name **one-and-a-half syndrome** (Figs. 17.14 and 17.15). Patients with this condition may have an exotropia when attempting to look straight ahead; the eye opposite the side of the lesion deviates outward. This strabismus is thought to be caused by the unopposed drives of the intact pontine gaze center. Thus, the condition is often called **paralytic pontine exotropia.**

Many patients, however, have an esotropia or no deviation in primary position (as with many cases of INO). The spared abduction saccades of the contralateral eye are followed by centripetal drift, so a nystagmus similar to that of the abducting eye in INO is present.

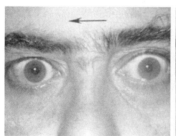
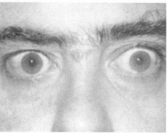
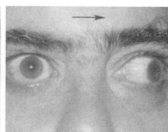

Figure 17.15. One-and-a-half syndrome in a 23-year-old man with multiple sclerosis. Arrows indicate direction of attempted gaze. All ocular motor signs cleared within 3 months after onset.

Table 17.4. *Etiology of Slow Saccades*

1. Olivopontocerebellar atrophy and related spinocerebellar degenerations
2. Huntington's disease
3. Progressive supranuclear palsy
4. Parkinson's disease (advanced cases) and related diseases; Lytico-Bodig
5. Whipple's disease
6. Lipid storage diseases
7. Wilson's disease
8. Drug intoxications: anticonvulsants, benzodiazepines
9. Tetanus
10. Dementia: Alzheimer's disease (stimulus-dependent) and AIDS-associated
11. Lesions of the paramedian pontine reticular formation
12. Internuclear ophthalmoplegia
13. Peripheral nerve palsy; diseases affecting the neuromuscular junction and extraocular muscle; restrictive ophthalmopathy
14. Paraneoplastic syndromes

Occasionally, the ipsilateral horizontal vestibular responses are preserved when voluntary gaze is abolished, suggesting that the pontine lesion is more rostral in the PPRF or more discrete in the caudal PPRF, thus sparing the vestibular projections to the abducens nucleus. Although attempts at conjugate (version) movements elicit no adduction, vergence movements may be preserved in such cases. Ocular bobbing may accompany the one-and-a-half syndrome.

The one-and-a-half syndrome may result from brainstem ischemia, hemorrhage, tumor infiltration, trauma, or demyelination.

SLOW SACCADES FROM PONTINE LESIONS

Certain metabolic, toxic, and degenerative conditions can cause selective deficits of ocular motility suggestive of predominant loss of one population of brainstem neurons concerned with eye movements. Such a process may explain both slow saccades and saccadic oscillations in patients with lesions in the pons.

Slow saccades are characteristic of many degenerative and metabolic diseases (Table 17.4). Horizontal saccades may be slowed in patients with spinocerebellar or olivopontocerebellar degenerations; vertical saccades are often relatively less affected in such patients. In diseases that principally affect the midbrain, such as progressive supranuclear palsy (PSP), vertical saccades are the first to become slow. Patients with spinocerebellar degenerations usually make saccades that have normal amplitudes despite their low velocity. PSP, however, causes both slow and small horizontal saccades. Patients with slow saccades may use a variety of strategies of eye-head coordination to move their eyes more quickly to the target.

OCULAR MOTOR SYNDROMES CAUSED BY LESIONS OF THE MESENCEPHALON

SITES AND MANIFESTATIONS OF LESIONS

Disturbances of vertical eye movements from midbrain lesions usually are caused by damage to one or more of three main structures: the posterior commissure, the rostral interstitial nucleus of the medial longitudinal fasciculus (riMLF), and the interstitial nucleus of Cajal (Fig. 17.13).

Posterior Commissure

Lesions of the **posterior commissure** cause a syndrome characterized by loss of upward gaze and a number of other associated findings (Table 17.5 and Figs. 17.16 through 17.18). The condition is known by a variety of names: Parinaud's syndrome, pretectal

Table 17.5. *Features of the Dorsal Midbrain Syndrome*

1. Limitation of upward eye movements (Parinaud's syndrome):
   Saccades
   Smooth pursuit
   Vestibulo-ocular reflex
   Bell's phenomenon
2. Lid retraction (Collier's sign); occasionally ptosis
3. Disturbances of downward eye movements:
   Downward gaze preference ("setting sun" sign)
   Downbeating nystagmus
   Downward saccades and smooth pursuit may be impaired, but vestibular movements are relatively preserved
4. Disturbances of vergence eye movements:
   Convergence-retraction nystagmus (Koerber-Salus-Elschnig syndrome)
   Paralysis of convergence
   Spasm of convergence
   Paralysis of divergence
   "A" or "V"-pattern exotropia
   Pseudo-abducens palsy
5. Fixation instability (square-wave jerks)
6. Skew deviation
7. Pupillary abnormalities (light-near dissociation)

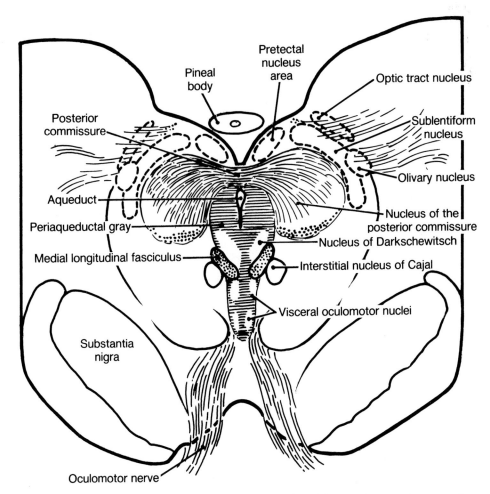

Figure 17.16. Drawing of the major pretectal nuclei. Note relationship of the posterior commissure to other structures. (Reprinted from: Carpenter MB, Pierson RJ. Pretectal region and the pupillary light reflex: an anatomical analysis in the monkey. *J Comp Neurol.* 1973;149:271–300, with permission.)

syndrome, dorsal midbrain syndrome, and the sylvian aqueduct syndrome. Unilateral midbrain lesions can also create the same ocular motor syndrome, but probably by interrupting the afferent and efferent connections of the posterior commissure.

The dorsal midbrain syndrome is also characterized by disturbances of horizontal eye movements, especially vergence. In some patients, convergence is paralyzed, whereas in others it is excessive, resulting in **convergence spasm.** During horizontal saccades, the abducting eye may move more slowly than its adducting fellow eye. This finding is called **pseudo-abducens palsy** and may reflect an excess of convergence tone.

Convergence-retraction nystagmus may occur in patients with disease of the midbrain. This disorder presumably results from damage to the posterior

commissure, because it can be produced by experimental lesions restricted to this structure. Convergence-retraction nystagmus is best regarded as a saccadic disorder because it consists of asynchronous, opposed saccades.

Eyelid abnormalities occur in patients with dorsal midbrain lesions. The most common is eyelid retraction (Collier's tucked lid sign), but ptosis may occasionally occur (Fig. 17.17).

Pupillary size and reactivity are commonly abnormal in patients with lesions of the midbrain in the region of the posterior commissure. The pupils are usually large and react better to an accommodative stimulus than to light (i.e., light-near dissociation).

A variety of disease processes can affect the region of the posterior commissure (Table 17.6). Pineal

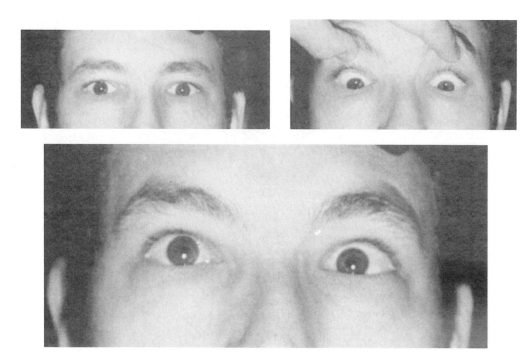

Figure 17.17. Appearance of a patient with Parinaud's dorsal midbrain syndrome. The eyes are straight in primary position (**above left**). Note bilateral upper eyelid retraction. Downward gaze is normal (**above right**). There is marked limitation of upward gaze bilaterally, worse on the left, producing a right hypertropia (**below**). (Reprinted from: Bajandas FJ, Aptman M, Stevens S. The sylvian aqueduct syndrome as a sign of thalamic vascular malformation. In: Smith JL, ed. *Neuro-Ophthalmology Focus 1980*. New York: Masson; 1979:401–406, with permission.)

tumors produce the dorsal midbrain syndrome either by direct pressure on the posterior commissure or by causing obstructive hydrocephalus. Hydrocephalus may produce this syndrome by enlarging the aqueduct and 3rd ventricle or the suprapineal recess, thus stretching or compressing the posterior commissure. Shunt dysfunction may produce Parinaud's syndrome before dilation of the ventricles is apparent on neuroimaging or measures of ICP are consistently high.

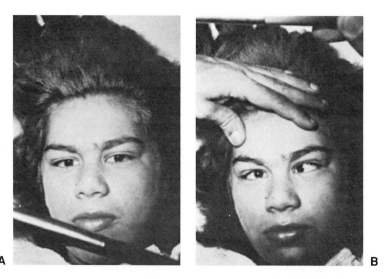

Figure 17.18. Dorsal midbrain syndrome. **A:** Gaze straight ahead. **B:** On attempted upward gaze, the patient develops convergence-retraction nystagmus.

Table 17.6. *Etiology of Disorders of Vertical Gaze*

1. **Tumor.** Classically, pineal germinoma or teratoma in an adolescent male; also pineocytoma, pineoblastoma, glioma, metastasis
2. **Hydrocephalus.** Usually aqueductal stenosis leading to dilation of the 3rd ventricle and aqueduct or enlargement of the suprapineal recess with pressure on the posterior commissure
3. **Vascular.** Midbrain or thalamic hemorrhage or infarction; subdural hematoma
4. **Metabolic.** Lipid storage disease: Niemann-Pick variants, Gaucher's disease, Tay-Sachs disease; maple syrup urine disease; Wilson's disease; kernicterus
5. **Drug-induced.** Barbiturates, carbamazepine, neuroleptic agents
6. **Degenerative.** Progressive supranuclear palsy, Huntington's disease, cortical basal degeneration, Lytico-Bodig syndrome, diffuse Lewy body disease; miscellaneous degenerations
7. **Miscellaneous.** Multiple sclerosis, Whipple's disease, hypoxia, encephalitis, syphilis, aneurysm, neurosurgical procedure, mesencephalic clefts, tuberculoma, trauma, benign transient form of childhood

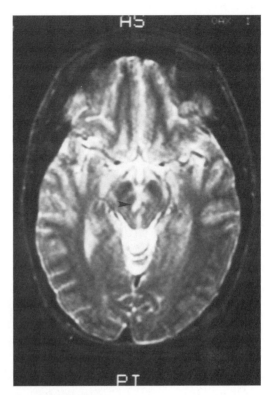

Figure 17.19. Neuroimaging of a lesion in a patient with bilateral conjugate vertical saccadic gaze palsy and cognitive dysfunction. T2-weighted axial MRI shows a hyperintense midline lesion (*arrowhead*) affecting the region of the rostral interstitial nucleus of the medial longitudinal fasciculus.

Rostral Interstitial Nucleus of the Medial Longitudinal Fasciculus

The **rostral interstitial nucleus of the medial longitudinal fasciculus,** which lies in the prerubral fields of the mesencephalon, contains the burst neurons that generate vertical and torsional saccades (Fig. 17.13). The riMLF lies dorsomedial to the rostral half of the red nucleus, medial to the fields of Forel, lateral to the periventricular gray and the nucleus of Darkschewitsch, and immediately rostral to the INC. The right and left riMLF are connected, probably via the posterior commissure dorsally and perhaps also by a commissure that lies ventral to the aqueduct. Bilateral experimental lesions of the riMLF abolish all vertical and torsional saccadic movements.

Lesions of the riMLF are usually infarcts in the distribution of a small perforating vessel (the posterior thalamosubthalamic paramedian artery) that arises between the bifurcation of the basilar artery and the origin of the posterior communicating artery (Fig. 17.19). This vessel may be paired or single. It supplies structures that include the riMLF, rostromedial red nucleus, adjacent subthalamus, the posterior inferior portion of the dorsomedial nucleus, and the parafascicular nucleus of the thalamus. Lesions of the riMLF usually produce a downgaze palsy, mainly affecting saccades. Rarely, they cause a complete vertical gaze palsy.

Unilateral lesions of the riMLF produce slowed or abolished saccades in the vertical plane. Unilateral lesions also cause a contralaterally beating torsional nystagmus, a tonic torsional deviation to the contralateral side, and a deficit in generating ipsilateral directed torsional quick phases (top pole rolling to the side of the lesion).

Bilateral lesions of the riMLF are more common than unilateral lesions. They cause either loss of downward saccades or loss of all vertical saccades (Fig. 17.20). Although vertical smooth pursuit and the VOR may be affected with lesions in this area, this probably reflects damage to nearby structures, such as the MLF and INC.

The vertical one-and-a-half syndrome consists of loss of all downward movements and selective loss of upward movements in one eye or impairment of all upward eye movements and a selective deficit of downward saccades in the eye on the side of the lesion. Unilateral lesions of the midbrain can produce combined upgaze and downgaze palsies, isolated upgaze palsies, or a monocular elevator palsy, as well as the

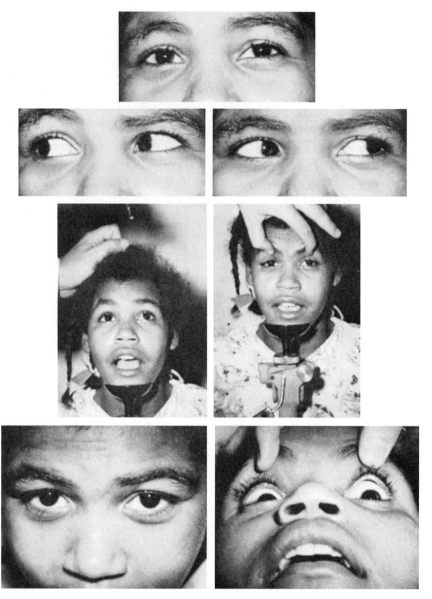

Figure 17.20. Supranuclear vertical ophthalmoplegia in a patient with a metabolic storage disease (DAF syndrome). In primary position, the patient's eyes are straight. She is also able to make normal voluntary horizontal eye movements **(top)**. The patient cannot make voluntary upward or downward vertical eye movements **(middle)**. On oculocephalic testing, full vertical ocular excursions are elicited **(bottom)**. (Reprinted from: von Noorden GK, Maumenee AE. *Atlas of Strabismus*. 2nd ed. St Louis: CV Mosby; 1973:161, with permission.)

vertical one-and-a-half syndrome. Lesions of the adjacent **periaqueductal gray matter** of the midbrain may cause an imbalance of the vertical gaze-holding mechanism.

Interstitial Nucleus of Cajal

Lesions restricted to the **interstitial nucleus of Cajal** may produce two distinct deficits: an ocular tilt reac-

tion and a defect in vertical pursuit and vertical gaze holding. In the OTR, there is a contralesional tonic torsional deviation and a contralesional beating torsional nystagmus. A jerk seesaw nystagmus may occur in patients with lesions that damage the INC, and the INC may also contribute to dynamic properties of the VOR, so-called velocity storage. Lesions in the midbrain produce a change in the phase of the VOR, and electric stimulation of the INC in humans produces torsional nystagmus and the OTR.

NEUROLOGIC DISORDERS THAT PRIMARILY AFFECT THE MESENCEPHALON

Progressive Supranuclear Palsy

Progressive supranuclear palsy is a degenerative disease of later life characterized by disturbances of tone and posture leading to falls, difficulties with swallowing and speech, and mental slowing. The disturbance of eye movements is usually present early in the course of the disease, but it occasionally is noted late or not at all. The condition is usually fatal within 6 years of onset, death commonly being caused by aspiration pneumonia. The disease is usually sporadic.

A variety of eyelid abnormalities occur in patients with PSP. These include typical blepharospasm, apraxia of eyelid closing or opening, lid retraction, and lid lag. More than one of these abnormalities may coexist in a single patient.

The initial ocular motor deficit of PSP consists of **impairment of vertical saccades and quick phases.** Downward saccades are usually affected first and are usually more severely impaired than upward saccades, at least in the early stages of the disease. Impaired saccades are at first slow and later also small, with eventual complete loss of voluntary vertical refixations. Vertical smooth pursuit is usually relatively preserved, and the VOR is intact until later in the disease, although a characteristic nuchal rigidity may make the vertical doll's head maneuver difficult.

Many patients with PSP first complain of visual difficulties related to the disturbance of vertical, and particularly downward, saccades. These complaints include problems with near tasks, particularly reading and eating. Such patients can be helped by providing them with a separate set of reading glasses so that they don't have to use bifocal or progressive-lens glasses, which require them to look downward through a small lower area of the spectacle lens for near viewing.

Horizontal eye movements also show characteristic disturbances in patients with PSP. Typical abnormalities include impaired fixation with square-wave jerks, impaired pursuit, impaired vestibular cancellation, and saccades and quick phases that are small and eventually slow. Late in the disease, the ocular motor deficit may progress to a complete ophthalmoplegia.

PSP is a diffuse brainstem disorder, although cortical involvement may also be important. Histologically, neuronal loss, neurofibrillary tangles, and gliosis principally affect the brainstem reticular formation and the ocular motor nuclei. The midbrain may bear the brunt of the early pathology, accounting for the relative vulnerability of vertical saccades.

Whipple's Disease

Whipple's disease is a rare, multisystem infectious disorder characterized by weight loss, diarrhea, arthritis, lymphadenopathy, and fever that may involve and even be confined to the central nervous system (CNS). This disease can cause a defect of ocular motility that may mimic PSP. Initially, vertical saccades and quick phases are abnormal; eventually, however, all eye movements may be lost. A highly characteristic finding is pendular vergence oscillations and concurrent contractions of the masticatory muscles, **oculomasticatory myorhythmia.** The pendular vergence oscillations are always associated with a vertical saccade palsy. Ophthalmoplegia may occur in association with myorhythmia of the leg, but not of the eyes or jaw. Whipple's disease can be diagnosed using molecular analysis and can be treated with antibiotics.

OCULAR MOTOR SYNDROMES CAUSED BY LESIONS OF THE THALAMUS

Thalamic lesions are characterized by disturbances of both horizontal and vertical gaze. Conjugate deviation of the eyes **contralateral** to the side of the lesion (also called wrong-way deviation) may occur with hemorrhage affecting the medial thalamus (Fig. 17.21). The cause of this contraversive deviation is unclear, but it may be an irritative phenomenon.

Forced downward deviation of the eyes, with convergence and miosis, is another common feature of thalamic hemorrhage; affected patients appear to peer at their noses. In autopsied cases, the hemorrhage usually extends into or compresses the midbrain. Hence, forced downward deviation of the eyes may represent either an irritant effect of the hemorrhage on structures responsible for downward gaze or an imbalance created by an acute upgaze palsy. Resolution of the downward deviation occurs after treatment of raised ICP; thus, traction on mesencephalic structures or hydrocephalus may be responsible for the condition in some patients.

Esotropia occurs in patients with caudal thalamic lesions and may be quite marked. Although it is usually associated with downward gaze deviation, it may occur as an isolated finding. The esotropia that occurs with thalamic lesions may reflect a disturbance of vergence inputs to the oculomotor nuclei.

Combined lesions of the thalamus and midbrain may cause paresis of convergence. Patients in whom this occurs are usually orthophoric in primary position during distance viewing but develop a significant exotropia during attempted near viewing.

Patients with posterolateral thalamic infarctions may have disturbances of the subjective visual vertical

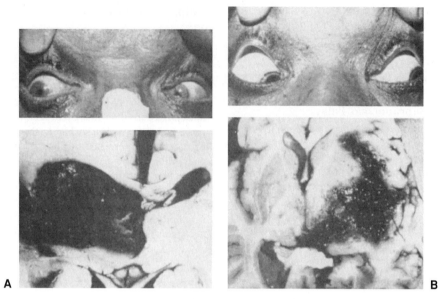

A   **B**

Figure 17.21.   Contralateral ("wrong-side") gaze deviation with supratentorial, thalamic-basal ganglia hemorrhage. *A, top:* The patient's eyes are deviated to the right **(top)**. **A:** Coronal section immediately posterior to the mammillary bodies shows a left intracerebral hemorrhage involving the thalamus, internal capsule, and basal ganglia **(bottom)**. **B:** In another patient, the eyes are deviated down and left **(top)**. **B:** Horizontal section through the mid-diencephalon reveals a right intracerebral hemorrhage involving the pretectum, thalamus, posterior limb of the internal capsule, globus pallidus, and putamen **(bottom)**. In both patients, the hemorrhage also involved the lateral midbrain tegmentum. (Reprinted from: Keane JR. Contralateral gaze deviation with supratentorial hemorrhage: three pathologically verified cases. *Arch Neurol.* 1975;32:119–122, with permission.)

(either ipsilateral or contralateral). The ocular tilt reaction is not present, however, unless the rostral midbrain is also damaged. Associated disturbances of arousal and short-term memory occur in some patients with thalamic lesions and may be caused by damage to specific thalamic nuclei.

Patients with central thalamic lesions show defects in double-step saccade paradigms, suggesting that information for saccades programmed using extraretinal information about eye position must pass through the thalamus and possibly the internal medullary lamina.

Patients with lesions of the pulvinar develop difficulties in shifting attention and gaze into the contralateral hemifield, manifested by a paucity and prolonged latency of visually guided saccades. These results indicate the importance of this thalamic nucleus in directing visual attention.

OCULAR MOTOR ABNORMALITIES AND DISEASE OF THE BASAL GANGLIA

A number of diseases characterized by damage to the basal ganglia are associated with specific disturbances of ocular motility and alignment.

PARKINSON'S DISEASE

Patients with Parkinson's disease may show a number of ocular findings. Steady fixation is often disrupted by square-wave jerks, and upward gaze is often moderately restricted, although this abnormality frequently is observed in normal, elderly persons. Convergence insufficiency is a particularly common and often symptomatic disturbance.

Saccades in Parkinson's disease are characteristically hypometric, particularly when patients are asked to perform rapid, self-paced refixations between two stationary targets. Saccades made in anticipation of the appearance of a target light or to a remembered target location are also hypometric, and patients with Parkinson's disease have difficulty in generating sequences of memory-guided saccades to all types of stimuli. In contrast, saccades made **reflexively** to novel visual stimuli are of normal amplitude and usually promptly initiated. Patients with mild Parkinson's disease perform normally on the antisaccade task, but with advanced disease, errors increase, especially when patients are also taking anticholinergic drugs.

Oculogyric crises, once encountered mainly in patients with postencephalitic parkinsonism, now occurs primarily as a side effect of drugs, especially neuroleptic agents. A typical attack begins with feelings of fear or

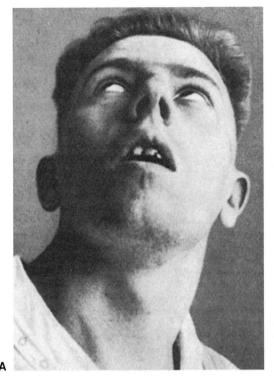
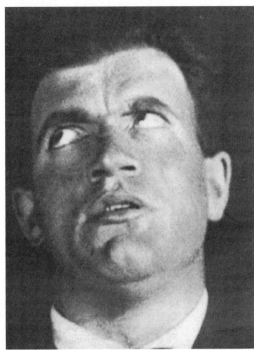

A   **B**

Figure 17.22. Oculogyric crisis in patients with postencephalitic parkinsonism. **A:** In a young man. Note hyperextension of neck, opening of the mouth, and conjugate deviation of the eyes up and to the right. **B:** In a middle-aged man. Again, the eyes are conjugately deviated up and to the right. (Reprinted from: Kyrieleis W. Die Augenveränderungen bei entzündlichen Erkrankungen des Zentralnervensystems. III. Die nichteitrigen entzündlichen Erkrankungen des Zentralnervensystems. A. Die nichteitrige epidemische Encephalitis (Encephalitis epidemica, lethargica). In: Schieck F, Brückner A, eds. *Kurzes Handbuch der Ophthalmologie.* Vol 6. Berlin: Julius Springer; 1931:712–738, with permission.)

depression, which give rise to an obsessive fixation of a thought. The eyes typically deviate upward and sometimes laterally (Fig. 17.22); they rarely deviate downward. Anticholinergic drugs promptly terminate both the thought disorder and the ocular deviation.

Oculogyric crises are distinct from the brief upward ocular deviations that occur in Tourette's syndrome, Rett's syndrome, and in most patients with tardive dyskinesia. In some patients with tardive dyskinesias, however, the upward eye deviations are longer lasting and also have the characteristic neuropsychologic features of oculogyric crises, thus making the differentiation between the two entities difficult, if not impossible.

In general, treatment of Parkinson's disease with dopaminergic drugs such as L-dopa does not seem to improve the ocular motor deficits, except for saccadic accuracy (i.e., saccades become larger). Occasionally, reversal of saccadic slowing occurs with treatment, and newly diagnosed patients with idiopathic Parkinson's disease may experience improved smooth pursuit after institution of dopaminergic therapy.

HUNTINGTON'S DISEASE

Huntington's disease produces disturbances of voluntary gaze, particularly **saccades.** The disease is caused by a genetic defect of the IT15 gene (the "Huntington" gene) on chromosome 4, producing a CAG triplet repeat. Initiation of saccades in patients with Huntington's disease may be difficult. Such patients show prolonged latencies, especially when the saccade is to be made on command or in anticipation of a target moving in a predictable fashion. An obligatory blink or head turn may be used to start the eye moving. Saccades may be slow in the horizontal or vertical plane. This deficit can often be detected early in the disease if eye movements are measured, but it may not be evident clinically until late in the course.

Smooth pursuit may be impaired with decreased gain in patients with Huntington's disease, but it often is relatively spared compared with saccades. By contrast, gaze holding and the VOR are preserved. Late in the disease, rotational stimulation causes the eyes to deviate tonically with few or no quick phases. **Fixation**

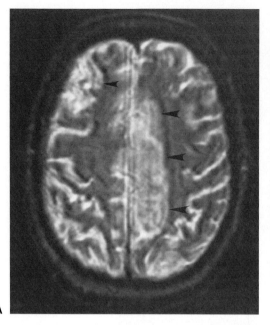
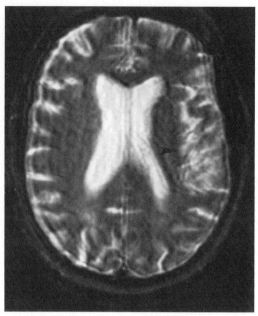

A

B

Figure 17.23. Neuroimaging of an acute infarct in the territory of the left anterior cerebral and middle cerebral arteries. **A:** T2-weighted axial MRI shows diffuse hyperintensity in the distribution of the left anterior cerebral artery (*large arrowheads*). Note also small area of hyperintensity in the right frontal region, consistent with an old infarct (*small arrowhead*). **B:** T2-weighted MRI at a lower plane reveals an area of hyperintensity in the region of the left middle cerebral artery (*arrowhead*). The patient had a supranuclear conjugate gaze paresis to the left side and right hemineglect. He also had difficulty generating rightward saccades. The ocular motor signs were transient as expected from a left-sided cerebral lesion.

is abnormal in some patients with Huntington's disease because of saccadic intrusions. Thus, these patients have difficulty initiating voluntary saccades but show an excess of extraneous saccades during attempted fixation.

Despite the nearly ubiquitous finding of abnormal eye movements in patients with Huntington's disease, some persons with the disease who are evaluated before they become symptomatic show normal eye movements. Thus, routine testing of eye movements cannot be regarded as a reliable method for determining which offspring of affected patients will go on to develop the disease. The abnormal eye movements that occur in patients with Huntington's disease may improve in patients treated with sulpiride.

OCULAR MOTOR SYNDROMES CAUSED BY LESIONS IN THE CEREBRAL HEMISPHERES

ACUTE UNILATERAL LESIONS

Following an acute destructive lesion of one cerebral hemisphere, the eyes usually deviate conjugately toward the side of the lesion (Prevost's or Vulpian's sign). Gaze deviations are more common after large strokes involving predominantly the right post-Rolandic cortex (Fig. 17.23). Visual hemineglect often accompanies such gaze deviations. Gaze deviation that occurs after a stroke usually resolves within a few days to a week. Persistence of gaze deviation in this setting occurs only if there is a previous lesion in the contralateral frontal lobe. In general, for comparably sized lesions, ocular motor defects—both pursuit and saccades—are more profound when the lesion is in the nondominant hemisphere.

In the acute phase, patients may not voluntarily direct their eyes toward the side of the intact hemisphere, in part because of neglect. Shortly thereafter, however, vestibular stimulation usually produces a full range of horizontal movement (with the slow phase), in contrast to most gaze palsies associated with pontine lesions (see the previous text).

When acute right cerebral hemisphere lesions cause conjugate deviation of the eyes, the lesions are located predominantly in the subcortical frontoparietal region and the internal capsule. In the left hemisphere, the lesions are usually larger, covering the entire frontotemporoparietal area. The larger the lesion, the more persistent the conjugate deviation. Both the pursuit and the saccade deficits associated with conjugate deviation of the eyes are predominantly contralateral, but as

Table 17.7. *Persistent Effects of Large Unilateral Lesions of the Cerebral Hemispheres upon Ocular Motor Function*

Fixation	In darkness, eyes usually drift away from the side of the lesion. This may also be evident during fixation (on ophthalmoscopic examination[a]) as nystagmus with quick phases toward the side of the lesion; square-wave jerks.
Saccades	Slower saccades to both sides, especially contralaterally; latency longer for small saccades directed contralateral to the side of the lesion; inaccurate (hypometric and hypermetric) saccades into the "blind" hemifield.
Smooth pursuit	Reduced pursuit gain toward the side of the lesion; smooth pursuit gain away from the side of the lesion may be increased for low-velocity targets.
Optokinetic	Reduced gain for stimuli directed toward the side of the lesion; impaired optokinetic afternystagmus; may be relatively preserved compared with pursuit, with prolonged build-up of slow-phase velocity.[b]
Vestibular	During sinusoidal rotation, VOR gain in darkness may be slightly asymmetric (greater for eye movements away from the side of the lesion); with attempted fixation of an imagined or real stationary target, the asymmetry is increased.
Forced eyelid closure	Eyes usually deviate conjugately away from the side of the lesion ("spasticity of conjugate gaze").

[a] Remember that the direction of eye movements appears inverted during ophthalmoscopy.
[b] Recorded in patients with parietal lobe lesions.

the conjugate deviation resolves, an ipsilateral pursuit defect becomes more apparent.

Conjugate eye deviation is occasionally "wrong way"—contralateral to the side of the lesion. The lesions are almost always hemorrhagic, most commonly in the thalamus (see above). Affected patients usually have signs of rostral brainstem dysfunction and a shift of midline structures. Epileptic phenomena, impairment of ipsilateral pursuit pathways, and more caudal damage to descending pathways near the brainstem are evoked as explanations. Acute hemisphere lesions may cause epileptic seizures with contralateral deviation of the eyes or nystagmus, often with an associated head turn.

PERSISTENT DEFICITS CAUSED BY LARGE UNILATERAL LESIONS

Persistent ocular motor deficits caused by lesions such as hemidecortication for intractable seizures are summarized in Table 17.7. Although there may be no resting deviation of the eyes, forced eyelid closure may cause a contralateral **spastic** conjugate eye movement, the mechanism of which is not understood (Fig. 17.24). This tonic deviation (Cogan's sign) differs from the tonic deviation associated with Wallenberg's syndrome; in the former, active or attempted eyelid closure is necessary to cause the eyes to deviate, whereas in the latter, the deviation occurs even with eyes open in darkness. Cogan's sign occurs most frequently in patients with parietotemporal lesions.

In primary position, a small-amplitude nystagmus may be present that is best seen during ophthalmoscopy. It is characterized by slow phases directed toward the side of the intact hemisphere and may represent an imbalance in smooth pursuit tone. Horizontal pursuit gain (eye velocity/target velocity) is low for tracking of targets moving toward the side of the lesion for all stimulus velocities. For targets moving slowly toward the intact hemisphere, the eye movements may be too fast (pursuit gain >1); for higher target velocities, pursuit gain toward the intact side is normal. This disturbance of smooth pursuit probably reflects loss of both posterior (occipital-parietal-temporal) and frontal influences.

A convenient way to demonstrate the asymmetry of smooth pursuit that occurs with large hemisphere lesions is with a handheld "optokinetic" tape or drum. The response is decreased when the stripes are moved or the drum is rotated toward the side of the lesion. At the bedside, this response is usually judged by the frequency and amplitude of quick phases; but because these quick-phase variables also depend on slow-phase

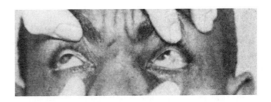

Figure 17.24. Conjugate lateral deviation of the eyes on forced closure of the eyelids in a patient with a tuberculoma of the left occipitoparietal region. (Reprinted from: Cogan DG. Neurologic significance of lateral conjugate deviation of the eyes on forced closure of the lids. *Arch Ophthalmol.* 1948;39:37–42, with permission.)

velocity, a decreased response may reflect impaired slow-phase generation, impaired quick-phase generation, or a combination of the two.

FOCAL LESIONS

Ocular motor disturbances that occur from focal lesions of the cerebral hemispheres depend on a variety of factors, including the location and size of the lesion and whether the lesion is unilateral or bilateral.

Occipital Lobe Lesions

A small, unilateral lesion of either occipital lobe causes a contralateral homonymous visual field defect without any significant disturbance of ocular motor function; however, a large, unilateral lesion of either occipital lobe usually causes a contralateral homonymous hemianopia and an ocular motor deficit (saccadic dysmetria) that is related primarily to the field defect. Saccades into the hemianopic visual field are dysmetric, usually hypometric.

Parietal Lobe Lesions

Unilateral lesions of the parietal lobes, especially those involving the inferior parietal lobule and underlying deep white matter, cause abnormalities of ocular tracking of moving targets, including an asymmetry of smooth pursuit and of optokinetic nystagmus as tested at the bedside with handheld drums or tapes. Lesions at the temporoparietooccipital junction probably affect secondary visual areas that are important for motion processing and for programming of smooth-pursuit eye movements. One such area is likely to be the human homologue of what in monkeys is called the middle temporal (MT) visual area.

Lesions of MT in monkeys impair the ability to estimate the speed of a moving target that is within the affected visual field, although stationary objects can be seen and accurately localized. The ocular motor consequences of this **scotoma for motion** are that saccades made to targets moving in the affected, contralateral hemifield are inaccurate and that the initiation of smooth pursuit is impaired. Such a behavior deficit occurs in patients with lesions affecting the temporoparietooccipital cortex.

Lesions of adjacent cortex (including Brodmann areas 19 and 39), which probably correspond to the medial superior temporal (MST) visual area and underlying white matter lead to a **directional defect** in smooth pursuit that is characterized by impaired tracking (reduced gain) for targets moving toward the side of the lesion, irrespective of the visual hemifield in which the target lies.

In some patients, pursuit gain away from the side of the parietal lobe lesion is also somewhat reduced, especially when the eyes move into the contralateral field of gaze. This phenomenon probably results from contralateral neglect. In other patients, contralateral pursuit gain is increased. Subcortical, thalamic, and brainstem lesions may cause an ipsilateral defect from damage to the descending pathway for smooth pursuit. In human patients with parietal lesions, optokinetic nystagmus is often impaired in response to stimuli moving toward the side of the lesion, although it may be relatively spared compared with foveal tracking. Optokinetic afternystagmus and circularvection (the sensation of self-rotation) may also be impaired.

Unilateral lesions of the parietal lobe may affect saccadic initiation, causing an increase in saccadic latencies, either bilaterally or only for saccades to contralateral targets. These changes are independent of any visual field defect. The latency defects are enhanced when the fixation target remains on and a new target appears in the periphery (the "overlap" task) and are diminished when the fixation target is extinguished before the presentation of the new target in the periphery (the "gap" task).

Bilateral parietal lobe lesions may cause acquired ocular motor apraxia, particularly if the lesions are large (see later). When smooth pursuit is possible, it is particularly limited with higher acceleration target motion.

Temporal Lobe Lesions

In patients with posterior temporal lesions, fixation-suppression of caloric-induced nystagmus is impaired when slow phases are directed away from the side of the lesion. This abnormality may reflect impairment of visual-motion or smooth-pursuit pathways rather than any effect on vestibular nystagmus per se. Patients with homonymous hemianopia and lesions affecting the temporal lobes may lack the sensation of self-rotation (circularvection) that normally occurs during full-field optokinetic stimulation, compared with patients who have an homonymous hemianopia from occipital lesions and who do experience circularvection. These findings support the localization of the vestibular cortex to the superior temporal gyrus and, perhaps, the adjacent parietal cortex. Patients with parieto-insular lesions may have tilts of the subjective visual vertical, usually contraversive. This is not associated with a skew deviation, although occasionally there is some monocular torsion. Patients with lesions in the same area may also have a defect in generating memory-guided saccades after a vestibular (rotational) stimulus. Finally, patients with lesions in the medial temporal lobe—the hippocampus—show marked impairment of generating sequences of saccades, whereas their spatial memory is intact.

Frontal Lobe Lesions

Lesions of the frontal lobe may produce an ipsilateral conjugate deviation of the eyes that resolves with time. Rarely, contralateral deviation occurs with acute frontal lesions or frontoparietal lesions. Enduring deficits after frontal lobe lesions include abnormalities of saccades and smooth pursuit. Three areas within the frontal lobes that play an important role in the control of eye movements are: (a) the frontal eye fields, (b) the supplementary eye fields (SEF) in the supplementary motor area, and (c) the prefrontal cortex (PFC) (Fig. 17.13).

Unilateral FEF lesions lead to a slight increase in saccade latency to reflexively triggered saccades with a predominantly contralateral hypometria. Latencies are greatest in the overlap task (when the initial fixation target remains on, even after the peripheral target appears), suggesting a role for the FEF in disengagement from central fixation. Saccades may show a prolonged latency to predictable target jumps, particularly in patients with right-sided frontal lesions. Patients with this condition show a bilateral deficit in latency and accuracy for saccades to a remembered visual target but not for remembered saccades after a vestibular (rotation) input. With attempted vertical saccades, a horizontal component directed toward the side of the lesion often causes an oblique movement. Mild slowing of contralateral saccades occurs in some patients. Deep, unilateral frontal lobe lesions cause increased latency for contralateral saccades. This deficit is probably caused by damage of efferent and afferent connections of the FEF.

Patients with unilateral frontal lobe lesions also show pursuit deficits. The FEF, SEF, and perhaps the PFC play a role in this abnormality. The defects are in both initiation and maintenance (more so at higher target speeds and frequencies). If lesions are in the SEF, defects are ipsilateral; if lesions are in the FEF, defects are bilateral but usually are greater for ipsilateral tracking. Patients with SEF lesions may have delayed reversal with periodic constant-velocity stimuli, implying impaired anticipation of the target trajectory. Saccades to moving targets are also inaccurate in some of these patients. Patients with lesions affecting the FEF may also show craniotopic as well as directional (ipsilateral) defects in pursuit. Tracking in the field contralateral to the lesion is worse than in the ipsilateral field. Visual exploration deficits may also play a role in some of the eye movement deficits seen with frontal lesions.

Acute bilateral frontal or frontoparietal lesions may produce a striking disturbance of ocular motility that is called **acquired ocular motor apraxia.** It is characterized by loss of voluntary control of eye movements, both saccades and pursuit, with preservation of reflex movements, including the VOR and quick phases of nystagmus. There is also relative preservation of saccades made to visual targets compared with internally guided saccades made on command and with blinking or head movements. Voluntary movements of the eyes are limited in the horizontal and usually also in the vertical plane. The defect of voluntary eye movements probably reflects disruption of descending pathways both from the FEF and the parietal cortex so that the superior colliculus and brainstem reticular formation are bereft of their supranuclear inputs.

OCULAR MOTOR APRAXIA

Ocular motor apraxia is characterized by an impaired ability to generate saccades on command (Fig. 17.25). In congenital ocular motor apraxia (COMA), an abnormality in eye movements may be recognized shortly after birth, when the child does not appear to fixate upon objects normally and may be thought to be blind. Between ages 4 to 6 months, characteristic thrusting

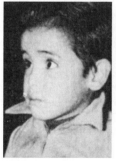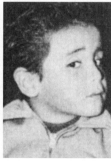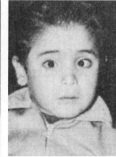

Figure 17.25. Congenital ocular motor apraxia. The patient was looking to the right **(left)** when he was told to glance at the camera. His head rapidly moved to the left, while the eyes remained deviated toward the right. As a result, the patient's head had to turn farther to the left in order to permit fixation ahead **(center)**. After the patient was able to fixate on the camera, his head turned slowly back to the right until it was straight **(right)**. (Reprinted from: Urrets-Zavalia A, Remonda C. Congenital ocular motor apraxia. *Ophthalmologica.* 1957;134:157–167, with permission.)

horizontal head movements develop, sometimes with prominent blinking or even rubbing the eyelids, when the child attempts to change fixation. In children with poor head control, development of head thrusting may be delayed or absent. Almost all patients also show a defect in generating quick phases of nystagmus, which can usually be appreciated at the bedside by manual spinning of the patient, either when holding the child out at arm's length or by rotating the child on a swivel chair (if necessary sitting in an adult's lap). Despite difficulties in shifting horizontal gaze, vertical voluntary eye movements are normal, an important differential diagnostic point because **most acquired cases of ocular motor apraxia cause defects in both the horizontal and vertical planes.**

The head thrusts made by patients with COMA probably reflect one of several adaptive strategies to facilitate changes in gaze. Younger patients appear to use their intact VOR, which drives their eyes into an extreme contraversive position in the orbit. As the head continues to move past the target, the eyes are dragged along in space until they become aligned with the target. The head then rotates backward, and the eyes maintain fixation as they are brought back to the primary position in the orbit by the VOR. In contrast, older patients appear to use the head movement alone to trigger the generation of a saccadic eye movement that cannot normally be made with the head still. This strategy may reflect the use of a phylogenetically old linkage between head and saccadic eye movements that occurs reflexively in afoveate animals when they desire to redirect their center of visual attention.

A variety of disorders that directly damage the brainstem mechanisms for generating saccades—including structural or degenerative processes within the pontine and mesencephalic reticular formations—are characterized by the development of a strategy of head thrusting or blinking to shift the gaze that superficially resembles COMA. These disorders usually can be differentiated from COMA because all types of saccades and quick phases (both horizontal and vertical) are typically affected, and because saccades may be slow. In the early stages of these diseases, however, the ocular motor apraxia may be indistinguishable from COMA. Thus, patients with ataxia telangiectasia (Louis-Bar syndrome, 11q22-23) and its variants (ataxia-oculomotor apraxia syndrome of Aicardi), Gaucher's disease (types 2 and 3, 1q21-31), Niemann-Pick disease type 2s, Pelizaeus-Merzbacher disease, Cockayne's syndrome, Huntington's disease, hepatolenticular degeneration, vitamin E deficiency, some of the peroxisome disorders, Whipple's disease, and many other storage diseases and aminoacidurias may appear to have COMA or at least COMA-like eye movements (Fig. 17.20).

ABNORMAL EYE MOVEMENTS AND DEMENTIA

Patients with various dementing processes have abnormal eye movements, reflecting either disturbances in cerebral cortical structures or in other subcortical structures that may also be affected by that particular disease. Excessive errors on the antisaccade test, particularly when associated with a "visual grasp reflex," are a useful indicator of an organic process when pseudodementia is a diagnostic consideration in a patient with a possible cognitive decline.

Patients with Alzheimer's disease have excessive numbers of square-wave jerks and defects in saccade latency and, occasionally, accuracy and velocity. Alzheimer's disease patients show longer mean fixation durations and a reduced number of exploring saccades when viewing simple but not complex scenes, perhaps reflecting a motivation deficit. Impairment of spatially directed attention may also be reflected in eye-movement abnormalities, and a Balint-like syndrome may develop. Pursuit abnormalities also occur in patients with Alzheimer's disease.

Patients with Creutzfeldt-Jakob disease may show limitation of vertical gaze and slow vertical saccades as well as two rare forms of nystagmus, periodic alternating nystagmus and centripetal nystagmus. Cerebellar eye signs are typically found in another prion disorder, Gerstmann-Sträussler-Scheinker disease.

OCULAR MOTOR MANIFESTATIONS OF SEIZURES

Abnormal eye and head movements are common manifestations of epileptic seizures. A variety of eye movements can occur in this setting, including horizontal or vertical gaze deviation and conjugate, retractory, or monocular nystagmus. Epileptic convergence nystagmus also occurs with periodic lateralizing epileptiform discharges and with burst-suppression patterns. The seizure focus may arise from any lobe, although the lesions usually are more posterior. Epileptic nystagmus occurs with typical absence seizures and with infantile spasms.

Patients with epileptic foci affecting the temporoparietooccipital cortex may show either ipsiversive or contraversive eye deviation and nystagmus. Overall, contraversive deviation of the eyes is more common than ipsiversive deviation during seizures. In cases with posterior foci (temporal, parietal, or occipital lobes), experimental studies suggest that eye movements may be mediated by projections via either the superior colliculus or the FEF. Thus, saccades may be generated by more than one of the descending parallel pathways. Frontal lobe foci are also reported to cause contraversive deviations unless they are bilateral, in which case vertical deviations also may occur.

EYE MOVEMENTS IN STUPOR AND COMA

The ocular motor examination is especially useful for evaluating the unconscious patient, because both arousal and eye movements are controlled by neurons in the brainstem reticular formation. Comatose patients do not make eye movements that depend upon cortical visual processing. Voluntary saccades and smooth pursuit are in abeyance, and quick phases of nystagmus also may be absent. The ocular motor examination of the unconscious patient, therefore, consists of observing the resting position of the eyes, looking for any spontaneous movements, and reflexively inducing eye movements.

Gaze Deviations

Conjugate, horizontal deviation of the eyes is common in coma. When the coma is caused by a lesion above the brainstem ocular motor decussation between the midbrain and pons, the eyes are usually directed toward the side of the lesion and away from the hemiparesis that typically is present. A vestibular stimulus, however, can usually drive the eyes across the midline. If the conjugate deviation is caused by a lesion below the ocular motor decussation, the eyes will be directed away from the side of the lesion and toward the hemiparesis. The latter is typically seen with pontine lesions, but also in some patients with thalamic and, rarely, hemispheric disease above the thalamus (so-called wrong-way deviations).

Intermittent deviation of the eyes and head is usually caused by seizure activity. At the onset of each attack, gaze is usually deviated contralateral to the side of the seizure focus and may be followed by nystagmus with contralaterally directed quick phases. Toward the end of the seizure, gaze drifts to an ipsilateral (paretic) position.

Tonic downward deviation of the eyes, often accompanied by convergence, occurs in patients with thalamic hemorrhage and with lesions affecting the dorsal midbrain. It may be induced by unilateral caloric stimulation, after the initial horizontal deviation subsides, in patients with coma induced by sedative drugs. Forced downward deviation of the eyes can also be seen in patients with nonorganic (feigned) coma or seizures.

Tonic upward deviation of the eyes is uncommon in coma, but it may occur following an hypoxic-ischemic insult, even when no pathologic lesions are found in the midbrain. Patients who survive after manifesting this ocular motor disturbance typically develop downbeating nystagmus, the upward drift of which is thought to be caused by loss of inhibition on the upward vertical VOR. Upward deviation of the eyes also occurs as a component of oculogyric crisis, which usually occurs as a side effect of certain drugs, especially neuroleptic agents. Tonic uninhibited elevation of the lids **(eyes-open coma)** may also occur in unconscious patients and may be related to pontomesencephalic dysfunction.

Spontaneous Eye Movements

Spontaneous eye movements that occur in unconscious patients may help establish the etiology of the coma (Table 17.8). **Slow conjugate or disconjugate roving**

Table 17.8. *Spontaneous Eye Movements Occurring in Unconscious Patients*

Term	Description	Causes
Ocular bobbing	Rapid, conjugate, downward movement; slow return to primary position	Pontine strokes; other structural, metabolic or toxic disorders
Ocular dipping or inverse ocular bobbing	Slow downward movement; rapid return to primary position	Unreliable for localization; follows hypoxic-ischemic insult or metabolic disorder
Reverse ocular bobbing	Rapid upward movement; slow return to primary position	Unreliable for localization; may occur with metabolic disorders
Reverse ocular dipping or converse bobbing	Slow upward movement; rapid return to primary position	Unreliable for localization; pontine infarction and with AIDS
Ping-pong gaze	Horizontal conjugate deviation of the eyes, alternating every few seconds	Bilateral cerebral hemispheric dysfunction
Periodic alternating gaze deviation	Horizontal conjugate deviation of the eyes, alternating every 2 minutes	Hepatic encephalopathy; disorders causing periodic alternating nystagmus and unconsciousness
Vertical myoclonus	Vertical pendular oscillations (2–3 Hz)	Pontine strokes
Monocular movements	Small, intermittent, rapid monocular horizontal, vertical, or torsional movements	Pontine or midbrain destructive lesions, perhaps with co-existent seizures

eye movements are similar to the eye movements of light sleep but slower than the rapid eye movements (REM) of paradoxic or REM sleep. Their presence indicates that brainstem gaze mechanisms are intact.

Other types of spontaneous eye movements consist of various forms of vertical to-and-fro movements, often called "bobbing." Typical **ocular bobbing** consists of intermittent, usually conjugate, rapid downward movement of the eyes followed by a slower return to the primary position. Reflex horizontal eye movements are usually absent. Ocular bobbing is a classic sign of intrinsic pontine lesions, usually hemorrhage, but it also occurs in patients with cerebellar lesions that compress the pons and in some cases of metabolic or toxic encephalopathy. **Inverse bobbing** also occurs in this setting. This eye movement abnormality, which is also called **ocular dipping,** is characterized by a slow downward movement, followed by a rapid return to midposition. **Reverse bobbing** consists of rapid deviation of the eyes upward and a slow return to the horizontal, whereas **converse bobbing** (also called **reverse dipping**) is characterized by a slow upward drift of the eyes that is followed by a rapid return to primary position. These variants of ocular bobbing are less reliable for localization than is straightforward ocular bobbing. Nevertheless, the occurrence in some patients of several different types of ocular bobbing during the course of their illness suggests a common underlying pathophysiology. Because the pathways that mediate upward and downward eye movements differ anatomically, and probably pharmacologically, it seems likely that these movements represent a varying imbalance of mechanisms for vertical gaze in the setting of bilateral horizontal gaze paralysis.

Rarely, large-amplitude pendular vertical oscillations occur in the acute phase of a brainstem stroke. This **vertical myoclonus** may have a pathogenesis similar to that of acquired pendular nystagmus.

Repetitive vertical eye movements, including variants of ocular bobbing, may contain **convergent-divergent** components. Such movements are usually caused by disease affecting the dorsal midbrain.

Monocular bobbing movements may occur as a synkinesis with jaw movement. Such movements are similar to those seen in the congenital condition called the Marcus Gunn jaw-winking phenomenon and primarily involve the neural pathways to the inferior rectus muscle.

Ping-pong gaze consists of slow, horizontal, conjugate deviations of the eyes that alternate every few seconds. Although ping-pong gaze can occur in patients with posterior fossa hemorrhage, it is usually a sign of bilateral infarction of the cerebral hemispheres. Sometimes, oscillations with a periodicity similar to that of ping-pong gaze can be induced transiently by a rapid head rotation in patients with bilateral hemisphere disease.

Rapid, small-amplitude, vertical eye movements may be the only manifestation of epileptic seizures in patients with co-existent brainstem injury. Rapid, monocular eye movements with horizontal, vertical, or torsional components, which occur in coma, may also indicate brainstem dysfunction.

Identification of patients who are conscious but quadriplegic—the **locked-in syndrome** or de-efferented state—depends on identifying preserved voluntary vertical eye movements. The syndrome is typically caused by pontine infarction and is characterized in part by a variable loss of voluntary and reflex horizontal movements, such that eyelid or vertical eye movements may be the only means of communication during the acute illness. The locked-in syndrome also occurs with midbrain lesions, in which case ptosis and ophthalmoplegia may be present.

Reflex Eye Movements

Reflex eye movements may be elicited in unconscious patients either by head rotation (the oculocephalic or doll's head maneuver) or by caloric stimulation. Head rotation, with the patient supine, stimulates the labyrinthine semicircular canals, the otoliths, and neck muscle proprioceptors. However, eye rotations induced by head rotation in unconscious individuals principally result from the effects of the semicircular canals and their central connections (Fig. 17.26). Head rotations should not be used in unconscious patients unless it is certain that no neck injury or abnormality is present.

Caloric irrigation of the external auditory meatus causes convection currents of the vestibular endolymph that displace the cupula of a semicircular canal; thus, this procedure also tests the VOR. The canal stimulated depends on the orientation of the head; for example, with the head elevated 30° from the supine position, the horizontal canals are principally stimulated. Before caloric stimulation, the physician should always check that the tympanic membrane is intact. Usually only about 5 mL of ice water need be introduced into the external auditory meatus, but large quantities (100 mL or more) may be necessary to induce a response in some comatose patients.

In testing reflex eye movements in unresponsive patients, it is important to note: (a) the magnitude of the response, (b) whether the ocular deviation is conjugate, (c) the dynamic response to position-step head rotations, and (d) the occurrence of any quick phases of nystagmus, particularly during caloric stimulation. Impaired abduction suggests an abducens nerve palsy. Impaired adduction usually indicates either an INO or an oculomotor nerve palsy, although occasionally

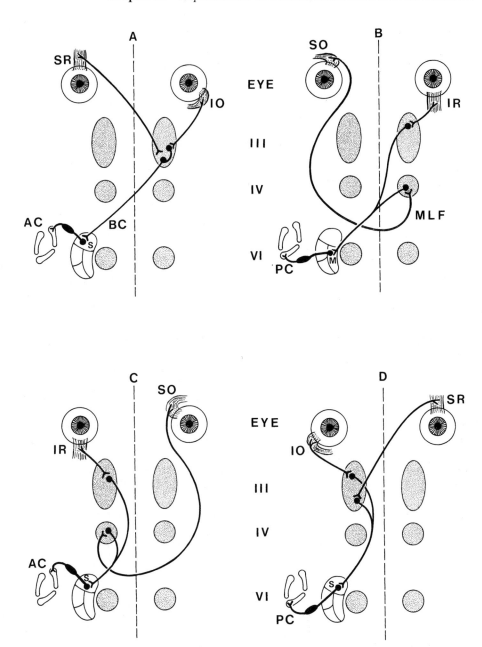

Figure 17.26. Direct vertical vestibulo-ocular projections from the vertical semicircular canals. **A and B:** Excitatory connections. **C and D:** Inhibitory connections. **A:** Excitatory afferents from the anterior semicircular canals *(AC)* synapse in the superior vestibular nucleus *(S)*, and their signals are relayed via the brachium conjunctivum *(BC)* to ocular motor subnuclei that drive the ipsilateral superior rectus *(SR)* and contralateral inferior oblique *(IO)* muscles. **B:** Excitatory afferents from the posterior semicircular canals *(PC)* synapse in the medial vestibular nucleus *(M)*, and their signals are relayed via the contralateral medial longitudinal fasciculus *(MLF)* to the ocular motor subnuclei that drive the ipsilateral superior oblique *(SO)* and contralateral inferior rectus *(IR)* muscles. **C:** Inhibitory afferents from the anterior semicircular canals. *D,* Inhibitory afferents from the posterior semicircular canals. (Redrawn from: Ghelarducci B, Highstein SM, Ito M. In: Baker R, Berthoz A, eds. *Control of Gaze by Brain Stem Neurons.* New York: Elsevier/North-Holland Biomedical Press; 1977:167–175.)

impaired adduction to vestibular stimulation may be observed in patients with metabolic coma or drug intoxication. Vertical responses may be impaired with disease of the midbrain or bilateral lesions of the MLF. Pontine lesions may abolish the reflex eye movements in the horizontal plane but spare the vertical responses. When reflex eye movements are present in an unresponsive patient, the brainstem is likely to be structurally intact. When reflex eye movements are abnormal or absent, the cause may be structural disease, profound metabolic coma, or drug intoxication.

If reflex eye movements are intact in an unconscious patient, the eyes are carried into a corner of the orbit when the head is rapidly rotated horizontally to a new position (velocity step stimulus). If the head is held stationary in its new position, the eyes may slowly drift back to the midline. This implies that the gaze-holding mechanism (neural integrator) is not functioning normally. Patients with more rapid centripetal drift may have more severe brain injury.

Quick phases of nystagmus are usually absent in acutely unconscious patients. Their presence, without a tonic deviation of the eyes, should raise the possibility of nonorganic (i.e., feigned) coma. In patients who are stuporous but uncooperative, caloric nystagmus may be a useful way of inducing eye movements that cannot be initiated voluntarily. Patients who survive coma but who are left in a persistent vegetative state, with severe damage of the cerebral hemispheres but preservation of the brainstem, regain nystagmus with caloric or rotational stimulation.

During syncope, normal subjects develop downbeat nystagmus and tonic upward deviation of the eyes. Most also exhibit an increased amplitude of the VOR. These findings are most compatible with cerebellar hypoperfusion.

OCULAR MOTOR MANIFESTATIONS OF SOME METABOLIC DISORDERS

Some babies who ultimately develop normally show transient ocular motor disturbances, including upward or downward deviation of the eyes (but with a full range of reflex vertical movement), intermittent opsoclonus, and skew deviation. However, abnormal eye movements also occur in many metabolic diseases that affect the nervous system, particularly inborn errors of metabolism, in infants, children, and adults.

The **lipid storage diseases** are often characterized by gaze palsies. Tay-Sachs disease impairs vertical and, subsequently, horizontal eye movements. Adult-onset hexosaminidase deficiency also preferentially affects vertical gaze. Variants of Niemann-Pick disease that begin after the first year of life (e.g., the sea-blue histiocyte syndrome or juvenile dystonic lipidosis) are characterized by deficits of voluntary vertical eye movements, particularly saccades and smooth pursuit; vertical vestibular and horizontal eye movements are relatively preserved (Fig. 17.20). Gaucher's disease is associated with a prominent deficit of horizontal gaze, and slow saccades may be a prominent finding in adults with this condition.

Pelizaeus-Merzbacher disease is an X-linked recessive leukodystrophy with severe cerebellar signs, including saccadic dysmetria. Some patients with this condition also show difficulty initiating saccades and pendular nystagmus.

Wernicke's encephalopathy is characterized by the triad of ophthalmoplegia, mental confusion, and gait ataxia. It is caused by thiamine deficiency and is most commonly encountered in alcoholics. The ocular motor findings include weakness of abduction, gaze-evoked nystagmus, primary-position vertical nystagmus, impaired vestibular responses to caloric and rotational stimulation, INO, the one-and-a-half syndrome, and horizontal and vertical gaze palsies that may progress to total ophthalmoplegia. The ophthalmoplegia is almost always bilateral but may be asymmetric. Lesions are found in the ocular motor and vestibular nuclei, as well as in the paraventricular regions of the thalamus, the hypothalamus, periaqueductal gray matter, superior vermis of the cerebellum, and dorsal motor nucleus of the vagus.

Most likely, affected areas of the brain contain neurons that use high amounts of glucose and, therefore, are particularly dependent upon thiamine, an important coenzyme in glucose metabolism. Administration of thiamine usually causes rapid improvement of the ocular motor signs, although complete recovery may take several weeks. Co-existent magnesium deficiency should also be treated. In patients with Wernicke's disease who go on to develop Korsakoff's syndrome, which is primarily characterized by a severe and enduring memory loss, ocular motor abnormalities may persist. The ocular motor abnormalities include slow and inaccurate saccades, impaired smooth pursuit, and gaze-evoked nystagmus.

Leigh's syndrome is a subacute necrotizing encephalopathy of infancy or childhood characterized by psychomotor retardation, seizures, and brainstem abnormalities, including eye movements. It is invariably fatal. It is an inherited disorder of mitochondrial function and can be caused either by abnormalities of mitochondrial DNA or by chromosomal disease. Both the disturbances of ocular motility and the pathologic findings resemble those caused by experimental thiamine deficiency or Wernicke's encephalopathy.

Deficiency of vitamin E may cause a progressive neurologic condition characterized by areflexia, cerebellar ataxia, and loss of joint position sense. Ocular

Table 17.9. *Effects of Drugs on Eye Movements*

Drug	Reported Effects
Amphetamines	Reduced saccadic latency
	Increased AC/A ratio
Baclofen	Reduced VOR time constant
	Complete paralysis of gaze
Benzodiazepines	Reduced velocity and increased duration of saccades
	Impaired smooth pursuit
	Decreased gain and increased time constant of VOR
	Divergence paralysis
Beta-adrenergic blocking agents	Internuclear ophthalmoplegia
Carbamazepine	Decreased velocity of saccades
	Impaired smooth pursuit
	Gaze-evoked nystagmus
	Oculogyric crisis
	Downbeat nystagmus
	Complete paralysis of gaze
Chloral hydrate	Impaired smooth pursuit
Ethyl alcohol	Reduced peak velocity of saccades
	Increased latency of saccades
	Hypometric saccades
	Impaired smooth pursuit and VOR suppression
	Gaze-evoked nystagmus
	Position-induced nystagmus
	Reversed compensation of cerebellar lesions
Lithium carbonate	Saccadic dysmetria
	Impaired smooth pursuit
	Gaze-evoked nystagmus
	Downbeat nystagmus
	Oculogyric crises
	Internuclear ophthalmoplegia
	Complete paralysis of gaze
	Opsoclonus
Methadone	Hypometric saccades
	Impaired smooth pursuit
Nitrous oxide	Reduced peak velocity of saccades
	Impaired smooth pursuit
Phenobarbital and other barbiturates	Reduced peak saccadic velocity
	Gaze-evoked nystagmus
	Impaired vergence
	Decreased VOR gain
	Perverted caloric responses
	Vertical nystagmus
	Partial or complete paralysis of gaze
Phenothiazines	Oculogyric crises
	Internuclear ophthalmoplegia
Phenytoin	Impaired smooth pursuit and VOR suppression
	Gaze-evoked nystagmus
	Downbeat nystagmus
	Periodic alternating nystagmus
	Complete paralysis of gaze
	Convergence spasm
Tobacco	Upbeat nystagmus in darkness (cigarettes)
	Square-wave jerks (nicotine)
	Impaired pursuit (nicotine)
Toluene	Pendular nystagmus
	Internuclear ophthalmoplegia
Tricyclic antidepressants	Internuclear ophthalmoplegia
	Complete paralysis of gaze
	Opsoclonus

motor involvement includes progressive gaze restriction, sometimes with strabismus. There usually is a dissociated ophthalmoplegia and nystagmus in which adduction is fast but with a limited range and abduction is slow but with a full range (the posterior INO of Lutz). The combination of ocular motor findings in patients with vitamin E deficiency probably reflects a mixture of central and peripheral pathology. Vitamin E deficiency is more common in children, in whom it may be caused by abetalipoproteinemia (Bassen-Kornzweig disease). It is also reported in adults who have bowel or liver diseases that interfere with fat absorption or as part of an inherited ataxia caused by a defect of chromosome 8q13, the site of the α-tocopherol transfer protein gene.

Hepatolenticular degeneration, also called Wilson's disease, is an inherited disorder of copper metabolism that is transmitted in an autosomal-recessive fashion. The defect is in a copper-transporting ATPase gene at q14.3 on chromosome 14. The classic clinical picture is a movement disorder with psychiatric symptoms and associated liver disease. Ocular motor disorders in hepatolenticular degeneration include a distractibility of gaze with inability to voluntarily fix upon an object unless other competing visual stimuli are removed. Slow saccades and apraxia of eyelid opening can also occur.

Amyotrophic lateral sclerosis is associated with various eye movement disorders, including nystagmus, saccade disturbances that suggest a frontal lobe disturbance, and pursuit impairment. However, the existence of multisystem diseases in which motor neuron degeneration is just one neurologic feature makes specific clinical diagnoses difficult.

EFFECTS OF DRUGS ON EYE MOVEMENTS

Many substances affect eye movements (Table 17.9). In some cases, the drug induces abnormalities of eye movements at therapeutic concentrations (e.g., anticonvulsants). In other cases, abnormalities of eye movements develop only when concentrations of the drug in the CNS are inappropriately elevated. In still other cases, the eye movement abnormalities are caused by substances not meant for internal use.

Patients with drug-induced abnormalities of eye movements most often complain of diplopia, caused by ocular misalignment, or oscillopsia, caused by spontaneous nystagmus or an inappropriate VOR. Many drugs have their effect on central vestibular and cerebellar connections, and they cause ataxia and gaze-evoked nystagmus.

Although all classes of eye movements may be affected by **therapeutic doses** of various drugs, smooth pursuit, eccentric gaze holding, and convergence are particularly susceptible. For example, diazepam, methadone, phenytoin, barbiturates, chloral hydrate, and alcohol all impair smooth-pursuit tracking.

At **toxic levels,** neuroactive drugs can impair all eye movements, particularly when consciousness is also impaired. Phenytoin may cause a complete ophthalmoplegia in an awake patient, and therapeutic levels may cause ophthalmoplegia in patients in stupor. Phenytoin and diazepam can lead to opsoclonus. The tricyclic antidepressants may cause complete ophthalmoplegia or an INO in stuporous patients. Lithium causes a variety of abnormalities, including fixation instability and downbeat nystagmus.

In addition to drugs, certain **toxins** can cause abnormal eye movements. Some, such as chlordecone and thallium, cause saccadic oscillations. Intoxication with hydrocarbons can cause a vestibulopathy, and exposure to trichloroethylene and other solvents may affect pursuit, suppression of the VOR, and saccades. Prolonged exposure to toluene, especially in glue-sniffing addiction, may lead to a variety of ocular motor disturbances, including pendular and downbeat nystagmus, saccadic oscillations, and INO. Tobacco has a number of ocular motor effects. It causes upbeat nystagmus, impaired pursuit, decreased saccade latency, and increased square-wave jerks during pursuit, although performance is normal on the antisaccade test. Cocaine can affect eye movements, with opsoclonus being the most dramatic abnormality.

Ototoxicity, especially that associated with administration of aminoglycosides, is an important cause of loss of the VOR. Intravenous gentamicin is most often responsible. Its toxicity may be insidious, occurring without hearing symptoms and even with normal blood levels and relatively short periods of administration. Some patients who develop ototoxicity may be genetically predisposed to its toxic side effects. Topical (intratympanic) gentamicin is used to purposefully ablate labyrinthine function as part of the treatment of intractable Ménière's syndrome or Tullio's phenomenon, but it may occasionally lead to unwanted labyrinthine loss when used to treat external ear infections. Cisplatin is probably not as vestibulotoxic as originally thought.

FOR FURTHER INFORMATION

See *Walsh & Hoyt's Clinical Neuro-Ophthalmology*, 6th edition, Volume 1, Chapter 19, pages 907–967.

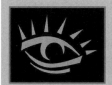

CHAPTER **1 8**

Nuclear and Infranuclear Ocular Motility Disorders*

The ocular motor system is separated anatomically and physiologically into infranuclear (peripheral), nuclear, internuclear, and supranuclear components. In this chapter, we consider ocular motor disturbances caused by congenital and acquired lesions of the nuclear and infranuclear neural structures—the lesions of the ocular motor nuclei and nerves.

Disorders that produce dysfunction of the oculomotor, trochlear, and abducens nerves may be located anywhere from the ocular motor nuclei to the termination of the nerves in the extraocular muscles within the orbit. Ocular motor nerve palsies may present in one of four ways:

1. As isolated partial or complete nerve palsies without any other neurologic signs and without symptoms except those related to the palsy itself.
2. In association with symptoms other than those related to the palsy (e.g., pain, dysesthesia, paresthesias) but without any signs of neurologic or systemic disease.
3. In association with other ocular motor nerve palsies (e.g., the simultaneous onset of an oculomotor palsy and an abducens palsy) but without any other neurologic signs.
4. In association with neurologic signs other than the ocular motor nerve palsy.

---

*Adapted from: Sargent JC. Nuclear and infranuclear ocular motility disorders. In: Miller NR, Newman NJ, Biousse V, Kerrison JB, eds. *Walsh & Hoyt's Clinical Neuro-Ophthalmology.* 6th ed. Vol. I. Philadelphia: Lippincott Williams & Wilkins; 2005:969–1040.

OCULOMOTOR (THIRD) NERVE PALSIES

CONGENITAL

Congenital oculomotor nerve palsies constitute nearly half of the oculomotor nerve pareses seen in children (Fig. 18.1). Most cases are unilateral. As a general rule, patients with congenital oculomotor nerve palsies have no other neurologic or systemic abnormalities. Usually, these patients have some degree of amblyopia.

All patients with congenital oculomotor nerve palsy have some degree of ptosis, ophthalmoparesis, and pupillary involvement. In most of these cases, the pupil is miotic rather than dilated, presumably because of misdirected oculomotor nerve regeneration. Abnormalities of the oculomotor nerve that are present at birth may be caused by absent or incomplete development of the nucleus, nerve, or both. Injury to the oculomotor nerve during gestation or at the time of delivery may produce a congenital oculomotor nerve palsy. Such patients may or may not have other physical signs of trauma or other neurologic signs.

In addition to simple congenital oculomotor nerve palsy, several congenital syndromes implicate oculomotor maldevelopment with anomalous or paradoxic innervation of the extraocular muscles. These syndromes include (a) congenital adduction palsy with synergistic divergence, (b) atypical vertical retraction syndrome, and (c) cyclic oculomotor nerve paresis with cyclic spasm.

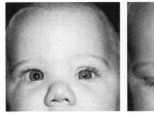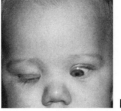

A   **B**

Figure 18.1. Congenital left oculomotor nerve palsy with aberrant regeneration in a child with a history of birth trauma. **A:** In primary position, there is a left hypotropia. Note the miotic left pupil. **B:** On attempted downward gaze, there is retraction of the left upper eyelid (pseudo-Graefe sign).

Congenital Adduction Palsy with Synergistic Divergence

Patients with this syndrome have congenital unilateral paralysis of adduction associated with simultaneous bilateral abduction on attempted gaze into the field of action of the paretic medial rectus muscle (Fig. 18.2). Most patients with congenital adduction palsy with synergistic divergence have no other neurologic abnormalities.

Electromyographic studies in patients with this condition suggest that it is caused by absent oculomotor nerve innervation of the affected medial rectus

muscle, combined with absent or minimal innervation of the lateral rectus muscle by the abducens nerve but with a branch of the oculomotor nerve innervating the lateral rectus muscle (Fig. 18.3).

Vertical Retraction Syndrome

The main clinical feature of the vertical retraction syndrome is limitation of movement of the affected eye on elevation or depression, associated with a retraction of the globe and narrowing of the palpebral fissure. There may be an associated esotropia or exotropia, more marked in the direction of the restricted vertical field of action. The condition is usually unilateral. The results of both electro-oculography and electromyography in patients with this condition are consistent with anomalous oculomotor innervation of the vertical rectus muscles of the affected eye.

Oculomotor Paresis with Cyclic Spasms (Cyclic Oculomotor Paresis)

Cyclic oculomotor paresis is usually unilateral and is, in the majority of cases, present from birth. The typical patient with this condition has an oculomotor nerve paresis with ptosis, mydriasis, reduced accommodation, and ophthalmoparesis. About every 2 minutes, the ptotic eyelid elevates, the globe begins to adduct, the pupil constricts, and accommodation increases.

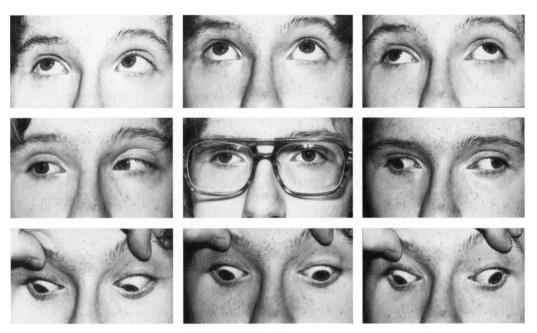

Figure 18.2. Congenital right adduction palsy and synergistic divergence. Extraocular movements in nine fields of gaze. The right eye abducts somewhat on attempted right lateral gaze, but also abducts on right lateral gaze. (Reprinted from: Wilcox LM Jr, Gittinger JW Jr, Breinin GM. Congenital adduction palsy and synergistic divergence. *Am J Ophthalmol.* 1981;91:1–7, with permission.)

Synergistic divergence

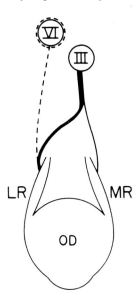

Figure 18.3. Anomaly of peripheral innervation that may explain synergistic divergence with congenital limitation of adduction. The oculomotor nerve provides major innervation of the lateral rectus muscle (which may or may not also be innervated by the abducens nerve). The thickness of the line representing the nerve represents quantitative innervation. Dashed lines indicate hypoplasia or aplasia of the abducens nucleus and/or nerve. *OD*, right eye; *LR*, lateral rectus muscle; *MR*, medial rectus muscle; *III*, oculomotor nucleus; *VI*, abducens nucleus. (Redrawn from: Wilcox LM Jr, Gittinger JW Jr, Breinin GM. Congenital adduction palsy and synergistic divergence. *Am J Ophthalmol.* 1981;91:1–7, with permission.)

These spasms last 10 to 30 seconds and then give way to the paretic phase. Cyclic oculomotor palsy usually continues throughout life.

Most patients with unilateral cyclic oculomotor paresis have reduced visual acuity in the affected eye because of amblyopia. The syndrome is occasionally associated with other pathologic conditions, including birth trauma and congenital infections. Rarely, cases occur after an acquired oculomotor nerve palsy, such as from a posterior fossa tumor. However, patients with true congenital oculomotor nerve paresis with cyclic spasms do not require any workup unless they have other evidence of neurologic disease, or they give a history of progressive neurologic dysfunction.

ACQUIRED

Acquired dysfunction of the oculomotor nerve is far more common than its congenital counterpart, being caused by nearly every pathologic process.

Lesions of the Oculomotor Nucleus

Lesions that damage the oculomotor nucleus are not uncommon. When they occur, they often produce bilateral defects in ocular motility, eyelid position, or both. The bilaterality of involvement is explained by the anatomy of the nucleus and its fibers. Both levator palpebrae superioris muscles are innervated by a single, midline subnucleus located at the caudal end of the oculomotor nerve complex (Fig. 18.4). A lesion that damages this region thus produces a bilateral, symmetric ptosis. In some cases, the ptosis is isolated, whereas in others, there is associated ophthalmoplegia.

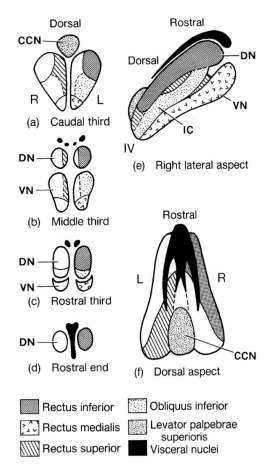

Rectus inferior	Obliquus inferior
Rectus medialis	Levator palpebrae superioris
Rectus superior	Visceral nuclei

Figure 18.4. Warwick's schema of topographic organization within the oculomotor nucleus. Note the caudal dorsal midline position of caudal central nucleus (CCN), the motor pool for the levator palpebrae superioris. The motor pool of the superior rectus (*hashed area*) is **contralateral** to the extraocular muscle it innervates. The visceral (parasympathetic) nuclei are shown in black. *DN*, dorsal nucleus; *IC*, intermediate column; *IV*, tegion of the trochlear nucleus; *VN*, ventral nucleus. (Reprinted from: Warwick R. Representation of the extra-ocular muscles in the oculomotor nuclei of the monkey. *J Comp Neurol.* 1953;98:449–504, with permission.)

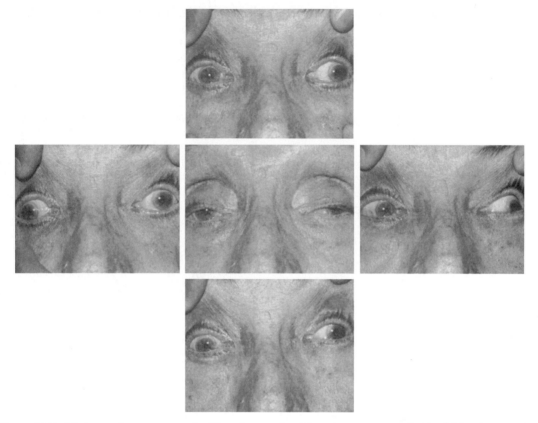

Figure 18.5. Nuclear oculomotor nerve palsy. There is a complete left oculomotor nerve palsy. In addition, however, there is absence of elevation of the right eye. The right eye also has marked limitation of depression, suggesting that the lesion is not limited to the left oculomotor nerve nucleus but also involves the right nucleus as well. Neither oculocephalic nor caloric stimulation produced any improvement in vertical gaze.

Lesions of the oculomotor nuclear complex may spare the central caudal nucleus. Patients with such lesions have fixed, dilated pupils and ophthalmoparesis affecting one or more of the muscles innervated by the oculomotor nerve but no ptosis.

A second anatomic feature of the oculomotor nuclear complex that results in bilateral ocular damage is the course of the nerve to the superior rectus muscle, which is crossed. The subnucleus for superior rectus function on either side of the brainstem gives rise to fibers that pass through the contralateral superior rectus subnucleus without synapse and innervate the **contralateral** superior rectus muscle. Lesions that affect this region thus cause not only ipsilateral weakness of superior rectus, medial rectus, inferior rectus, inferior oblique, or a combination of these muscles, but also limitation of elevation in the contralateral eye from impairment of superior rectus function on that side. Such patients have bilateral limitation of upward gaze, occasionally worse on the contralateral side (Figs. 18.5 and 18.6).

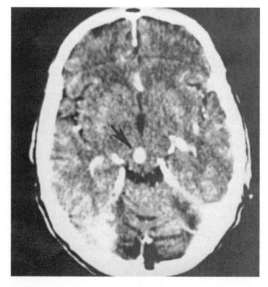

Figure 18.6. Computed tomographic scan in the patient whose appearance is seen in Figure 18.5. Note the enhancing lesion in the dorsal mesencephalon (*arrow*).

Lesions of the oculomotor nucleus are most often caused by ischemia, usually from embolic or thrombotic occlusion of small, dorsal perforating branches of the mesencephalic portion of the basilar artery or, less often, from occlusion of the distal portion of the basilar artery itself ("top of the basilar syndrome"). Other etiologies include hemorrhage, infiltration by tumor, inflammation, and brainstem compression.

Involvement of the immediate premotor mesencephalic structures located adjacent to the oculomotor nuclei complex may produce difficulties with ocular motility that may initially appear indistinguishable from direct damage to the nucleus itself. Such supranuclear defects can usually be distinguished from their nuclear and infranuclear counterparts by stimulation of the vestibular system using oculocephalic or caloric testing.

Lesions of the Oculomotor Nerve Fascicle

Fascicular lesions of the oculomotor nerves produce both complete and incomplete palsies that cannot be differentiated clinically from palsies caused by lesions outside the brainstem. Although most lesions that affect the fascicle produce an oculomotor nerve palsy with pupillary involvement, occasionally the pupil is spared. A fascicular oculomotor nerve palsy may occur as an isolated finding or in association with other neurologic signs (Fig. 18.7).

Fascicular oculomotor nerve palsies that are associated with other neurologic manifestations produce several characteristic syndromes. Lesions in the area of the brachium conjunctivum may produce ipsilateral oculomotor nerve palsy and cerebellar ataxia **(Nothnagel's syndrome)**. The syndrome of ipsilateral oculomotor nerve palsy combined with contralateral involuntary movements is known as **Benedikt's syndrome** and

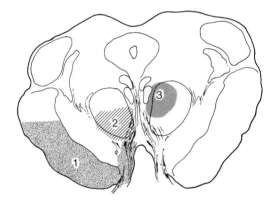

Figure 18.7. Diagram of a section through the mesencephalon showing regions in which the oculomotor nerve fascicle may be injured causing specific neurologic syndromes. **1.** Weber's syndrome. **2.** Benedikt's syndrome. **3.** Claude's syndrome.

reflects damage to the red nucleus, especially its dorsocaudal portion, through which the oculomotor fascicle passes (Fig. 18.7). Mesencephalic lesions ventral to the red nucleus may damage fascicular oculomotor fibers and motor fibers in the cerebral peduncle, producing an oculomotor nerve palsy with contralateral hemiplegia or hemiparesis, including the lower face and tongue **(Weber's syndrome)** (Figs. 18.7 through 18.9). Simultaneous damage in the mesencephalon to the red nucleus *and* the brachium conjunctivum produces a syndrome with the features of both Benedikt's and Nothnagel's syndromes—oculomotor nerve paresis, contralateral asynergia, ataxia, dysmetria, and dysdiadochokinesia—called **Claude's syndrome** (Fig. 18.7). The majority of mesencephalic syndromes is vascular in origin and are caused by occlusion or other injury to the vascular area of the basilar artery or perforating branches of the posterior cerebral artery; however, Claude's syndrome can result from thrombosis of the medial interpeduncular branch of the posterior cerebral artery.

Although divisional oculomotor nerve pareses are often caused by lesions in the cavernous sinus or posterior orbit, anatomic separation into superior and inferior divisions begins in the brainstem. Thus, lesions of the oculomotor fascicles can cause isolated dysfunction of either the superior or inferior division of the oculomotor nerve. It is likely that fascicular lesions can also cause isolated weakness of only one of the muscles innervated by the oculomotor nerve.

As with nuclear oculomotor palsies, fascicular lesions may be ischemic, hemorrhagic, compressive, infiltrative, traumatic, or rarely, inflammatory. Because the fascicles are white matter tracts, demyelinating disease may also cause an oculomotor nerve paresis that may occur as an isolated phenomenon or associated with other neurologic manifestations.

Lesions of the Oculomotor Nerve in the Subarachnoid Space

Lesions that damage the oculomotor nerve in the interpeduncular fossa may be located anywhere from the emergence of the nerve at the ventral surface of the mesencephalon to the point at which the nerve penetrates the dura beside the posterior clinoid process to enter the cavernous sinus (Figs. 18.10). Interpeduncular damage to the oculomotor nerve may be partial or complete. In some cases, the palsy is initially incomplete but progresses over hours, days, weeks, or even months. In most cases, there is some degree of accommodative paresis, but pupillary involvement is variable and depends primarily on the nature of the lesion. Oculomotor nerve dysfunction that is produced by damage to its subarachnoid portion may occur as (a) isolated pupillary dilation with a reduced or absent light reaction, (b) ophthalmoplegia with pupillary

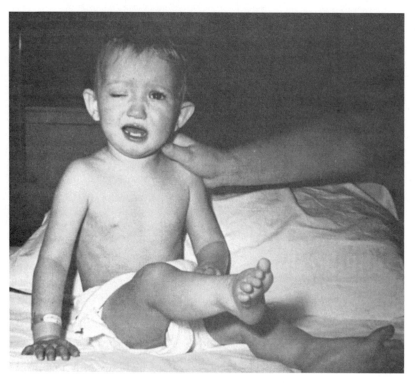

Figure 18.8. Weber's syndrome produced by a brainstem glioma infiltrating the mesencephalon. Note the oculomotor nerve palsy on the right, and the hemiplegia on the left.

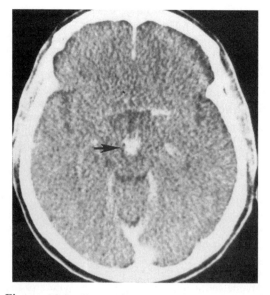

Figure 18.9. Computed tomogram in a patient with Weber's syndrome showing an enhancing lesion in the ventral mesencephalon (*arrow*). The lesion was thought to be a solitary metastasis from a breast carcinoma.

involvement, or (c) ophthalmoplegia with normal pupillary size and reactivity.

Isolated Fixed, Dilated Pupil as the Sole Manifestation of Subarachnoid Oculomotor Nerve Palsy

Many different lesions that compress the oculomotor nerve from above and medially rarely may produce isolated pupillary dilation. Intracranial aneurysms, particularly those at the junction of the internal carotid artery and the posterior communication artery, are capable of producing a fixed dilated pupil in the early stages of oculomotor nerve involvement, but *other signs of oculomotor nerve palsy usually develop within a few hours*. Basilar artery aneurysms can produce an isolated mid-dilated nonreactive or poorly reactive pupil that may be the only sign of an oculomotor nerve palsy for days or even weeks. Other extrinsic lesions in the interpeduncular cistern, such as cysts, can also produce this condition, as can intrinsic lesions of the oculomotor nerve, such as schwannomas or angiomas. Basal meningitis may damage the oculomotor nerve in the interpeduncular fossa and produce unilateral or bilateral internal ophthalmoplegia.

Truly isolated pupillary dilation from involvement of the interpeduncular portion of the oculomotor

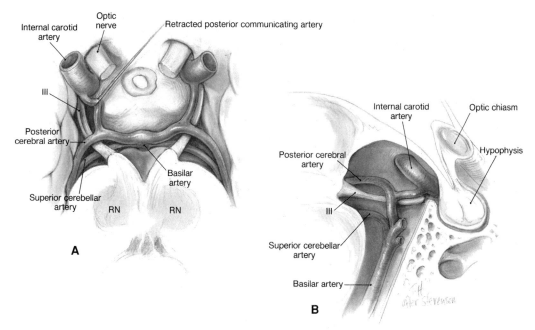

Figure 18.10. The relationship of the oculomotor nerve to the intracranial arteries in the subarachnoid space. **A:** The oculomotor nerves (III) are viewed from above. On the left, the posterior communicating artery has been retracted to show the groove that it may produce through its contact with the oculomotor nerve. *RN*, red nucleus. **B:** Lateral view of the left oculomotor nerve (III) showing its arterial relationships.

nerve is *exceptionally rare*. The occurrence of a widely dilated, nonreactive pupil in an otherwise healthy patient, even a patient complaining of headache, is far more likely to be caused by either ciliary ganglion involvement (i.e., a tonic pupil) or direct pharmacologic blockade, both of which can be diagnosed easily by pharmacologic testing.

Subarachnoid Oculomotor Nerve Palsy with Pupillary Involvement

Intracranial aneurysms are the most common cause of isolated oculomotor nerve palsy with pupillary involvement, particularly when the patient has a history of sudden severe pain in or around the eye (Figs. 18.11 and 18.12). The aneurysms usually arise from the

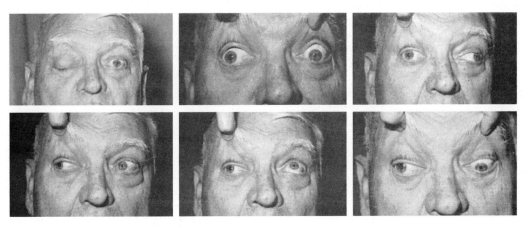

Figure 18.11. Complete right oculomotor nerve palsy with involvement of the pupil. The patient also complained of severe right-sided retro-orbital pain.

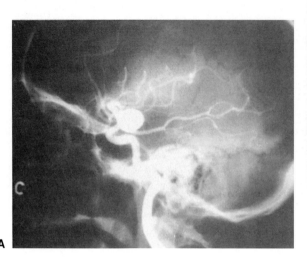

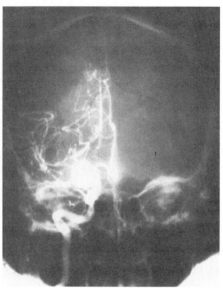

A

B

Figure 18.12. Selective right internal carotid arteriogram showing large aneurysm at the junction of the right internal carotid and right posterior communicating arteries in the patient whose appearance is shown in Figure 18.11. **A:** Lateral view. **B:** Anteroposterior view.

junction of the internal carotid and posterior communicating arteries; however, aneurysms located at the top of the basilar artery and aneurysms located at the junction of the basilar artery and superior cerebellar artery may produce a similar clinical picture. Such aneurysms may injure the oculomotor nerve by direct compression, from a small hemorrhage, or at the time of a major rupture. Trauma to the oculomotor nerve may occur during aneurysm surgery.

A painful oculomotor nerve palsy with pupillary involvement may result from a posteriorly draining, low-flow carotid-cavernous sinus fistula. Tumors and other compressive lesions, such as ectatic posterior cerebral or basilar artery vessels, can occasionally stretch or compress the oculomotor nerve in the interpeduncular fossa. Intrinsic lesions of the oculomotor nerve, such as schwannomas or cavernous angiomas, can also produce an acute or progressive oculomotor nerve paresis (Fig. 18.13).

Vascular diseases, particularly diabetes mellitus, often produce an oculomotor nerve palsy that spares the pupil. Nevertheless, the pupil is involved in many cases.

Subarachnoid Oculomotor Nerve Palsy with Pupillary Sparing

Ischemia is the most frequent cause of pupil-sparing oculomotor nerve palsies, particularly those that are unassociated with any other neurologic signs or symptoms (Fig. 18.14). In most instances, the patient has diabetes mellitus, but systemic hypertension, atheroscle-

rosis, and migraine can all produce a similar clinical picture. In cases of ischemic oculomotor nerve palsy, the lesion is most often located in the oculomotor nerve fascicle, where the pupillary efferent fibers are anatomically separate from the fibers to the extraocular

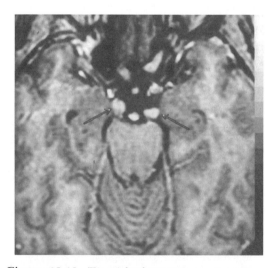

Figure 18.13. T1-weighted magnetic resonance image (axial view) in a 31-year-old-woman with progressive bilateral pupillary-involved oculomotor pareses and neurofibromatosis. There are bilateral enhancing lesions in the interpeduncular cistern (*arrows*) consistent with schwannomas of the oculomotor nerves.

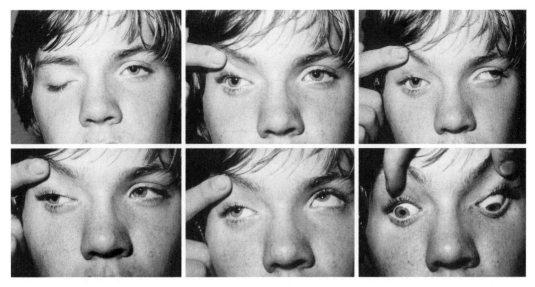

Figure 18.14. Pupil-sparing oculomotor nerve palsy in a patient with diabetes mellitus.

muscles, or in the subarachnoid portion of the nerve, where the pupillary fibers occupy a peripheral location and receive more collateral blood supply than the main trunk of the nerve.

Patients with oculomotor nerve pareses caused by ischemia often have severe pain regardless of whether or not the pupil is involved. Ischemic oculomotor nerve palsies characteristically resolve within 4 to 16 weeks without treatment. The resolution is almost always complete, and there is almost never evidence of aberrant regeneration.

Although most pupil-sparing oculomotor nerve palsies (with or without associated pain) are caused by ischemia, such palsies may also be produced by subarachnoid compressive lesions, particularly aneurysms, ipsilateral temporal lobe astrocytomas and ipsilateral acute subdural hematomas. Such palsies are nearly always **incomplete** and are often accompanied by ocular or orbital pain. Patients with a painful, incomplete, pupil-sparing oculomotor nerve paresis should undergo MRI as well as either computed tomographic angiography (CTA) or MR angiography (MRA). Depending on the results of these studies, conventional angiography may be appropriate.

Subarachnoid Oculomotor Nerve Palsy from Involvement at or near Its Entrance to the Cavernous Sinus

The oculomotor nerve is particularly vulnerable to stretch and contusion injuries where it is firmly attached to the dura adjacent to the posterior clinoid process just posterior to the cavernous sinus. Frontal head trauma, aneurysms, and surgery in the parasellar region are common causes of injury at this site.

Herniation of the hippocampal gyrus compresses the oculomotor nerve where it passes over the ridge of the dura associated with the attachment of the free edge of the tentorium to the clivus. As the herniating hippocampal gyrus descends into the tentorial incisura, it presses upon the upper surface of the ipsilateral oculomotor nerve that is running beneath it and pulls the oculomotor nerve more firmly into contact with the posterior clinoid process. The herniating cerebral mass ultimately reaches and impinges on the dorsal surface of the pons on the same side. The posterior cerebral arteries are also drawn tightly down across the dorsal surface of the oculomotor nerves, producing even more compression (Fig. 18.10). Pupillary dilation is often the first sign of increasing cerebral edema or of an ipsilateral, expanding, supratentorial mass. This initial pupillary sign is caused by pressure on the peripheral portion of the nerve. With increasing compression, additional signs of impaired oculomotor nerve function appear.

Lesions of the Oculomotor Nerve within the Cavernous Sinus and Superior Orbital Fissure

Lesions within the cavernous sinus or superior orbital fissure may produce isolated oculomotor nerve dysfunction but more often cause a cranial polyneuropathy. Because the cavernous sinus contains structures that continue through the superior orbital fissure, it is often impossible to determine with certainty if the lesion is confined to the sinus, is in the fissure, or involves both structures. It is reasonable to consider damage in

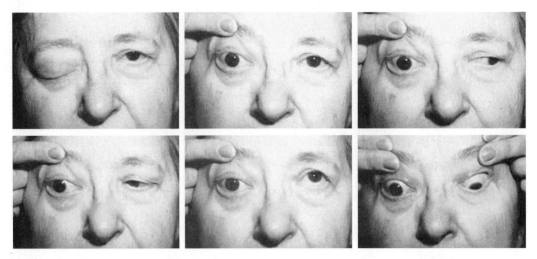

Figure 18.15. Patient with cavernous sinus syndrome from basal meningioma. The patient has right proptosis associated with a complete right oculomotor nerve palsy, a right abducens nerve paresis, and a right Horner's syndrome. Note that the right pupil is slightly smaller than the left pupil.

this region as a single entity, the **sphenocavernous syndrome.** This syndrome is characterized by paralysis or paresis of the oculomotor, trochlear, and abducens nerves, usually associated with involvement of the ophthalmic division (and in the cavernous sinus, the maxillary division) of the trigeminal nerve (Fig. 18.15). Involvement of the optic nerve either within the orbit or intracranially often causes visual loss. Because of the frequent involvement of the trigeminal nerve by lesions of the cavernous sinus and superior orbital fissure, patients with such lesions often complain of severe pain when they develop ophthalmoplegia. In many cases, there is oculosympathetic paresis, and there may be proptosis, edema of the eyelids, and chemosis of the conjunctiva. In patients with combined oculomotor paresis and sympathetic denervation, the pupil may be small or midposition and poorly reactive. This appearance is almost pathognomonic of a cavernous sinus lesion.

The sphenocavernous syndrome may be produced by primary or secondary lesions within the cavernous sinus or superior orbital fissure or by lesions within the orbit or intracranial cavity that compress the cranial nerves that pass through these structures. Common lesions capable of producing the sphenocavernous syndrome include aneurysms, meningiomas, pituitary tumors, craniopharyngiomas, nasopharyngeal tumors, metastatic tumors, lymphoma, and infectious and inflammatory processes.

Idiopathic granulomatous inflammation may produce a painful ophthalmoplegia from involvement of the cranial nerves within the cavernous sinus and su-

perior orbital fissure: the **Tolosa-Hunt syndrome.** Patients with this syndrome typically improve rapidly and dramatically when treated with systemic corticosteroids; however, both spontaneous and steroid-induced remissions of symptoms and signs, sometimes of prolonged duration, occur in cases of painful ophthalmoplegia caused by tumors and aneurysms. Thus, because of the similarity of the symptoms, signs, and response to therapy of both inflammatory and noninflammatory lesions of the cavernous sinus (including ischemic lesions), patients with the syndrome of painful ophthalmoplegia require a complete assessment, including neuroimaging, a systemic evaluation for an underlying vascular or inflammatory disorder, and, in most cases, a lumbar puncture (Fig. 18.16).

Vascular processes can produce a painful ophthalmoplegia from damage to structures in the cavernous sinus and superior orbital fissure. Cavernous sinus thrombosis and carotid-cavernous sinus fistulas can produce typical cavernous sinus syndromes. Painful ophthalmoplegia also occurs in patients with syphilis, giant cell (temporal) arteritis, diabetes mellitus, rheumatoid arthritis, and systemic lupus erythematosus.

The ischemia that produces oculomotor nerve dysfunction in patients with diabetes mellitus is, at least in some instances, caused by a lesion in the intracavernous portion of the nerve. Similar lesions may be responsible for the isolated oculomotor nerve palsies that develop in patients with systemic hypertension, ophthalmoplegic migraine, herpes zoster ophthalmicus, and giant cell arteritis.

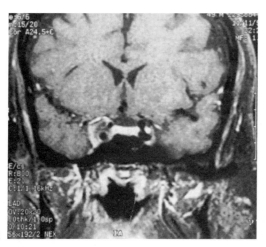
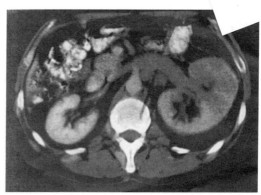

A **B**

Figure 18.16. Neuroimaging in a patient with painful ophthalmoplegia. The patient was a 49-year-old man with right retrob-ulbar pain and generalized limitation of movement of the right eye. The patient was thought to have the Tolosa-Hunt syndrome and was treated with oral corticosteroids without improvement. The ophthalmoparesis progressed to a complete ophthalmo-plegia associated with loss of vision in the eye. **A:** T1-weighted, coronal magnetic resonance image (MRI) after intravenous injection of paramagnetic contrast material reveals enlargement of the right cavernous sinus. **B:** CT scan of the abdomen reveals a left renal mass. The patient was found to have a metastatic renal cell carcinoma. (Reprinted from: Mehelas TJ, Kosmorsky GS. Painful ophthalmoplegia syndrome secondary to metastatic renal cell carcinoma. *J Neuroophthalmol.* 1996;16:289–290, with permission.)

Trauma to the cavernous sinus and superior or-bital fissure may produce an isolated oculomotor nerve palsy. Such palsies are usually associated with skull frac-ture and are caused by intraneural and perineural hem-orrhage in the cavernous sinus or superior orbital fis-sure.

Lesions of the Oculomotor Nerve within the Orbit

The sphenocavernous syndrome is characterized by a painful ophthalmoplegia and is generally unassociated with visual loss from an optic neuropathy. Conversely, lesions in the apex of the orbit produce ophthalmople-gia that may or may not be painful but that are usually associated with loss of vision from optic neuropathy and variable proptosis. The distinction between these two entities—the sphenocavernous syndrome and the orbital apex syndrome—can thus often be made both on clinical grounds and by neuroimaging.

The oculomotor nerve enters the orbit as two sep-arate divisions: the superior division, which innervates the levator palpebrae superioris and the superior rectus muscle; and the inferior division, which innervates the medial and inferior rectus muscle, the inferior oblique muscle, and the motor root of the ciliary ganglion. Thus, an incomplete oculomotor nerve paresis in the distribution of either division is often caused by a le-sion of either the sphenocavernous region or the or-

bital apex. However, as noted previously, the oculo-motor nerve has a divisional topographic arrangement beginning in the brainstem. Thus, divisional oculomo-tor nerve pareses may result from lesions not only in the cavernous sinus and orbital apex but also from le-sions in the brainstem or subarachnoid space. It is often impossible to determine if such a paresis is caused by a lesion within the orbit or the cavernous sinus un-less there are other clinical signs of cavernous sinus or orbital disease, or unless neuroimaging studies are performed.

Processes within the orbit that can produce an ocu-lomotor nerve palsy include inflammation, ischemia, infiltration, and compression. Trauma can also pro-duce such a palsy. Oculomotor nerve palsies produced by orbital lesions may be complete or incomplete and usually involve the pupil. Other signs of orbital dis-ease, including loss of vision, proptosis, and other oc-ular motor nerve pareses, are often but not invariably present.

Recovery from Acquired Oculomotor Nerve Palsy

Oculomotor nerve paralysis, whether complete or in-complete, may have several outcomes. First, complete recovery may occur. In such cases, recovery may be complete within 1 to 2 weeks after the onset of symp-toms. In other instances, notably those associated with diabetes mellitus and systemic hypertension, recovery does not begin for a month or more but is usually complete within 3 months. In still other cases, recovery can take much longer, sometimes as long as 3 years.

In some cases of oculomotor nerve palsy, the paralysis persists completely unchanged. In such cases, the nerve has usually been transected by trauma or chronic compression or has been infiltrated by tumor.

Finally, some patients with oculomotor nerve pareses experience partial recovery of oculomotor nerve function. This occurs especially after damage to the fascicular portion of the nerve. Partial recovery may be characterized by evidence of oculomotor nerve synkinesis. In most cases, this synkinesis becomes apparent within 9 weeks after injury, but in other cases, there is no evidence of aberrant regeneration for as long as 3 to 6 months.

Acquired Oculomotor Synkinesis: Misdirection of Regenerating Fibers in the Oculomotor Nerve

Peripheral motor and sensory nerves, including the autonomic nerves, can regenerate. The regenerative process produces more axons than were present before the nerve was interrupted. Axons sprout from the proximal end of the severed nerve and from collateral nerves that have not been severely damaged. Cords of Schwann cells form in the peripheral segment of the nerve so that the new nerve fibers are conducted to the end organ. The newly formed neurons reach the empty tubes (Schwann's tubes) that contained functioning neurons before degeneration. Regenerating axons have the capacity to bridge long gaps in damaged nerves.

In peripheral nerves that innervate more than one muscle, misdirection of regenerating nerve fibers may occur. Thus, regenerating sprouts from axons that previously innervated one muscle group may ultimately innervate a different muscle group with a different function.

Following injury to the oculomotor nerve at any point along its pathway from the brainstem to the orbit, a syndrome of oculomotor nerve synkinesis may occur. In adults, evidence of synkinesis first appears about 9 weeks after injury, whereas in infants with oculomotor nerve palsy from birth trauma, such signs may be observed from 1 to 6 weeks following birth. Oculomotor nerve synkinesis is thought to occur from misdirection of regenerated axons in the nerve. Thus, the levator palpebrae superioris may receive fibers that were originally destined for the medial rectus muscle, or fibers originally intended for the superior rectus muscle may reach the inferior oblique, inferior rectus, or medial rectus muscles. The active elevation of the eyelid during attempted downward eye movement is called the **pseudo-Graefe sign** to distinguish it from the lid lag

on downward gaze that occurs in patients with thyroid eye disease (Graefe's sign) (Fig. 18.17).

Fibers originally destined for any of the muscles innervated by the oculomotor nerve may reach the ciliary ganglion to synapse with the postganglionic parasympathetic fibers that innervate the iris sphincter muscle, the ciliary body muscle, or both. Often, this anomalous reinnervation of the pupil is easily observed because the pupil constricts only when the patient is asked to look in a direction requiring oculomotor nerve function (Fig. 18.18). In other cases, the pupil may appear to be permanently paralyzed in the mid-dilated position, but slit lamp biomicroscopy will enable the examiner to observe subtle abnormalities of pupillary movement that reflect misregeneration of the iris sphincter (Fig. 18.19).

The signs of aberrant regeneration of the oculomotor nerve may be summarized as follows:

1. Horizontal gaze-eyelid synkinesis—elevation of the involved eyelid in attempted adduction of the eye.
2. Pseudo-Graefe sign—retraction and elevation of the eyelid on attempted downward gaze.
3. Limitation of elevation and depression of the eye with occasional retraction of the globe on attempted vertical movement.
4. Adduction of the involved eye on attempted elevation or depression.
5. Pseudo–Argyll Robertson pupil—the involved pupil does not react or reacts poorly and irregularly to light stimulation but does constrict on adduction during conjugate gaze.
6. Monocular vertical optokinetic responses—the normal eye responds normally, but the involved eye has suppressed vertical responses.

The phenomenon of **secondary oculomotor nerve synkinesis** occurs in nearly all patients with congenital oculomotor nerve palsy; however, the majority of patients with this syndrome have experienced a primary, acute event that has produced a complete oculomotor nerve palsy. Secondary oculomotor nerve synkinesis occurs commonly following oculomotor nerve palsy from intracranial aneurysms, trauma (including surgical trauma), syphilis, and basal meningitis. As a general rule, synkinetic movements *do not occur* after ischemic insults to the nerve. Thus, in a patient suspected of having an ischemic oculomotor nerve palsy, particularly if there have been no previous episodes, the development of oculomotor synkinesis should suggest an alternative etiology, such as compression or inflammation.

Although the syndrome of acquired oculomotor nerve synkinesis occurs most frequently after acute oculomotor nerve palsy, it also occurs as a "primary" phenomenon; that is, without a preexisting acute oculomotor nerve paresis. Patients with **primary**

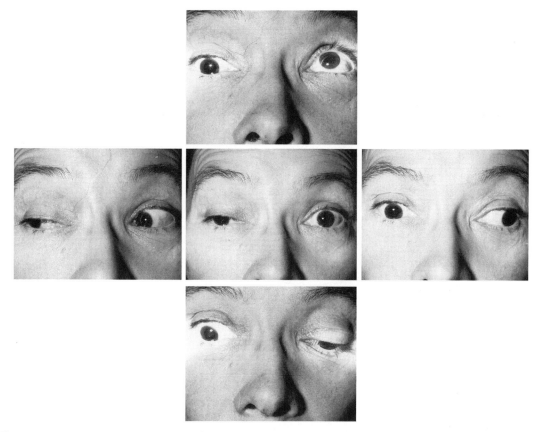

Figure 18.17. Misdirected regeneration of the right oculomotor nerve following trauma (secondary aberrant regeneration). Note elevation of the right upper eyelid on attempted downward gaze and on attempted adduction of the right eye (pseudo-Graefe sign). Although the right pupil was markedly dilated and poorly reactive to light, it constricted slightly on attempted adduction of the eye.

oculomotor nerve synkinesis usually harbor slowly growing lesions of the cavernous sinus, usually meningiomas or aneurysms but also trigeminal schwannomas. Slowly growing lesions in the subarachnoid space, including unruptured aneurysms, can also produce primary oculomotor nerve synkinesis. Lesions that cause primary aberrant regeneration grow so slowly that the mild oculomotor nerve damage that results does not produce major visual difficulties and allow regeneration to occur.

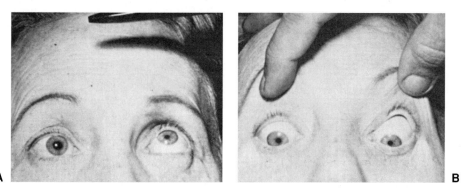

Figure 18.18. Aberrant regeneration of the right oculomotor nerve with involvement of the pupil. **A:** During attempted elevation of the eyes, the right pupil remains mid-dilated. **B:** During depression of the eyes, the right pupil constricts.

BEFORE INJURY

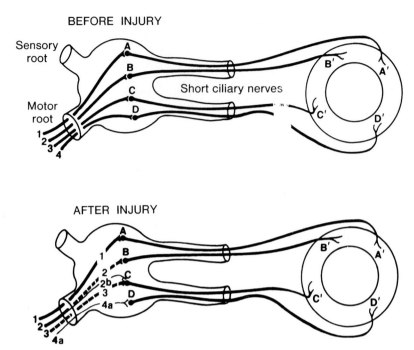

Figure 18.19. Diagram of aberrant regeneration of the oculomotor nerve as it affects pupillary function. Before injury, preganglionic fibers serving the pupillary light reaction synapse in the ciliary ganglion with axons that then proceed along short ciliary nerves to supply specific sectors of the iris sphincter **(above)**. Thus preganglionic fiber 1 synapses with postganglionic fiber *A* to supply sector *A'* of the iris sphincter. After injury to the preganglionic pathway, several phenomena may occur **(below)**. A fiber may be undamaged (fiber 1). A fiber may be completely destroyed and may never grow (fibers 3 and 4), or it may be damaged, and regeneration may occur (fibers 2 and 2*b*). In such a scenario, a collateral sprout could grow from a preganglionic fiber other than that originally intended for the iris sphincter. If fiber 4*a* grew from a nerve originally destined for the inferior rectus muscle, then segment *D'* of the iris sphincter would constrict whenever the patient attempted to look downward. (Redrawn from: Czarnecki JSC, Thompson HS. The iris sphincter in aberrant regeneration of the third nerve. *Arch Ophthalmol.* 1978;96:1606–1610.)

EVALUATION AND MANAGEMENT OF PATIENTS WITH OCULOMOTOR NERVE PALSY

The evaluation of a patient with a congenital oculomotor nerve palsy is minimal. Generally, a careful systemic and neurologic assessment is all that is required. Such patients are at risk to develop amblyopia and must be managed with occlusion therapy. The decision to surgically correct ocular misalignment is based on the goals of the patient and the severity of the condition.

The evaluation of a patient with a congenital oculomotor nerve palsy depends on the associated symptoms and signs, the pattern of oculomotor nerve involvement, and the age of the patient.

Acquired oculomotor nerve dysfunction may present in one of five ways:

1. *With a dilated, nonreactive or poorly reactive pupil without ophthalmoplegia or ptosis.* This presentation is **extremely rare** and usually occurs in the setting

of a comatose or obtunded patient with an expanding supratentorial mass lesion. In the awake, alert patient with a widely dilated pupil, pharmacologic blockade or a tonic pupil are far more likely etiologies than compressive oculomotor nerve palsy. Nevertheless, it may be appropriate in some patients to obtain MRI, MRA, or CTA. Conventional angiography is rarely indicated in such patients, unless noninvasive neuroimaging reveals abnormalities consistent with an aneurysm or other vascular lesion.

2. *With complete or incomplete ophthalmoparesis, ptosis, and a dilated, poorly reactive or nonreactive pupil.* This presentation may be produced by any pathologic process at any point along the pathway of the oculomotor nerve, but an intracranial aneurysm must be suspected and appropriate diagnostic studies immediately performed. Tests include CT scanning without (looking for blood in the subarachnoid space) and with (looking for an intracranial aneurysm

or other mass lesion) intravenous contrast, MRI, MRA, CTA, conventional angiography, or a combination of these techniques. None of these tests is 100% sensitive in detecting small intracranial aneurysms; however, both MRA and CTA, when performed correctly, can probably detect 95% of aneurysms 3 mm or greater in diameter. Nevertheless, conventional angiography remains the most sensitive test for detecting an intracranial aneurysm and should be performed in any patient in which this possibility is considered likely. The decision to perform conventional angiography if noninvasive neuroimaging (e.g., MRI, MRA, CTA) reveals no abnormalities must be made on a case by case basis.

3. *With ophthalmoplegia and ptosis, but without any pupillary involvement.* Pupil-sparing oculomotor nerve palsies are most commonly caused by ischemia, but compression and inflammation may also produce them. Patients in this setting must be individualized; however, we believe that almost all cases of **complete but pupil-sparing** oculomotor nerve pareses are caused by ischemia and that patients with such pareses do not necessarily require neuroimaging. Conversely, patients with an **incomplete, pupil-sparing** oculomotor nerve paresis may require—in addition to measurement of systemic blood pressure, serum glucose, and sedimentation rate—noninvasive neuroimaging, such as standard MRI, MRA, CTA, or a combination of these studies, especially when pain accompanies the palsy. A lumbar puncture may also be appropriate in some of these patients. If these studies are negative, some patients may require arteriography to eliminate the possibility of an intracranial aneurysm. However, most older patients with incomplete, pupil-sparing oculomotor nerve pareses can be followed after a workup has been performed to determine if there is an underlying ischemic or inflammatory process (e.g., diabetes mellitus, giant cell arteritis, systemic hypertension). It must also be remembered that whenever the pupils are normal, an ophthalmoplegia may represent the effects of myopathic or neuromuscular disease (e.g., myasthenia gravis), rather than a neuropathy.

4. *With ophthalmoplegia, ptosis, and a small or midpositioned pupil.* Patients with this clinical picture usually have lesions in the cavernous sinus that have damaged not only the oculomotor nerve but also the oculosympathetic fibers.

5. *With misdirected (aberrant) regeneration.* Patients with **primary** aberrant regeneration have slowly growing mass lesions compressing or infiltrating the oculomotor nerve in the cavernous sinus or, less often, in the subarachnoid space.

Following diagnosis and treatment of the underlying disorder that has produced an oculomotor nerve palsy, one must wait to see if recovery will occur, and, if so, to what degree. Once it is clear that recovery of oculomotor nerve function will not be complete, the patient may have several choices.

In patients with partial recovery, various strabismus procedures may be of benefit in providing binocular single vision, at least in primary position, and ptosis surgery may also be used to improve the position of the affected eyelid. Botulinum toxin injections of the lateral rectus can realign the eyes for better fusion in patients with mild oculomotor nerve palsy who are awaiting improvement. Other patients seem content to simply patch the affected eye or are able to ignore the double image. An opaque contact lens provides a cosmetically acceptable means to alleviate subjective diplopia in these patients.

The management of patients with complete oculomotor nerve palsy is more difficult. Despite reports of cosmetic and functional success using surgical procedures that involve transposing or transplanting the superior oblique tendon, surgery rarely produces a satisfactory result from the standpoint of either the patient or the surgeon.

TROCHLEAR (FOURTH) NERVE PALSIES

Paralysis of the trochlear nerve is far less commonly recognized than paralysis of either the oculomotor or abducens nerves. However, trochlear nerve palsy is the most common cause of acquired vertical strabismus in the general population, other causes being ocular myopathies (e.g., dysthyroid eye disease), disorders of the neuromuscular junction (e.g., myasthenia gravis), incomplete oculomotor nerve paresis, and skew deviation. Trochlear nerve palsy causes partial or complete paralysis of the superior oblique muscle, usually associated over time with overaction of its antagonist, the ipsilateral inferior oblique muscle (Figs. 18.20 and 18.21). Patients with this disorder complain of vertical diplopia that is greatest in downgaze and to the opposite side. Such patients also have excyclotorsion when tested with double Maddox rods or Lancaster red-green glasses, particularly when the eye is in abduction, and this feature helps to distinguish trochlear nerve palsy from skew deviation, in which the higher eye is invariably intorted. The ability of the superior oblique muscle to intort the eye is particularly important when assessing superior oblique function in patients with an oculomotor nerve palsy. In such cases, the absence of intorsion when the patient attempts to depress the eye while it is abducted indicates lack of superior oblique function as well.

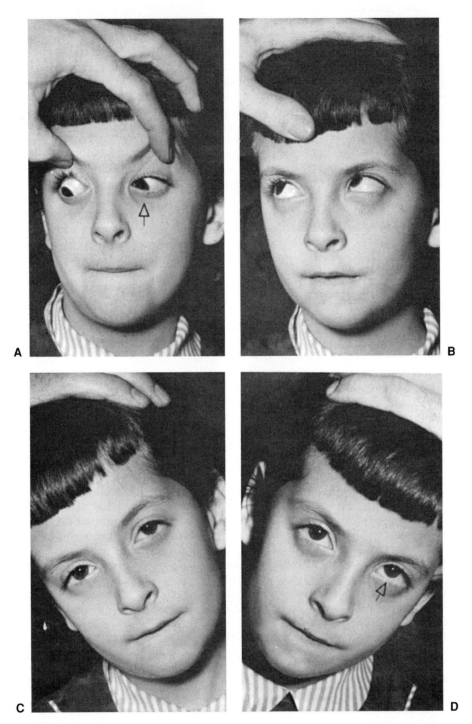

Figure 18.20. Left trochlear nerve palsy. **A:** Downward movement of the left eye (*arrow*) is limited in gaze down and right. **B:** Upward gaze to the right shows secondary overaction of the left inferior oblique muscle, the antagonist of the left superior oblique muscle. **C:** Head tilt to the right produces orthophoria and eliminates diplopia. **D:** Head tilt to the left results in upward deviation of the left eye (*arrow*). (Courtesy of Dr. R.D. Harley.)

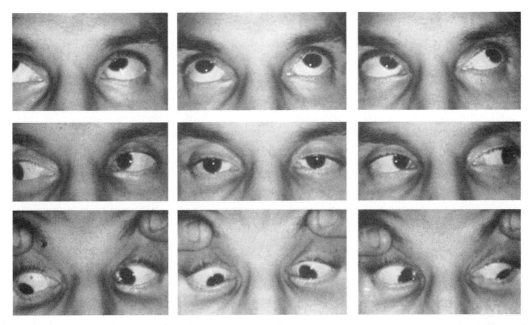

Figure 18.21. Bilateral trochlear nerve palsies in a 28-year-old man following a motorcycle accident. The patient suffered a severe blow to the vertex of his head. Note the patient's inability to depress either eye fully in adduction. There is bilateral overaction of both inferior oblique muscles. (Courtesy of Jacqueline Morris, C.O.)

Most patients with trochlear nerve palsy have torticollis. Such patients typically tilt the head to the side opposite the paralyzed superior oblique muscle. This spontaneous ocular torticollis is absent in patients with poor vision in either eye and in patients with large vertical fusional amplitudes that allow them to fuse in all positions of gaze. In addition, some patients with trochlear nerve palsy tilt their heads to the side of the palsy. This results in greater separation of images, thus allowing one of the images to be ignored.

CONGENITAL

Congenital trochlear nerve palsy is common. The etiology of congenital trochlear palsy is unknown; however, aplasia of the trochlear nerve nucleus appears to be responsible in some cases, and hypoplasia in others. Most congenital trochlear nerve palsies are sporadic. Most patients with congenital trochlear nerve palsy are neurologically normal, and many have some degree of facial asymmetry.

Patients with congenital trochlear nerve palsy usually develop large vertical fusion amplitudes that, in association with a head tilt, allow them to compensate for their muscle weakness. Such patients may, however, develop diplopia from decompensation of the palsy after a minor head injury. When these patients are evaluated, a review of old photographs often reveals a pre-existing head tilt. In addition, direct measurement of vertical fusion amplitudes may also establish the diagnosis. Normal persons have a vertical fusion range of only 3 to 6 prism diopters, whereas patients with congenital superior oblique paresis may have 10 to 25 prism diopters of vertical fusion amplitude.

Congenital superior oblique palsy may be bilateral. In some instances, the patients appear to have a unilateral palsy until they undergo surgical correction, at which time the contralateral palsy becomes apparent. In most cases, however, careful measurements of both vertical and torsional deviation permit differentiation between unilateral and bilateral palsies.

ACQUIRED

When an etiology can be determined, blunt head trauma, usually a direct orbital, frontal, basal, or oblique cranial blow, is the most common cause of isolated, acquired, unilateral and bilateral trochlear nerve palsy in both adults and children. As with other ocular motor nerve palsies, almost any pathologic process can damage the trochlear nerve at any point from its nucleus to its termination in the orbit where it innervates the superior oblique muscle.

Lesions of the Trochlear Nerve Nucleus

Lesions of the brainstem that damage the trochlear nerve nucleus cannot be localized with certainty on clinical grounds unless there are other neurologic signs suggesting intrinsic mesencephalic damage. Even when such signs are present, distinguishing nuclear from fascicular involvement is almost impossible. In addition, extrinsic lesions that compress the dorsal mesencephalon may damage the trochlear nerves as they emerge from the brainstem and at the same time produce damage to intrinsic brainstem structures. Cells of the trochlear nucleus are often damaged by lesions that involve the tegmentum at the junction of the pons and mesencephalon, particularly contusion and hemorrhage caused by impact against the tentorial margin. Other lesions that can produce intrinsic damage to the trochlear nerve nuclei include ischemia, primary and metastatic tumors, and vascular malformations. However, paresis of the superior oblique muscle with such lesions can be obscured by associated conjugate or internuclear gaze defects. In such patients, the recognition of a trochlear nerve palsy becomes possible only after the supranuclear difficulties resolve.

Both unilateral and bilateral superior oblique paresis can be associated with Parinaud's dorsal midbrain syndrome from pineal tumors, aqueductal stenosis, and hydrocephalus; vertical diplopia in this setting is far more commonly caused by trochlear nerve dysfunction than previously recognized. Trochlear nerve palsy also can follow neurosurgical procedures in the posterior fossa.

Lesions of the Trochlear Nerve Fascicle

Fascicular involvement of the trochlear nerves can be caused by the same processes that cause damage to the trochlear nuclei. These processes include compression, infiltration, ischemia, hemorrhage, trauma, and inflammation, particularly multiple sclerosis.

Because of the dorsal location of the trochlear fascicles, associated neurologic signs are of less help in the topographic diagnosis of such lesions than are neuroimaging studies. Nevertheless, two important associated signs that suggest that the site of a trochlear nerve paresis is the trochlear nucleus or fascicle are a central Horner's syndrome and a relative afferent pupillary defect (RAPD) unassociated with evidence of an optic neuropathy or optic tract syndrome.

The Horner's syndrome is caused by damage to descending sympathetic fibers in the dorsal brainstem, which are usually adjacent to the trochlear nerve nucleus. Thus, the Horner's syndrome is usually on the side opposite the trochlear nerve paresis (because the trochlear nerves are crossed). The only exception is if the lesion affects the postdecussation portion of the trochlear nerve fascicle, in which case both the trochlear nerve paresis and the Horner's syndrome are on the same side.

The RAPD is caused by damage to afferent pupillary fibers in the brachium of the superior colliculus. If the trochlear nerve paresis is caused by a lesion of the predecussation portion of the fascicle (or the trochlear nerve nucleus), the RAPD is on the same side as the trochlear nerve paresis, whereas if the paresis is caused by damage to the postdecussation portion of the fascicle, the RAPD is on the side opposite the trochlear nerve paresis (Fig. 18.22).

Lesions of the Trochlear Nerve in the Subarachnoid Space

The trochlear nerve is particularly susceptible to injury or compression as it emerges from the dorsal surface of the brainstem. Injuries in this location may avulse the rootlets of the emerging nerve, or there may be stretching or contusion injury from hemorrhage within the nerve.

When damage occurs to the trochlear nerves at their exit from the brainstem, both nerves are often involved. The presence of bilateral palsies may first become apparent after the patient undergoes surgical correction of the apparent unilateral palsy. Trauma that is insufficient to produce a skull fracture or loss of consciousness may cause a trochlear nerve palsy because of the extremely fragile nature of the nerve and its long subarachnoid course. The subarachnoid portion of the trochlear nerve can occasionally be damaged by posterior fossa aneurysms. In most cases, the aneurysm arises from the junction of the basilar and superior cerebellar arteries.

The subarachnoid portion of the trochlear nerve may also become affected in patients with basal meningitis. Syphilis, tuberculosis, sarcoidosis, and Lyme disease are the most common causes.

Schwannomas of the trochlear nerve may produce diplopia from trochlear nerve palsy by involvement of the nerve in the subarachnoid space. Other intrinsic lesions of the subarachnoid portion of the trochlear nerve include cavernous angiomas and arteriovenous malformations.

Patients with posteriorly draining dural carotid-cavernous sinus fistulas may develop an acute, painful trochlear nerve paresis. Because the fistula is draining posteriorly, such patients have none of the orbital congestive manifestations usually associated with carotid-cavernous sinus fistulas, such as conjunctival chemosis, dilation of conjunctival vessels, or proptosis.

The association of trochlear nerve palsy and elevated ICP is well documented. Some of these patients have pseudotumor cerebri, whereas others have hydrocephalus related to a variety of different processes, including blocked ventriculoperitoneal shunts. Indeed, bilateral trochlear nerve paresis may be a localizing sign

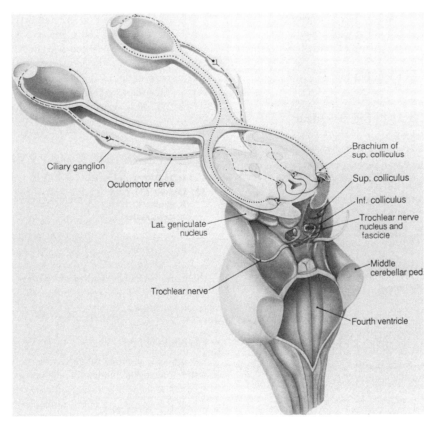

Figure 18.22. Presumed site of damage in a young woman who developed a left trochlear nerve paresis and was found to have a left relative afferent pupillary defect unassociated with any visual sensory deficit. The shaded portion of the illustration indicates a lesion involving the brachium of the right superior colliculus and the right dorsal mesencephalon, including the right trochlear nucleus or the predecussation portion of the right trochlear nerve fascicle. The patient was found to have an anaplastic astrocytoma of the brainstem. (Reprinted from: Eliott D, Cunningham ET Jr, Miller NR. Fourth nerve paresis and ipsilateral relative afferent pupillary defect without visual sensory disturbance: a sign of contralateral dorsal midbrain disease. *J Clin Neuroophthalmol.* 1991;11:169–171, with permission.)

of involvement of the superior medullary velum by a dilated sylvian aqueduct or downward pressure from an enlarged 3rd ventricle.

Lesions of the Trochlear Nerve within the Cavernous Sinus and Superior Orbital Fissure

Lesions that produce a cavernous sinus syndrome are discussed previously. When such lesions produce combined ocular motor nerve palsies, the trochlear nerve is often involved. It is unusual, however, for isolated trochlear nerve palsy to occur from cavernous sinus disease, although ischemic conditions (e.g., diabetes mellitus) may conceivably affect the trochlear nerve in this location as they do the oculomotor nerve. In this respect, it is also possible that the isolated trochlear nerve palsy that occurs in some patients with herpes zoster may be produced by a local granulomatous angiitis that originates in the ophthalmic division of the trigeminal

nerve and spreads to the sphenocavernous portion of the trochlear nerve. This cannot be the only mechanism, however, because trochlear nerve palsy also occurs in patients with geniculate herpes zoster (i.e., the Ramsay-Hunt syndrome).

Lesions of the Trochlear Nerve within the Orbit

Trauma (including surgical injury) may damage the trochlear nerve within the orbit; however, in many cases, it is impossible to ascertain if the damage has occurred to the nerve, the trochlea, the superior oblique muscle or tendon, or several of these structures. A similar problem arises in assessing patients with orbital inflammation, ischemia, or vascular malformations that are associated with superior oblique dysfunction. The superior oblique paralysis that occurs in patients with Paget's disease of the orbit and with hypertrophic arthritis may also be caused by mechanical disruption of the superior oblique tendon within the trochlea and not by damage to the trochlear nerve itself. The orbital portions of both the oculomotor and trochlear nerves may become ischemic after dental anesthesia.

Recovery from Acquired Trochlear Nerve Palsy

Following the development of a trochlear nerve palsy, superior oblique function may:

*   Recover completely, particularly in cases of ischemia or closed injury or after relief of compression from tumor or aneurysm.
*   Recover incompletely, leaving the patient with mild but persistent vertical diplopia, torsional diplopia, or both.
*   Show no recovery, as occurs primarily after mesencephalic injury or with transection of the trochlear nerve by trauma or compression.

EVALUATION AND MANAGEMENT OF TROCHLEAR NERVE PALSY

The diagnosis of a trochlear nerve palsy is made primarily by performing the "three-step test." It must be emphasized that this test is only useful if the paresis is of a single cyclovertical muscle. Furthermore, although we believe the three-step test is extremely useful in patients with presumed trochlear nerve palsies, its reliability in the diagnosis of pareses of other vertical muscles is questionable. In addition, restrictive ophthalmoplegia, myasthenia gravis, and skew deviation can mimic a trochlear nerve palsy when they are evaluated using the three-step test.

The easiest method of treating the vertical or torsional diplopia experienced by patients awaiting resolution of an acquired or a decompensated congenital trochlear nerve palsy is occlusion of one eye with a patch or an opaque contact lens. In other cases, particularly those with mild vertical displacement, the use of a vertical press-on (Fresnel) prism may be of benefit, although some degree of diplopia in extremes of gaze is almost always present. In cases of acquired trochlear nerve palsy, no attempt at surgical correction should be considered until at least 8 to 12 months have elapsed without improvement in superior oblique function, unless the physician knows with certainty that the trochlear nerve has been severed.

When a trochlear nerve palsy has been stable over an appropriate period of time, one may attempt to correct persistent diplopia using any one of several operative procedures. These procedures are designed to (a) strengthen all or a portion of the superior oblique muscle, (b) weaken its antagonist, the ipsilateral infe-

rior oblique muscle, or (c) weaken its yoke muscle, the contralateral inferior rectus muscle. The decision to use one or another of these procedures or to use several in combination depends on the results of a careful orthoptic examination. Similar considerations apply for the treatment of bilateral trochlear nerve palsies. The results of surgery for both congenital and acquired trochlear nerve palsies are usually excellent.

ABDUCENS (SIXTH) NERVE PALSIES AND NUCLEAR HORIZONTAL GAZE PARALYSIS

The abducens nerve is unique in that damage to its nucleus results not in ipsilateral abduction weakness but in horizontal gaze paralysis toward the side of the lesion. In addition, the precise anatomic location of the nerve produces syndromes that are different from those seen with damage to either the oculomotor or trochlear nerves.

CONGENITAL

Congenital absence of abduction as an isolated phenomenon is exceedingly rare but may occur from injury to the abducens nerve shortly before or during birth. That birth trauma is a significant factor indicated by an incidence of congenital abduction weakness in infants that increases progressively from 0% for deliveries by caesarean section, to 0.1% for spontaneous vaginal delivery, to 2.4% for forceps delivery, and to 3.2% for vacuum extraction.

Congenital paralysis of conjugate horizontal eye movements occurs more frequently than does unilateral or bilateral abduction weakness. Congenital horizontal gaze palsy may occur as an isolated sporadic finding or it may be familial. Histologic findings in patients with isolated bilateral horizontal gaze palsy include absent or hypoplastic abducens nuclei and absent abducens nerves.

Far more common are congenital disturbances of horizontal gaze associated with two conditions: Möbius syndrome and Duane's retraction syndrome (DRS).

Möbius Syndrome (Congenital Bulbar Paralysis)

Characteristically, this defect involves the face and horizontal gaze mechanisms bilaterally. Affected patients have a mask-like facies, with the mouth constantly held open. The eyelids often cannot be completely closed. Some patients have only an esotropia associated with unilateral or bilateral limitation of abduction, and some may even be able to converge. In most cases, however,

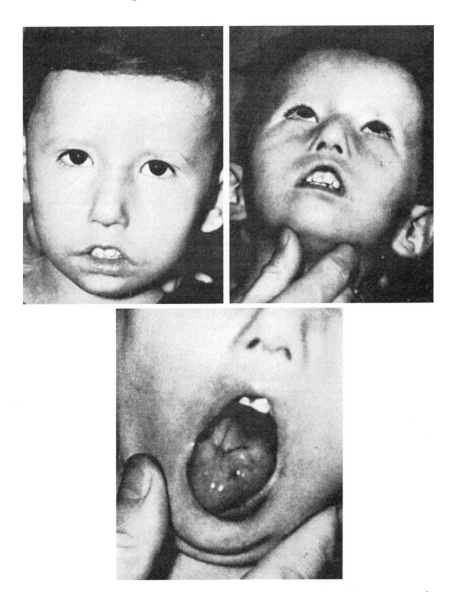

Figure 18.23. Möbius syndrome in a 3-year-old boy. The boy had spontaneous vertical eye movements but no horizontal eye movements. Note bilateral facial palsy and atrophy of the tongue.

the eyes are straight and do not move horizontally in either direction (Fig. 18.23).

Other congenital defects that are found in patients with this syndrome include deafness, webbed fingers or toes, supernumerary digits, atrophy of the muscles of the chest, neck, and particularly the tongue, and absence of the hands, feet, fingers, or toes. Nearly all patients with Möbius syndrome have some degree of mental retardation.

The diversity of brainstem pathologic findings in patients with Möbius syndrome suggests that the syndrome actually is a heterogeneous group of congenital disorders that in some cases are caused by developmental defects, and in others, by acquired hypoxic or other insults. Most cases of Möbius syndrome are sporadic.

Duane's Retraction Syndrome (Stilling-Turk-Duane Syndrome)

Duane's retraction syndrome is a predominantly congenital eye movement disorder characterized by marked limitation or absence of abduction, variable limitation of adduction, and palpebral fissure narrowing and globe retraction on attempted adduction.

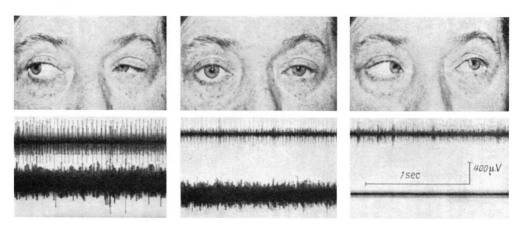

Figure 18.24. Electromyogram in left Duane's retraction syndrome. Simultaneous recording from left lateral rectus **(A)** and medial rectus **(B)** muscles shows *paradoxic innervation* of the lateral rectus muscle during attempted adduction of the left eye. In fact, the lateral rectus muscle receives its maximal innervation during adduction and its minimal innervation during attempted abduction **(upper right)**. The innervation pattern of the left medial rectus is normal. Note its inhibition during abduction of the eye. (Reprinted from: Huber A, Esslen E, Kloti R, et al. Zum problem des Duane syndromes. *Albrecht von Graefes Arch Klin Exp Ophthalmol.* 1964;167:169–191, with permission.)

Vertical ocular movements are often noted on adduction, most frequently in an upward direction.

A disorder of horizontal eye movements is common to all patients with DRS. In most cases, the abnormalities are unilateral, but bilateral Duane's syndrome occurs in 15% to 20% of affected patients. In most patients, gaze is directed toward the side of the unaffected eye, and in some instances, the face is turned toward the affected side to allow binocular single vision. Vision is almost always normal. Thus, in the majority of cases, no treatment is necessary unless the patient has a marked head turn.

Electromyographic studies show that DRS is a neurogenic disorder in which branches of the oculomotor nerve innervate the lateral rectus muscle (Fig. 18.24). Retraction of the globe is produced by a co-contraction of horizontal rectus muscles. Autopsy studies have confirmed anomalous innervation of the extraocular muscles. Abducens nuclei and nerves are absent and the lateral rectus muscle is innervated by branches from the oculomotor nerve. Interestingly, in the region of the abducens nuclei, cell bodies representing internuclear neurons typically remain intact.

There are three types of DRS: Duane I type consists of limited or absent abduction with relatively normal adduction; Duane II consists of limited or absent adduction with relatively normal abduction; and Duane III is characterized by limited abduction and adduction. In all cases, an anomaly of ocular motor innervation involving the oculomotor and abducens nerves is thought to be responsible.

Although some cases may be caused by birth trauma, 30% to 50% of patients with DRS have as-sociated congenital defects involving ocular, skeletal, and neural structures. The differentiation of these frequently affected structures occurs between the fourth and eighth weeks of gestation, coincident with the development of the ocular motor nerves. Thus, a teratogenic event during the second month of gestation may cause DRS. Given the multitude of associated anomalies seen in DRS, multiple etiologies, including chromosomal disorders and trauma, may produce DRS. Most cases of DRS are sporadic, but familial unilateral and bilateral cases occur and constitute about 10% of observed cases.

ACQUIRED

Lesions of the Abducens Nerve Nucleus

The abducens nucleus contains not only motoneurons that innervate the ipsilateral lateral rectus but also cell bodies of internuclear neurons that cross the midline and ascend in the contralateral medial longitudinal fasciculus (MLF) to synapse in the medial rectus subnucleus on that side (Fig. 18.25). Thus, lesions that damage the abducens nucleus produce a **conjugate gaze palsy** to the ipsilateral side, and lesions of both abducens nuclei completely eliminate conjugate horizontal gaze. **Neither unilateral nor bilateral isolated abduction weakness ever occurs from a lesion of the abducens nucleus.** In most but not all cases in which the abducens nucleus is damaged, an ipsilateral, peripheral, facial nerve palsy is also present. This palsy occurs because the facial nerve fascicle loops around the abducens nucleus before exiting from the brainstem.

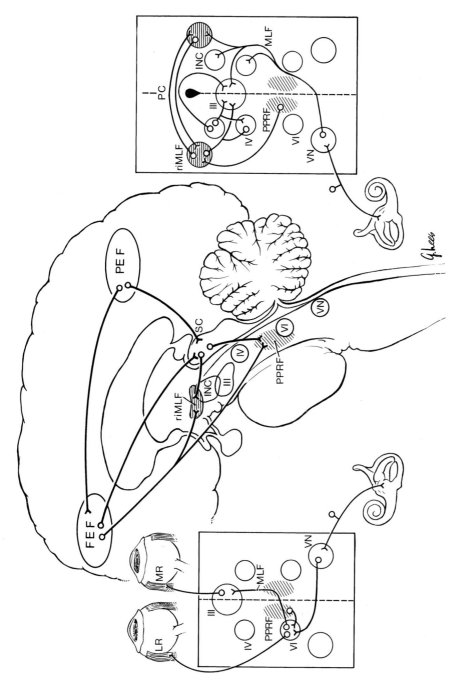

Figure 18.25. Diagram on left shows that the abducens nucleus (VI) contains not only motoneurons that innervate the ipsilateral lateral rectus (LR) but also cell bodies of internuclear neurons that cross the midline and ascend in the contralateral medial longitudinal fasciculus (MLF) to synapse in the medial rectus subnucleus on that side (III). *MR*, medial rectus muscle; *PPRF*, paramedian pontine reticular formation; *VN*, vestibular nucleus; *IV*, trochlear nerve nucleus.

The horizontal gaze palsy that occurs from damage to the abducens nucleus is not always symmetric, perhaps because the cell bodies of the abducens motoneurons are more vulnerable than those of the internuclear neurons to certain insults, thus producing an asymmetric horizontal gaze paralysis that is worse in the abducting eye. Lesions of the abducens nucleus sometimes damage the ipsilateral MLF, producing the **one-and-a-half syndrome.** This syndrome consists of a horizontal gaze palsy combined with an internuclear ophthalmoplegia (INO).

Lesions that produce intrinsic brainstem damage and cause acquired unilateral or bilateral paralysis of horizontal gaze from damage to the abducens nuclei include ischemia, infiltration, trauma, inflammation, and compression (Figs. 18.26 and 18.27).

Patients with the Wernicke-Korsakoff syndrome often develop paralysis of conjugate gaze, presumably from a metabolic insult to the abducens nuclei. Neuronal loss and gliosis can occur in the abducens nuclei of patients with ALS.

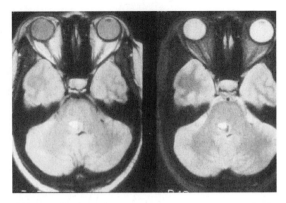

Figure 18.26. MRI in a 62-year-old woman with a slowly progressive right horizontal gaze paresis and ipsilateral facial weakness. Axial proton-density **(left)** and T2-weighted **(right)** images demonstrate a lesion in the region of the right abducens nerve nucleus. An evaluation revealed breast carcinoma with evidence of systemic metastases, and the lesion was thought to be a metastasis.

Lesions of the Abducens Nerve Fascicle

When an abducens nerve palsy coexists with a gaze palsy to the same side from damage to both the abducens nucleus and the ipsilateral abducens nerve fascicle, identification of the peripheral nerve element in the gaze palsy cannot be assessed unless there is a marked asymmetry between the two eyes, with the abducting eye being more limited in movement than the adducting eye. In other instances, fascicular involvement of the abducens nerve produces an isolated abduction weakness that cannot be differentiated clinically from involvement outside the brainstem. However, most lesions that damage the abducens fascicle produce distinctive clinical syndromes from damage to the surrounding neurologic tissue.

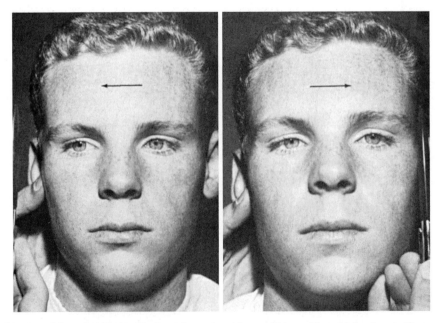

Figure 18.27. Acute bilateral paralysis of horizontal gaze in a 16-year-old boy with multiple sclerosis. Two weeks after this photograph was obtained, all neurologic signs had resolved.

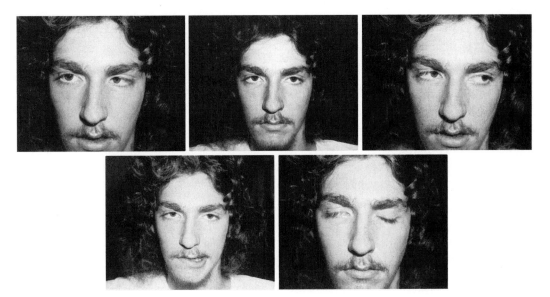

Figure 18.28. Millard-Gubler syndrome in a 23-year-old man with an intrapontine hemorrhage. The patient has a right abducens nerve paresis, a right peripheral facial nerve paresis, and a left (contralateral) hemiparesis.

A lesion in the pontine tegmentum may damage the abducens and facial nerve fascicles, the nucleus of the tractus solitarius, the central tegmental tract, the spinal tract of the trigeminal nerve (and its nucleus), the superior olivary nucleus, or a combination of these structures. Such a lesion may produce ipsilateral paralysis of abduction, ipsilateral facial palsy (flaccid), loss of taste from the anterior two-thirds of the tongue, ipsilateral central Horner's syndrome, ipsilateral analgesia of the face, and ipsilateral peripheral deafness. Together, these signs comprise the syndrome of the anterior inferior cerebellar artery—**Foville's syndrome.** The clinical expression of this syndrome is rarely complete, and many of its features may occur in association with ipsilateral paralysis of horizontal gaze rather than ipsilateral paralysis of abduction, indicating nuclear, rather than fascicular, involvement.

A lesion in the ventral paramedian pons may damage, in addition to the ventral portion of the abducens fascicle, the corticospinal tract, the ventral portion of the facial nerve fascicle, or both. Such a lesion produces an ipsilateral abducens palsy and a contralateral hemiplegia, with **(Millard-Gubler syndrome)** or without **(Raymond-Cestan syndrome)** ipsilateral peripheral facial paralysis (Fig. 18.28).

Fascicular lesions of the abducens nerve may be produced by ischemia, tumor compression or infiltration, infection, demyelination, and other inflammation. For example, although the abducens nerve palsies that occur in association with diabetes mellitus are usually assumed to occur from involvement of the subarachnoid or cavernous sinus portion of the nerve, some patients with isolated abducens nerve pareses in the setting of diabetes mellitus have MRI evidence of small hemorrhagic or ischemic brainstem lesions. The most common inflammation causing a fascicular abducens nerve paresis is demyelination.

Lesions of the Abducens Nerve in the Subarachnoid Space

Causes of abducens nerve damage in the subarachnoid space are many and varied. The long course of the nerve is usually cited as an explanation for its frequent involvement; however, the course of the trochlear nerve is longer and yet trochlear nerve pareses occur less frequently than do abducens nerve pareses. In fact, the location and course of the abducens nerve, rather than its length, are the major factors that lead to an abducens nerve paresis. The abducens nerve lies along the ventral surface of the pons and is bound to that structure by the anterior inferior cerebellar artery. The nerve may therefore be compressed by this vessel, the posterior inferior cerebellar artery, or the basilar artery, particularly when the vessel is atherosclerotic or dolichoectatic. Aneurysms of these vessels may also cause abducens paralysis. In most of these cases, there are no other cranial nerve findings, but there may be severe headache.

After its exit from the pons, the abducens nerve passes almost vertically through the subarachnoid space to pierce the dura overlying the clivus. During its course, it is vulnerable to damage from a variety of processes in the posterior fossa, including descent of the brainstem associated with vertex blows,

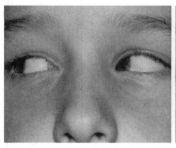
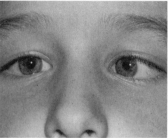
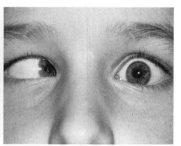

Figure 18.29. Left abducens nerve palsy in a 7-year-old boy with aseptic meningitis. It was assumed that the palsy was caused by damage to the abducens nerve in the subarachnoid space. The palsy cleared without treatment.

space-occupying masses above the tentorium (transtentorial herniation), posterior fossa masses, and structural abnormalities (e.g., Chiari malformations). In these settings, the abducens nerve may be stretched and injured at its attachment at either the pons or the clivus. Trauma may be direct, including neurosurgical, or indirect from blunt, closed head injury. Both unilateral and bilateral abducens paralysis, usually associated with other neurologic signs and symptoms, have been reported in patients placed in halo-pelvic traction.

Meningitis may produce abducens nerve paralysis (Fig. 18.29). As with other ocular motor nerve palsies produced by meningitis, abducens nerve palsies are often bilateral. Both unilateral and bilateral abducens nerve paresis can also occur in patients with idiopathic hypertrophic cranial pachymeningitis, a condition characterized by chronic, nongranulomatous inflammation of the meninges (Fig. 18.30).

Basal tumors may directly damage the subarachnoid portion of the abducens nerve. Meningioma and chordoma may produce both unilateral and bilateral abducens palsies without any other neurologic signs and symptoms. Vestibular schwannomas (acoustic neuromas) may cause abducens palsy but almost never as their sole manifestation. Similarly, although the abducens nerve may be damaged by exophytic spread of intrinsic posterior fossa tumors such as glioma, medulloblastoma, or ependymoma, patients with these tumors almost always have other neurologic symptoms and signs. Cavernous angiomas of the nerve may produce a similar clinical picture.

Changes in ICP may produce abducens palsy. Patients with increased ICP commonly develop both unilateral and bilateral abducens palsies. In such instances, the palsies may represent false localizing signs of intracranial tumors. A unilateral (and occasionally bilateral) abducens palsy may develop after a lumbar puncture, whether or not there is increased ICP.

Lesions of the Extradural Portion of the Abducens Nerve at the Petrous Apex

After the abducens nerve penetrates the dura overlying the clivus, it passes beneath the petroclinoid (Gruber's) ligament. In this region, it is adjacent to the mastoid air cells. In patients with severe mastoiditis, the inflammatory process may extend to the tip of the petrous bone, producing localized inflammation of the meninges in the epidural space and a classic condition called **Gradenigo's syndrome.** The adjacent abducens nerve becomes inflamed and paretic. In addition, because the gasserian ganglion and facial nerve are also nearby, such patients have severe pain on the ipsilateral side of the face and around the eye and may also develop facial paralysis. Abducens paresis may not occur until 2 to 3 days following the onset of pain. Photophobia and lacrimation are often present, and corneal sensation may be diminished. In some patients, meningitis develops, whereas in others, only a localized inflammation occurs. Because of the prompt and almost

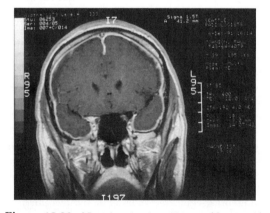

Figure 18.30. Neuroimaging in a 39-year-old man with a slowly progressive right abduction deficit associated with headache. Axial T1-weighted MRI shows diffuse meningeal enhancement as well as inflammatory changes in the right cavernous sinus. Biopsy of the meninges established a diagnosis of idiopathic hypertrophic cranial pachymeningitis. The disease was arrested with cranial irradiation and immunotherapy.

universal use of antibiotics in children with known or presumed acute otitis media, the incidence of Gradenigo's syndrome is extremely low.

Lesions other than inflammation can involve the petrous apex and produce symptoms suggesting Gradenigo's syndrome. These lesions include tumors and aneurysms of the intrapetrosal segment of the internal carotid artery. Thus, patients presenting with the petrous apex syndrome should be carefully evaluated with appropriate neuroimaging studies before it is concluded that the involvement is inflammatory.

When lateral sinus thrombosis or phlebitis extends into the inferior petrosal sinus, the abducens nerve may become paretic. A similar situation may occur when one jugular vein (particularly the right jugular) is ligated during radical neck dissection. Thrombosis of the inferior petrosal sinus may explain the abducens nerve palsy that sometimes occurs in patients with mastoiditis. In other cases, however, a pseudotumor cerebri syndrome develops, and the abducens palsy is secondary to increased ICP.

Lesions of the Abducens Nerve in the Cavernous Sinus and Superior Orbital Fissure

Abducens nerve paralysis, either isolated or in combination with other cranial neuropathies, may occur from lesions within the cavernous sinus. The location of the abducens nerve within the body of the sinus itself—rather than in the deep layer of the lateral sinus wall where the oculomotor, trochlear, and ophthalmic nerves are located—predisposes it to damage from intracavernous vascular lesions, including aneurysms, direct and dural carotid-cavernous fistulas, and rarely internal carotid artery dissection.

Tumors that infiltrate the cavernous sinus as well as those that compress the structures within it may produce isolated abducens palsy. These include meningioma, metastatic carcinoma, nasopharyngeal carcinoma, Burkitt's lymphoma, pituitary adenoma with and without apoplexy, craniopharyngioma, and a variety of other rare lesions in the region of the optic chiasm and cavernous sinus, including suprasellar germinomas, osteogenic sarcomas, teratomas, and multiple myeloma or plasmacytoma. When such lesions are sufficiently large, they may involve both cavernous sinuses and produce bilateral abducens nerve palsies.

Ischemic conditions, such as hypertension, diabetes mellitus, giant cell arteritis, systemic lupus erythematosus, and migraine, may damage the abducens nerve within the cavernous sinus, as may both granulomatous (e.g., tuberculosis, sarcoidosis, or the Tolosa-Hunt syndrome) and nongranulomatous (e.g., sphenoid sinus abscess or idiopathic hypertrophic pachymeningitis) inflammation. Herpes zoster may also produce abducens palsy from involvement of the abducens nerve in the cavernous sinus.

Although isolated involvement of the abducens nerve by cavernous sinus pathology is not rare, it is far more common for such involvement to be associated with other neurologic signs and symptoms, even if there are no other ocular motor nerve palsies. One of the more important of these cavernous sinus syndromes consists of the combination of isolated abducens paralysis and ipsilateral postganglionic Horner's syndrome. This syndrome can occur in association with primary and traumatic intracavernous aneurysms and with both benign and malignant tumors that arise in or invade the cavernous sinus. The occurrence of this syndrome is explained by the anatomic course of the oculosympathetic fibers within the cavernous sinus which leave the internal carotid artery and join briefly with the abducens nerve before separating and fusing with the ophthalmic division of the trigeminal nerve.

Lesions of the Abducens Nerve within the Orbit

The abducens nerve has a very short course in the orbit, piercing the lateral rectus muscle only a few millimeters from the superior orbital fissure. For this reason, isolated involvement of this nerve within the orbit is rare, although it may occur in patients with a primary orbital schwannoma that originates from the sheath of the orbital portion of the abducens nerve. Abducens nerve paresis can also occur following injection of an anesthetic solution in preparation for mandibular surgery.

Chronic, Isolated Abducens Nerve Paralysis

Most patients who develop abducens nerve pareses either experience spontaneous improvement of the paresis or are found to have an underlying lesion that has caused the paresis. Some patients, however, do not recover and have no obvious lesion despite an extensive evaluation (see later). We follow such patients at regular intervals, obtaining an interval history and performing a complete examination each time the patient is seen. If, during this time, the patient develops other neurologic signs or the paresis worsens, a complete workup, including neuroimaging and an otolaryngologic evaluation, is performed. If no changes occur over a 3-month period, we perform or repeat a complete assessment of the patient. Although many patients with isolated, chronic abducens nerve palsies that last more than 6 months follow a completely benign course, a substantial number of such patients harbor basal tumors that may be amenable to treatment if identified at an early stage.

Spontaneous recovery of an abducens nerve palsy does not eliminate the presence of a neoplastic process.

The possible mechanisms for recovery in such cases include remyelination, axon regeneration, relief of transient compression (e.g., resorption of hemorrhage), restoration of impaired blood flow, slippage of a nerve previously stretched over the tumor, or immune responses to the tumor.

EVALUATION AND MANAGEMENT OF ABDUCENS NERVE PALSY

There is a tendency to assume that all patients with an esotropia associated with unilateral or bilateral abduction weakness have an abducens nerve paresis. In fact, the physician encountering such a patient should first consider the possibility that the condition is myopathic (e.g., thyroid eye disease) or neuromuscular (e.g., myasthenia gravis). A careful history and examination directed at these possibilities may be sufficient to eliminate them as etiologies. Alternatively, the physician may need to perform further studies, including orbital ultrasonography, orbital imaging, thyroid function studies, serum assay for antireceptor antibodies, and single-fiber electromyography.

Once the physician is satisfied that an abducens nerve paresis is likely, he or she should initiate an evaluation that, like the evaluation performed in patients with an oculomotor nerve palsy, depends on the associated symptoms and signs and the age of the patient. All patients with a presumed abducens nerve palsy *must* undergo a thorough neurologic assessment, particularly with respect to the first eight cranial nerves and the integrity of the oculosympathetic pathway. If other neurologic signs (e.g., trigeminal sensory neuropathy, facial paresis, hearing loss, Horner's syndrome) are present, such patients should undergo neuroimaging. If patients have mild redness, swelling, or proptosis of the affected eye, an evaluation for a spontaneous dural carotid-cavernous sinus fistula or even cavernous sinus thrombosis should be performed. Patients with septic cavernous sinus thrombosis nearly always have prominent systemic manifestations of sepsis.

If a patient with an apparent abducens nerve paresis has no other findings and has underlying systemic vascular disease or is in the vasculopathic age group (i.e., over age 60), and if the onset of the palsy is sudden, the patient should be followed at regular intervals, with an interval history obtained and a complete examination performed each time the patient is seen. If, during this time, the patient develops other neurologic signs or the paresis worsens, a complete workup, including neuroimaging and an otolaryngologic evaluation, is performed. If no changes occur over a 3-month period, a complete reassessment of the patient should be performed. On the other hand, if the patient is under age 60 and has no risk factors for ischemic or inflammatory disease, we perform MRI with careful attention to the

pathway of the abducens nerve from the brainstem to the orbit. A lumbar puncture may be indicated in some patients, as may MRA or CTA and an otolaryngologic assessment.

Abducens nerve paralysis may or may not resolve, and the resolution may be complete or incomplete. Ischemic pareses patients almost always recover completely, usually within 2 to 4 months, whereas some degree of spontaneous recovery of traumatic abducens pareses occurs in 30 to 54% of patients and may take more than 1 year. Among patients who do not recover, serious pathology (e.g., tumor, stroke, aneurysm) is often present, emphasizing the importance of performing an evaluation in patients whose abducens nerve palsy does not recover within 3 to 6 months.

As is the case with trochlear nerve function, patients whose abducens nerve is transected during a neurosurgical procedure may recover abducens nerve function if the cut ends of the nerve are rejoined with sutures at the time of surgery.

Strabismus surgery should not be considered to correct an abducens nerve palsy until at least 8 to 10 months have passed without improvement, unless it is known that the abducens nerve is no longer intact. During this period, some patients prefer to occlude one eye, whereas others are able to ignore their diplopia or visual confusion. Although a patch is the simplest manner in which to occlude one eye, an opaque contact lens can also be used. Patients under 8 years old should undergo alternate patching of the eyes to prevent amblyopia. In most patients with unilateral abducens paresis, prisms are not of great benefit, although they are occasionally useful in achieving binocular single vision in primary position.

Chemodenervation of the antagonist medial rectus muscle with botulinum toxin can be used to treat patients with both acute and chronic abducens nerve palsy. We believe that early use of botulinum toxin in patients with acute abducens nerve palsy does not affect the eventual outcome of the condition and that chemodenervation therapy is generally less beneficial than surgery in the treatment of chronic abducens nerve palsy.

Surgery, when required, usually consists of either weakening of the ipsilateral medial rectus muscle combined with strengthening of the ipsilateral lateral rectus muscle or some type of vertical muscle transposition procedure, often combined with chemodenervation of the ipsilateral medial rectus muscle with botulinum toxin.

HYPERACTIVITY OF THE OCULAR MOTOR NERVES

Several ocular motor syndromes are characterized by hyperactivity, rather than hypoactivity, of one or more

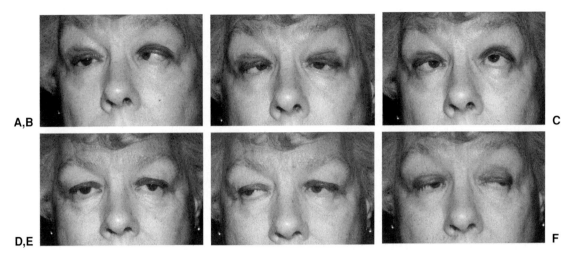

Figure 18.31. Ocular neuromyotonia. Appearance of a 62-year-old woman who had been treated with whole brain radiation for a pituitary tumor 15 years prior to her presentation. The patient had paroxysmal spasms of adduction of the right eye, left eye (**A**), or both eyes (**B**), lasting several seconds. The pupils remained normal during the spasms, and there was no evidence of accommodation spasm as might be expected if the patient was experiencing spasm of the near response. In addition, there was occasional spasm of elevation of the left eye (**C**). Between episodes of spasm, the eyes were straight (**D**) and horizontal gaze to the right (**E**) and left (**F**) was normal. The spasms initially responded to quinine (tonic water) but later required carbamazepine.

of the ocular motor nerves. The most common of these are ocular neuromyotonia and superior oblique myokymia (SOM).

OCULAR NEUROMYOTONIA

Ocular neuromyotonia is characterized by brief, episodic contractions of muscles supplied by the oculomotor, trochlear, or abducens nerves. The condition is usually unilateral, but bilateral cases occur. In most cases, the extraocular muscles corresponding to only one of the ocular motor nerves are affected; however, some patients have involvement of muscles innervated by more than one of the ocular motor nerves on one side (Fig. 18.31). In most patients, ocular neuromyotonia is permanent; however, it resolves spontaneously in some patients and disappears with treatment in others.

Most patients who develop ocular neuromyotonia have previously received radiation therapy to the base of the skull. This is not always the case, however. For example, some patients have received radiation indirectly, as occurred in a patient who develop ocular neuromyotonia many years after he underwent myelography with iophendylate (Pantopaque, Thorotrast), a substance that is weakly radioactive. Other patients have developed the condition in the setting of dysthyroid orbitopathy.

The evaluation of patients with ocular neuromyotonia, particularly those without a history of prior radiation therapy, should include MRI of the brain, with

particular attention to the suprasellar region and posterior fossa. Carbamazepine is often effective in treating this condition.

SUPERIOR OBLIQUE MYOKYMIA (SUPERIOR OBLIQUE MICROTREMOR)

Superior oblique myokymia is characterized by typical symptoms of monocular blurring of vision or tremulous sensations in the eye. Patients typically experience brief episodes of vertical or torsional diplopia, vertical or torsional oscillopsia, or both. Attacks usually last less than 10 seconds but may occur many times per day. The attacks may be brought on by looking downward, by tilting the head toward the side of the affected eye, or by blinking. The eye movements of SOM are often difficult to appreciate on gross examination, although they are usually apparent during examination with the ophthalmoscope or slit lamp biomicroscope. They consist of spasms of cyclotorsional and vertical movements.

The majority of patients with SOM have no underlying disease, although cases have been reported following trochlear nerve palsy, after mild head trauma, in the setting of multiple sclerosis, after brainstem stroke, in a patient with a dural arteriovenous fistula, and in patients with cerebellar tumor. The etiology of SOM may be neuronal damage and subsequent regeneration, leading to desynchronized contraction of muscle fibers.

Superior oblique myokymia spontaneously resolves in some patients. Other patients are not bothered by their symptoms and thus do not need treatment. For patients whose symptoms are particularly distressing, both medical and surgical therapies are available. Individual patients may respond to a number of drugs, including carbamazepine, baclofen, and topically or systemically administered β-adrenergic blocking agents. Patients who do not respond to drug therapy, who develop side effects from the drugs, or who do not wish to take drugs for their condition may experience complete relief of symptoms after extraocular muscle surgery, the most successful of which is tenectomy of the affected superior oblique muscle combined with ipsilateral inferior oblique myectomy.

SYNKINESES INVOLVING THE OCULAR MOTOR AND OTHER CRANIAL NERVES

A *synkinesis* is a simultaneous movement or a coordinated set of movements of muscles supplied by different nerves or different branches of the same nerve. Normally occurring cranial synkineses are exemplified by sucking, chewing, conjugate eye movements, and Bell's phenomenon.

Abnormal cranial nerve synkineses occur most commonly in DRS (see the previous text) and in the Marcus Gunn jaw-winking phenomenon (trigemino-ocular motor synkinesis). Similar synkineses involving various facial and neck muscles and the extraocular muscles occur in rare patients. A synkinesis between the superior oblique muscle (innervated by the trochlear nerve) and one of the muscles elevating the tongue and hyoid (innervated by the trigeminal, facial, or hypoglossal nerve) can cause double vision produced by swallowing. Similarly, bobbing movements of the eyes may be associated with jaw movements, suggesting a complex form of trigemino-ocular motor synkinesis similar to the classic Marcus Gunn jaw-winking phenomenon but involving more than just the levator muscle.

FOR FURTHER INFORMATION

See *Walsh & Hoyt's Clinical Neuro-Ophthalmology*, 6th edition, Volume 1, Chapter 20, pages 969–1040.

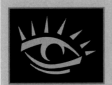

CHAPTER **19**

Disorders of Neuromuscular Transmission*

NORMAL NEUROMUSCULAR TRANSMISSION

Acetylcholine (ACh), the natural transmitter, is synthesized chiefly in the motor nerve terminals and is stored in vesicles for subsequent release. Neurotransmission begins with the release of the contents of the vesicles by a process of exocytosis that occurs at specialized release sites located directly opposite the areas of highest concentration of ACh receptors on the postsynaptic membranes (Fig. 19.1), thus minimizing the distance that the transmitter must travel to reach the receptor site. When ACh combines with its receptor, a transient increase of permeability to sodium and potassium ions occurs, resulting in membrane depolarization. When a nerve impulse arrives at the motor nerve terminal, the amplitude of the depolarization is normally sufficient to trigger an action potential that is propagated along the muscle membrane. The muscle action potential, in turn, initiates the sequence of events that leads to muscle contraction. The entire process of neuromuscular transmission is rapid, on the order of a millisecond. It is terminated by the removal of ACh, in part by its diffusion away from the neuromuscular junction (NMJ), but mostly by the action of acetylcholinesterase, which rapidly hydrolyzes ACh.

MYASTHENIA GRAVIS

MG is a disease characterized clinically by muscle weakness and fatigability, caused by a reduction in the number of available ACh receptors at NMJs. Receptor depletion is mediated by one or more antibodies directed against ACh receptors or other NMJ postsynaptic membrane constituents, resulting in impaired neuromuscular transmission. Such antibodies, which

either degrade or block the receptors, are found in the serum of 80% to 90% of patients with MG. Some patients with MG who have no antireceptor antibodies have an immunoglobulin (Ig) G antibody that binds to muscle specific kinase (MuSK). Finally, there is a subpopulation of patients who are seronegative for both anti-ACh receptor antibodies and anti-MuSK antibodies, estimated at about 9% of MG patients overall. These doubly seronegative patients often have purely ocular disease.

EPIDEMIOLOGY

Autoimmune MG affects all races and ages, with an incidence of 4 to 5 per 100,000. There is a female predominance overall, but the sex predilection is age-dependent, with women predominating among younger patients and men among those who are older at diagnosis.

SYMPTOMS AND SIGNS

The hallmark clinical feature of MG is variability in the strength of the affected muscles. Weakness varies from day to day and from hour to hour, typically increasing toward evening. Transient weakness is often associated with physical exertion. Affected muscles fatigue if contraction is maintained or repeated, with the most commonly affected muscles being the levator palpebrae superioris, the extraocular muscles, and the orbicularis oculi. Indeed, the levator palpebrae superioris and extraocular muscles are initially affected in about 70% of cases, and these muscles are eventually affected in over 90% of patients. When weakness of these muscles is combined with weakness of the orbicularis oculi, the combination is highly suggestive of MG.

Ptosis and Other Signs of the Levator Palpebrae Superioris

Ptosis may occur as an isolated sign or in association with extraocular muscle involvement. It is

---

*Adapted from Chapter 21 by Preston C. Calvert, Disorders of Neuromuscular Transmission.

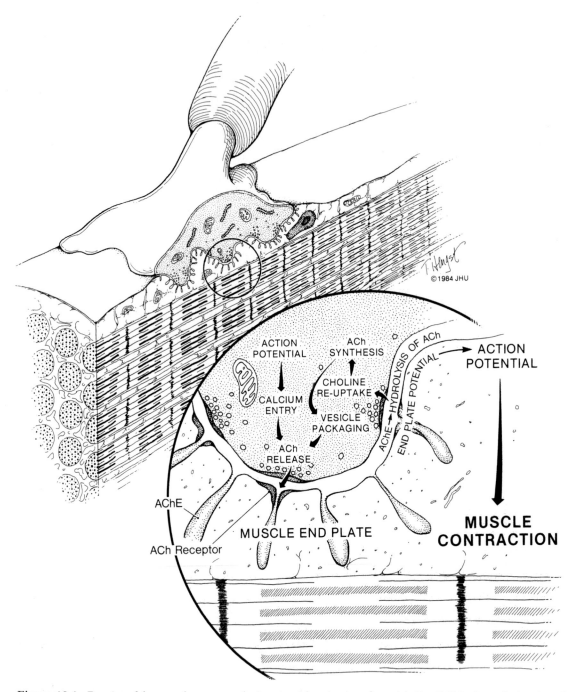

Figure 19.1. Drawing of the normal neuromuscular junction. Note the sites of acetylcholine (ACh) release, the location of acetylcholine receptors, and the location of acetylcholinesterase (AChE).

characterized by its fluctuating nature and frequently shifts from one eye to the other. Ptosis is often initially unilateral but eventually almost always becomes bilateral. When ptosis is bilateral, it is usually asymmetric, but severe symmetric ptosis may occur, particularly in patients with severe ophthalmoplegia. The ptosis is frequently absent when the patient awakens, but it appears later in the day, becoming most pronounced in the evening. Repeated closure of the eyelids may make ptosis appear or may worsen it when it is initially

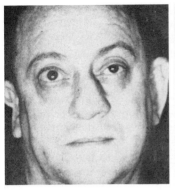
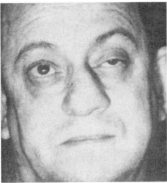
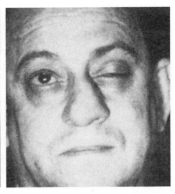

A,B   **C**

Figure 19.2. Increasing ptosis on maintained upward gaze in a patient with myasthenia gravis. **A–C:** represent three frames from a movie showing progressive ptosis over a 3-minute period as the patient maintained fixation above the horizontal meridian. (Reprinted from: Cogan DG. Myasthenia gravis: a review of the disease and a description of lid twitch as a characteristic sign. *Arch Ophthalmol.* 1965;74:217–221, with permission.)

minimal. Prolonged upward gaze also will often result in gradual lowering of the eyelids (Fig. 19.2), but fatigability of bilateral ptosis does not exclude a nonmyasthenic cause, such as dorsal midbrain compression by a mass lesion.

Patients with MG-related ptosis often have worsening of ptosis on one side when the opposite eyelid is elevated and held in a fixed position (Fig. 19.3). The explanation of this "seesaw" phenomenon is Hering's law of equal innervation, which relates to the levator muscles as it does to the extraocular muscles. Manual eyelid elevation decreases the effort required for eyelid elevation ipsilaterally and thus results in relaxation of the contralateral levator and consequent worsening ptosis on that side. Enhancement of ptosis is not pathognomonic for MG, however. It can be seen in patients with congenital ptosis and in patients with acquired ptosis from causes other than MG. Nevertheless, in a patient with an appropriate history, the observation of enhancement of ptosis is highly suggestive of MG.

Cogan's lid twitch is another important sign that suggests MG. When the patient's eyes are directed downward for 10 to 20 seconds and the patient is then instructed to make a vertical saccade back to primary position, the upper eyelid elevates and either slowly begins to droop or else twitches several times before settling into a stable position (Fig. 19.4). This eyelid twitch phenomenon is caused by the rapid recovery and easy fatigability of myasthenic muscle.

Ophthalmoparesis and Other Abnormalities of Eye Movement

Involvement of the extraocular muscles, like ptosis, is extremely common in patients with MG, although the reason for this is unknown. In most cases, disturbances of ocular motility and alignment are associated with ptosis; however, cases without clinical involvement of

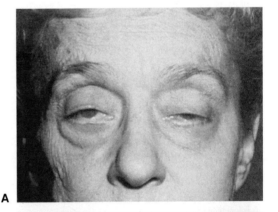

A

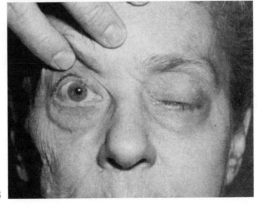

B

Figure 19.3. Enhanced ptosis in a 78-year-old woman with myasthenia gravis. **A:** The patient has bilateral ptosis. **B:** When the right eyelid is elevated, the patient develops increased (enhanced) ptosis on the opposite side.

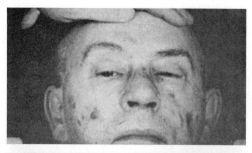
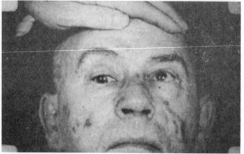
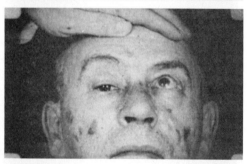
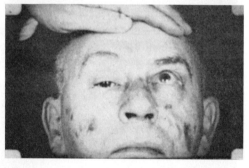

Figure 19.4. Cogan's eyelid twitch phenomenon in a patient with myasthenia gravis. The photograph is made from successive frames of a movie. As the patient looks upward, the left eyelid elevates fully while the right eyelid elevates only partially. The right eyelid then immediately becomes successively more ptotic. The entire process takes only a few seconds. In motion, this transient eyelid elevation gives the appearance of a twitch. (Reprinted from: Cogan DG. Myasthenia gravis: a review of the disease and a description of lid twitch as a characteristic sign. *Arch Ophthalmol.* 1965;74:217–221, with permission.)

the levator muscles occur. There is no set pattern to extraocular muscle involvement. All degrees of ocular motor dysfunction, from apparent involvement of a single isolated muscle to complete external ophthalmoplegia, occur. Thus, the abnormalities may mimic such neurologic disturbances as ocular motor nerve palsies, unilateral or bilateral internuclear ophthalmoplegia, or vertical or horizontal gaze palsies (Fig. 19.5). Unlike patients with neurologic ophthalmoparesis in whom saccadic (fast) eye movements have reduced velocities, however, patients with MG-related ophthalmoparesis have saccades with normal velocities or velocities that are increased relative to the extent of the saccade, and patients with MG-related complete ophthalmoplegia may show tiny "quiver movements" on attempted eccentric gaze.

Orbicularis Oculi Involvement

Patients with MG often have involvement of the orbicularis oculi muscles that may not be apparent when ptosis or ophthalmoplegia predominates. The combination of ptosis, ocular motility disturbances, and weakness of the orbicularis oculi is found in only a few disorders, including MG, myotonic dystrophy, oculopharyngeal dystrophy, and mitochondrial myopathy. Of these, MG is the most common. Patients suspected of having MG should therefore have testing of orbicularis oculi strength by having the patient forcefully shut the eyes while the examiner manually attempts to open the eyelids against the forced lid closure (Fig. 19.6). Some patients with MG exhibit a "peek" sign caused by orbicularis fatigue. In such patients, upon gentle eyelid closure, the orbicularis oculi muscle contracts, initially achieving eyelid apposition; however, the orbicularis muscle rapidly fatigues and the palpebral fissure widens, thereby exposing the sclera. The patient thus appears to "peek" at the examiner.

Pupillary Function

Patients with MG do not have clinically abnormal pupillary reactions to light or near stimulation. Thus, when ocular motor disturbances occur in the setting of a dilated, poorly reactive pupil, MG should not be considered a likely cause. Conversely, any patient in whom an ocular motor disturbance, ptosis, or both are associated with normally reactive pupils may have MG.

Nonocular Features

In patients with generalized involvement of skeletal muscles, the facies may be characteristic, showing a generalized weakness of expression. Weakness frequently affects the neck extensors (head "ptosis") and proximal limb muscles. When the muscles of expression, phonation, articulation, swallowing, and chewing

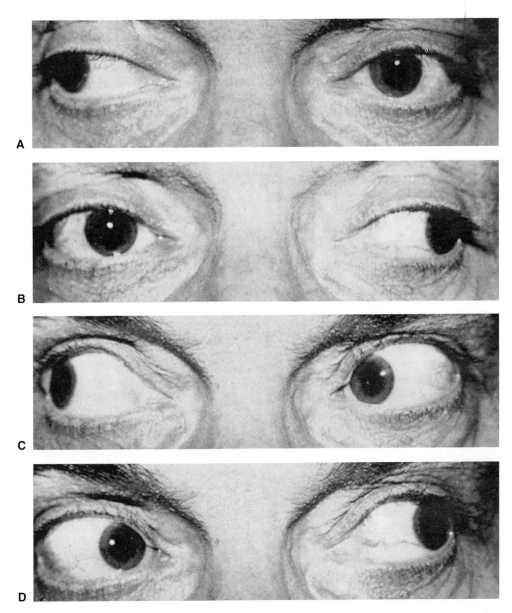

Figure 19.5. Bilateral pseudo-internuclear ophthalmoplegia in a patient with myasthenia gravis. **A:** On attempted rightward gaze, there is adduction lag of the left eye. Note bilateral ptosis. **B:** On attempted leftward gaze, there is adduction lag of the right eye. Following intravenous administration of edrophonium chloride (Tensilon®), there is marked improvement of adduction of both the left eye **(C)** and the right eye **(D)**. (Reprinted from: Glaser JS. Myasthenic pseudo-internuclear ophthalmoplegia. *Arch Ophthalmol.* 1966;75:363–366, with permission.)

are affected, there may be a characteristic facial "snarl," dysarthric speech, nasal regurgitation of liquids, and the need to prop the jaw closed. When the muscles of respiration or swallowing are involved, the term "myasthenic crisis" indicates the gravity of the disease. Rarely, MG presents with respiratory insufficiency alone. On physical examination, the findings are limited entirely to the lower motor unit, without loss of reflexes or altered sensation or coordination.

DIAGNOSTIC TESTING

The tests used to diagnose MG include clinical tests, assays for circulating antibodies to components of the NMJ, pharmacologic tests, repetitive nerve stimulation, and single-fiber electromyography.

Clinical Tests

Two simple office tests are particularly helpful in supporting the clinical diagnosis of MG: the sleep test and

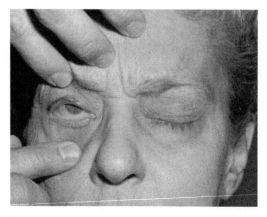

Figure 19.6. Orbicularis oculi weakness in myasthenia gravis. The patient is attempting to close her eyes tightly Note that she is unable to bury the lashes on the left and that the examiner is easily able to open the eyelids on the right.

the ice test. These tests have generally supplanted pharmagologic testing and are particularly useful in elderly or ill patients for whom such testing may be potentially dangerous.

Sleep Test   The sleep test is based on the observation that when many patients with MG awaken in the morn-

ing, they have little or no ptosis or diplopia; however, these manifestations appear or worsen during the day. The sleep test is performed as follows: The patient first undergoes a complete ocular examination and external photographs. The patient is then taken to a quiet, darkened room and instructed to close the eyes and try to sleep. Thirty minutes later, the patient is awakened, immediately photographed, and measurements taken of his or her palpebral fissures, ocular alignment, and ocular motility. Most patients with MG show marked improvement in ptosis, ocular motor dysfunction, or both immediately upon awakening from sleep (Fig. 19.7). The improvement lasts 2 to 5 minutes, following which the ptosis and ophthalmoparesis recur. Patients with ptosis and ophthalmoparesis caused by disorders other than MG show no such improvement after sleep. In our opinion, the sleep test is a safe, moderately sensitive, and specific way to confirm a presumptive diagnosis of MG.

Ice Test   The strength of myasthenic muscles often improves when the muscles are cooled, probably because lowering the temperature reduces the effects of acetylcholinesterase. In patients with ptosis in whom the diagnosis of MG is considered, the use of local cooling to eliminate or reduce the ptosis is a rapid, simple, and inexpensive test with a high degree of specificity

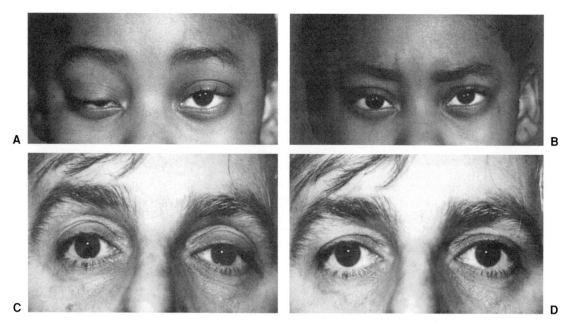

Figure 19.7. The sleep test for myasthenia gravis. **A:** A 10-year-old girl has right ptosis. Note use of the frontalis to help elevate the eyelid. **B:** After 30 minutes of sleep, the ptosis has resolved. The frontalis is no longer contracted. **C:** A 48-year-old man has bilateral symmetric ptosis. **D:** After 30 minutes of sleep, the ptosis has resolved. (Reprinted from: Odel JG, Winterkorn JMS, Behrens MM. The sleep test for myasthenia gravis: a safe alternative to Tensilon. *J Clin Neuroophthalmol.* 1991;11:288–292, with permission.)

and sensitivity for MG. The ice test is performed as follows: the sizes of the palpebral fissures are measured, photographed, or both. The patient is instructed to close the eyes for 2 minutes, following which the palpebral fissures are again assessed. A surgical glove containing crushed ice or ice cubes is then applied to the ptotic (if unilateral) or more ptotic (if bilateral) eyelid for 2 minutes, with the opposite lid serving as a control. After 2 minutes, the glove is removed, and the size of the palpebral fissure is immediately measured or photographed. The test is considered positive if the size of the palpebral fissure is greater after cooling than after the rest period; this difference is usually greater than 2 mm in patients with MG, with the improvement in ptosis typically lasting about 1 minute (Fig. 19.8). The ice test is over 95% sensitive and 100% specific for the diagnosis of MG, making it one of the most useful tests for the clinician. Interestingly, the ice test is most likely to give false-negative results in those patients with MG in whom there is complete or nearly complete ptosis. The ice test is not clinically useful in patients with ophthalmoparesis but no ptosis.

Specific Autoantibody Assays

A radioimmunoassay to detect antireceptor antibodies is one of the standard diagnostic tests for MG; however, although this test detects antibodies in about 85% of all patients with MG, such antibodies are detected in no more than 50% of patients with weakness confined to

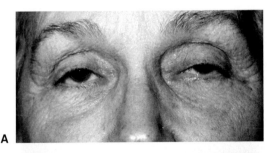

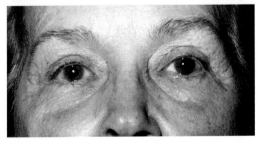

Figure 19.8. The ice test for myasthenia gravis. **A:** Before placement of ice, patient has severe bilateral ptosis. **B:** After placement of ice for 2 minutes, the ptosis has resolved.

the levator and extraocular muscles. In addition, anti-MuSK antibodies are only very rarely found in patients with ocular myasthenia. Thus, should a patient with a clinical diagnosis of MG show no evidence of either antireceptor or anti-MuSK antibodies, the diagnosis should not necessarily be abandoned.

Pharmacologic Tests

The abnormal fatigability of skeletal muscles may be evaluated by observing or quantifying their strength before and after the injection of anticholinesterase agents. Anticholinesterase pharmacologic testing has a sensitivity of about 50% to 75% in MG. Thus, when MG is strongly suspected, and the ice or sleep tests are negative, these tests may be useful.

Edrophonium (Tensilon®) Test Edrophonium chloride (usually supplied as the chloride salt under the trade name Tensilon®) is a rapidly acting and quickly hydrolyzed anticholinesterase that competes with ACh for acetylcholinesterase and thus allows prolonged and repetitive action of ACh at the synapse. It is commonly chosen because of the rapid onset (≤30 seconds) and short duration (about 5 min) of its effects. The edrophonium test is performed as follows: the position of the eyelids is verified as is any ocular misalignment and restriction of movement. A total of 10 mg (1 cc) of edrophonium is drawn up in a 1 cc syringe (if performing the test with an intravenous line in place) or a 3 cc syringe (if a direct venous injection if being performed). A test dose of 2 mg of edrophonium is injected intravenously, and the patient is observed carefully for improvement in ptosis, ocular alignment, range of movement, or a combination of these, lasting 2 to 5 minutes (Fig. 19.9). If definite improvement occurs, the test is considered positive and is terminated. If no such changes occur within 30 seconds, the remainder of the dose (8 mg) is injected either as a single bolus or in 2-mg boluses at 30-second intervals and the patient is observed for improvement in ptosis, ocular alignment, and/or range of movement. Because patients with diplopia and strabismus may not appreciate changes in their ocular alignment, when performing the edrophonium test on a patient with strabismus but without ptosis, it may be helpful to have them hold a red glass over one eye (or use red-green glasses), fixate a distant white light, and describe the relative positions of the two lights seen (red and white or green). Edrophonium is then injected, and the patient is asked to describe any change in the position of the two lights. Another option is to use the Lancaster red-green test or the Hess screen to plot the position of the two eyes before and after the injection of edrophonium. This technique provides an extremely accurate determination of eye position and is much more reliable than asking the

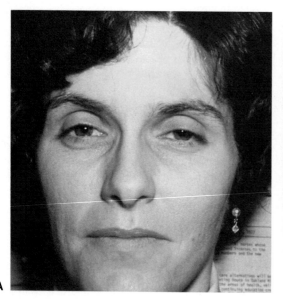
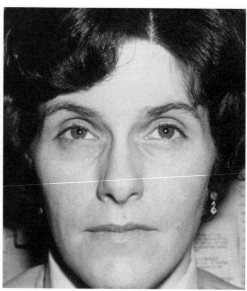

A   **B**

Figure 19.9. The edrophonium (Tensilon®) test for myasthenia gravis. **A:** Before injection of edrophonium, the patient has bilateral ptosis and weakness of facial musculature. **B:** One minute following an intravenous injection of 2 mg of edrophonium, the patient's ptosis has disappeared and her facial muscles appear to function more normally.

patient if he or she sees any improvement in his or her diplopia. The alternate prism-cover test can also be used to document the effects of edrophonium on ocular motor alignment, but this test may be better suited to the more prolonged effects of neostigmine (see later).

Occasionally, a paradoxical reaction (e.g., worsening of ptosis) occurs following administration of edrophonium. This should not be considered a positive response. Similarly, virtually all patients experience transient quivering of the eyelids, lacrimation, and salivation. These responses also do not constitute a positive test.

Because edrophonium is a peripheral anticholinesterase agent, it allows ACh to accumulate briefly in ganglia, at parasympathetic nerve endings, and at NMJs in all types of muscle: cardiac, smooth, and striated. It is the transient excess of ACh at nicotinic synapses that produces a positive test in patients with MG, but this same excess also may produce muscarinic cholinergic side effects from a brief over-stimulation of the parasympathetic nervous system. Major side effects occur in about 1 in 1,000 persons and include bradycardia, asystole, syncope, and seizures. Less severe side effects include near-syncope, dizziness, and involuntary defecation. Although most side effects associated with the edrophonium test can probably be prevented by pretreating patients with an intramuscular injection of atropine sulfate, such reactions are sufficiently rare that it is not necessary to pretreat with atropine.

Nevertheless, it is prudent always to have the drug available during the test. In addition, great caution should be used in performing edrophonium (or neostigmine) tests in older patients, particularly those with known cardiac disease. Instead, the clinician may depend on the results of other features of the presentation, or the results of an ice or sleep test (see the previous text) to direct a further diagnostic evaluation. Should it be necessary to perform an edrophonium test in a patient with cardiac disease, the patient should always have an intravenous line in place and be hooked up to an electrocardiograph machine, in an environment with advanced cardiac life support immediately available.

A positive edrophonium test is usually, but not always, indicative of MG. No reliable quantitative estimates of the specificity of the test are available, but the specificity is believed to be fairly high. Nevertheless, on rare occasions, patients with intracranial lesions producing pupil-sparing oculomotor nerve palsies and other ocular motor disorders may show transient improvement of their findings when tested with edrophonium. Some of these patients may have both MG and an intracranial lesion. In others, however, there is no other evidence of MG, and the response to edrophonium is thought to be falsely positive. For this reason, it is advisable to perform neuroimaging in all patients with isolated, unilateral, pupil-sparing ophthalmoparesis and in selected patients with other ocular muscle pareses, even when the diagnosis of MG seems certain. Other neuromuscular disorders that may produce a positive edrophonium test include Lambert-Eaton myasthenic syndrome, botulism, envenomation by snakes, Guillain-Barré syndrome, amyotrophic lateral sclerosis, and postpoliomyelitis syndrome.

A negative edrophonium test does out eliminate the possibility of MG. The sensitivity of the test in patients with generalized MG ranges from 73% to 96%, whereas its sensitivity in ocular MG ranges from 60% to 95%. Most experienced neuro-ophthalmologists have seen patients in whom several edrophonium tests were unequivocally negative but who had other evidence of MG. Patients may have several negative edrophonium tests before a positive edrophonium test is observed. In patients suspected of having MG, a negative edrophonium test should be followed either by a neostigmine test or by other nonocular diagnostic tests (see later).

Neostigmine (Prostigmin®) Test Because of the transient nature of the ocular (and systemic) changes in muscle strength that occur following the administration of edrophonium, the neostigmine bromide (Prostigmin®) test remains an exceptionally valuable method of diagnosing MG, particularly in patients with diplopia but without ptosis. The longer duration of the effects of this drug is sufficient to permit repeated testing of muscle strength and evaluation of ocular motility. In adults with obvious ptosis and ophthalmoparesis, it is appropriate to mix 0.6 mg of atropine sulfate with 0.5 to 1.5 mg of neostigmine in a 3-cc syringe and inject the mixture into a deltoid or gluteus muscle. A change in ocular motility and ptosis is usually apparent within 15 minutes and is most obvious 30 to 45 minutes following the injection (Fig. 19.10). The sensitivity of this test ranges from 70% to 94%.

The neostigmine test may be particularly helpful in the diagnosis of MG in children, in whom intravenous injection of edrophonium may be accompanied by crying and lack of cooperation, precluding any meaningful assessment of its effect. In such patients, neostigmine is injected, and by the time the neostigmine takes effect, the child usually has stopped crying and can be observed and the eye movements

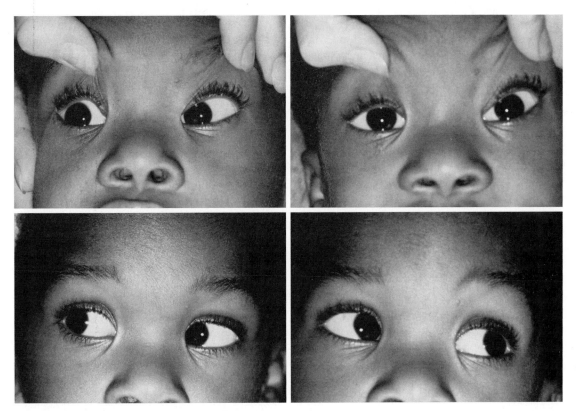

Figure 19.10. The neostigmine (Prostigmin®) test for myasthenia gravis. The 10-year-old boy has moderate limitation of eye movement on attempted right horizontal gaze **(top left)**. His eyelids are being manually elevated because of his ptosis. There is almost no horizontal eye movement on attempted left lateral gaze **(top right)**. Thirty minutes after intramuscular injection of neostigmine, the child's ptosis has resolved **(bottom)**. Horizontal eye movements to the right **(bottom left)** and left **(bottom right)** are almost normal.

measured if necessary. In children, the amount of neostigmine given is related to body weight and is 0.025 to 0.04 mg/kg, not exceeding a total dose of 1.5 mg (the adult dose). The dose of atropine in children is adjusted to 0.011 mg/kg, up to a maximum of 0.4 mg.

Adverse effects of neostigmine testing include bradycardia, syncope, near-syncope, and paradoxical tachycardia (especially at low doses). The combined muscarinic autonomic effects of neostigmine and atropine are often not completely balanced, and if neostigmine predominates, the patient may transiently experience increased salivation, tearing, borborygmi, and the urge to defecate or urinate. Atropine predominance produces dry mouth, tachycardia, and so forth. The relative balance of these competing effects may change over time during the test period. In addition, fasciculations are almost always induced in normal subjects as well as myasthenic patients by the administration of neostigmine. Fasciculations are a useful marker of neostigmine pharmacologic effect and are not blocked by atropine.

As with edrophonium, a positive neostigmine test usually, but not always, indicates MG. Positive responses have been reported in patients with multiple sclerosis, brain stem tumors, and congenital ptosis. Isolated, nonreproducible positive neostigmine tests may thus occur in nonmyasthenics.

Electrophysiologic Tests

Repetitive nerve stimulation has long been used to diagnose MG. In recent years, however, single-fiber electromyography has been shown to be a much more sensitive and specific technique.

Repetitive Nerve Stimulation   The primary technique used by most clinical electrophysiologists in the diagnosis of MG consists of eliciting a decremental response between the first and fourth or fifth response to repetitive supramaximal motor nerve stimulation. Supramaximal electric stimuli are delivered at a rate of 2 to 3 Hz to the appropriate nerves, and compound muscle action potentials are recorded from muscles. A decrement in amplitude of 10% or more is usually considered abnormal. The sensitivity of repetitive nerve stimulation in diagnosing generalized MG has been reported to vary from 51% to 100%, depending on the technique used and the severity of myasthenia in sampled patients. The wide range of sensitivity of the test implies that a normal test does not exclude MG.

Single-Fiber Electromyography   Endplate potentials in the postsynaptic membrane of the NMJ reach the threshold for triggering an action potential of the muscle fiber with random variability, resulting in a variable latency between a nerve stimulus and the action potential of the responding muscle fiber. The latencies of responses of fibers belonging to the same motor unit are therefore not quite synchronous. The variability between any fiber and a reference fiber from the same unit is called "jitter." When the safety factor for transmission is low, these latency variabilities (jitters) are increased. There are also more response failures ("blocking"), in which an action potential of the muscle fiber is not triggered by arrival of a nerve terminal action potential. Jitter and blocking can be detected in human muscles using suitably selective electrodes, and the latencies can be studied statistically during either voluntary contraction or indirect stimulation in a technique called collectively single-fiber electromyography (single-fiber EMG). In patients undergoing evaluation for MG who are antibody-negative and in whom repetitive nerve stimulation is negative or equivocal, single-fiber EMG is an extremely useful diagnostic test, being positive in 88% to 99% of all patients with MG, although an experienced electrophysiologist is required to perform this test.

Like the edrophonium and neostigmine tests, single-fiber EMG may be negative initially only to be positive several months later. Thus, a negative single-fiber EMG test in a muscle with normal strength is not absolute evidence that the patient does not have MG. However, if a clinically weak muscle has normal jitter at all endplates, the diagnosis of MG can be excluded. Conversely, single-fiber EMG abnormalities are frequently seen in other disorders of neuromuscular transmission, including the Lambert-Eaton myasthenic syndrome, congenital myasthenic syndromes, and botulism. Increased jitter may have causes other than defective neuromuscular transmission, such as denervation of many causes, amyotrophic lateral sclerosis, mitochondrial cytopathy, and oculopharyngeal dystrophy, and the results are considered positive only in the context of normal fiber density and routine EMG.

Additional Tests

Because a thymic tumor is found in about 10% of patients with MG, the evaluation of a patient with suspected or proven MG should include CT scanning or MR imaging of the anterior mediastinum. Chest radiographs have such a low sensitivity as to make them useless for such screening.

A complete blood count, erythrocyte sedimentation rate, antinuclear antibody test, and thyroid function tests should be performed in all patients diagnosed with MG because of the increased prevalence of other autoimmune diseases in these patients. Any patient who may be a candidate for corticosteroid treatment should be screened for diabetes mellitus, and all patients should undergo a skin test for tuberculosis prior to institution of chronic immunosuppression.

OCULAR MYASTHENIA GRAVIS

About 60% of patients with MG initially present with ocular manifestations, but up to 87% of these individuals eventually develop other signs and symptoms, including proximal muscle weakness, difficulty with speech, and difficulty swallowing, usually within 2 years of symptom onset. Thus, less than 10% of patients with MG have manifestations that remain limited to the eyelids and extraocular muscles for more than 2 years and thus have the condition known as "ocular MG." Patients in whom MG has been diagnosed on the basis of isolated ocular manifestations should be warned about the tendency for generalization, and the symptoms of generalization should be reviewed with them.

TREATMENT

Most patients with MG can lead full and productive lives with proper therapy. Treatment includes cholinesterase inhibitors, thymectomy, immunosuppressive drugs, and, for selected patients with ocular manifestations, local therapy. Although cholinesterase inhibitors tend to be the primary therapy for patients with MG, the ocular manifestations of the disease are often refractory o these drugs, being more responsive to systemic corticosteroids or thymectomy. In addition, there is some evidence that early treatment of "ocular" MG with systemic corticosteroids prevents generalization of the disease. The choice of therapy for a given patient with MG who has ocular manifestations, is best left to a specialist in neuromuscular diseases with appropriate input from the ophthalmologist.

CONGENITAL MYASTHENIC SYNDROMES

Once thought to be a single clinical and pathologic entity, congenital MG is now known to be a heterogeneous group of genetic neuromuscular transmission disorders. These conditions can be differentiated from acquired autoimmune MG on the basis of clinical, electromyographic, electrophysiologic, cytochemical, structural, and molecular genetic grounds. Many but not all cases present neonatally or in infancy with ptosis, fluctuating ophthalmoparesis, poor feeding, and respiratory difficulty. Symptoms may be episodic or may demonstrate fatigability that is worsened by crying, activity, or fever. Persistence of symptoms, rather than a transient monophasic course, distinguishes a congenital myasthenic syndrome from neonatal MG. Some syndromes may not even present until adolescence or adulthood. Serum anti-ACh receptor antibodies are absent. In many cases, siblings or parents are affected, but a negative family history does not exclude autosomal-recessive inheritance. The edrophonium test, which relies on intact acetylcholinesterase and normal channel open times for its effect, is negative in many congenital myasthenic syndromes. Thus, a negative test does not exclude the diagnosis, and a positive test cannot distinguish any of the congenital myasthenic syndromes from autoimmune myasthenia. The diagnosis instead rests on the results of electrophysiologic testing and other key features.

Congenital myasthenic syndromes may be separated into those in which the defect is primarily presynaptic and those in which the defect is primarily postsynaptic. The major syndromes in which the defect is presynaptic are related to defects in ACh synthesis, mobilization, or release. Postsynaptic syndromes are mainly those caused by endplate acetylcholinesterase deficiency and ACh receptor deficiency, as well as disorders of the ACh receptor kinetics, including the fast- and slow-channel syndromes. Nevertheless, almost any gene or process involved in neuromuscular transmission is a potential target for these rare genetic mutations.

ACQUIRED DISORDERS OF NEUROMUSCULAR TRANSMISSION OTHER THAN MYASTHENIA GRAVIS

As with congenital "myasthenic" syndromes, acquired disorders of neuromuscular transmission other than MG may be caused by presynaptic or postsynaptic abnormalities. In addition, some syndromes are characterized by both pre- and postsynaptic abnormalities. Most of the acquired disorders of neuromuscular transmission other than MG are caused by the effects of exogenous agents on the NMJ.

LAMBERT-EATON MYASTHENIC SYNDROME

Lambert-Eaton myasthenic syndrome is characterized primarily by weakness but also by fatigability, hyporeflexia, and autonomic dysfunction. Weakness is proximal and more prominent in legs and truncal muscles than in arms. Ocular and bulbar muscles are sometimes affected but mildly so, in contrast to their prominent involvement in MG.

Lambert-Eaton myasthenic syndrome is most commonly a paraneoplastic syndrome associated with small-cell lung cancer and occasionally with non-Hodgkin's lymphoma, leukemia, and other malignancies. Paraneoplastic Lambert-Eaton myasthenic syndrome presents before the discovery of the neoplasm in 86% of patients, with the vast majority of patients being found to have a tumor within 2 years of onset of neurologic symptoms. Although most affected patients are adults, the disorder can also occur in children. The Lambert-Eaton myasthenic syndrome may also develop in patients with other autoimmune disorders including pernicious anemia, thyroid disease, systemic lupus erythematosus, celiac disease, type I diabetes mellitus, ulcerative colitis, Addison's disease, rheumatoid arthritis, and Sjögren's syndrome.

Pathophysiology

The neuromuscular transmission defect in Lambert-Eaton myasthenic syndrome is presynaptic. It is caused by impaired release of ACh at motor nerve terminals because of antibodies directed against voltage-gated calcium channels in the motor nerve terminal and cholinergic autonomic nerve terminals. These antibodies reduce the number of calcium channels and thus the probability of synaptosomal release of ACh at active zones. Small-cell lung carcinomas enriched in voltage-gated calcium channels provide the shared antigenic stimulus in paraneoplastic Lambert-Eaton myasthenic syndrome. Close to 100% of patients with the myasthenic syndrome associated with small-cell lung carcinoma have antibodies to voltage-gated calcium channels. In patients with the Lambert-Eaton syndrome without underlying cancer, 8% to 90% have voltage-gated calcium channel antibodies. A small residual percentage of patients with clinical and electrophysiologic evidence of Lambert-Eaton myasthenic syndrome, usually without associated cancer, have no detectable antibodies to voltage-gated calcium channels.

Acetylcholine synthesis and mobilization are unimpaired in Lambert-Eaton myasthenic syndrome, and the amount of depolarization produced by single quanta is normal. The impaired ACh release results in compound endplate potentials that may be too small to trigger muscle action potentials. As a result, muscles fatigue and evoked compound muscle action potentials are low in amplitude. The normally increased mobilization of calcium that occurs in the nerve terminal immediately following exercise or electric activation of motor nerves at rates above 10 Hz transiently increases the release of ACh, the resultant endplate potential amplitude, and therefore muscle strength. This facilitation is the basis for the electrophysiologic diagnosis.

Ocular Manifestations

Ocular symptoms and signs are less common in Lambert-Eaton syndrome than in MG, but ptosis and both clinical and subclinical ocular motor involvement do occur. Nevertheless, a patient with obvious ptosis and ocular motor dysfunction is very unlikely to have Lambert-Eaton myasthenic syndrome.

Therapy

In general, the Lambert-Eaton myasthenic syndrome responds to therapy somewhat less well than does MG. An individualized, combined approach to therapy includes treatment of any underlying cancer, pharmacotherapy of the neuromuscular transmission defect, and immunosuppression. Because the syndrome may precede the discovery of a tumor by several years, the evaluation should include not only an initial extensive search for underlying malignancy, including chest CT or MRI, but also frequent surveillance if the initial evaluation is negative. Partial but rarely complete remission may be achieved by removal or control of the underlying small-cell cancer with surgery, radiation therapy, or chemotherapy.

NEUROMUSCULAR DISORDERS CAUSED BY DRUGS OR TOXINS

Substances that cause neuromuscular disturbances do so by affecting presynaptic mechanisms, postsynaptic mechanisms, or both. These substances are primarily drugs and toxins.

The common settings in which the effects of drugs appear are (a) in a patient at increased risk because of abnormally increased drug concentration; (b) as part of a drug-induced generalized immunologic disorder; (c) with delayed recovery of strength following general anesthesia during which neuromuscular blocking agents may have been used; and (d) unmasking or worsening of MG or the myasthenic syndrome. Drug-induced disturbances of neuromuscular transmission usually resemble naturally occurring MG, causing prominent ptosis and ophthalmoparesis as well as variable degrees of facial, bulbar, and extremity muscle weakness. Respiratory difficulties may occur early and are often severe. Treatment consists of discontinuing the offending agent and reversing the block with various agents, including calcium gluconate, potassium, and anticholinesterases.

Toxins that disturb neuromuscular transmission may be acquired from many sources, including bacteria, arthropods, and snakes. Treatment depends on the recognition of the specific toxin, the availability of antitoxin, and supportive therapy.

Drug-Induced Autoimmune Damage to the Neuromuscular Junction

A myasthenic syndrome may develop in patients receiving D-penicillamine for rheumatoid arthritis or Wilson's disease. The syndrome may consist of ocular symptoms and signs alone or may be associated with generalized muscle involvement. It mimics true MG not only in its clinical features but also in that affected patients have the same histocompatibility antigens and anti-ACh receptor antibodies that either block or

Table 19.1. *Drugs that Interfere with Function of the Neuromuscular Junction*

Drug	Site of Action
Neuromuscular blocking agents (pancuronium, vecuronium, alcuronium)	Postsynaptic
Acetylcholinesterase inhibitors:	Postsynaptic
Medications—pyridostigmine, neostigmine	
Pesticides—organophosphates, carbamates	
Biowarfare agents—Sarin, VX	
Phenothiazines	Postsynaptic
Trimethaphan	Postsynaptic
D,L-Carnitine	Postsynaptic
Inhalational anesthetics (ether, ketamine, halothane)	Postsynaptic
Amphetamine	Presynaptic
Corticosteroids	Pre- and postsynaptic
Antiarrhythmics (procainamide, quinidine)	Pre- and postsynaptic
Antibiotics:	Pre- and postsynaptic
Aminoglycosides (e.g., gentamicin)	
Polymyxins (e.g., polymyxin B)	
Penicillins (e.g., ampicillin)	
Macrolides (e.g., erythromycin)	
Tetracyclines (e.g., minocycline)	
Quinolones (e.g., ciprofloxacin)	
Monobasic amino acids (e.g., clindamycin)	
Anticonvulsants (e.g., phenytoin)	Pre- and postsynaptic
Beta-adrenergic blocking agents	Pre- and postsynaptic
Chloroquine	Pre- and postsynaptic
Cis-platinum	Unknown
Lithium	Pre- and postsynaptic
Magnesium	Pre- and postsynaptic
Iodinated radiographic contrast agents	Unknown

increase the degradation of ACh receptors, just as they do in true MG. D-penicillamine thus has no direct neuromuscular blocking effect but produces a myasthenic syndrome in much the same way that MG occurs naturally. The onset averages 8 months after the onset of therapy, and the syndrome is unrelated to D-penicillamine dosage or cumulative dosage.

Drugs that Affect Neuromuscular Transmission through Presynaptic or Postsynaptic Effects

A variety of drugs act at both pre- and postsynaptic sites of the NMJ to disturb neuromuscular transmission in humans. Such drugs can "unmask" subclinical MG or worsen known MG. Table 19.1 lists some of the drugs that interfere with the function of the NMJ.

Toxins that Damage Presynaptic Neuromuscular Transmission

Arthropod Envenomation Envenomation by a variety of arthropods, including the female black widow spider (*Latrodectus mactans*), the brown widow spider (*Latrodectus geometricus*), several species of scorpions, and a variety of ticks such as *Dermacentor, Amblyomma, and Ixodes holocyclus* species cause a variety of systemic and ocular disturbances related to the effects of the venom on the presynaptic portion of the NMJ. Treatment of this type of envenomation is generally supportive.

Botulism Botulism occurs in three forms: food-borne, wound, and infantile. The disease is produced by a polypeptide toxin elaborated by the organism *Clostridium botulinum*. In food-borne botulism, symptoms begin 8 to 36 hours after food containing the preformed toxin is eaten. The toxin is intact because proper cooking that normally would denature the toxin has not been performed. In wound botulism, organisms contaminating wounds produce toxin that is absorbed systemically. Nearly all cases develop either from extremity wounds that occur outside the home or intravenous drug abuse. Symptoms begin 4 to 17 days after the injury, with an average incubation time of 7 days. Wounds that cause botulism may appear clinically uninfected; however, when the wound is carefully explored and cultured, the organism is usually found.

In infantile botulism, organisms in the gastrointestinal tract produce toxin that is systemically absorbed.

At least eight types of botulinum toxin are characterized (A, B, Cα, Cβ, D, E, F, and G). Types A and B are the most common causes of botulism in the United States, although type E should be suspected when seafood is eaten. All of these toxins impair neuromuscular transmission presynaptically by interfering with the exocytotic release of ACh vesicles after the stimulus-induced influx of calcium into the nerve terminal. Recovery eventually occurs when nerve fibers sprout, and new NMJs are established, but the process may take months to years.

The diagnosis of botulism depends on clinical, epidemiologic, and electrophysiologic findings and may be confirmed by the discovery of the toxin or the organism in food, stool, or a wound. Signs of infantile botulism are constipation, listlessness, poor suck, regurgitation, and generalized weakness. In children and adults, the symptoms of botulism include nausea, vomiting, blurred vision, dysphagia, and pooling of secretions in the mouth and pharynx, followed by generalized weakness mostly proximal in the upper extremities and diplopia. Examination of affected patients reveals facial, pharyngeal, and generalized proximal weakness but normal sensation.

Ophthalmologic findings in patients with botulism include dilated pupils with little or no pupillary light reaction, accommodation weakness or paralysis, decreased lacrimation, and ptosis that usually is bilateral and symmetric as is ophthalmoparesis or ophthalmoplegia (Fig. 19.11).

The diagnosis of botulism should be suspected by the history and may be confirmed by electromyography which shows findings consistent with a presynaptic disorder analogous to Lambert-Eaton myasthenic syndrome. Motor and sensory nerve conduction velocities are normal. The amplitude of the evoked muscle action potential is usually reduced. There may be no decrement at low rates of stimulation. Following exercise or at high stimulus frequencies, significant facilitation is present. Single-fiber EMG shows increased jitter and blocking.

Botulism is treated with bivalent (A and B) or trivalent (A, B, and E) antitoxin in addition to removal of stomach and intestinal contents if ingestion was the likely route of entry. In patients with wound botulism, the most important treatment is to open and extensively debride the wound. Penicillin or another antibiotic should be given, with the choice of the antibiotic being based on sensitivities from wound culture. Regardless of the apparent severity of the disease when the patient is first seen, full respiratory and nutritional support may be required. Patients with botulism do not normally respond to treatment with anticholinesterase agents.

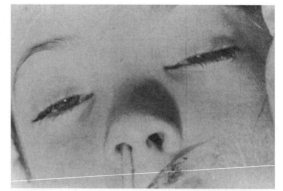
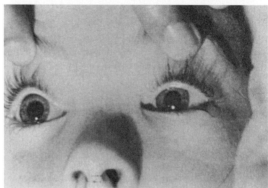
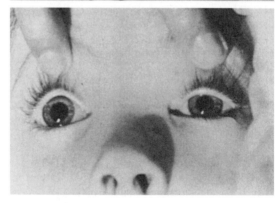

Figure 19.11. Clinical appearance of an 8-year-old girl who developed wound botulism after she fell from a horse and sustained a compound fracture of the humerus. Although the wound appeared clean, *Clostridium botulinum* was cultured from it. The patient has severe bilateral ptosis **(top)**. On attempted rightward gaze, there is marked limitation of movement of both eyes **(middle)**. Note dilated pupils. On attempted leftward gaze, there is almost no movement of the eyes. The patient was quadriparetic but was awake and alert **(bottom)**. She recovered completely within several months.

Tetanus Like *Clostridium botulinum*, *Clostridium tetani* produces a neurotoxin that blocks the calcium-dependent release of ACh at NMJs, but this effect is overshadowed by its effects on the CNS.

Toxins that Damage Both Pre- and Postsynaptic Neuromuscular Transmission

Envenomation by poisonous snakes is an important problem around the world. Of the four largest families of poisonous snakes (*Elapidae*, cobras, coral snakes, mambas, kraits; *Hydrophiidae*, sea snakes; *Viperidae*, Old World vipers; and *Crotalidae*, rattlesnakes and related species), only the first two have venom with potent neuromuscular blocking properties. In most cases of *Elapidae* envenomation, neuromuscular blocking activity of the venoms is a major cause of death and disability. Envenomation is followed in minutes to hours by signs of neuromuscular blockade resembling that caused by competitive neuromuscular blocking drugs. Patients initially develop bilateral ptosis, ophthalmoparesis, and dysphagia, followed by tongue, laryngeal, and pharyngeal weakness. Respiratory paralysis eventually occurs, leading to death if patients are not treated. Ophthalmoparesis and ptosis are frequent components, related to both pre- and postsynaptic effects on neuromuscular transmission. Sea snakes, members of *Hydrophiidae*, produce a neurotoxic venom that can also produce ptosis and ophthalmoplegia. Many of the symptoms show improvement with anticholinesterase agents, although antivenom administration and ventilatory and cardiocirculatory support are the mainstays of treatment.

FOR FURTHER INFORMATION

See *Walsh & Hoyt's Clinical Neuro-Ophthalmology*, 6th edition, Volume 1, Chapter 21.

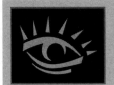

CHAPTER 20

Myopathies Affecting the Extraocular Muscles*

I n this chapter, we consider disorders that produce ocular motor dysfunction from involvement of the extraocular muscles. Some of these disorders affect only the extraocular muscles, whereas others are multisystem disorders in which various organ systems are also affected.

DEVELOPMENTAL DISORDERS OF EXTRAOCULAR MUSCLE

Anomalous development of extraocular muscles is probably more common than the literature would indicate. Many of these anomalies are recognized only during surgical procedures or at autopsy. The most common congenital anomalies of the extraocular muscles are agenesis, anomalous insertions or origins, and the adherence and fibrosis syndromes.

AGENESIS OF THE EXTRAOCULAR MUSCLES

Most cases of agenesis of the extraocular muscles involve only a single muscle. Isolated agenesis of the lateral rectus muscle, medial rectus muscle, inferior rectus muscle, superior rectus muscle, and superior oblique muscle are all well described, particularly in children with craniostenosis. In some patients, agenesis of more than one muscle occurs.

ANOMALIES OF EXTRAOCULAR MUSCLE ORIGIN, INSERTION, AND STRUCTURE

Abnormal origins of extraocular muscles are quite rare. They appear to affect the inferior oblique muscle more than any of the other muscles. Somewhat more commonly responsible for ocular motor dysfunction is an abnormal insertion of an extraocular muscle. Abnormal insertions of extraocular muscles, like agenesis of the muscles, often occur in children with craniostenosis.

Occasionally, an extraocular muscle shows underaction because of an abnormally increased length. In other instances, an anomalous muscle slip or fibrous band may be present. This phenomenon appears to be responsible for most of the congenital cases of superior oblique tendon dysfunction called Brown syndrome. Patients with this syndrome show absence of elevation in adduction, improvement of elevation in the primary position, and normal or near-normal elevation in abduction (Fig. 20.1). Forced duction testing (see Chapter 16) shows mechanical limitation of motion upward and inward in the involved eye, but upward saccadic velocities are normal.

CONGENITAL ADHERENCE AND FIBROSIS SYNDROMES

Congenital fibrosis of the extraocular muscles (CFEOM) is the term used to describe several hereditary disorders characterized by (a) ophthalmoplegia, (b) ptosis, (c) fibrosis of all the extraocular muscles, (d) fibrosis of Tenon's capsule, (e) adhesions between muscles,

---

*Adapted from Chapter 22 by Paul N. Hoffman, Myopathies Affecting Extraocular Muscles.

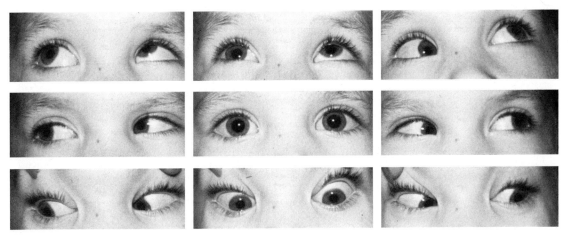

Figure 20.1. Four-year-old child with congenital Brown's superior oblique tendon sheath syndrome. Note marked limitation of upward movement of the right eye when the eye is adducted, compared to mild limitation of upward movement of the eye when it is abducted. The patient was able to fuse in the primary position. (Courtesy of Jacqueline E. Morris, C.O.)

Tenon's capsule, and globe, and (f) inelasticity and fragility of the conjunctiva (Fig. 20.2). CFEOM is associated with mutations at three distinct loci, FEOM1, FEOM2, and FEOM3, located on chromosomes 12, 11, and 16, respectively (Table 20.1). FEOM1 and FEOM3 mutations produce autosomal-dominant CFEOM, whereas the FEOM2 mutation produces autosomal-recessive CFEOM. Most patients with these disorders have only ocular dysfunction, but some patients have facial diparesis, and individual patients have been described who also had inguinal hernias and cryptorchidism or a cleft palate.

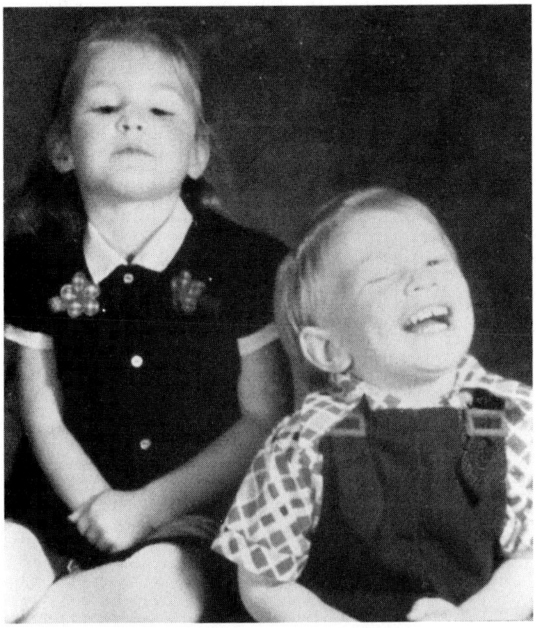

Although histopathologic findings in some patients with CFEOM include replacement of muscle tissue with fibrous tissue and degenerative changes in the muscles, these findings are secondary to maldevelopment of the oculomotor (III) nerve, trochlear (IV) nerve, or both. Thus, CFEOM is actually a disorder similar in origin to Duane and Möbius syndromes.

CONGENITAL MYOPATHIES

Two types of congenital, primarily nonprogressive myopathies can affect the extraocular and eyelid muscles, producing bilateral ptosis, ophthalmoparesis, and facial weakness (Fig. 20.3). One group consists of disorders that are similar to one another clinically but have distinctive histopathologic features. They are called collectively **structurally defined congenital myopathies** and include: (a) central core myopathy, (b) nemaline myopathy, (c) centronuclear (or myotubular) myopathy, (d) multicore disease, and (e) congenital fiber-type disproportion.

A second group of congenital myopathies remains to be characterized fully. These disorders generally present with congenital hypotonia or with early onset generalized weakness that does not progress. Some have ocular features; others do not. Skeletal deformities, such as high-arched palate, scoliosis, and a slender body habitus may be present.

Most congenital myopathies are mild and nonprogressive or slowly progressive. Some cases, however,

Figure 20.2. Congenital fibrosis syndrome in a brother and sister. Because of the bilateral ptosis and ophthalmoplegia, both children have adopted a head posture with the chin elevated. (Courtesy of Dr. Stewart M. Wolff.)

Table 20.1. *Syndromes of Congenital Fibrosis of the Extraocular Muscles*

Phenotype	Inheritance	Locus (Chromosome)	Gene	Clinical Presentation
CFEOM1	AD	FEOM1 (12cen)	Unknown	Bilateral ptosis and ophthalmoplegia; eye is primarily hypotropic, may also be eso- or exotropic; unable to elevate eyes above midline
CFEOM2	AR	FEOM2 (11q13)	ARIX	Bilateral ptosis and ophthalmoplegia; eye is primarily exotropic but may also be hypo- or hypertropic
CFEOM3	AD	FEOM3 (16qter)	Unknown	Unilateral or bilateral ptosis and motility deficits range from mild to severe; phenotypes overlap with CFEOM1 and CFEOM2

AD, autosomal dominant; AR, autosomal recessive.

are severe, relentlessly progressive, or both, resulting in substantial debilitation.

Congenital myopathies must be differentiated from other causes of congenital hypotonic weakness such as various forms of spinal muscular atrophy. This distinc-tion usually is fairly simple, however, as most of these latter conditions are not associated with either pto-sis or ophthalmoparesis/plegia. Thus, an infant with congenital hypotonia associated with ptosis, external ophthalmoplegia, or both almost always has a my-opathy. Nevertheless, conditions other than congenital myopathies, including neonatal myasthenia gravis and infant botulism, can also cause hypotonia, weakness, facial paresis, and ophthalmoparesis.

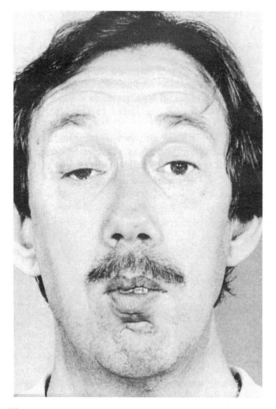

Figure 20.3. Appearance of a 45-year-old man with a con-genital (nemaline) myopathy. Note bilateral asymmetric pto-sis. The patient must use the frontalis muscle to help raise the eyelids. (Reprinted from: Wright RA, Plant GT, Landon DN, et al. Nemaline myopathy: an unusual cause of ophthalmo-paresis. *J Neuroophthalmol.* 1997;17:39–43, with permission.)

MUSCULAR DYSTROPHIES

The term *muscular dystrophy* covers a group of ge-netically determined disorders that cause **progressive** weakness and wasting of the skeletal muscles and that are assumed to affect the muscle cell directly. Some forms cause death after 15 to 20 years, whereas oth-ers are compatible with a normal life expectancy. The distinction between the terms *myopathy* and *dystro-phy* breaks down, however, when it is realized that some glycogenolytic myopathies, like acid maltase de-ficiency, can progress inexorably like dystrophies, and some dystrophies, like Becker dystrophy, may hardly progress at all. Nevertheless, the diagnostic category is a tradition. Although the diagnosis of this group of dis-orders cannot be established by morphology alone, his-tologic examination of an affected muscle can exclude other myopathies (e.g., the congenital myopathies and the mitochondrial myopathies). In others, molecular genetic testing can provide the correct diagnosis.

Muscular dystrophies are historically subdivided on the basis of age of onset, mode of inheritance, and clin-ical features as follows:

1. The dystrophin-deficient dystrophies, including the severe X-linked pseudohypertrophic muscu-lar dystrophy of Duchenne, with its more benign "Becker" variant
2. The dystrophin-associated glycoprotein disorders that may resemble Duchenne or Becker dystrophy,

including mutations of merosin and the α-, β-, γ-, or δ-sarcoglycans
3. Various limb-girdle dystrophies, including severe childhood-onset autosomal-recessive (chromosome 13) muscular dystrophy, juvenile scapulohumeral dystrophy of Erb, pelvifemoral dystrophy of Leyden and Möbius, and adult-onset autosomal-dominant limbgirdle dystrophy
4. The fascioscapulohumeral dystrophy of Landouzy and Déjérine
5. Distal dystrophies (myopathies) of Welander, Miyoshi, and others
6. Congenital muscular dystrophies, including Fukuyama dystrophy, muscle-eye-brain disease, and Walker-Warburg syndrome
7. Myotonic muscular dystrophy
8. Proximal myotonic myopathy
9. Oculopharyngeal muscular dystrophy.

Only the last four of these disorders are of neuro-ophthalmologic importance and are discussed below.

CONGENITAL MUSCULAR DYSTROPHIES

A number of patients have dystrophic muscle pathology associated with symptoms that are present at birth and a variable clinical course. These patients are said to have congenital muscular dystrophy (CMD).

Patients with CMD show generalized muscle involvement at birth. Muscle atrophy and weakness are symmetric and predominate in proximal muscles. In addition, non-muscular ocular involvement is common in three congenital dystrophy syndromes that are really multisystemic disorders of eye, brain, and skeletal muscle. These three, the Fukuyama type of CMD, so-called muscle-eye-brain disease, and the Walker-Warburg syndrome, are associated with mutations that result in protein glycosylation defects

Fukuyama Congenital Muscular Dystrophy

The Fukuyama type of CMD is transmitted as an autosomal-recessive trait with no sex predilection, a high incidence of consanguinity, and a high frequency of affected siblings. The mutant gene, located on chromosome 9q31, encodes fukutin, a putative glycosyltransferase.

Patients with Fukuyama dystrophy have CMD associated with central nervous system (CNS) involvement, including mental retardation and convulsions. Children are severely weak from birth, and only a few children can walk without assistance. Most survive beyond infancy to remain relatively stable, but the average life span is only 8 to 10 years. Serum levels of creatinine kinase (CK) are elevated, and the muscle biopsy shows myopathic and fibrotic changes. Ventricular enlargement and hypoplasia of the cerebellar vermis are seen with computed tomographic (CT) scanning, and

magnetic resonance (MR) imaging shows severe signal abnormalities in white matter.

The neuropathologic findings in Fukuyama dystrophy include polymicrogyria of the cerebrum and cerebellum, loss of cerebral cytoarchitecture with demyelination and proliferation of interstitial tissue, occasionally absent or hypoplastic corpus callosum, and brainstem pyramidal tract abnormalities. Chronic meningeal thickening, lymphocytic infiltration of intracranial tissues, and proliferation of meningeal tissue and blood vessels are less common.

Ocular involvement in Fukuyama CMD is inconsistent, but it is milder than that in muscle-eye-brain disease and Walker-Warburg syndrome (see the subsequent text). Reported findings include occasional optic nerve hypoplasia and optic atrophy, as well as high myopia, cataracts, weakness of the orbicularis oculi muscles, and retinal abnormalities that may be mild or severe, including mottling of the retinal pigment epithelium, abnormal retinal vessels, incomplete retinal vascularization with temporally displaced foveas, and dysplasia.

Muscle-Eye-Brain Disease

This autosomal-recessive disorder is associated with homozygous mutations in O-mannose beta-1,2–N-acetylglucosaminyltransferase (POMGnT1), an enzyme that participates in O-mannosyl glycan synthesis. It is characterized by severe congenital hypotonic weakness from both progressive CNS disease and CMD. Though the cerebral and visual abnormalities are severe, most patients reach adulthood (average age of death, 18). As in Fukuyama dystrophy, levels of serum CK are elevated, and muscle biopsy shows mild myopathy with fibrosis.

Ocular abnormalities are more consistent and severe in muscle-eye-brain disease than in Fukuyama dystrophy, but they are less uniform than in Walker-Warburg syndrome. High myopia is common. Other ocular findings include severe generalized loss of retinal ganglion cells, retinochoroidal scars, a pronounced preretinal membrane and gliosis, mottled retinal pigment epithelium, and mild optic nerve and chiasm atrophy with reactive gliosis. The microscopic and macroscopic features of the cortex in these cases may be highly abnormal, showing argyric areas, coarse and nodular gyri, or total disorganization. The cerebellar vermis and brainstem may be hypoplastic.

Walker-Warburg Syndrome

The Walker-Warburg syndrome is an autosomal-recessive disorder with more severe findings than either Fukuyama dystrophy or muscle-eye-brain disease. The Walker-Warburg syndrome is associated with homozygous mutations in the gene encoding O-mannosyltransferase 1 (POMT1), which like POMGnT1 (the mutant protein in muscle-eye-brain disease) participates in O-mannosyl glycan synthesis. Although the neuropathologic features of Walker-Warburg syndrome are the same as those of muscle-eye-brain disease, they are more extensive and include the macroscopic features of arrhinencephaly: cephalocele, hemispheric fusion, agenesis of the corpus callosum, or a combination of these manifestations.

The ocular malformations in Walker-Warburg syndrome, like the neuropathologic features, are also more severe than in muscle-eye-brain disease. Typical ocular features include retinal dysplasia and nonattachment, persistent hyperplastic primary vitreous, optic nerve atrophy, microphthalmia, corneal opacities, congenital cataract, and congenital glaucoma.

The skeletal muscle biopsy changes in Walker-Warburg syndrome are similar to those of muscle-eye-brain disease and less severe than those in Fukuyama dystrophy. Levels of serum CK are elevated in this disorder as it is in the other two.

MYOTONIC MUSCULAR DYSTROPHIES

Myotonic dystrophy (dystrophia myotonica 1 [DM1]) and the less severe proximal myotonic myopathy (PROMM [DM2]) are autosomal-dominant disorders associated with nucleotide repeat expansions in untranslated regions of the respective target genes. The genetic defect in DM1 is amplification of an unstable trinucleotide CTG repeat located in the 3′ untranslated region of the gene that encodes dystrophia myotonica protein kinase (DMPK) on chromosome 19. DM1 is highly variable in severity and age of onset, and it exhibits "anticipation," the phenomenon of increasing severity of inherited disease in successive generations of an affected family. The number of CTG repeats ranges from about 50 in patients who are mildly affected to thousands in severely affected patients. Amplification of the CTG repeat is the molecular basis for genetic anticipation. Although the mutation does not alter the protein-coding region of the DMPK gene, the CTG repeats can disrupt RNA splicing and cellular metabolism by interacting with RNA-binding proteins.

PROMM/DM2 is caused by a CCTG expansion (approximately 5,000 repeats) in intron 1 of the gene encoding zinc finger protein 9 (ZNF9). Like the CTG expansion of the DMPK gene in DM1, the CCTG expansion does not alter the protein-coding region of the ZNF9 gene. However, the CCTG repeats can also disrupt RNA splicing and cellular metabolism by interacting with RNA-binding proteins.

Myotonic Dystrophy (DM1)

Myotonic dystrophy (DM1) is the most common inherited neuromuscular disease in adults, with a prevalence of approximately 5 per 100,000 and men and

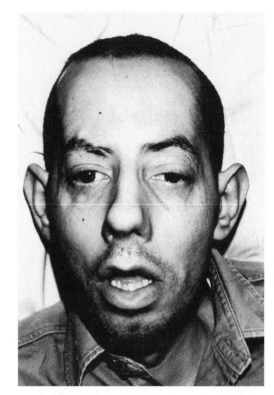

Figure 20.4. Cliincal appearance of a 56-year-old man with myotonic dystrophy (DM1). Note bilateral ptosis, exotropia, myopathic facies, and frontal baldness typical of this disorder.

women being equally affected. It is a multisystem disorder characterized by progressive wasting and weakness of distal muscles and myotonia.

Systemic and Ocular Manifestations   Many patients can be recognized instantly by their characteristic frontal balding, long face, ptosis, hollowing of the masseter and temporalis muscles, slackened mouth, facial weakness, and thin neck and limbs (Fig. 20.4). Other features include intellectual impairment, testicular atrophy, excessive daytime somnolence, insulin resistance, and cardiac conduction defects. The most important finding on physical examination is myotonia—involuntary delayed relaxation following a contraction, such as after sustained handgrip. However, most patients with DM1 complain of weakness, not the myotonia.

Cataract is the most common ocular abnormality in patients with DM1, occurring in nearly 100% of patients with the disease. The severity of the cataract is not related to the severity of the disease. Even if lens changes are not visible by ophthalmoscope, slit-lamp biomicroscopy will usually reveal some lens opacification. Myotonic cataracts may be of two types. The

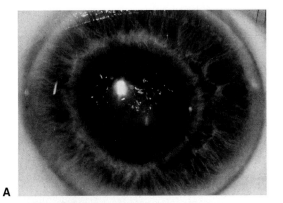

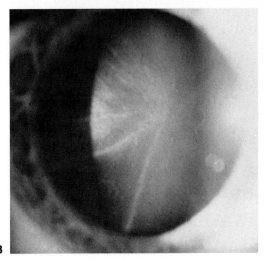

Figure 20.5. The typical appearance of cataracts in myotonic dystrophy (DM1). **A:** Numerous dot opacities, each having a different color, located primarily in the posterior subcortical region of the lens. **B:** Spoke-like opacities of the posterior subcortical region of the lens.

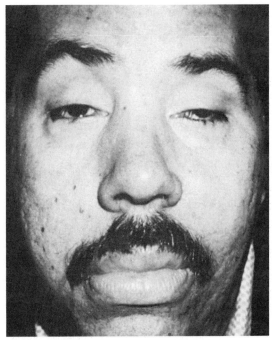

Figure 20.6. Severe ptosis in a 49-year-old man with myotonic dystrophy (DM1). (Courtesy of Dr. Thomas L. Slamovits.)

first consists of tiny opaque, white, or—most often—iridescent, colored (usually red, green, or blue) crystals that are located in a thin band of anterior and posterior cortex just beneath the lens capsule (Fig. 20.5A). The second type is a stellate grouping of opacities at the posterior pole along the posterior suture lines, producing a spoke-like appearance (Fig. 20.5B).

In addition to cataracts, ptosis is frequently present in patients with DM1 and may be mild or profound (Figs. 20.4 and 20.6). In addition, there may be weakness of the orbicularis oculi muscles, producing infrequent blinking and difficulty closing the eyes. When the orbicularis is affected, there may be bilateral lower lid retraction or delayed opening of the eyes after forceful closure.

Abnormal eye movements are present in many patients with DM1. In its mildest form, the ocular motor involvement consists of slowed saccades in patients who have a full range of eye movements and no visual complaints. In other patients, however, there are varying degrees of ophthalmoparesis (Fig. 20.7). The ophthalmoparesis, particularly when combined with ptosis and orbicularis weakness, may suggest a diagnosis of myasthenia gravis or chronic progressive external ophthalmoplegia (CPEO), the two disorders with which DM1 is most often confused.

The pupils in patients with DM1 tend to be miotic, react sluggishly and incompletely to both light and near stimuli, react normally to psychosensory stimuli, and do not tend to fatigue on repeated stimuli any more than normal pupils. Despite these abnormalities, most patients with DM1 appear clinically to have normally reactive pupils.

Vascular abnormalities of the iris occur in many patients with DM1. These iris neovascular tufts can usually be identified by slit-lamp biomicroscopy. In most cases, they are of no consequence, but they can bleed spontaneously or after mild ocular trauma, resulting in a hyphema.

The ciliary processes may be short and depigmented in patients with DM1. These abnormalities may explain the finding of ocular hypotony in many patients with this disorder.

Retinal abnormalities occur in patients with DM1. The involvement ranges from abnormalities of dark

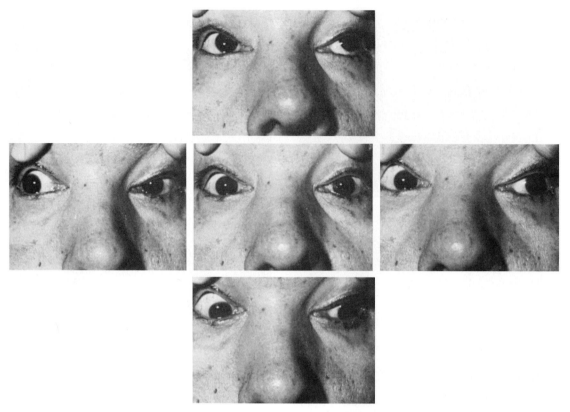

Figure 20.7. Severe ophthalmoparesis in a patient with myotonic dystrophy (DM1). (Courtesy of Dr. Thomas L. Slamovits.)

adaptation and electroretinography in patients with no visual complaints and normal-appearing fundi to decreased vision with pigmentary retinopathy involving the macula, peripheral retina, or both (Fig. 20.8). Regardless of the degree of retinopathy, it is not as severe as retinitis pigmentosa and does not cause blindness. Indeed, the retinopathy observed in patients with DM1 is similar in appearance, electrophysiologic dysfunction, and visual prognosis to that in patients with the Kearns-Sayre variant of CPEO.

Abnormal visual evoked potentials may be found in patients with DM1 who have no visible retinal abnormalities and a normal electroretinogram (ERG), suggesting that at least some patients with DM1 have dysfunction in the visual sensory conducting system other than at the retinal level.

Pathology   Nearly every pathologic change possible in skeletal muscle occurs in DM1; however, the characteristic features are a marked variation in the caliber of the fibers, myofiber degeneration and regeneration, ringed fibers ("ringbinden") or myofibrils with an aberrant course, sarcoplasmic masses of tightly packed disordered myofilaments, focal areas of myofibrillar disruption and Z-band streaming, and associated secondary changes in mitochondria or the sarcotubular system. In the advanced stages of the disease, a large proportion of the total fiber population is lost and is replaced by connective tissue and fat cells. This pathologic end stage is indistinguishable from the advanced stage of other muscular dystrophies.

In patients with DM1 who have ophthalmoparesis, the extraocular muscles may undergo changes similar to those of striated muscle. In addition, some patients show a proliferation of mitochondria in the extraocular muscles.

The iridescent crystals that comprise some myotonic cataracts are not crystals at all but represent whorls of lens fiber plasma membrane.

Pathologic changes in the iris and ciliary body in patients with DM1 are nonspecific and consist of hyalinization, vacuole degeneration, and interstitial proliferation. Whether these changes are responsible for the pupillary abnormalities observed in patients with DM1 is unclear.

The retinal lesions observed in patients with DM1 are many and varied. Atrophy of the inner retinal layers with preservation of photoreceptors occurs, particularly in the peripheral retina. In the macula, increased pigmentation with a granular, striate, or stellate pattern

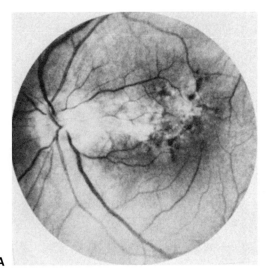
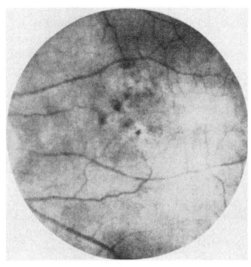

A   B

Figure 20.8. Chorioretinopathy in myotonic dystrophy (DM1). **A:** Posterior pole of the left eye in a 50-year-old man. Note the streak-like arrangement of the pigment clumps radiating from the fovea as well as the white streak extending between the disc and the macula. **B:** Posterior pole of the left eye in a 36-year-old woman. Note pigment clumps and surrounding white streaks in the macula. (Reprinted from: Burian HM, Burns CA. Ocular changes in myotonic dystrophy. *Am J Ophthalmol.* 1967;63:22–24, with permission.)

may occur. Foci of pigmented cells in the outer plexiform layer and macular edema over subretinal fluid are also observed.

Diagnosis The diagnosis of DM1 may be suspected by a combination of a patient's external appearance, the presence of an external ophthalmoplegia, the observation of multihued subcortical iridescent crystals and/or spoke-like posterior cataracts on slit-lamp biomicroscopy, hypotony revealed by tonometry, and retinal changes on funduscopy. The diagnosis can be confirmed by findings of myotonia on EMG, and testing of DNA for the CTG repeat can be performed when the diagnosis is not clinically obvious, thus eliminating the need for a muscle biopsy.

Treatment When troublesome, myotonia can be treated with phenytoin or other drugs, but few patients require such therapy. Distal weakness causing foot drop is treated with ankle-foot orthoses. Cardiac conduction defects may require pacemakers.

Treatment of ophthalmoparesis usually is unnecessary because the limitation of eye movement in patients with DM1 is usually symmetric. Thus, such patients do not commonly report diplopia. Prisms can be used to treat patients with diplopia in primary position. Extraocular muscle surgery usually is unwarranted but may be appropriate in rare instances of ocular misalignment.

Treatment of ptosis is somewhat problematic in patients with DM1 because of the commonly associated orbicularis weakness. If the eyelids are raised to a "normal" level, such patients may develop severe tearing and irritation from exposure keratopathy, and some patients may even develop corneal ulceration, leading to blindness. Thus, the eyelids should be raised only when ptosis is interfering with function and only as high as needed to improve vision.

Proximal Myotonic Myopathy (PROMM/DM2)

Proximal myotonic myopathy (PROMM/DM2) has certain features in common with DM1 but has a different clinical presentation. The clinical features of PROMM/DM2 are muscle stiffness, myotonia, weakness, muscle pain, and cataracts. These problems can occur singly or in various combinations. Initial symptoms usually develop between 20 and 60 years of age. Many patients first complain of intermittent stiffness in the thigh muscles of one or both legs and of intermittent grip myotonia. In other patients, cataracts are the first manifestation of the disorder. These may appear in late childhood or early adolescence and are indistinguishable from those in DM1, being posterior subcapsular, iridescent, multicolored opacities. Cardiac arrhythmias occur in some patients.

EMG usually reveals myotonic discharges in affected patients, including those without obvious clinical myotonia. However, these discharges are scarce and difficult to detect. Muscle biopsy usually reveals a

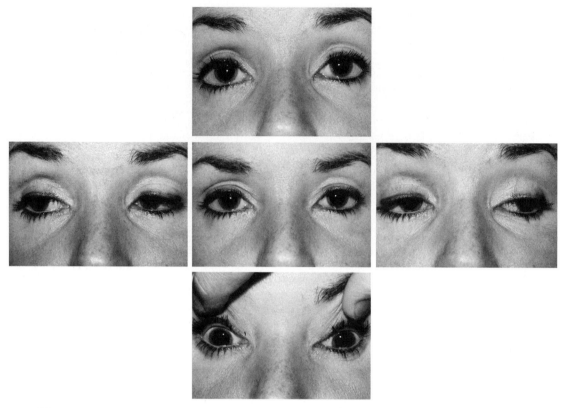

Figure 20.9. Ptosis and ophthalmoparesis in a 23-year-old woman with oculopharyngeal dystrophy (OPMD).

nonspecific myopathy. In contrast to DM1, there are no ringbinden or subsarcolemmal masses, and there is no evidence of selective type 1 fiber atrophy.

The prognosis of PROMM/DM2 is more favorable than that of DM1. Most patients do not show any deterioration of mental status, dysarthria, dysphagia, or respiratory failure. Nonsteroidal anti-inflammatory drugs and muscle relaxants can be used to treat the muscle pain experienced by these patients, and antimyotonia therapy, including mexiletine, phenytoin, and acetazolamide, can be used in patients with severe myotonic stiffness and grip myotonia. Cataract surgery is warranted in some patients.

OCULOPHARYNGEAL MUSCULAR DYSTROPHY

Oculopharyngeal muscular dystrophy (OPMD) is a hereditary disorder that is transmitted in most cases in an autosomal-dominant fashion, although rare autosomal-recessive cases have been reported. The mutation is located on chromosome 14q11 and increases the length of a polyalanine sequence located at the N terminus of the polyadenylate binding protein nuclear 1 (PABPN1).

The two essential clinical characteristics of OPMD are ptosis and dysphagia (Fig. 20.9). Neither manifestation usually presents until late in life, but mild ptosis usually precedes any significant dysphagia, often by several years. The ptosis eventually becomes bilateral but is rarely complete. It usually is symmetric, although one lid may become ptotic weeks or months before the other. External ophthalmoplegia is present in most but not all patients. The pupils are never clinically abnormal.

Dysphagia may be disabling in patients with OPMD. At first there is difficulty only in swallowing solid foods, but eventually swallowing liquids also becomes difficult, and several attempts at swallowing may be necessary to empty the upper pharynx. Examination of the swallowing mechanisms in affected patients usually reveals weak movements in the pharynx and larynx. The pharyngeal musculature cannot propel the bolus of food into the upper esophagus, partly because of dysfunction of the pharyngeal musculature and partly because of the absence of reflex relaxation of the cricopharyngeal muscle. Degeneration of the pharyngeal striated musculature evidently results in uncoordinated activity, with material pooling in the pyriform sinuses and regurgitating into the nasopharynx rather than passing into the esophagus. Ingested material may thus be aspirated, resulting in recurrent pneumonitis. Some patients with severe dysphagia are treated successfully with cricopharyngeal myotomy, but a percutaneous feeding gastrostomy is a more practical treatment and is more commonly used.

The morphologic hallmark of OPMD is intranuclear filamentous inclusions that contain PABPN1, sequestered polyadenylated RNA, and ubiquitin and that are confined to muscle cells, where PABPN1 plays a specific role in differentiation. It is believed that the reduced solubility of mutant PABPN1 and its tendency to form intranuclear aggregates play a direct role in the pathogenesis of OPMD.

As in other dystrophies, biopsies from affected muscles show advanced degenerative changes, fibrosis, abundant central nuclei, altered myofibrils and Z-bands, and other nonspecific changes. "Ragged red" fibers with mitochondrial proliferation and other mitochondrial abnormalities are sometimes found, but these are probably the result of age-related mitochondrial DNA mutations, phenomena unrelated to the pathogenesis of OPMD.

ION CHANNEL DISORDERS (MYOTONIA)

Myotonia is a phenomenon in which muscle fibers have a pathologically persistent activity after a strong contraction or are continuously active when they should be relaxed. Myotonia is identified physiologically as a delay in muscle relaxation after percussion or electric stimulation of a muscle, or after a voluntary contraction. The phenomenon is caused by mutations affecting chloride, sodium, and calcium ion channels in surface membranes. It persists after blockage of either the peripheral nerve or the neuromuscular junction. In patients with myotonia, the spontaneous action potentials as recorded in the EMG are high-frequency discharges of single muscle fibers that wax and wane in both amplitude and frequency. When translated into sound, these discharges produce a noise resembling that of a dive-bomber or a motorcycle engine.

Clinical myotonia is a common feature of a number of different genetically determined, primary muscle diseases, including autosomal-dominant and autosomal-recessive myotonia congenita, paramyotonia congenita, the familial periodic paralyses, and chondrodystrophic myotonia.

Myotonia Congenita

Autosomal-dominant and autosomal-recessive myotonia congenita result from allelic mutations of the chloride channel gene encoded on chromosome 7q35. Myotonic symptoms, noted in the first years of life and often worse in males than females, frequently lessen by the 20s or 30s. Myotonia of limb muscles is more likely to occur when strenuous exertion is initiated after a period of rest; myotonia is then followed by transient weakness. Unlike paramyotonia, the myotonia is not aggravated by cooling, and long-lasting paralysis does not occur. This is one of a few neuromuscular disorders in which prominent hypertrophy can occur, particularly in the masseter, proximal arms, thighs, calves, and extensor digitorum brevis.

Patients with myotonia congenita often have eyelid myotonia. At the very least, lid lag is usually present, and blepharospasm may occur in some patients after forced closure of the eyelids. Strabismus is said to occur in some patients, but not ptosis or generalized ophthalmoplegia. Swallowing and voice are spared, but chewing is sometimes affected.

Needle EMG shows typical myotonic runs. Muscle biopsy is nonspecific. Specific genetic diagnosis is possible.

The pathophysiology of the myotonia is thought to be caused by both low chloride channel conductance and abnormal reopening of sodium channels. Treatment, which is most often successful with mexiletine or quinine, and less so with procainamide or phenytoin, is best undertaken several days before vigorous activity rather than on a regular basis.

Paramyotonia Congenita

Paramyotonia congenital is a condition characterized by autosomal-dominant inheritance, paradoxic myotonia (i.e., myotonia that worsens with exercise), exacerbation of myotonia by cold, and periodic attacks of weakness. The disorder is caused by mutations in the sodium channel gene and is allelic to hyperkalemic periodic paralysis, accounting for the great overlap between the two syndromes. Neither ptosis nor ophthalmoplegia occurs in patients with this disease; however, some patients show myotonic lid lag similar to that observed in other myotonic disorders, including myotonia congenita.

Familial Periodic Paralysis

Familial periodic paralysis is a rare syndrome characterized by abnormal flux of potassium across muscle membranes and by spells of severe flaccid weakness in the limb muscles. The spells last minutes to hours and are provoked by rest following exercise. Bulbar and ocular muscles are rarely affected; thus, patients with this disorder do not often present to the ophthalmologist. Respiratory muscles are almost never affected. The syndrome is subdivided into hyper-, hypo-, and normokalemic types, but all three types are characterized by presentation in the 3rd decade of life, greater severity in males, autosomal-dominant inheritance, and oliguria preceding attacks. In rare patients, hypo- or hyperkalemia causes a complicating cardiac arrhythmia. Examination shows normal strength between attacks, but if the attacks are frequent and not treated, mild fixed proximal weakness may develop. Myotonia, especially eyelid myotonia, may be seen, manifesting as intermittent lid lab or staring episodes. During paralytic attacks, muscles are inexcitable and deep tendon reflexes are hypoactive or absent. The histologic hallmark is a vacuolar myopathy most consistently associated with the permanent myopathy that develops after repeated attacks.

Chondrodystrophic Myotonia (Schwartz-Jampel Syndrome)

This rare syndrome of dwarfism, abnormalities of long bones and the face, blepharospasm, and myotonic symptoms is caused by mutation of a gene that is located on chromosome 1p34–36.1. This gene encodes perlecan, a heparan sulfate proteoglycan component of the basement membrane that is responsible for the localization of acetylcholinesterase in the postsynaptic clefts of the neuromuscular junction.

The facial appearance of blepharospasm, puckered lips, myokymic twitching of the chin, low-set ears, receding chin, a high-pitched forced voice, and high-arched palate is distinctive. Frequent ophthalmologic features include myopia, cataract, strabismus, and nystagmus. Serum CK levels are usually normal. Although muscle biopsies show many changes, none are specific. This condition is not a true myotonia, because EMG discharges from affected muscles are abolished by *d*-tubocurarine. Instead, the abnormal activity of affected muscles appears to reflect prolonged activation of postsynaptic receptors resulting from the impaired degradation of acetylcholine at the neuromuscular junction.

MITOCHONDRIAL MYOPATHIES

The mitochondrial myopathies are a genetically and biochemically diverse set of disorders that are defined by structural abnormalities of mitochondria on muscle biopsy. The histologic hallmark of these disorders is the abnormal accumulation of increased numbers of enlarged mitochondria beneath the sarcolemma of affected muscle fibers. Because of their irregular appearance and their strikingly dark-red color when stained with the modified Gomori trichrome stain, these abnormal muscle fibers are called **ragged-red fibers** (RRF) (Fig. 20.10). In patients with ophthalmoplegia, RRFs are present not only in skeletal muscles but also in the orbicularis oculi and in the extraocular muscles.

When viewed with the electron microscope, the mitochondria in affected muscle fibers appear more numerous and more variable in size than in normal muscle fibers. The mitochondria are often enlarged, with distorted or disorganized cristae that are sometimes arranged concentrically. Paracrystalline inclusions are

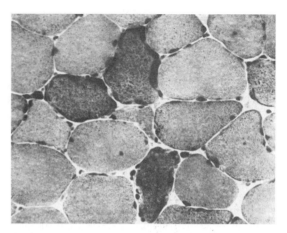

Figure 20.10. "Ragged red" fibers in chronic progressive external ophthalmoplegia. A group of three "ragged red" fibers surround an atrophic, angulated muscle fiber. Modified Gomori trichrome stain. (Reprinted from: Morgan-Hughes JA. Mitochondrial myopathies. In: Mastaglia FL, Walton J, eds. *Skeletal Muscle Pathology.* Edinburgh: Churchill Livingstone; 1982:309, with permission.)

invariably present within the cristae, and similar inclusions may be observed outside the cristae. Similar mitochondrial inclusions may be observed in liver cells, in sweat glands, and in the granular and Purkinje cells of the cerebellum of affected patients.

The most common mitochondrial myopathy in which ophthalmoplegia is a prominent feature is chronic progressive external ophthalmoplegia (CPEO) and its variant, the Kearns-Sayre syndrome (KSS).

CHRONIC PROGRESSIVE EXTERNAL OPHTHALMOPLEGIA

The syndrome known as chronic progressive external ophthalmoplegia or CPEO is by far the most common of the mitochondrial myopathies. Most patients with CPEO also have generalized skeletal muscle weakness. Nevertheless, some patients with CPEO have either no evidence of weakness elsewhere or their weakness is sufficiently mild as to be overlooked by patient and physician alike.

Ptosis is usually the first evidence of involvement and may precede ophthalmoparesis by months to years (Fig. 20.11). The ptosis is slowly progressive and tends to become complete in most cases. Characteristically, it is bilateral, but unilateral ptosis can be present for years before the opposite side becomes involved or ophthalmoparesis is observed. As ptosis progresses, it eventually interferes with vision, and the patient must tilt the head backward and use the frontalis muscles to elevate the eyelids. The ptosis in patients with CPEO is

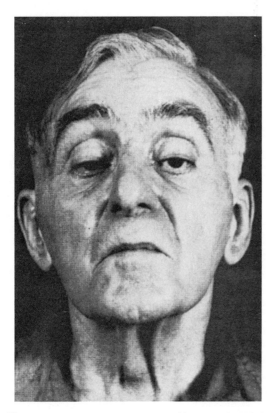

Figure 20.11. Ptosis in a 63-year-old man with CPEO. Note also flat, expressionless facial features associated with continuous wrinkling of the frontalis muscles and a posterior head tilt in order to compensate for bilateral ptosis. (Courtesy of Dr. I. Lewis and the Canadian Medical Association Journal.)

fixed, unlike the variable, fatigable ptosis in myasthenia gravis.

Although ptosis usually is the earliest sign of CPEO, rare patients develop progressive ophthalmoparesis or even complete external ophthalmoplegia months to years before ptosis develops, and some of these patients never develop ptosis.

Because limitation of ocular movements is generally symmetric, most patients with CPEO do not report diplopia and are not aware of a problem with ocular motility until it is of such severity that it limits peripheral vision or until someone points it out to them. For this reason, immobility of the eyes is often severe when such patients are first examined (Fig. 20.12). In many cases, downward movements are relatively intact compared with upward and horizontal movements.

Both ultrasonography and CT scanning in patients with CPEO show thin, presumably atrophic, extraocular muscles (Fig. 20.13). The thinning usually is symmetric.

Because most patients with CPEO have generalized symmetric limitation of eye movement and have no diplopia, they do not require surgical realignment of the eyes. In the rare patients who have asymmetric limitation of movement and complain of double vision, prism therapy or surgery may be used to improve ocular alignment, at least temporarily. Surgery to raise the eyelids can be performed in patients with severe ptosis that prevents them from functioning normally, but because such patients may also have weakness of the orbicularis oculi muscles, care must be taken to avoid raising the eyelids so much that the patient develops exposure keratopathy from inability to close the eyes.

KEARNS SAYRE SYNDROME

The Kearns Sayre syndrome is a variant of CPEO characterized by a typical external ophthalmoplegia associated with a bilateral pigmentary retinopathy, and cardiac conduction abnormalities including complete heart block. Most patients develop these manifestations before the age of 20 years.

In contrast to retinitis pigmentosa, which usually initially affects the peripheral and midperipheral retina, the retinopathy of KSS usually occurs initially in the posterior fundus (Fig. 20.14). In advanced cases, a metallic sheen or mottled fluorescent appearance surrounds the optic nerve. "Bone spicule" pigment formation, a common feature of retinitis pigmentosa, rarely occurs. Examination of affected fundi usually shows diffuse depigmentation of the retinal pigment epithelium with a characteristic mottled "salt-and-pepper" pattern of pigment clumping similar to that seen in patients with congenital rubella. This appearance may be most marked around the macula. Pallor of the optic disc, attenuation of retinal vessels, visual field defects, and posterior cataracts—all common in patients with retinitis pigmentosa—rarely if ever occur. As might be expected, visual symptoms such as night blindness or diminished visual acuity are generally mild and occur in only about 40% to 50% of patients. Thus, the retinopathy of KSS is similar to that in DM1. There are, however, rare cases of KSS with CNS involvement in which bone spicule formation and pigment clumping in the macula are associated with profound loss of visual acuity.

As might be expected, the results of electrophysiologic tests performed on patients with KSS also differ from those in patients with retinitis pigmentosa. Although exceptional cases exist, dark adaptometry and electroretinography are usually normal or only mildly abnormal.

The cardiac conduction disturbances that are occur in patients with KSS typically do so years after the onset of ptosis and ophthalmoplegia. Thus, any patient with CPEO and a pigmentary retinopathy or neurologic dysfunction but with a normal ECG should

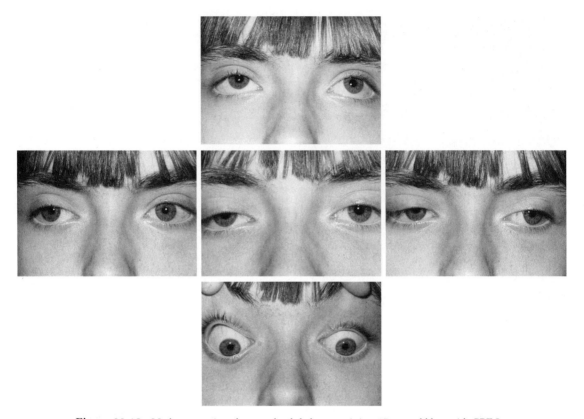

Figure 20.12. Moderate ptosis and external ophthalmoparesis in a 15-year-old boy with CPEO.

be warned of the possibility of future cardiac disease, and the symptoms of such disease should be explained. In addition, such patients should undergo cardiac examinations at regular intervals, regardless of their age.

Although the cardiac dysfunction that occurs in patients with KSS can often be managed effectively with an artificial pacemaker, patients may die suddenly, even after insertion of a pacemaker, because of a decreased ventilatory response to hypoxia and hypercarbia caused by deficient brain stem respiratory control mechanisms. Cardiac failure in patients with KSS also can be successfully treated with cardiac transplantation.

Cardiac abnormalities other than conduction defects occur uncommonly in patients with KSS but include intraventricular septal hypertrophy of the idiopathic hypertrophic subaortic stenosis type and mitral valve prolapse with mitral regurgitation.

Some patients with KSS have weakness of skeletal muscles in addition to ptosis and ophthalmoplegia. Facial muscles, particularly the orbicularis oculi muscles, may be affected. Patients in whom this occurs may be unable not only to open the eyelids but also to close them tightly (Fig. 20.15). With involvement

of the frontalis muscle, there is an increasing inability to wrinkle the forehead and use the frontalis to help open the eyelids. This results in an apparent worsening of ptosis. All muscles of the face may eventually become affected, and the face thus becomes thin and expressionless. In some patients, the muscles of mastication become involved, and the patients report difficulty chewing.

With progression of the disease, there is often weakness and wasting of the neck and shoulder muscles. Although the muscles of the extremities may be involved, the weakness is often mild.

Patients with KSS usually have evidence of neurologic dysfunction. Abnormalities include cerebellar ataxia, pendular nystagmus, vestibular dysfunction, hearing loss, impaired intellectual function, and peripheral neuropathy. In addition, in many patients there is elevation of CSF protein content. Spongiform changes in the brain are present in almost every patient in whom an autopsy is performed.

CNS involvement in KSS is reflected in MR imaging abnormalities with high signal intensity for proton density, T2-weighted, and T2-weighted fluid attenuated inversion recovery (FLAIR) sequences. These abnormalities are present in the brainstem, globus

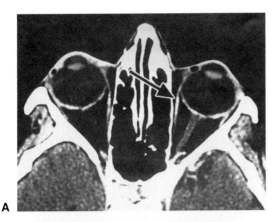

A

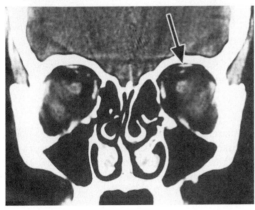

B

Figure 20.13. CT scanning of extraocular muscles in a patient with CPEO. **A:** Axial view shows marked thinning of left medial rectus muscle (*arrow*). **B:** Coronal view shows similar thinning of left superior rectus muscle (*arrow*). (Reprinted from: Wallace DK, Sprunger DT, Helveston EM, et al. Surgical management of strabismus associated with chronic progressive external ophthalmoplegia. *Ophthalmology.* 1997;104:695–700, with permission.)

pallidus, thalamus, and white matter of the cerebrum and cerebellum. In addition, regional abnormalities of brain metabolism are demonstrated in patients with KSS using MR spectroscopy (MRS). These changes include an increase in the lactate/creatine resonance intensity ratio (an index of impairment of oxidative metabolism) in resting occipital cortex, as well as a significant decrease in N-acetylaspartate/creatine (a measure of neuron loss or dysfunction) in cerebral cortex.

Endocrine dysfunction is common in patients with KSS. In addition to short stature, other manifestations include hypoparathyroidism with tetany as a presenting symptom, gonadal dysfunction, and diabetes mellitus.

There is no adequate treatment for KSS, although rare patients appear to respond to controlled carbohydrate intake and coenzyme Q10 therapy. As is the case with CPEO, some patients with diplopia benefit from treatment with prisms or strabismus surgery. Ptosis may also be treated surgically.

GENETICS

Although most cases of CPEO and KSS are sporadic, some are hereditary, being transmitted in an autosomal-dominant or autosomal-recessive fashion. Most of the sporadic cases of CPEO and KSS are caused by single deletions of mtDNA. Deleted mtDNAs appear to be distributed to a wider variety of tissues in KSS than CPEO. Furthermore, duplications of mtDNA appear to be present in all cases of KSS but are absent in CPEO. Deletions of mtDNA impair mitochondrial protein synthesis, with the severity of dysfunction within an affected cell correlating with the proportion of deleted mtDNA. The close association between deletions of mtDNA and dysfunction of the extraocular muscles may be related to the relatively high metabolic activity of these muscles, which are tonically active while the eyes are maintained in primary position.

Most autosomal-dominantly inherited cases of CPEO (as well as some sporadic cases) are caused by mutations in three main nuclear genes: (a) the adenine nucleotide translocator-1 (ANT1) located on chromosome 4q35 and that encodes an isoform of ATP-ADP translocator common to muscle, heart, and brain. This gene regulates the adenine nucleotide pool within mitochondria and is a structural element of the mitochondrial permeability pore; (b) the chromosome 10 open reading frame 2 (C10 *orf* 2) gene that produces Twinkle, an adenine nucleotide-dependent mtDNA helicase, alterations in which may impair mtDNA replication; and (c) POLG, a gene located on chromosome 15q22-26 that produces the α subunit of polymerase γ, an enzyme required for mtDNA replication.

A number of different clinical phenotypes are associated with autosomal-dominant ophthalmoplegia. In one lineage, they included dysphagia, exercise intolerance, lactic acidosis, cataract formation, and early death; in another, affected family members had muscle atrophy, proximal muscle weakness, hearing loss, and ataxia; in another pedigree, affected individuals had cataracts, ataxia, tremor, peripheral neuropathy, mental retardation, or a combination of these manifestations.

An autosomal-recessive form of CPEO is associated with a mutation in the gene on chromosome 22 that encodes the enzyme thymidine phosphorylase (TP). This enzyme is responsible for the thymidine salvage pathway in mitochondria, which are incapable of de novo thymidine synthesis. Another autosomal-recessively

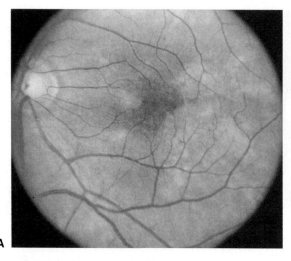 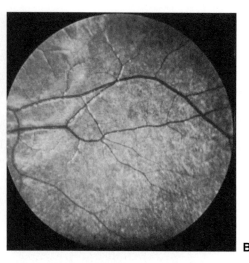

Figure 20.14. Pigmentary retinopathy in Kearns-Sayre syndrome. **A:** Posterior pole of a 17-year-old male shows mild pigmentary disturbance with pigment clumping overlying white streaks. Note resemblance to retinopathy of myotonic dystrophy (Fig. 20.8). **B:** Stippled retinal pigmentary disturbance in a 35-year-old woman with Kearns Sayre syndrome.

inherited form—one without ptosis—has been linked to a genetic defect at chromosome 17p13.1-p12, the nature of which has not yet been clarified.

Autosomal-recessive CPEO may occur as part is associated with the **MNGIE syndrome** (mitochondrial neurogastrointestinal encephalomyopathy). Patients with the MNGIE syndrome also have mild peripheral neuropathy, leukoencephalopathy, and gastrointestinal symptoms (recurrent nausea, vomiting,

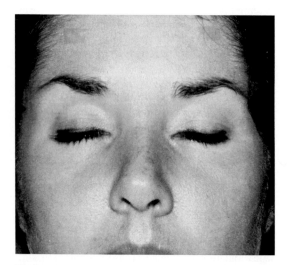

Figure 20.15. Orbicularis weakness in a patient with Kearns Sayre syndrome. The patient is attempting to close her eyelids as tightly as possible. Note that she is unable to bury the lashes.

or diarrhea) with intestinal dysmotility. By contrast, a disablingly severe sensory ataxic neuropathy with dysarthria and ophthalmoplegia (SANDO) occurs as a sporadic disorder in association with multiple mitochondrial DNA deletions.

DIAGNOSIS

It is important to distinguish the mitochondrial myopathies from autosomal-dominant oculopharyngeal muscular dystrophy (see the previous text) and myasthenia gravis, because these disorders have distinct therapeutic and genetic implications. Muscle biopsy is the single most useful diagnostic tool for evaluating patients with suspected mitochondrial disease. The presence of RRFs on muscle biopsy, in excess of what can be accounted for by age, establishes the diagnosis of mitochondrial myopathy, and mutations of mtDNA (both deletions and point mutations) can be detected in muscle, blood, and other biopsied tissue.

The diagnosis of KSS is aided by the finding of elevated levels of lactic acid in blood or CSF and by low-density lesions in the basal ganglia on MR imaging. MRS is a valuable tool for diagnosing abnormalities of energy metabolism in brain and other tissues, but it is not available for generalized screening of patients with suspected mitochondrial mutations.

All patients with known or presumed CPEO should undergo a careful ophthalmologic assessment, including a dilated ophthalmoscopic examination to determine whether a pigmentary retinopathy is present. In addition, patients with CPEO with pigmentary retinopathy or neurologic dysfunction should undergo an immediate assessment of cardiac function, and patients in whom no disturbances are found should nevertheless be monitored with periodic ECGs.

ENCEPHALOMYOPATHY WITH OPHTHALMOPLEGIA FROM VITAMIN E DEFICIENCY

Abetalipoproteinemia, also called the Bassen-Kornzweig syndrome, is characterized by acanthocytosis, pigmentary retinopathy, progressive ataxia, and neuropathy. The disorder results from the lack of apolipoprotein B, which is essential to the transport of fat-soluble vitamins and is caused by lack of vitamin E because of impaired intestinal absorption of lipids and lipid-soluble vitamins. In fact, the neurologic disorder of abetalipoproteinemia is identical with that observed in other forms of human vitamin E deficiency, whether caused by malabsorption, cholestatic liver disease with impaired secretion of bile salts, bowel resection, or cystic fibrosis. The neurologic signs in patients with vitamin E deficiency include ataxia, areflexia, and loss of vibratory sensation due both to demyelinating neuropathy and neuronal degeneration of the cerebellum. The ocular motor abnormalities in patients with this disorder include abnormally slow voluntary saccades, slow or absent fast components of vestibular and optokinetic nystagmus, strabismus, pseudo-internuclear ophthalmoplegia with dissociated nystagmus in the adducting eye on attempted horizontal gaze, moderate to severe progressive external ophthalmoplegia, and internuclear ophthalmoplegia of abduction (e.g., the posterior internuclear ophthalmoplegia of Lutz).

Many patients with vitamin E deficiency syndromes develop pigmentary retinopathy in addition to ocular motor abnormalities. This retinopathy is similar in appearance and visual outcome to the retinopathies observed in patients with mitochondrial cytopathies (see the previous text).

Vitamin E deficiency produces a true multisystem disorder. The disease appeared initially to be a pure myopathy, because biopsy specimens from affected patients showed distinctive autofluorescent inclusions in muscle fibers. However, there is also extensive involvement of peripheral and central nerve tissue, including dystrophic changes in the brain, spinal cord, and dorsal roots.

In patients with the vitamin E deficiency syndrome, the neurologic defects, including the ocular motor disturbances, can be improved if the serum vitamin E level is restored to normal with supplemental vitamin E therapy, administered via either an oral or parenteral route. Other fat-soluble vitamins should also be administered.

INFLAMMATORY MYOPATHIES

The term *myositis* can be used for any disorder in which inflammation affects muscle. The inflammation may be confined to a single muscle or may be diffuse. Inflammatory myopathies may be separated into two major categories: myopathies caused by an identified infective agent and idiopathic inflammatory myopathies.

INFECTIVE MYOSITIS

Infective myositis may be caused by bacteria, viruses, parasites, or fungi. The most common bacteria that produce pyomyositis are *Staphylococcus aureus*, *Streptococcus pyogenes*, and *Clostridium welchii*. These and other bacteria usually produce ophthalmoparesis indirectly when there is a generalized, suppurative orbital inflammation with swelling of soft tissues. On rare occasions, however, true extraocular myositis occurs from direct muscle invasion by bacteria. The bacteria usually gain entrance to the orbit from infected paranasal sinuses, often after trauma. Recognition is important because of the immediate need for antibiotics.

Viruses associated with an infective myopathy include the influenza virus and the Coxsackie A and B viruses. The extraocular muscles are not involved in most cases.

Although many parasites can theoretically involve the extraocular muscles, the most frequent and best-known form of parasitic infestation of muscle in general and extraocular muscle in particular is **trichinosis**. The causative agent, *Trichinella spiralis*, is a nematode that usually is acquired in humans as the result of ingesting raw or incompletely cooked pork, bear meat, or horse meat. After penetration of the small intestine, the larvae enter the lymphatic system and the bloodstream and are disseminated widely throughout the body. Involvement of the extraocular muscles is common, occurring second in frequency after involvement of the diaphragm. The clinical course has three stages. The first, the invasion period or intestinal stage, commences with the liberation of encysted larvae from the infected meat. It is characterized by diarrhea, vomiting, fever, and weakness. This stage persists for about 7 days. The second phase begins about 1 week after ingestion of tainted meat and is the period during which the disease is disseminated throughout the body. It is characterized by fever, peripheral leukocytosis and eosinophilia, headache, urticaria, muscle pain, weakness, edema of the eyelids and face, conjunctivitis, and headache. It is during this period that myocardial and skeletal muscle involvement become evident, and in some cases there is severe kidney involvement. Convalescence, the third stage, begins about 5–8 weeks after the onset of symptoms.

Patients with trichinosis often develop ocular signs early in the course of the disease. Chemosis of the

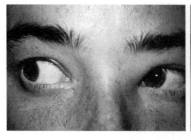
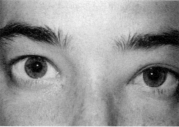
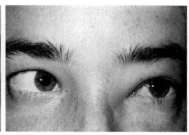

Figure 20.16. Orbital myositis affecting one muscle of one eye. The patient has involvement of the left medial rectus muscle. The nasal conjunctiva of the left eye is chemotic and injected, and the patient cannot fully abduct the eye.

conjunctiva is characteristic and primarily occurs over the extraocular muscles. There is a varying degree of ophthalmoparesis from muscle involvement, and movement of the eyes is painful. Other ocular signs include proptosis, optic neuritis, and retinal ischemia.

Other parasites that produce infective myopathies include *Cysticercus*, *Echinococcus*, *Toxoplasma gondii*, *Sarcocystis*, and *Trypanosoma*. These parasites produce ophthalmoparesis by direct invasion of the extraocular muscles.

A variety of **fungi** can produce orbital inflammation with limitation of ocular motility. As with other infective agents, the inflammatory response may be granulomatous or nongranulomatous and may produce ophthalmoplegia through inflammation of ocular motor nerves, extraocular muscles, or soft tissue. The fungi most commonly responsible for orbital inflammation include organisms from the class Phycomycetes (mucormycosis) and *Aspergillus*.

Neither tuberculosis nor syphilis commonly involves the orbit. Nevertheless, tubercles and syphilitic gummas may occur in the orbital nerves, the optic nerve, and the extraocular muscles.

IDIOPATHIC MYOSITIS

Idiopathic myositis affecting the extraocular muscles usually occurs as an isolated phenomenon unassociated

with systemic disease. In some cases, however, orbital myositis is part of a systemic process.

Orbital Myositis

Orbital myositis may affect one or more muscles in one or both orbits. Patients with orbital myositis typically experience sudden diplopia associated with unilateral or bilateral orbital pain that ranges from mild to excruciating, conjunctival chemosis and injection, and occasionally proptosis (Figs. 20.16 and 20.17). Ultrasonography, CT scanning, and MR imaging show enlargement of one or more extraocular muscles, and biopsies of involved muscles show infiltration with chronic inflammatory cells. Orbital myositis may occur not only as an isolated phenomenon but also in association with systemic disorders characterized by vasculitis or granulomatous inflammation, including systemic lupus erythematosus, rheumatoid arthritis, sarcoidosis, and Wegener's granulomatosis.

Local inflammatory disorders within the orbit also may produce limitation of ocular motility. Such conditions may be focal, as in the acquired form of Brown's superior oblique tendon sheath syndrome. The acquired form of this syndrome differs from its congenital counterpart in that it is often intermittent and is associated with inflammation and scarring, either within the superior oblique tendon or next to the anterior sheath. It may occur following superior oblique

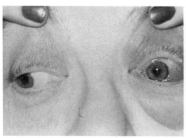
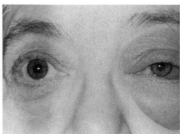
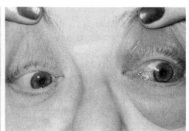

Figure 20.17. Orbital myositis affecting more than one muscle of one eye. The patient has left proptosis, diffuse eyelid edema, conjunctival chemosis, and ophthalmoparesis.

surgery, retinal detachment surgery, or trauma; in association with paranasal sinus disease; or with either the adult or juvenile forms of rheumatoid arthritis. Most cases of acquired Brown's syndrome are intermittent. Although persistent cases imply predominant scarring and contracture rather than inflammation, some respond to local injections of corticosteroids.

Systemic Myositis

Dermatomyositis is a systemic vasculopathic autoimmune disorder with histopathologic abnormalities and disease mechanisms distinct from polymyositis. Fever, skin lesions, arthritis, Raynaud's phenomenon, gastrointestinal manifestations, and even cardiac dysfunction may occur in this disease, but weakness of proximal limb-girdle muscles is most often the dominant feature. The skin signs are distinctive—heliotrope orbital/malar rash, Gottron's nodules and periungual erythema, and extensor surface rash. Ophthalmoplegia almost never occurs in patients with dermatomyositis, but at least two cases have been described.

In polymyositis, signs are limited to the skeletal muscle, and proximal weakness predominates in the legs over the arms. Less than 25% of patients have either muscle pain or dysphagia. Although the face and jaw may be weak, ptosis and ophthalmoplegia are uncommon. If they occur, one should consider myasthenia gravis as an overlapping second autoimmune disease.

ENDOCRINE MYOPATHIES

By far the most common endocrine myopathy that affects the extraocular muscles and eyelids is that associated with dysthyroidism; however, other, less common, forms exist.

DYSTHYROID ORBITOPATHY

The most common disorder associated with diplopia, ophthalmoparesis, and enlargement of extraocular muscles is the orbitopathy of dysthyroidism. In many but not all cases, there are other signs, including eyelid retraction and proptosis (Fig. 20.18). The orbitopathy may occur months or years before there is any clinical or laboratory evidence of thyroid dysfunction or it may develop shortly after radioablation of the thyroid gland in patients with primary hyperthyroidism, particularly if those patients are allowed to develop significant secondary hypothyroidism.

The extraocular muscles are the primary focus of dysthyroid orbitopathy. Both imaging studies (i.e., ultrasonography, CT scanning, MR imaging) and pathologic examination of affected muscles demonstrate involvement only of the muscle tissue, with sparing of the muscle tendons (Fig. 20.19A). This finding is in contrast to involvement of the muscles by idiopathic or-

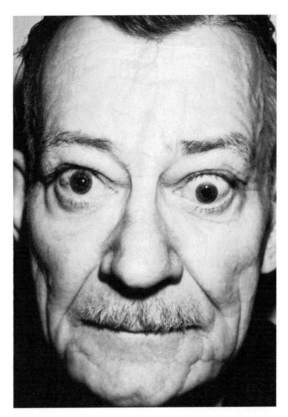

Figure 20.18. External appearance of a 65-year-old man with dysthyroid orbitopathy. Note marked upper and lower eyelid retraction, bilateral proptosis, and marked left hypotropia.

bital inflammation (i.e., orbital myositis), which tends to involve the muscle **and** the tendon (Fig. 20.19B).

Ultrasonography, CT scanning, and MR imaging can all be used to diagnose dysthyroid orbitopathy. For ultrasonography to be useful, the test must be performed by an experienced ultrasonographer who can perform the scan in both B- and standardized A-modes. CT scanning must include axial and direct coronal views of the extraocular muscles. MR imaging must concentrate on the orbit.

Pathologic examination of extraocular muscles in patients with dysthyroid orbitopathy reveals lymphocyte and plasma cell infiltration along with edema within the endomysium of the extraocular muscles. The primary autoimmune target in dysthyroid orbitopathy appears to be the orbital fibroblasts rather than muscle cells. The nature of the orbital antigen recognized by the infiltrating T lymphocytes is unknown, but cytokines (i.e., interleukin-1α, transforming growth factor β, and interferon-γ) released by T lymphocytes appear to stimulate the proliferation of orbital fibroblasts and increase their synthesis of

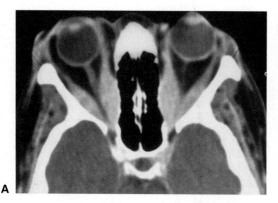 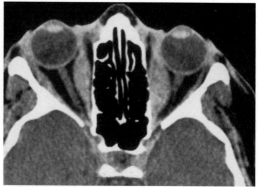

A   B

Figure 20.19. Appearance of the extraocular muscles in dysthyroid orbitopathy compared with orbital myositis. **A:** CT scan, axial view, in a patient with dysthyroid orbitopathy shows generalized enlargement of the medial rectus muscles with sparing of the tendons. **B:** CT scan, axial view, in a patient with bilateral orbital myositis involving the medial rectus muscles shows diffuse enlargement of the medial rectus muscles (left more than right) as well as their tendons.

glycosaminoglycans. In addition to diplopia, involvement of extraocular muscles may produce proptosis, swelling of the conjunctiva and eyelid, and compression optic neuropathy.

In the early stages of extraocular muscle involvement, the muscles become enlarged, resulting in limitation of ocular motility. If this limitation is symmetric among the muscles of both eyes, patients will not report diplopia even though they may have severe limitation of ocular motility. In most cases, however, asymmetric involvement of the two eyes or of the extraocular muscles in one eye causes diplopia that may be vertical, horizontal, or oblique. The most common clinically affected muscles are the inferior and medial recti (Fig. 20.20). The superior rectus is affected somewhat less often and the lateral rectus virtually never. Indeed, if a patient with known or suspected dysthyroid orbitopathy develops an exotropia, the patient either has co-existent myasthenia gravis or a decompensated phoria until proven otherwise.

As thyroid eye disease progresses, the infiltration and edema of the extraocular muscles produce loss of muscle tissue, and the muscles become fibrotic. In such cases, proptosis may be minimal despite severe diplopia. Ultrasonography, CT scanning, and MR imaging may show normal or thinned extraocular muscles, and only a fibrous band may be found at surgery.

In patients suspected of having dysthyroid orbitopathy, ultrasonography, CT scanning, and MR imaging are the most important tests to obtain. Although orbital myositis, tumor infiltration, orbital venous congestion, and trichinosis may all produce large extraocular muscles, imaging when combined with a careful history and clinical examination and when performed in the appropriate manner and interpreted correctly,

will usually differentiate among these conditions without difficulty.

Patients with clinical and imaging evidence of dysthyroid orbitopathy should undergo appropriate tests of thyroid function. Patients with systemic evidence of dysthyroidism who have evidence of orbitopathy should have an aggressive approach aimed at normalization of their thyroid function. About 50% of patients with dysthyroid orbitopathy improve, some substantially, when their thyroid function is normalized. For those who do not improve or improve incompletely, medication (e.g., systemic corticosteroids, lubricating drops and gels), low-dose radiation therapy, surgery or a combination of these modalities can be used to address virtually all the features of the condition.

MYOPATHY OF CUSHING SYNDROME

Some patients with Cushing syndrome develop ophthalmoparesis and mild exophthalmos. Because most of these patients harbor microadenomas that are too small to damage the intracranial portions of the ocular motor nerves, it is likely that the limitation of ocular motility is caused by direct involvement of the extraocular muscles; indeed, ultrasonography and other imaging studies in such patients often show enlargement of the extraocular muscles.

CORTICOSTEROID MYOPATHY

Proptosis and limitation of ocular motility may occur in patients on long-term systemic corticosteroid therapy. It is possible that the orbital tissue changes in these patients represent a local toxic myopathy similar to that observed in Cushing syndrome. Eye signs are extraordinarily rare in this condition.

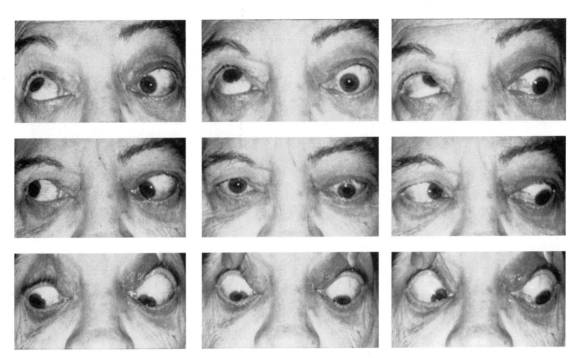

Figure 20.20. Marked vertical strabismus in a 63-year-old woman with dysthyroid orbitopathy. Note inability of the left eye to elevate above the midline. Despite the marked extraocular muscle involvement, the patient has almost no proptosis. (Courtesy of Jacqueline E. Morris, C.O.)

OTHER ENDOCRINE MYOPATHIES

Endocrine myopathies occur with hyperparathyroidism, hypoparathyroidism, acquired hypothyroidism, adrenal insufficiency, and acromegaly. The myopathic features tend to be mild and similar in all cases. Extraocular muscle involvement is rare.

TRAUMATIC MYOPATHIES

Trauma is probably the most common cause of isolated extraocular muscle damage. When the injury is not associated with orbital fracture, ocular motor dysfunction may be caused by intramuscular edema and hemorrhage, by muscle laceration, or by avulsion of the muscle origin or insertion (Fig. 20.21). When there is associated orbital fracture, the same mechanisms of injury may occur. In addition, however, the extraocular muscles and surrounding tissue may be injured by bone fragments or become entrapped within the fracture site, producing restriction of ocular motility (Figs. 20.22, 20.23).

Iatrogenic trauma to the orbit may also produce ocular motor dysfunction by direct muscle injury. Extraocular muscle imbalance occurs occasionally after retinal detachment surgery, usually related to the size and location of the silicone material used during a scleral buckling procedure. Inadvertent injury to the ex-

traocular muscles may occur during both cataract and glaucoma surgery. The superior rectus muscle may be injured by a bridle suture placed to stabilize the eye during surgery; however, the most common injury is damage to the inferior rectus muscle, inferior oblique muscle, or both from the toxic effects of the local anesthetic (usually lidocaine or Marcaine). Both transient and permanent extraocular muscle imbalance after blepharoplasty are well recognized. The mechanism of such damage is thought to be edema and hemorrhage into and around the extraocular muscles with secondary muscle contracture. Injury to the extraocular muscles may occur during surgery on the paranasal sinuses, particularly during endoscopic surgery.

OTHER MYOPATHIES

Acute necrotizing myopathy in association with carcinoma is so rare that it is best considered an uncertain entity. Nevertheless, at least one patient with this entity who had an external ophthalmoplegia has been described.

Any local orbital process that acts as a space-occupying lesion can cause limitation of ocular motility simply by its mass effect. **Primary tumors** within the muscle cone typically produce limitation of motion in this manner. In addition, rhabdomyosarcoma

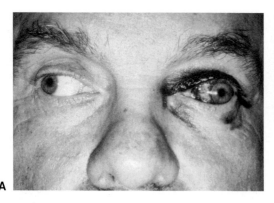
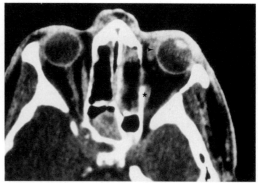

A   B

Figure 20.21. Iatrogenic strabismus from laceration of the left medial rectus muscle during transnasal endoscopic surgery. **A:** the patient cannot adduct the left eye. **B:** Axial CT scan shows a lacerated left medial rectus muscle. One can see separate proximal (*asterisk*) and distal (*arrowhead*) segments.

occasionally arises in one or more of the extraocular muscles, usually in childhood or adolescence, producing limitation of motion and rapidly progressive proptosis.

Discrete and diffuse **metastases** of carcinomas and lymphomas to the extraocular muscles are common. In such cases, CT scanning and MR imaging may show focal or generalized enlargement of the infiltrated extraocular muscle or muscles (Fig. 20.23).

Infiltration of extraocular muscles can occur in patients with **amyloidosis.** Amyloidosis is classified on the basis of its clinical features into three general categories: (a) primary (systemic or localized; familial or sporadic), (b) secondary, and (c) amyloidosis associated with multiple myeloma. Although only small, clinically insignificant deposits of amyloid in the eye occur in secondary amyloidosis, extraocular muscle infiltration is common in primary amyloidosis and also occurs

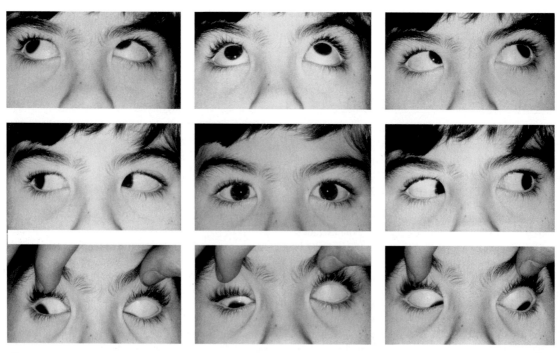

Figure 20.22. Clinical appearance of a 10-year-old boy with a right orbital floor fracture. Note inability of the right eye to fully elevate or depress.

malformations often develop enlargement of the extraocular muscles because of the greatly **increased venous pressure** within the orbit. Similarly, in rare patients, tumors or aneurysms in the anterior temporal fossa may compress draining orbital veins and produce a similar picture. The diagnosis is established by neuroimaging.

Localized **ischemia of extraocular muscles** such as that which can occur in patients with giant cell arteritis, ipsilateral occlusion or severe atherosclerotic stenosis of the internal carotid artery, or compression of the orbital structures during spine surgery with the patient in the prone position can produce limitation of ocular motility that ranges from mild ophthalmoparesis to complete ophthalmoplegia.

A skeletal myopathy is occasionally a presenting feature of **celiac disease;** however, an ocular myopathy may occasionally occur in such patients and may even be the presenting feature of the disease.

Patients with **skeletal muscle storage diseases** generally present with exercise-induced weakness or fixed muscle weakness. Regardless of the presentation, most have no disturbance of ocular motility or alignment, although exceptions have been reported.

Drug-induced toxic myopathies are rare without the superimposition of another risk factor, such as renal insufficiency, hepatic insufficiency, malnutrition, or a concomitant drug interaction, that elevates levels of the offending drug. Undoubtedly, drug-induced myotoxic reactions occur in extraocular muscles, but there are few well-documented cases.

The **venom of the common sea snake,** *Enhydrina schistosa,* produces an unusual myotoxic reaction that apparently can involve the extraocular muscles. The primary clinical manifestations of this type of poisoning are trismus, flaccid paresis of the extremities, and myoglobinuria. In severe poisoning, there may be ptosis and limitation of ocular motility. It is likely, although not proven histologically, that the ocular motor weakness is myopathic in origin and not caused by damage to ocular motor nuclei or nerves.

FOR FURTHER INFORMATION

See *Walsh & Hoyt's Clinical Neuro-Ophthalmology,* 6th edition; Volume 1, Chapter 22.

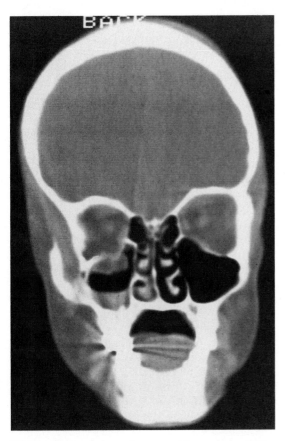

Figure 20.23. Computed tomographic scan, coronal view, of an orbital floor fracture. The scan shows a dehiscence in the floor of the right orbit with prolapse of tissue into the maxillary sinus. There is a soft tissue density in the floor of the sinus, indicating either swollen mucosa or blood. (Courtesy of Dr. Nicholas T. Iliff.)

in patients with amyloidosis associated with multiple myeloma. In some patients, the involvement is subclinical, producing no ocular motor dysfunction, whereas in other cases, varying degrees of proptosis and ophthalmoparesis are present, depending on the extent of extraocular muscle load.

Patients with anteriorly draining, high-flow carotid-cavernous sinus fistulas or arteriovenous

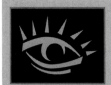

CHAPTER 21

Nystagmus and Related Ocular Motility Disorders*

GENERAL CONCEPTS AND CLINICAL APPROACH

This chapter concerns abnormal eye movements that disrupt steady fixation and thereby degrade vision. In the first section, the mechanisms by which gaze is normally held steady to achieve clear and stable vision are discussed. Next are described the pathogenesis and clinical features of each of the disorders that

*Adapted from Chapter 23 by R. John Leigh and Janet C. Rucker, Nystagmus and Related Ocular Motility Disorders.

disrupt steady gaze, including the various forms of pathologic nystagmus and saccadic intrusions. Finally, currently available treatments for these abnormal eye movements are summarized.

NORMAL MECHANISMS FOR GAZE STABILITY

In order for a person to see an object best, its image must be held steady over the foveal region of the retina. Although the visual system can tolerate some motion of images on the retina, if this motion becomes excessive, vision declines. Furthermore, if the image is moved from the fovea to peripheral retina, it will be seen less clearly.

In healthy persons, three separate mechanisms work together to prevent deviation of the line of sight from the object of regard. The first is fixation, which has two distinct components: (a) the visual system's ability to detect retinal image drift and program corrective eye movements; and (b) the suppression of unwanted saccades that would take the eye off target. The second mechanism is the vestibulo-ocular reflex (VOR), by which eye movements compensate for head perturbations at short latency and thus maintain clear vision during natural activities, especially locomotion. The third mechanism is the ability of the brain to hold the eye at an eccentric position in the orbit against the elastic pull of the suspensory ligaments and extraocular muscles, which tend to return it toward central position. For all three gaze-holding mechanisms to work effectively, their performance must be tuned by adaptive mechanisms that monitor the visual consequences of eye movements.

TYPES OF ABNORMAL EYE MOVEMENTS THAT DISRUPT STEADY FIXATION: NYSTAGMUS AND SACCADIC INTRUSIONS

The essential difference between nystagmus and saccadic intrusions lies in the **initial** eye movement that takes the line of sight off the object of regard. For nystagmus, it is a slow drift (or "slow phase"), as opposed to an inappropriate saccadic movement that intrudes on steady fixation. After the initial movement, corrective or other abnormal eye movements may follow. Thus, nystagmus may be defined as a repetitive, to-and-fro movement of the eyes that is initiated by a slow phase (drift). Saccadic intrusions, on the other hand, are rapid eye movements that take the eye off target. They include a spectrum of abnormal movements, ranging from single saccades to sustained saccadic oscillations.

DIFFERENCES BETWEEN PHYSIOLOGIC AND PATHOLOGIC NYSTAGMUS

Not all nystagmus is pathologic. **Physiologic nystagmus** preserves clear vision during self-rotation. Under most circumstances, (e.g., during locomotion), head movements are small and the VOR is able to generate eye movements that compensate for them. Consequently, the line of sight remains pointed at the object of regard. In response to large head or body rotations, however, the VOR alone cannot preserve clear vision because the eyes are limited in their range of rotation. Thus, during sustained rotations, quick phases occur to reset the eyes into their working range: **vestibular nystagmus.** If rotation is sustained for several seconds, the vestibular afferents no longer accurately signal head ro-

tation, and visually driven or **optokinetic nystagmus** takes over to stop excessive slip of stationary retinal images. In contrast to vestibular and optokinetic nystagmus, **pathologic nystagmus** causes excessive drift of stationary retinal images that degrades vision and may produce illusory motion of the seen world: **oscillopsia.** An exception is congenital nystagmus, which may be associated with normal visual acuity and which seldom causes oscillopsia.

Nystagmus, both physiologic and pathologic, may consist of alternating slow drifts (slow phases) in one direction and corrective, resetting saccades (quick phases) in the other: **jerk nystagmus** (Fig. 21.1A). Pathologic nystagmus may, however, also consist of smooth to-and-fro oscillations: **pendular nystagmus** (Fig. 21.1D). Conventionally, jerk nystagmus is described according to the direction of the quick phase. Thus, if the slow movement is drifting up, the nystagmus is called "downbeating;" if the slow movement is to the right, the nystagmus is "left beating." Although it is convenient to describe the frequency, amplitude, and direction of the quick phases of the nystagmus, it is the slow phase that reflects the underlying abnormality.

Nystagmus may occur in any plane, although it is often predominantly horizontal, vertical, or torsional. Physiologic nystagmus is essentially conjugate. Pathologic nystagmus, on the other hand, may have different amplitudes in the two eyes (dissociated nystagmus), may go in different directions leading to different trajectories of nystagmus in the two eyes, or may have different temporal properties; that is, phase shift between the two eyes, leading to movements that are sometimes in opposite directions (disconjugate nystagmus).

METHODS OF OBSERVING, ELICITING, AND RECORDING NYSTAGMUS

It is often possible to diagnose the cause of nystagmus through careful history and systematic examination of the patient. History should include duration of nystagmus, whether it interferes with vision and causes oscillopsia, and accompanying neurological symptoms. The physician should also determine if nystagmus and attendant visual symptoms are worse with viewing far or near objects, with patient motion, or with different gaze angles (e.g., worse on right gaze). If the patient habitually tilts or turns the head, the physician should determine if these features are evident on old photographs.

Before assessing eye movements, the physician must examine the visual system to determine if the patient has any congenital or acquired afferent deficits that may indicate the cause of the nystagmus. The stability of fixation should be assessed with the eyes close to central position, viewing near and far targets, and at eccentric gaze angles. It is often useful to record the direction and amplitude of nystagmus for each of the cardinal gaze positions. If the patient has a head turn or tilt, the eyes should be observed in various directions of gaze when the head is in that position as well as when the head is held straight. During fixation, each eye should be occluded in turn to check for latent nystagmus. The presence of pseudo-nystagmus and oscillopsia in patients with head tremor who have lost their VOR must be differentiated from true nystagmus.

Subtle forms of nystagmus, due to low amplitude or inconstant presence, require prolonged observation over 2 to 3 minutes. Low amplitude nystagmus may be detected only by viewing the patient's retina with an ophthalmoscope. Note, however, that the direction of horizontal or vertical nystagmus is inverted when viewed through the ophthalmoscope. The effect of **removal of fixation** should always be determined. Nystagmus caused by peripheral vestibular imbalance may be apparent **only** under these circumstances. Removal of fixation is often achieved by eyelid closure; nystagmus is then evaluated by recording eye movements, by palpating the globes, or by auscultation with a stethoscope. Lid closure itself may affect nystagmus, however, and it is better to evaluate the effects of removing fixation with the eyelids open. Several clinical methods are available, such as Frenzel goggles: 10- to 20-diopter spherical convex lenses placed in a frame that has its own light source. The goggles defocus the patient's vision, thus preventing fixation of objects, and also provide the examiner with a magnified, illuminated view of the patient's eyes. An alternative is to use two high-plus spherical lenses from a trial case, or to determine the effect of transiently covering the viewing eye during ophthalmoscopy in an otherwise dark room.

Evaluation of nystagmus is incomplete without a systematic examination of each functional class of eye movements (vestibular, optokinetic, smooth-pursuit, saccades, vergence) and their effect on the nystagmus, because different forms of nystagmus can be directly attributed to abnormalities of some of these movements. For example, the vestibular system can be assessed with the oculocephalic maneuver or by rotating the patient in a swivel chair for 30 seconds, then stopping the rotation and observing the eyes for the development of postrotational nystagmus. The optokinetic system can be assessed by rotating a small drum or moving a tape on which is printed a repetitive pattern. The slow phases generated with this technique represent visual tracking, including smooth pursuit, whereas the resetting quick phases are saccadic in origin.

It is often helpful to **determine the nystagmus waveform** because the shape of the slow phase often provides a pathophysiological signature of the underlying disorder. To properly characterize nystagmus, it is important to measure eye position and velocity, as well as target position, during attempted fixation at

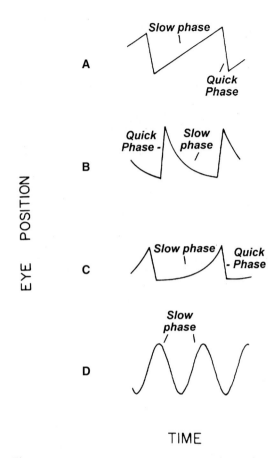

Figure 21.1. Four common slow-phase waveforms of nystagmus. **A:** Constant velocity drift of the eyes. This occurs in nystagmus caused by peripheral or central vestibular disease and also with lesions of the cerebral hemisphere. The added quick-phases give a "saw-toothed" appearance. **B:** Drift of the eyes back from an eccentric orbital position toward the midline (gaze-evoked nystagmus). The drift shows a negative exponential time course, with decreasing velocity. This waveform reflects an unsustained eye position signal caused by a "leaky" neural integrator. **C:** Drift of the eyes away from the central position with a positive exponential time course (increasing velocity). This waveform suggests an unstable neural integrator and is usually encountered in congenital nystagmus. **D:** Pendular nystagmus, which is encountered as a type of congenital nystagmus and with acquired brainstem disease. (Reprinted from: Leigh RJ, Zee DS. *The Neurology of Eye Movements.* 3rd ed. New York: Oxford University Press; 1999, with permission.)

different gaze angles, in darkness, and during vestibular, optokinetic, saccadic, pursuit, and vergence movements. Common slow-phase waveforms of nystagmus are shown in Figure 21.1.

Conventionally, nystagmus is measured in terms of its amplitude, frequency, and their product: intensity; however, visual symptoms caused by nystagmus usually correlate best with the speed of the slow phase and displacement of the image of the object of regard from the fovea.

There are many different methods now available for recording eye movements. Because many patients with nystagmus cannot accurately point their eyes at visual targets, precise measurement is best achieved with the magnetic search coil technique. This is the only technique that permits precise measurement of horizontal, vertical, and torsional oscillations over an extended range of amplitudes and frequencies. Although originally introduced as a research tool, the technique is now widely used to evaluate clinical disorders of eye movements, and is well tolerated.

CLASSIFICATION OF NYSTAGMUS BASED ON PATHOGENESIS

The classification of nystagmus starts by relating the various forms of nystagmus to disorders of visual fixation, the VOR, or the mechanism for eccentric gaze-holding.

NYSTAGMUS ASSOCIATED WITH DISEASE OF THE VISUAL SYSTEM AND ITS PROJECTIONS TO BRAINSTEM AND CEREBELLUM

ORIGIN AND NATURE OF NYSTAGMUS ASSOCIATED WITH DISEASE OF THE VISUAL PATHWAYS

Disorders of the visual pathways are often associated with nystagmus. The most obvious example is the nystagmus that accompanies blindness. At least two separate mechanisms are responsible: dysfunction of the visual fixation mechanism itself and dysfunction of the visually mediated calibration mechanism that optimizes its action. The smooth visual fixation mechanism normally stops the eyes from drifting away from a stationary object of regard. This fixation mechanism depends upon the motion detection portion of the visual system that is inherently slow, with a response time of about 100 milliseconds that encumbers all visually mediated eye movements, including fixation, smooth pursuit, and optokinetic responses. If the response time is delayed further by disease of the visual system, the attempts by the brain to correct eye drifts may actually add to the retinal error rather than reduce it, thus leading to ocular oscillations.

Vision is also needed for recalibrating and optimizing all types of eye movements. These functions depend on visual projections to the cerebellum. Lesions at any part of this recalibration pathway can deprive the brain of signals that hold each of the eyes on the object of regard, the result being drifts of the eyes off target, leading to nystagmus.

CLINICAL FEATURES OF NYSTAGMUS WITH LESIONS AFFECTING THE VISUAL PATHWAYS
Disease of the Retina

Congenital or acquired retinal disorders causing blindness, such as Leber congenital amaurosis, lead to continuous jerk nystagmus with components in all three planes and that changes direction over the course of seconds or minutes. This nystagmus is associated with a drifting "null point"—the eye position at which nystagmus changes direction—that probably reflects inability to calibrate the ocular motor system. This type of nystagmus often shows an increasing-velocity waveform (Fig. 21.1C). Recent developments in gene therapy for retinal disorders suggest that if vision can be restored, this type of nystagmus will be suppressed.

Disease Affecting the Optic Nerves

Optic nerve disease is commonly associated with pendular nystagmus. With unilateral disease of the optic nerve, nystagmus largely affects the abnormal eye, resulting in monocular or markedly asymmetric nystagmus. When both optic nerves are affected, the amplitude of nystagmus is often greater in the eye with poorer vision (the Heimann-Bielschowsky phenomenon). This phenomenon also occurs in patients with profound amblyopia, dense cataract, and high myopia. Oscillations may disappear when vision is restored, supporting the contention that in such cases, the ocular oscillations are caused by loss of vision rather than by any primary disorder of the ocular motor system.

Disease Affecting the Optic Chiasm

Parasellar lesions such as pituitary tumors have traditionally, albeit rarely, been associated with **seesaw nystagmus** (see the subsequent text). Seesaw nystagmus also occurs in persons whose optic nerve axons do not cross in the optic chiasm, such as some patients with severe albinism. Thus, it is possible that visual inputs, especially crossed inputs, are important for optimizing vertical-torsional eye movements and if interrupted, lead to seesaw oscillations.

Disease Affecting the Postchiasmal Visual Pathway

Horizontal nystagmus is a documented finding in patients with unilateral disease of the cerebral hemispheres, especially when the lesion is large and posterior. Such patients show a constant-velocity drift of the eyes toward the intact hemisphere (i.e., quick phases directed toward the side of the lesion, which are often low amplitude) and also usually show asymmetry of horizontal smooth pursuit that can be brought out using an optokinetic tape or drum. The response is reduced

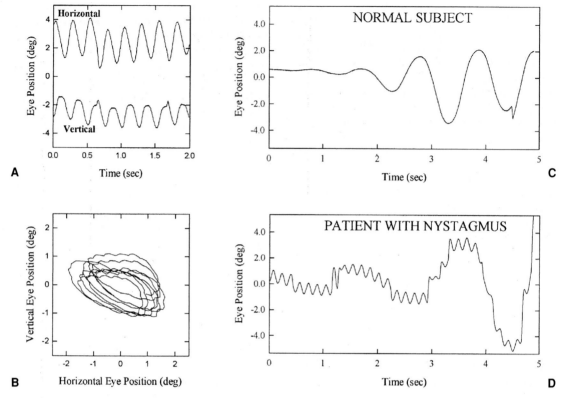

Figure 21.2. Acquired pendular nystagmus. Note both horizontal and vertical pendular waveforms.

when the stripes move, or the drum is rotated, toward the side of the lesion. Whether this asymmetry occurs primarily from impairment of parietal cortex necessary for directing visual attention or from disruption of cortical areas important for processing motion-vision is unclear.

ACQUIRED PENDULAR NYSTAGMUS AND ITS RELATIONSHIP TO DISEASE OF THE VISUAL PATHWAYS

Acquired pendular nystagmus (Fig. 21.2) is one of the more common types of nystagmus and is associated with the most distressing visual symptoms. Its pathogenesis is undefined, and more than one mechanism may be responsible. It is encountered in a variety of conditions (Table 21.1).

Acquired pendular nystagmus usually has horizontal, vertical, and torsional components with the same frequency, although one component may predominate. The temporal waveform usually approximates a sine wave, but more complex oscillations have been noted. The frequency of oscillations ranges from 1 to 8 Hz, with a typical value of 3.5 Hz. For any particu-

lar patient, the frequency tends to remain fairly constant; only rarely is the frequency of oscillations different in the two eyes. In some patients, the nystagmus stops momentarily after a saccade. This phenomenon is called postsaccadic suppression. Acquired pendular nystagmus may be suppressed or brought out by eyelid closure or evoked by convergence.

Table 21.1. *Etiology of Pendular Nystagmus*

Visual loss (including unilateral disease of the
  optic nerve)
Disorders of central myelin
  Multiple sclerosis
  Pelizaeus-Merzbacher disease
  Peroxisomal assembly disorders
  Cockayne's syndrome
  Toluene abuse
Oculopalatal myoclonus
Acute brainstem stroke
Whipple's disease
Spinocerebellar degenerations
Congenital nystagmus

Acquired Pendular Nystagmus with Demyelinating Disease

Acquired pendular nystagmus is a common feature of acquired and congenital disorders of central myelin, such as multiple sclerosis (MS), toluene abuse, Pelizaeus-Merzbacher disease, and peroxisomal disorders. Because optic neuritis often coexists in patients with MS who have pendular nystagmus, prolonged response time of the visual processing might be responsible for the ocular oscillations. However, the nystagmus often remains unchanged in darkness, when visual inputs should have no influence on eye movements. A more likely possibility is that visual projections to the cerebellum are impaired, leading to instability in the reciprocal connections between brainstem nuclei and cerebellum that are important for recalibration.

Oculopalatal Myoclonus (Oculopalatal Tremor)

Acquired pendular nystagmus may be one component of the syndrome of oculopalatal (pharyngo-laryngo-diaphragmatic) myoclonus. This condition usually develops several months after brainstem or cerebellar infarction, although it may not be recognized until years later. Oculopalatal myoclonus also occurs with degenerative conditions. The term *myoclonus* is misleading, because the movements of affected muscles are to and fro and are approximately synchronized, typically at a rate of about 2 cycles per second. The palatal movements thus may be termed *tremor* rather than myoclonus, and the eye movements are really a form of pendular nystagmus. Although the palate is most often affected, movements of the eyes, facial muscles, pharynx, tongue, larynx, diaphragm, mouth of the eustachian tube, neck, trunk, and extremities may occur.

The ocular movements typically consist of to-and-fro oscillations. They often have a large vertical component, although they may also have small horizontal or torsional components. The movements may be somewhat disconjugate (both horizontally and vertically), with some orbital position dependency, and some patients show cyclovergence (torsional vergence) oscillations. Occasionally, patients develop the eye oscillations without movements of the palate, especially following brainstem infarction. Eyelid closure may bring out the vertical ocular oscillations. The nystagmus sometimes disappears with sleep, but the palatal movements usually persist. The condition is usually intractable, and spontaneous remission is uncommon.

The main pathologic finding with palatal myoclonus is hypertrophy of the inferior olivary nucleus (Fig. 21.3), which may be seen using magnetic resonance (MR) imaging. There may also be destruction of the contralateral dentate nucleus. Histologically, the olivary nucleus has enlarged, vacuolated neurons with

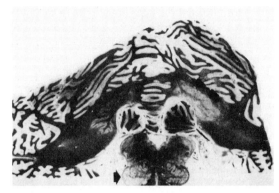

Figure 21.3. Pathology of oculopalatal myoclonus. Section through the cerebellum and medulla shows marked demyelination of the right dentate nucleus and restiform body (*double arrows*). The left inferior olive is hypertrophic and shows mild demyelination (*arrow*). (Reprinted from: Nathanson M. *Arch Neurol Psychiatr.* 1956;75:285–296, with permission.)

enlarged astrocytes. It has been postulated that the nystagmus of oculopalatal tremor results from instability in the projection from the inferior olive to the cerebellar flocculus, a structure thought to be important in the adaptive control of the VOR

Convergent-Divergent Pendular Oscillations

Vergence pendular oscillations occur in patients with MS, brainstem stroke, and cerebral Whipple's disease. In Whipple's disease, the oscillations typically have a frequency of about 1.0 Hz and are accompanied by concurrent contractions of the masticatory muscles, a phenomenon called oculomasticatory myorhythmia. Supranuclear paralysis of vertical gaze also occurs in this setting and is similar to that encountered in progressive supranuclear palsy.

At least two possible explanations have been offered to account for the convergent-divergent nature of vergence pendular oscillations: a phase shift between the eyes, produced by dysfunction in the normal yoking mechanisms, or an oscillation affecting the vergence system itself. The latter explanation is more likely, because patients who have been studied show no phase shift (i.e., are conjugate) vertically, and because the relationship between the horizontal and torsional components is similar to that occurring during normal vergence movements (excyclovergence with horizontal convergence).

NYSTAGMUS CAUSED BY VESTIBULAR IMBALANCE

Nystagmus related to imbalance in the vestibular pathway can be caused by damage to peripheral or central structures. Because the nystagmus varies, it usually is possible to distinguish nystagmus caused by peripheral vestibular imbalance from nystagmus caused by central vestibular imbalance.

NYSTAGMUS CAUSED BY PERIPHERAL VESTIBULAR IMBALANCE
Clinical Features of Peripheral Vestibular Nystagmus

Disease affecting the peripheral vestibular pathway (i.e., the labyrinth, vestibular nerve, and its root entry zone) causes nystagmus with linear slow phases (Fig. 21.1A). Such unidirectional slow-phase drifts reflect an imbalance in the level of tonic neural activity in the vestibular nuclei. If disease leads to reduced activity, for example, in the vestibular nuclei on the left side, then the vestibular nuclei on the right side will drive the eyes in a slow phase to the left. In this example, quick phases will be directed to the right—away from the side of the lesion. Two features of the nystagmus itself are useful in identifying the vestibular periphery as the culprit: its trajectory (direction) and whether it is suppressed by visual fixation.

The trajectory of nystagmus can often be related to the geometric relationships of the semicircular canals and to the finding that experimental stimulation of an individual canal produces nystagmus in the plane of that canal. Thus, complete unilateral labyrinthine destruction leads to a mixed horizontal-torsional nystagmus (the sum of canal directions from one ear), whereas in benign paroxysmal positional vertigo (BPPV), a mixed upbeat-torsional nystagmus reflects posterior semicircular canal stimulation. Pure vertical or pure torsional nystagmus almost never occurs with peripheral vestibular disease, because this would require selective lesions of individual canals from one or both ears, an unlikely event.

Nystagmus caused by disease of the vestibular periphery often is more prominent, or may only become apparent, when visual fixation is prevented. The reason for this is that when visually generated eye movements are working normally, as they usually are in patients with peripheral vestibular disease, they will slow or stop the eyes from drifting.

Another common, but not specific, feature of nystagmus caused by peripheral vestibular disease is that its intensity increases when the eyes are turned in the direction of the quick phase—**Alexander's law.** This probably reflects an adaptive strategy developed to counteract the drift of the vestibular nystagmus and so establish an orbital position (i.e., in the direction of the slow phases) in which the eyes are quiet and vision is clear. This phenomenon forms the basis for a common classification of unidirectional nystagmus. Nystagmus is called "first degree" if it is present only on looking in the direction of the quick phases, "second degree" if it is also present in the central position, and "third degree" if it is present on looking in all directions of gaze.

Although these clinical features help make the diagnosis of peripheral vestibular disease, it is important to realize that brainstem and cerebellar disorders may sometimes mimic peripheral disease and, especially in elderly patients or those with risk factors for vascular disease, careful observation is the prudent course.

Peripheral Vestibular Nystagmus Induced by Change of Head Position

Vestibular nystagmus is often influenced by changes in head position. This feature can be used to aid in diagnosis, especially of **benign paroxysmal positional vertigo** (BPPV). Patients with BPPV complain of brief episodes of vertigo precipitated by change of head position, such as when they turn over in bed or look up to a high shelf. The condition may follow head injury or viral neurolabyrinthitis.

To test for nystagmus and vertigo in a patient with possible BPPV, the examiner should turn the patient's head toward one shoulder and then quickly move the head and neck together into a head-hanging (down 30 to 45 degrees) position. About 2 to 5 seconds after the affected ear is moved to this dependent position, a patient with BPPV will report the onset of vertigo, and a mixed upbeat-torsional nystagmus, best viewed with Frenzel goggles, will develop. The direction of the nystagmus changes with the direction of gaze. Upon looking toward the dependent ear, it becomes more torsional; on looking toward the higher ear, it becomes more vertical. This pattern of nystagmus corresponds closely to stimulation of the posterior semicircular canal of the dependent ear (which causes slow phases mainly by activating the ipsilateral superior oblique and contralateral inferior rectus muscles). The nystagmus increases for up to 10 seconds, but it then fatigues and is usually gone by 40 seconds. When the patient sits back up, a similar but milder recurrence of these symptoms occurs, with the nystagmus being directed opposite to the initial nystagmus. Repeating this procedure several times will decrease the symptoms and make the signs more difficult to elicit. This habituation of the response is of diagnostic value, because a clinical picture similar to that of BPPV can be caused by cerebellar tumors, MS, or posterior circulation infarction. With such central processes, however, there is no latency to onset of nystagmus and no habituation of the response with repetitive testing.

Otolithic debris in the respective canals (canalolithiasis) interferes with the flow of endolymph or movement of the cupula and is probably responsible for BPPV. Neck movement causing vertebrobasilar kinking and vertigo as an isolated manifestation of transient brainstem ischemia is an uncommon mechanism; in such cases, associated neurologic symptoms are usually present.

Peripheral Vestibular Nystagmus Induced by Proprioceptive and Auditory Stimuli

The perception of passive body motion relies primarily on vestibular and visual information. However, an illusion of body rotation accompanied by a conjugate, horizontal, jerk nystagmus—**arthrokinetic nystagmus**—can be induced when the horizontally extended arm of a normal, stationary subject is passively rotated about a vertical axis in the shoulder joint. The slow phase of the nystagmus is in a direction opposite to that of the arm movement. The mean slow-phase velocity increases with increasing arm velocity, and the nystagmus continues for a short time following cessation of arm movement (arthrokinetic after-nystagmus). The existence of arthrokinetic circularvection and nystagmus suggests that there exists in normal humans a functionally significant somatosensory-vestibular interaction within the vestibular system, at least for afferent pathways carrying position and kinesthetic information from the joints.

Normal stationary subjects in darkness may experience illusory self-rotation when exposed to a rotating sound field. This illusion is generally accompanied by **audiokinetic nystagmus,** which is conjugate and horizontal, with the slow phase in the direction opposite to that of the experienced self-rotation. This nystagmus indicates that apparent, as well as actual, body orientation can influence ocular motor control. Neither the illusory self-rotation nor the nystagmus occurs when the subject is exposed to a rotating sound field in the light, i.e., when a stable visual environment is present, suggesting that visual information must dominate auditory information in determining apparent body orientation and sensory localization. Patients who develop vestibular symptoms and nystagmus when exposed to certain sounds—**Tullio's phenomenon**—often have dehiscence of the superior semicircular canal or pathologic stimulation of otolithic organs.

Peripheral Vestibular Nystagmus Induced by Caloric Stimulation

Nystagmus induced by caloric stimulation of one ear has all the features of that caused by unilateral or asymmetric peripheral vestibular disease. During caloric stimulation, a temperature gradient across the temporal bone induces a convection current in the endolymph of a semicircular canal if it is oriented vertical to the earth. Before attempting to induce caloric nystagmus, the physician must first check that the tympanic membrane is visible and intact. The subject is then placed supine and the neck is flexed 30 degrees. A cold stimulus (30°C) induces horizontal slow-phase components directed toward the stimulated ear (quick phases in the opposite direction). With a warm stimulus (44°C) and the same head orientation, quick phases are toward the stimulated ear (hence the mnemonic, **COWS:** cold-opposite, warm-same).

Caloric stimulation is an important way to test each peripheral labyrinth. Testing with ice-cold water is especially useful in the evaluation of the unconscious patient. In this setting, tonic eye deviation indicates preservation of pontine function. Induction of caloric nystagmus is also a useful way to confirm preservation of consciousness in patients feigning coma.

NYSTAGMUS CAUSED BY CENTRAL VESTIBULAR IMBALANCE

Clinical Features of Central Vestibular Nystagmus

In this section, we describe the clinical features of three common forms of nystagmus thought to be caused by imbalance of central vestibular connections: downbeat, upbeat, and torsional nystagmus. We also discuss the less common phenomenon of horizontal nystagmus caused by central vestibular imbalance. Finally, we offer a pathophysiologic scheme to account for these forms of central vestibular nystagmus.

Downbeat nystagmus occurs in a variety of disorders (Table 21.2), but it is most commonly associated with disease affecting the vestibulocerebellum—the flocculus, paraflocculus, nodulus, and uvula—and

Table 21.2. *Etiology of Downbeat Nystagmus*

Cerebellar degeneration, including familial episodic ataxia, and paraneoplastic degeneration
Craniocervical anomalies, including Chiari I malformation
Infarction of brainstem or cerebellum
Dolichoectasia of the vertebrobasilar artery
Multiple sclerosis
Cerebellar tumor, including hemangioblastoma
Syringobulbia
Encephalitis
Head trauma
Toxic-metabolic
Anticonvulsant medication
Lithium intoxication
Alcohol
Wernicke encephalopathy
Magnesium depletion
Vitamin B_{12} deficiency
Toluene abuse
Congenital
Transient finding in otherwise normal infants

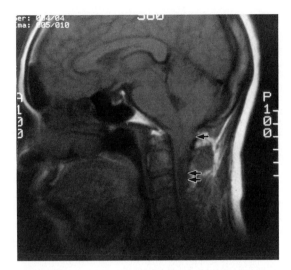

Figure 21.4. One cause of downbeat nystagmus. Sagittal MRI shows Chiari I malformation (*arrowhead*) associated with a syrinx (*double arrowheads*). Decompression of the malformation resulted in resolution of the nystagmus.

the underlying medulla. These include intrinsic brainstem and cerebellar lesions, such as MS and the Chiari I malformation (Fig. 21.4), and extrinsic lesions of the craniocervical junction such as meningioma. It may also be a manifestation of drug intoxication, notably by lithium. Downbeat nystagmus is usually present with the eyes in central position, but its amplitude may be so small that it can only be detected by viewing the ocular fundus with an ophthalmoscope. Generally, Alexander's law is obeyed in that the nystagmus intensity is greatest in downgaze and least in upgaze. Most often, it is enhanced by having the patient look down and to one side. Unlike patients with peripheral vestibular nystagmus, downbeat nystagmus does not change substantially with removal of fixation (e.g., with Frenzel goggles).

A variety of ocular motor abnormalities often accompany downbeat nystagmus and reflect coincident cerebellar involvement. These include abnormal vertical smooth pursuit and vertical VOR, skew deviation, and impairment of eccentric horizontal gaze-holding, smooth pursuit, and combined eye-head tracking.

Upbeat nystagmus that is present with the eyes close to central position occurs in many clinical conditions (Table 21.3). It is most commonly reported in patients with medullary lesions that affect the perihypoglossal nuclei and adjacent medial vestibular nucleus (structures important for gaze-holding) and the ventral tegmentum, which contains projections from the vestibular nuclei that receive inputs from the anterior semicircular canals (Fig. 21.5). It also occurs in patients with lesions affecting the caudal medulla, ante-

Table 21.3. *Etiology of Upbeat Nystagmus*

Cerebellar degenerations, including familial episodic ataxia
Multiple sclerosis
Infarction of medulla, midbrain, or cerebellum
Tumors of the medulla, midbrain, or cerebellum
Wernicke encephalopathy
Brainstem encephalitis
Behçet syndrome
Meningitis
Leber congenital amaurosis or other congenital disorder of the anterior visual pathways
Thalamic arteriovenous malformation
Organophosphate poisoning
Tobacco
Associated with middle ear disease
Congenital
Transient finding in otherwise normal infants

rior vermis of the cerebellum, or the adjacent brachium conjunctivum and midbrain. Regardless of the location or nature of the lesion, nystagmus intensity is usually greatest in upgaze (e.g., it obeys Alexander's law), it usually does not increase on right or left gaze, and removal of visual fixation has little or no effect on its waveform. Convergence may enhance or suppress upbeat nystagmus and may even convert it to downbeat nystagmus. As is the case with downbeat

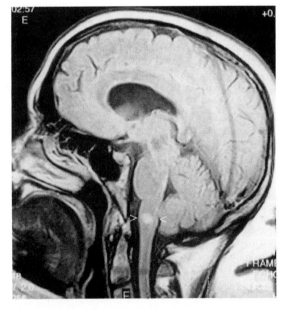

Figure 21.5. One cause of upbeat nystagmus. Axial MRI shows hyperintense signal in the medulla of a patient with upbeat nystagmus and multiple sclerosis.

Table 21.4. *Etiology of Torsional Nystagmus*

Syringobulbia, with or without syringomyelia and
   Chiari I malformation
Brainstem stroke (Wallenberg syndrome)
Brainstem arteriovenous malformation
Brainstem tumor
Multiple sclerosis
Oculopalatal myoclonus
Head trauma
Congenital
Associated with the ocular tilt reaction

Table 21.5. *Etiology of Periodic Alternating Nystagmus*

Chiari malformations and other hindbrain anomalies
Multiple sclerosis
Cerebellar degenerations
Cerebellar tumor, abscess, cyst, and other mass lesion
Creutzfeldt-Jakob disease
Ataxia telangiectasia
Brainstem infarction
Anticonvulsant medications
Lithium intoxication
Infections affecting cerebellum, including syphilis
Hepatic encephalopathy
Trauma
Following visual loss (from vitreous hemorrhage
   or cataract)
Congenital nystagmus

nystagmus, patients with upbeat nystagmus often show asymmetries of vertical vestibular and smooth pursuit eye movements, as well as associated cerebellar eye movement findings.

Torsional nystagmus is a much less common form of central vestibular nystagmus than downbeat or upbeat nystagmus. It is often difficult to detect except by careful observation of conjunctival vessels or by noting the direction of retinal movement on either side of the fovea, using an ophthalmoscope or contact lens. Although both peripheral vestibular and congenital nystagmus may have torsional components, purely torsional nystagmus, like purely vertical nystagmus, indicates disease affecting central vestibular connections (Table 21.4). Torsional nystagmus shares many of the features of downbeat and upbeat nystagmus, including modulation by head rotations, variable slow-phase waveforms, and suppression by convergence.

Horizontal nystagmus in central position from central vestibular imbalance is an uncommon but well-documented phenomenon. The underlying disorder usually is a Chiari malformation. The slow-phase waveform in this form of nystagmus may be of the increasing-velocity type, making distinction from congenital nystagmus potentially difficult. However, patients with acquired central vestibular horizontal nystagmus typically report recent onset of visual symptoms, such as oscillopsia, and measurements usually demonstrate an associated vertical component that is absent in congenital nystagmus. Patients with horizontal nystagmus that is present in the central position always should be observed continuously for 2 to 3 minutes to exclude the possibility that the nystagmus is actually periodic alternating nystagmus (see the subsequent text).

PERIODIC ALTERNATING NYSTAGMUS

Periodic alternating nystagmus is a spontaneous horizontal nystagmus, present in central gaze, that reverses direction approximately every 90 to 120 seconds. Because the period of oscillation is about 4 minutes, the disorder may be missed unless the examiner observes the nystagmus for several minutes. As the nystagmus finishes one half-cycle (e.g., of right-beating nystagmus), a brief transition period occurs during which there may be upbeating or downbeating nystagmus or saccadic movements before the next half-cycle (e.g., of left-beating nystagmus) starts. A congenital form of PAN also exists, but this is usually much less regular in the timing of reversal of direction and shows slow-phase waveforms typical of congenital nystagmus. PAN must be differentiated from "ping-pong gaze," an ocular deviation that reverses direction not over several minutes but every few seconds and that is encountered in unconscious patients with large bihemispheric lesions.

Acquired PAN occurs in association with a number of conditions (Table 21.5), many of which affect the nodulus and uvula of the cerebellum. Baclofen abolishes this nystagmus.

SEESAW NYSTAGMUS

In seesaw and hemi-seesaw nystagmus, one half-cycle consists of elevation and intorsion of one eye and synchronous depression and extorsion of the other eye; during the next half-cycle, the vertical and torsional movements reverse (Fig. 21.6A). Seesaw nystagmus may be congenital or acquired (Table 21.6), and the waveform may be pendular or jerk.

Jerk seesaw nystagmus is often referred to as "hemiseesaw" nystagmus and often occurs in patients with lesions in the region of the interstitial nucleus of Cajal (INC). Such patients also often have a contralateral **ocular tilt reaction.** With a right INC lesion, the reaction consists of a left head tilt, a skew deviation with a right hypertopia, tonic intorsion of the right eye and extorsion of the left eye, and misperception that earth-vertical is tilted to the left.

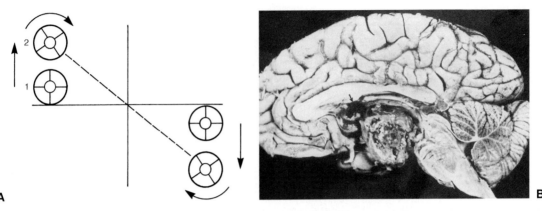

Figure 21.6. Appearance and pathology of seesaw nystagmus. **A:** Schematic drawing showing that as the right eye elevates, it also intorts. At the same time, the left eye depresses and extorts. The right eye then depresses and extorts, while the left eye elevates and intorts. **B:** Large craniopharyngioma in a patient with seesaw nystagmus. Note that the diencephalon and rostral mesencephalon are compressed and partially destroyed by the tumor.

Pendular seesaw nystagmus occurs most often in patients with large tumors in the region of the optic chiasm and diencephalon (Fig. 21.6B). Although these oscillations have been attributed to either compression of the diencephalon or to the effects of chiasmal visual field defects, both the jerk and pendular forms probably arise from imbalance or miscalibration of vestibular responses that normally function to optimize gaze during head rotations in roll.

NYSTAGMUS DUE TO ABNORMALITIES OF THE MECHANISM FOR HOLDING ECCENTRIC GAZE

GAZE-EVOKED NYSTAGMUS

Nystagmus that is induced by turning the eye to an eccentric position in the orbit is called **gaze-evoked nystagmus.** It is the most common form of nystagmus encountered in clinical practice. Although the terms *gaze-evoked nystagmus, end-point nystagmus,* and *gaze-paretic nystagmus* are often used synonymously, *gaze-evoked nystagmus* is a general term that includes both physiologic and pathologic nystagmus. When gaze-evoked nystagmus is physiologic, the term **end-point nystagmus** is appropriate (see the subsequent text). When gaze-evoked nystagmus is associated with a paresis of gaze, as in patients with ocular motor nerve palsies or weakness of the extraocular muscles, the term **gaze-paretic nystagmus** is appropriate.

Gaze-evoked nystagmus usually occurs on lateral or upward gaze, seldom on looking down. If fixation is impaired or prevented (e.g., in darkness), the slow phases consist of centripetal drifts that may have an exponentially decaying waveform (Fig. 21.1B). If visual fixation is possible, however, the slow phases have a more linear profile.

Gaze-evoked nystagmus is caused by a deficient step of innervation, such that the eyes cannot be maintained at an eccentric orbital position and are pulled back toward central position by the elastic forces of the orbital fascia. Corrective quick phases then move the eyes back toward the desired position in the orbit.

Gaze-evoked nystagmus may be caused by a variety of medications, including alcohol, anticonvulsants, and sedatives. It may also be caused by structural lesions that damage the gaze-holding neural network, particularly lesions of the nucleus prepositus hypoglossi/medial vestibular nucleus region.

Another cause of gaze-evoked nystagmus is familial episodic ataxia type 2 (EA-2), which is characterized by attacks of ataxia and vertigo lasting hours, with interictal nystagmus. The nystagmus is typically gaze-evoked, with a vertical component that can be downbeat or upbeat.

Table 21.6. *Etiology of Seesaw Nystagmus*

Meso-diencephalic disease[a]
Parasellar masses
Brainstem stroke
Septo-optic dysplasia
Chiari I malformation
Syringobulbia
Retinitis pigmentosa
Head trauma
Congenital form, including agenesis of optic chiasm, and as a transient finding in albinism

[a] Includes hemi-seesaw nystagmus.

Differences between Physiologic End-Point Nystagmus and Pathologic Gaze-Evoked Nystagmus

Gaze-evoked nystagmus is commonly encountered in normal subjects, in which case, as noted previously, it should be referred to as end-point nystagmus. End-point nystagmus typically occurs on looking far to the right or left and is poorly sustained. It usually is horizontal and symmetric, but it may be asymmetric, being more prominent on looking to one side than to the other. Most importantly, however, end-point nystagmus is not accompanied by any other ocular motor abnormalities, whereas pathologic gaze-evoked nystagmus tends to be accompanied by other defects of eye movements, such as impaired smooth pursuit.

Dissociated Nystagmus

A special type of pathologic gaze-evoked nystagmus is dissociated or "ataxic" nystagmus. This type of nystagmus is most commonly encountered in patients with an **internuclear ophthalmoplegia** (INO). In such cases, the nystagmus is present only in the abducting eye, not the adducting eye. Several explanations have been offered to account for dissociated nystagmus in INO, with the most plausible suggestion being that it represents an attempt by the brain to adaptively correct hypometric saccades due to the weak medial rectus muscle.

Dissociated nystagmus is, in fact, a series of saccades followed by postsaccadic drift that occurs when the patient attempts to look laterally away from the side of the lesion. Because the oscillations are initiated by saccades, this ocular motor abnormality is not a true nystagmus, but rather a series of saccadic pulses.

In addition to previous extraocular muscle surgery, both myasthenia gravis and the Miller Fisher variant of Guillain-Barré syndrome may produce a dissociated nystagmus similar to that seen in an INO.

Dissociated nystagmus characterized by larger movements in the **adducting** eye occurs when some patients with abducens nerve palsy look into the paretic field. Indeed, whenever a patient habitually prefers to fixate with a paretic eye, the normal eye will show a dissociated nystagmus while looking in the direction of action of the paretic muscle, regardless of the pathogenesis of the weakness.

Bruns' Nystagmus

Tumors in the cerebellopontine angle, such as meningiomas or schwannomas of the vestibulocochlear nerve, may produce a low-frequency, large-amplitude nystagmus when the patient looks toward the side of the lesion, and a high-frequency, small-amplitude nystagmus when the patient looks toward the side opposite the lesion. The nystagmus that occurs on gaze toward the side of the lesion is gaze-evoked nystagmus caused by defective gaze holding, whereas the nystagmus that occurs during gaze toward the side opposite the lesion is caused by vestibular imbalance. This special nystagmus is called **Bruns' nystagmus.**

CONVERGENCE-RETRACTION NYSTAGMUS

So-called convergence-retraction nystagmus is characterized by quick phases that converge or retract the eyes on attempts to look up. It is elicited either by asking the patient to make an upward saccade or by using a handheld optokinetic drum or tape and moving the stripes or figures down. This maneuver produces slow, downward, pursuit eye movements, but upward quick phases are replaced by rapid convergent movements, retractory movements, or both. Affected patients usually have impaired or absent upward gaze for both pursuit and saccadic eye movements; however, in some cases there is pursuit-saccadic dissociation: upward pursuit appears normal, whereas upward saccades are obviously slow or absent.

Convergence-retraction nystagmus is commonly produced by lesions of the mesencephalon that damage the posterior commissure, such as pineal tumors (Fig. 21.7). It may also occur with a Chiari malformation or during epileptic seizures.

Convergence-retraction nystagmus is usually intermittent, being determined by saccadic activity, and it thus can be differentiated from other more continuous forms of disjunctive nystagmus, such as convergent-divergent pendular nystagmus and the oculomasticatory myorhythmia characteristic of Whipple's disease.

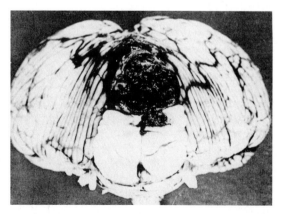

Figure 21.7. Pathology of convergence-retraction nystagmus. A pinealoma is compressing the dorsal midbrain of a 13-year-old boy who also had inability to elevate the eyes above the horizontal midline, limitation of downward gaze, and anisocoria.

DIVERGENCE NYSTAGMUS

Jerk-waveform **divergence nystagmus** is rare, but it may occur in patients with chronic cerebellar dysfunction, such as that which occurs in the Chiari malformation or MS. In such cases, slow phases are directed inward and fast phases outward.

CENTRIPETAL AND REBOUND NYSTAGMUS

If a patient with gaze-evoked nystagmus attempts to look eccentrically for a sustained period, the nystagmus may begin to decrease in amplitude and may even reverse direction, so that the eye begins to drift centrifugally ("centripetal nystagmus"). If the eyes are then returned to the central position, a short-lived nystagmus with slow drifts in the direction of the prior eccentric gaze occurs. This is called **rebound nystagmus**. Rebound nystagmus typically occurs in patients with chronic cerebellar disease, most often MS.

CONGENITAL FORMS OF NYSTAGMUS

In this section, we review those forms of nystagmus that develop during infancy. Three distinct syndromes are currently recognized: congenital (also called infantile) nystagmus, latent nystagmus, and spasmus nutans.

CONGENITAL (INFANTILE) NYSTAGMUS

Clinical Features

Congenital nystagmus is usually diagnosed during infancy, but occasionally presents during adult life when it may create a diagnostic problem, especially if the patient has other symptoms, such as headaches or dizziness. Certain clinical features usually differentiate congenital nystagmus from other ocular oscillations. It is almost always conjugate and horizontal, even on up or down gaze. A small torsional component to the nystagmus is common but difficult to identify clinically. Only rarely is congenital nystagmus purely vertical. Congenital nystagmus is usually accentuated by the attempt to visually fixate a distant object, whereas eyelid closure and convergence usually suppress it. Congenital nystagmus often decreases when the eyes are moved into a particular position in the orbit, called the "null" region.

Congenital nystagmus has one of three waveforms: jerk, pendular, or mixed. Frequently superimposed on these waveforms are **foveation periods**—the hallmark of congenital nystagmus. During each cycle, usually after a quick phase, there is a brief period when the eye is still and is pointed at the object of regard. Such periods probably are one reason (along with elevated thresholds for motion detection) that most patients with congenital nystagmus do not complain of oscil-

lopsia, despite otherwise nearly continuous movement of their eyes, and why many have normal visual acuity. Foveation periods are not invariably present in congenital nystagmus, however, and when they are absent or poorly developed, vision is usually impaired. Patients with acquired nystagmus almost never have foveation periods.

A commonly described finding in patients with congenital nystagmus is "inverted pursuit" or "reversed optokinetic nystagmus." With a handheld optokinetic drum or tape, quick phases are directed in the same direction as the drum rotates or the tape moves. This is different from normal persons who make pursuit movements in the direction of drum rotation or tape movement and quick phases in the opposite direction.

Head turns are common in patients with congenital nystagmus and are an adaptive strategy to bring the eyes close to the null position in the orbit, where nystagmus is reduced. The observation of such a head turn in childhood photographs is often helpful in diagnosing congenital nystagmus. Another strategy used by patients with either congenital or latent nystagmus is to purposely induce an esotropia to suppress the nystagmus. Such an esotropia requires a head turn to direct the viewing eye at the object of interest. This phenomenon is called the nystagmus blockage syndrome.

Some patients with congenital nystagmus also show head oscillations. Such head movements cannot act as an adaptive strategy to improve vision, however, unless the VOR is negated. Because most patients with congenital nystagmus have a normal VOR, their head movements are not compensatory but rather represent a pathologic process.

Pathogenesis of Congenital Nystagmus

Nystagmus developing early in life may occur in persons with normal afferent visual systems, in which case it is often referred to as "motor" nystagmus or in patients with a variety of afferent visual pathway disorders, in which case, it is called "sensory" nystagmus. Disorders associated with sensory congenital nystagmus include ocular and oculocutaneous albinism, achromatopsia, retinal cone dystrophy, optic nerve hypoplasia, Leber congenital amaurosis, retinal coloboma, aniridia, corectopia, congenital stationary night blindness, Chédiak-Higashi syndrome, Joubert syndrome, and peroxisomal disorders. Although both "motor" and "sensory" forms of congenital nystagmus have identical waveforms, this distinction is useful, because successful treatment of motor nystagmus is associated with improvement in visual sensory function, whereas elimination of sensory nystagmus does not result in improved vision. Because of the many diagnostic possibilities, a complete ophthalmologic evaluation and an electroretinogram should be performed in patients with congenital nystagmus associated with decreased visual acuity or visual dysfunction.

Congenital nystagmus, both with and without associated visual system abnormalities, may be familial. Several modes of inheritance have been reported, including autosomal-recessive, autosomal-dominant, and X-linked.

LATENT (OCCLUSION) NYSTAGMUS

Latent nystagmus is a horizontal jerk nystagmus that is absent when both eyes are viewing but appears when one eye is covered. This conjugate nystagmus is characterized by quick phases of both eyes that beat toward the side of the fixating eye. In most patients, a low-amplitude nystagmus is also present when both eyes are viewing, and is called "manifest latent nystagmus." Latent nystagmus usually reverses direction upon covering of either eye.

Latent nystagmus is usually associated with strabismus, typically esotropia. Amblyopia is frequent, whereas binocular vision with normal stereopsis is rare.

Latent nystagmus usually follows Alexander's law, with the nystagmus being greatest on looking in the direction of the quick phases, away from the covered eye. Thus, some patients turn the head to keep the viewing eye in an adducted position, where nystagmus is minimal. In addition to strabismus, patients with latent nystagmus frequently show an upward deviation of the covered eye (alternating sursumduction or dissociated vertical deviation). In such patients, the nystagmus often has a torsional component.

Latent nystagmus is thought to be caused by a defect in cortical motion processing that results from lack of development of binocular vision. A related theory is that latent nystagmus is caused by an imbalance in the subcortical optokinetic system, perhaps secondary to a loss of cortical motion detectors. Another theory is that latent nystagmus is caused by a defect in the influence of the internal representation of egocentric coordinates upon the direction of gaze. These proposed mechanisms may not be mutually exclusive.

Latent nystagmus is quite common, and accurate diagnosis is important to avoid inappropriate investigations.

SPASMUS NUTANS

Spasmus nutans is characterized by the triad of nystagmus, head nodding, and an anomalous head position, such as torticollis. It usually begins in the first year of life, although it may not be detected until the child is 3 or 4 years old. Neurologic abnormalities are absent, although strabismus or amblyopia may coexist. The syndrome is sometimes familial and has been reported in monozygotic twins. Spasmus nutans spontaneously remits, usually within 1 to 2 years after onset, although it may last for over 8 years.

The most consistent feature of spasmus nutans is the nystagmus, although head nodding may be the first abnormality to be noticed. Because the nystagmus is usually intermittent and has a small-amplitude, high-frequency (3 to 11 Hz) pendular waveform, it can easily be overlooked. When recognized, however, it has a "shimmering" quality.

The nystagmus of spasmus nutans almost always differs in the two eyes, and it may even be uniocular. Other features that differentiate it from simple congenital nystagmus are the variability of the amplitude of nystagmus in each eye and the difference in the phase relationship between the two eyes. Even over the course of a few seconds or minutes, the oscillations may variably be conjugate, disconjugate, dissociated, or purely monocular. The plane of the nystagmus is predominantly horizontal, but it may have vertical or torsional components. It may sometimes be brought out by evoking the near response.

The head nodding of spasmus nutans is irregular, with horizontal or vertical components. It is usually more prominent when the child attempts to inspect something of interest. About two-thirds of patients have an additional head tilt or turn. In some patients, the head nodding appears to turn off the nystagmus; however, it is unclear if head nodding, turning, or tilting are always adaptive strategies adopted to reduce the nystagmus or are simply another manifestation of the underlying abnormality in the central nervous system.

Two main clinical decisions must be made by the physician who sees a child with eye and head oscillations. The first is to determine if the ocular motor disturbance is really spasmus nutans, which will resolve over time, or congenital nystagmus, which probably will not. As noted previously, spasmus nutans usually can be differentiated from congenital and latent nystagmus by its intermittency, high frequency, and dissociated characteristics. The second, and perhaps most important, is to determine if the nystagmus is associated with retinal disease or a tumor of the visual pathway, particularly an optic chiasmal glioma. A careful ophthalmologic evaluation must be performed in all children, with particular emphasis on the anterior visual system. If there is any suggestion that the child has optic nerve or chiasmal dysfunction, neuroimaging studies must be performed, and some experts recommend that neuroimaging be performed on all children, given the difficulties inherent in eliciting a history of visual loss, and ophthalmoscopy, in small children.

SACCADIC INTRUSIONS

Several types of inappropriate saccadic eye movements may intrude upon steady fixation. These **saccadic intrusions** must be differentiated from nystagmus, in which a drift of the eyes from the desired position of gaze is the primary abnormality, and from saccadic

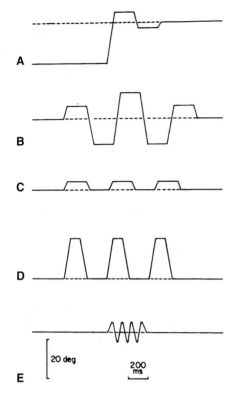

Figure 21.8. Schematic drawings of various saccadic oscillations. **A:** Saccadic dysmetria: Saccades with inappropriate amplitudes that occur in response to target jumps. **B:** Macrosaccadic oscillations: Hypermetric saccades about the position of the target. **C:** Square-wave jerks: Small, inappropriately occurring saccades away from and back to the position of the target. **D:** Macrosquare-wave jerks: Large, uncalled-for saccades away from and back to the position of the target. **E:** Ocular flutter: To-and-fro back-to-back saccades without an intersaccadic interval. (Reprinted from: Leigh RJ, Zee DS. *The Neurology of Eye Movements.* Ed 3. Philadelphia: FA Davis; 1991, with permission.)

dysmetria (Fig. 21.8A), in which the eye over- or undershoots a target, sometimes several times, before achieving stable fixation. In this section, we first describe the characteristics of each type of saccadic intrusion and then review possible mechanisms of pathogenesis.

SQUARE-WAVE JERKS

Square-wave jerks, also called Gegenrücke, are a common finding in healthy persons, particularly the elderly. They are best seen when the patient attempts to fixate a distant or near target and consist of small, conjugate saccades, ranging from 0.5 to 5.0 degrees in size, that take the eye away from fixation and return it after about 200 milliseconds (Fig. 21.8C). Their pro-

file on ocular motor recordings (the eyes move rapidly away from fixation, stay in a stable position for about 200 msec, and then return to fixation, thus producing a "square-wave" pattern) is the source of their name.

Square-wave jerks with an increased frequency (up to 2 Hz) occur in certain cerebellar syndromes, in progressive supranuclear palsy, and in cerebral hemispheric disease. When very frequent, they are called square-wave oscillations, and such movements may be mistaken for nystagmus. Cigarette smoking increases the frequency of square-wave jerks.

MACROSQUARE-WAVE JERKS (SQUARE-WAVE PULSES)

Macrosquare-wave jerks are large eye movements, typically greater than 5 degrees, that occur at a frequency of about 2 to 3 Hz. After taking the eye off the target, they return it after a latency of about 80 milliseconds (Fig. 21.8D). Macrosquare-wave jerks are present in both light and darkness, occur in bursts, and vary in amplitude. They are encountered in disease states that disrupt cerebellar outflow, such as MS.

MACROSACCADIC OSCILLATIONS

Macrosaccadic oscillations consist of horizontal saccades that occur in bursts, initially building up and then decreasing in amplitude, with intersaccadic intervals of about 200 milliseconds (Fig. 21.8B). Described originally in patients with cerebellar disease, macrosaccadic oscillations are thought to be an extreme form of saccadic dysmetria, in which the patient's saccades are so hypermetric that they overshoot the target continuously in both directions and thus oscillate around the fixation point. They usually are induced by a gaze shift, but they may also occur during attempted fixation and, thus, are often visually disabling. They may have vertical or torsional components and, occasionally, the former may be quite prominent clinically. Macrosaccadic oscillations are occasionally encountered in patients with myasthenia gravis after administration of edrophonium

SACCADIC PULSES, OCULAR FLUTTER, AND OPSOCLONUS

Saccadic pulses are brief intrusions upon steady fixation. They are produced when a saccadic pulse is unaccompanied by a step command. The eye movement thus consists of a saccade away from the fixation position, with a rapid drift back. Saccadic pulses may occur in series or as doublets. They are encountered in some normal subjects and in patients with MS.

Normally, there is a period of inactivity after a voluntary saccade. This intersaccadic interval usually lasts about 150 msec. Some saccadic pulses occur back-to-back without an intersaccadic interval. When these pulses occur in only one plane, usually the horizontal, they are called **ocular flutter** (Fig. 21.8E); when they are multivectorial, they are termed **opsoclonus** or **saccadomania.** The frequency of the oscillations of ocular flutter and opsoclonus is usually high, typically 10 to 15 cycles per second.

Sustained opsoclonus is a striking finding, in which multidirectional conjugate saccades, usually of large amplitude, interfere with steady fixation, smooth pursuit, or convergence. These movements may persist during sleep. Opsoclonus is often accompanied by myoclonus—brief jerky involuntary limb movements—hence the term *opsoclonus-myoclonus.* In children, this syndrome is called "dancing eyes and dancing feet." Ataxia and encephalopathy may also accompany opsoclonus.

The causes of ocular flutter and opsoclonus are summarized in Table 21.7. In children, about 50% of cases of opsoclonus are a paraneoplastic phenomenon, resulting from the distant effect of tumors of neural crest origin, such as neuroblastoma. The remaining cases occur after a known or presumed viral infection or are of unclear origin. In adults, opsoclonus is most often a paraneoplastic condition that is associated with small-cell lung carcinoma, breast carcinoma, or other malignancies but it also may follow a viral infection or occur spontaneously. Both children and adults with

Table 21.7. *Etiology of Ocular Flutter and Opsoclonus*[a]

Viral encephalitis
As a component of the syndrome of myoclonic encephalopathy of infants ("dancing eyes and dancing feet")
Paraneoplastic (occult tumor, especially small-cell lung and breast cancers)
Neuroblastoma
Other tumors
Trauma (in association with hypoxia and sepsis)
Meningitis
Intracranial tumors
Hydrocephalus
Thalamic hemorrhage
Multiple sclerosis
Hyperosmolar coma
Associated with systemic disease; e.g., viral hepatitis, sarcoid, AIDS
Side effects of drugs: lithium, amitriptyline, phenytoin, and diazepam
Toxins: chlordecone, thallium, strychnine, toluene, and organophosphates
Transient phenomenon of healthy neonates
Voluntary "nystagmus" or psychogenic flutter

[a]Not all case reports have documented the abnormality with eye movement recordings.

paraneoplastic opsoclonus have a variety of autoantibodies in their serum, CSF, or both, including anti-Ri, anti-Hu, and an antibody to neurofilaments.

The prognosis of idiopathic opsoclonus (including patients with manifestations of brainstem encephalitis) is generally good, although many children have persistent neurologic deficits. Patients with paraneoplastic opsoclonus-myoclonus syndrome may show spontaneous remissions, irrespective of the underlying tumor. In addition, those whose tumor can be identified and treated successfully may recover completely.

VOLUNTARY SACCADIC OSCILLATIONS OR VOLUNTARY NYSTAGMUS

About 5% to 8% of normal persons can voluntarily induce saccadic oscillations, usually by converging, a phenomenon called voluntary nystagmus. The oscillations are conjugate, with frequency and amplitude similar to those of ocular flutter and opsoclonus. Although usually confined to the horizontal plane, voluntary nystagmus can occasionally be vertical or torsional and may be accompanied by a head tremor. Voluntary nystagmus can be produced in the light or dark and with the eyes open or closed. It causes oscillopsia and reduced visual acuity and is often accompanied by eyelid flutter, a strained facial expression, and convergence. The clinical challenge is to distinguish voluntary forms of saccadic oscillations, which have no pathologic significance, from disorders such as ocular flutter and opsoclonus, which require a complete evaluation. Voluntary nystagmus may occur as a familial trait.

OSCILLATIONS WITH DISEASE AFFECTING OCULAR MOTONEURONS AND EXTRAOCULAR MUSCLE

SUPERIOR OBLIQUE MYOKYMIA (SUPERIOR OBLIQUE MICROTREMOR)

Superior oblique myokymia (SOM) is characterized symptomatically by monocular blurring of vision, tremulous sensations in the eye, brief episodes of vertical or torsional diplopia, and vertical or torsional oscillopsia. The eye movements themselves consist of monocular spasms of cyclotorsional and vertical movements that are often difficult to appreciate on gross examination, but that are usually apparent during ophthalmoscopy or slit-lamp biomicroscopy. The attacks last less than 10 seconds and may occur many times per day. They may be elicited on by looking downward, by tilting the head toward the side of the affected eye, and by blinking.

The majority of patients with SOM have no underlying disease, although cases have been reported following trochlear nerve palsy, after mild head trauma, in the setting of MS, after brainstem stroke, and in patients with cerebellar tumor.

The etiology of SOM is unknown but many authors believe it is a cranial nerve hyperfunction syndrome similar to trigeminal neuralgia and hemifacial spasm that is caused by vascular compression of the trochlear nerve.

Although SOM may spontaneously resolve, it usually is a chronic disorder with variable-length periods of remission. Many patients do not require treatment, but for those who do, some can be treated successfully with medication or extraocular muscle surgery (see the subsequent text).

OCULAR NEUROMYOTONIA

This rare, usually monocular disorder is characterized by episodes of diplopia that are usually precipitated by holding the affected eye in eccentric gaze. These symptoms are caused by involuntary contraction of the lateral rectus muscle, the superior oblique muscle, or one or more extraocular muscles innervated by the oculomotor nerve. Extraocular muscles innervated by more than one ocular motor nerve may occasionally be affected, and rare patients with bilateral ocular neuromyotonia have been reported.

Most patients with ocular neuromyotonia have undergone previous radiation to the parasellar region but rare cases have been reported in otherwise normal persons. The mechanism responsible for the condition is unknown, although both ephaptic neural transmission and changes in the pattern of neuronal transmission following denervation have been suggested.

The episodic nature of the diplopia associated with ocular neuromyotonia often suggests myasthenia gravis, but anticholinergic medicines are ineffective in this condition. Other conditions that may mimic ocular neuromyotonia include superior oblique myokymia, thyroid eye disease, and cyclic oculomotor palsy.

SPONTANEOUS EYE MOVEMENTS IN UNCONSCIOUS PATIENTS

The examination of eye movements often provides important diagnostic information in unconscious patients. For example, slow conjugate or disconjugate roving eye movements similar to the eye movements of light sleep but slower than the rapid movements of paradoxic or rapid eye movement (REM) sleep indicates that brainstem gaze mechanisms are intact.

Ocular bobbing consists of intermittent, usually conjugate, rapid downward movement of the eyes followed by a slower return to central position. Reflex-induced horizontal eye movements are usually absent. Classic ocular bobbing is a sign of intrinsic pontine lesions, usually hemorrhage (Fig. 21.9), but it has also

been reported in patients with cerebellar lesions that compress the pons and in patients with metabolic and toxic encephalopathies.

An inverse form of ocular bobbing is characterized by a slow downward movement and rapid return to midposition. This condition is called **ocular dipping.**

Reverse ocular bobbing is characterized by a rapid deviation of the eyes upward and a slow return to the horizontal, whereas **reverse ocular dipping** (also called converse bobbing) describes a slow upward drift of the eyes followed by a rapid return to central position. In general, the variants of ocular bobbing are less reliable for localization than is the classic form.

Ping-pong gaze consists of slow, horizontal, conjugate deviations of the eyes alternating every few seconds. Ping-pong gaze usually occurs with bilateral infarction of the cerebral hemispheres or of the cerebral peduncles.

Periodic alternating gaze deviation, in which conjugate gaze deviations change direction every 2 minutes, occurs in some patients with hepatic encephalopathy. This phenomenon is related to PAN (see the previous text).

TREATMENTS FOR NYSTAGMUS AND SACCADIC INTRUSIONS

Although a number of drugs have been reported to improve nystagmus in individual patients, few have been subjected to controlled clinical trials. When drug treatments fail or effective drugs cannot be tolerated by the patient, certain optical devices may be used to either suppress the nystagmus or negate its visual consequences. Finally, surgery can be performed to either weaken the extraocular muscles or reattach them to the globe in such a way that the resting position of the eyes is at the null position.

PHARMACOLOGIC TREATMENTS
Vestibular Nystagmus

Peripheral Vestibular Imbalance Nystagmus caused by peripheral vestibular lesions usually resolves spontaneously over the course of a few days. Present approaches use vestibular suppressants for 24–48 hours, primarily for severe vertigo and nausea. If the nystagmus persists after this time, exercises are used to accelerate the brain's ability to redress the imbalance. In the case of BPPV, maneuvers to displace otolithic debris from the affected semicircular canal and exercises to sustain recovery are usually effective.

Central Vestibular Nystagmus A number of drugs have been used to treat patients with downbeat nystagmus, including the GABA$_A$ agonist clonazepam, baclofen, intravenous scopolamine, trihexyphenidyl,

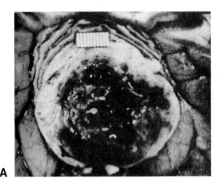
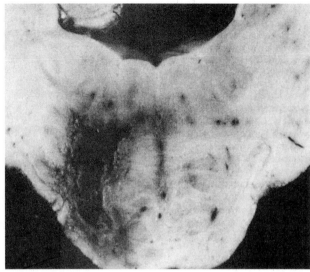

A   B

Figure 21.9. Pathology of ocular bobbing. **A:** Section through the midpons demonstrating a massive area of hemorrhage and necrosis in a 2-year-old girl with a pontine glioblastoma who developed a left hemiparesis, obtundation, seizures, and ocular bobbing. **B:** Organizing hematoma in the caudal portion of the basis pontis on the right side in a 57-year-old woman who developed a right gaze palsy, right facial palsy, and obtundation. (**A:** Reprinted from: Daroff RB, Waldman J. Ocular bobbing. *J Neurol Neurosurg Psychiatry.* 1965;28:375–377, with permission. **B:** Reprinted from: Katz B, Hoyt WF, Townsend J. Ocular bobbing and unilateral pontine hemorrhage. *J Clin Neuroophthalmol.* 1982;2:193–195, with permission.)

and the potassium channel blocking agent 3,4-diaminopyridine; however, none of these therapies is universally effective. A related drug, 4-aminopyridine, penetrates the blood-brain barrier better, has a longer half-life, and is generally better tolerated but its effect on downbeat nystagmus has not been assessed. The only drug that has been found to be effective in some cases of upbeat nystagmus is baclofen.

Periodic Alternating Nystagmus

Most cases of acquired PAN respond to baclofen. Indeed, this form of nystagmus is that which is most likely to respond to medical therapy.

Acquired Pendular Nystagmus

This type of nystagmus used to be treated with barbiturates, but their efficacy is limited by their sedative side effects. Other drugs that have been found to be useful in selected patients, including those with oculopalatal myoclonus, include trihexyphenidyl, intravenous scopolamine, valproate, isoniazid, gabapentin, and memantine (Fig. 21.10). In addition to these more-or-less "traditional" treatments, alcohol has been reported to suppress acquired pendular nystagmus as has smoking cannabis.

Seesaw Nystagmus

Improvement in seesaw nystagmus has been reported in some patients treated with alcohol. Clonazepam reduces this type of nystagmus and its associated oscillopsia in occasional patients, as does gabapentin.

Familial Episodic Ataxia with Nystagmus

The attacks of ataxia as well as the nystagmus that occur in patients with episodic ataxia type 2 (EA-2), a calcium channelopathy, respond well to treatment with acetazolamide, as do some cases of EA-1, a potassium channelopathy.

Square-Wave Jerks and Macrosaccadic Oscillations

Several benzodiazepines (diazepam, clonazepam) and the barbiturate phenobarbital may be effective in abolishing high-amplitude square-wave jerks and macrosaccadic oscillations. There is also evidence that amphetamines can suppress square-wave jerks in some patients.

Ocular Flutter and Opsoclonus

Patients with parainfectious opsoclonus-myoclonus often improve spontaneously, but intravenous immunoglobulin may speed recovery. Similarly, although

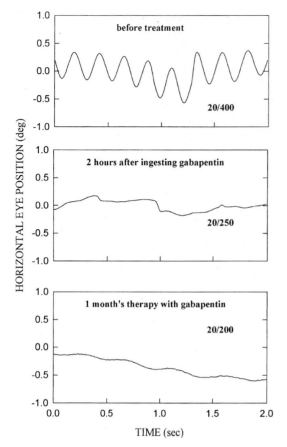

Figure 21.10. Effect of gabapentin on the horizontal component of pendular nystagmus in a 41-year-old woman with multiple sclerosis. After the initial recording **(top)**, the patient was given 300 mg of gabapentin, which reduced her oscillations and improved her vision **(middle)**. The effect was still present 2 months later, while she was taking a dose of 300 mg three times per day. Visual acuity measurements of the recorded eye are shown at the *right* in each panel.

Superior Oblique Myokymia and Ocular Neuromyotonia

As noted earlier, patients with SOM who request treatment may benefit from carbamazepine, propranolol, baclofen, or gabapentin given systemically or topically. Patients who do not respond to drug therapy, who develop side effects from the drugs, or who do not wish to take drugs for their condition, may experience complete relief of symptoms after extraocular muscle surgery (see the subsequent text).

Ocular neuromyotonia is usually responsive to carbamazepine.

OPTICAL TREATMENTS

Convergence prisms provide one optical approach for patients with congenital or acquired nystagmus whose nystagmus dampens when they view a near target. In some patients with congenital nystagmus, the resultant improvement of vision is sufficient for them to qualify for a driver's license. Patients whose nystagmus is worse during near viewing may benefit from wearing base-in (divergence) prisms.

Theoretically, it should be possible to use prisms to help patients whose nystagmus is reduced or absent when the eyes are moved into a particular position in the orbit: the null region. For patients with congenital motor nystagmus, there is usually some horizontal eye position in which the nystagmus is minimized, whereas downbeat nystagmus may decrease or disappear in upgaze. In practice, patients use head turns to bring their eyes to the optimum position and only rarely are prisms that produce a conjugate shift helpful.

Contact lenses sometimes suppress congenital nystagmus. This effect is not from the mass of the lenses but is probably mediated via trigeminal afferents.

The main optical therapy for latent nystagmus consists of measures to improve vision, particularly patching for amblyopia in children.

BOTULINUM TOXIN TREATMENT OF NYSTAGMUS

An approach to treatment of nystagmus that has gained some popularity is injection of botulinum toxin into either the extraocular muscles or the retrobulbar space. Although both techniques can result in dampening of the nystagmus and improvement in vision, ptosis is a potential major side effect, and the effect is only temporary, thus requiring repeated injections, with their attendant risks. Indeed, in one study, nystagmus was abolished or reduced in the treated eye for about 2 to 3 months, but no patient was pleased with the results because of ptosis, diplopia, an increase of nystagmus in the noninjected eye or, in one patient, filamentary keratitis, and no patient elected to continue the treatment. We do not recommend botulinum toxin for the

propranolol, verapamil, clonazepam, gabapentin, and thiamine have all been reported to diminish microsaccadic ocular flutter in such patients, the effect may have been due to spontaneous remission. Opsoclonus associated with neural crest tumors in children usually responds to corticosteroid treatment; however, as noted previously, up to 50% of such children have persistent neurological disabilities, including ataxia, poor speech, and cognitive problems. Similar responses to steroids may occur in children with parainfectious or idiopathic opsoclonus. Treatment with steroids is not uniformly successful in such cases nor are plasmapheresis, intravenous immunoglobulin, and immunoadsorption therapy.

treatment of congenital or acquired nystagmus of any type.

SURGICAL PROCEDURES FOR NYSTAGMUS

Two surgical procedures may be effective for certain patients with congenital nystagmus. One is the Anderson-Kestenbaum operation, which is designed to move the attachments of the extraocular muscles so that the new central position of the eyes is at the null position. It is performed after first making careful eye movement measurements of nystagmus intensity with the eyes in various positions of gaze and determining the approximate null position. The appropriate extraocular muscles are then weakened or strengthened as necessary to achieve the required shift in the position of the null. The Anderson-Kestenbaum procedure not only shifts and broadens the null region, but also results in decreased nystagmus outside the region. It is of uncertain value in the treatment of acquired forms of nystagmus.

The second procedure is an artificial divergence operation. It may be helpful in patients with congenital nystagmus that dampens or is suppressed during near viewing and who have stereopsis. Studies comparing these two methods indicate that the artificial divergence operation generally results in a better visual outcome than the Anderson-Kestenbaum procedure alone.

Several authors have recommended performing large recessions of all of the horizontal rectus muscles for treatment of patients with congenital nystagmus. Based on a long experience, Dell'Osso noted that any surgical procedure that detached and reattached the extraocular muscles tended to suppress congenital nystagmus. This led him to suggest that simply dissecting the perimuscular fascia and then reattaching the muscles at the same site on the globe might prove effective.

Preliminary results of a large, controlled clinical trial suggest that the operation is effective in some patients. The mechanism by which this type of procedure suppresses nystagmus is unclear.

The role of surgery in the treatment of acquired nystagmus is not well established, although individual patients may benefit from recession operations; however, it is clear that suboccipital decompression (with opening of the dura) improves downbeat nystagmus in patients with a Chiari malformation and also prevents progression of other neurologic deficits.

As noted previously, SOM that does not respond to treatment with medication may respond to extraocular muscle surgery. The procedure used by most surgeons is a superior oblique tenectomy combined with myectomy of the ipsilateral inferior oblique muscle.

OTHER FORMS OF TREATMENT

A variety of methods other than those described previously have been used to treat nystagmus, principally the congenital variety. Electrical stimulation or vibration over the forehead may suppress congenital nystagmus. It is thought that the suppressive effect on congenital nystagmus of this treatment, like that associated with contact lenses, may be exerted via the trigeminal system, which receives extraocular proprioception. Acupuncture administered to the neck muscles may suppress congenital nystagmus in some patients via a similar mechanism. Biofeedback has also been reported to help some patients with congenital nystagmus. The role of any of these treatments in clinical practice has yet to be demonstrated.

FOR FURTHER INFORMATION

See *Walsh & Hoyt's Clinical Neuro-Ophthalmology*, 6th edition, Volume 1, Chapter 23.

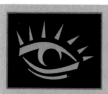

CHAPTER 22

Normal and Abnormal Eyelid Function*

EXAMINATION OF EYELID FUNCTION	Apraxia of Eyelid Opening
ANATOMY OF THE EYELIDS	Eyelid Retraction
Anatomy of the Muscles of Eyelid Opening	**ABNORMALITIES OF EYELID CLOSURE**
Anatomy of the Muscles of Eyelid Closure	Insufficiency of Eyelid Closure
ABNORMALITIES OF EYELID OPENING	Excessive or Anomalous Eyelid Closure
Ptosis	

Disorders of neuro-ophthalmologic significance may affect not only visual sensory, ocular motor, and pupil function but also the function of the eyelids. Indeed, the inability of a patient to fully open or close his or her eyelids may be the first sign of a more extensive process, the early diagnosis and treatment of which may be crucial to the ultimate well being of the patient. This chapter describes the elements that make up a complete assessment of eyelid function, the anatomy of the structures that provide normal eyelid function, and the various pathologic processes that impair eyelid opening and closure.

EXAMINATION OF EYELID FUNCTION

Detailed observation of eyelid position and movement is an important but often neglected part of the neuro-ophthalmologic examination (Table 22.1). In evaluating the eyelids, one should note the resting position of the upper and lower eyelids, assess the ability of the upper eyelid to open and close, and observe the various settings in which eyelid opening and closing occur, including voluntary, reflex, and spontaneous blinking, and lid movements accompanying eye movements.

Patients with eyelid dysfunction often complain of visual problems. Many of these problems are neurologic in origin. For example, laxity of the eyelids from a facial palsy can cause exposure keratopathy with associated blurring of vision, ocular pain, and tearing. However, the same clinical symptoms can also result from involutional changes in the elastic connective tissue supporting the lids. Ptosis, which also can be neurologic and non-neurologic in origin, can produce visual problems, even when incomplete, if the eyelashes or lid margin cover the pupil. When obtaining a history, it is important to inquire about the onset, duration and progression of the problem, and fluctuations of symptoms at different times of the day, in different seasons, and in different environmental conditions. Systemic diseases often affect eyelid function, but patients may have no reason to associate them with their eye problems. Therefore, a thorough medical history with particular attention to thyroid conditions, diabetes mellitus, systemic hypertension, myopathies, myasthenia gravis, sarcoidosis, and facial paresis should be obtained. In many situations, old photographs are useful in establishing the presence of a pre-existing condition such as ptosis or eyelid retraction which may have only recently become symptomatic or noticed by the patient.

The detailed examination of the eyelids should proceed as outlined in Table 22.1, with the examiner noting any abnormalities or asymmetries. In addition, because abnormalities of eyelid position, function, or both often are associated with other neuro-ophthalmic signs, a complete eyelid evaluation must be accompanied by an assessment of visual sensory function, ocular motility and alignment, pupil function, function of the trigeminal and facial nerves, and the status of the orbit, particularly for signs of orbital disease such as proptosis or enophthalmos.

All lid movements result from the interaction of four simple forces: (a) an active closing force produced by the orbicularis oculi muscle; (b) an active opening force generated by the levator palpebrae superioris muscle (often called the levator muscle or, simply, "the levator"); (c) an active opening force generated by a

---

*Adapted from Chapter 24 by Barry Skarf, Normal and Abnormal Eyelid Function.

Table 22.1. *Examination of the Eyelids*

1. General observation of contour, shape, and symmetry of eyelids.
2. Abnormal movements: Involuntary twitches, fasiculations, and synkinesis with other facial muscles.
3. The palpebral fissure (opening) is measured in primary position, and if an abnormality is suspected, in upgaze and downgaze, for each eye. If there is a strabismus or apparent retraction of the eyelid, these measurements are made with the contralateral eye occluded.
4. Upper eyelid position can also be documented and evaluated by measuring the distance between the upper eyelid margin and the corneal light reflex (marginal-reflex distance, or MRD).
5. Levator function is assessed by measuring difference in position of the eyelid margin between downgaze to upgaze while preventing contraction of the frontalis muscle by holding down the eyebrow.
6. Eyelid movement during slow pursuit of a target from upgaze to downgaze is observed for lid retraction or lid lag.
7. Fatigability of the levator is assessed by having the patient maintain maximal upgaze on a target for at least 1 minute. A progressive drooping of the eyelid during this test is a sign of ocular myasthenia gravis.
8. Cogan lid twitch, which is an upward overshoot of the eyelid on refixation from downgaze to primary position, is also a sign of myasthenia.
9. Synkinesis between the levator and other muscles (especially the ocular motor muscles, but, also occasionally with muscles innervated by cranial nerves V, VII, IX, and XI) is noted.
10. Abnormal spontaneous contractions of the orbicularis oculi, such as twitches, tics, fasciculation, blepharospasm, and synkinesis with other facial muscles and may also be signs of disease.
11. The strength and function of the orbicularis oculi is evaluated by observing normal blinking for frequency (rate) and completeness, and by testing the strength of closure by attempting to pry open the forcibly closed eyes.

smooth muscle—Müller's muscle (also called the superior tarsal muscle); and (d) passive lid-closing forces produced by stretching of ligaments and tendons of the eyelid. For example, normal blinks result from a cessation of the tonically active levator followed by a transient burst of the normally quiescent orbicularis oculi. The active orbicularis oculi force combined with passive lid-closing forces rapidly lower the lid. When the orbicularis oculi activity terminates, the tonic levator activity resumes. This action slowly raises the eyelid until the passive closing forces match the active opening forces generated by the levator. Moving the lid in conjunction with vertical eye movements involves changes only in the activity of the levator. This muscle receives an eye movement input qualitatively identical with that of its developmental progenitor, the superior rectus muscle. As the eye elevates, the tonic activity on the levator increases and raises the eyelid. With decreases in levator activity, the passive downward forces pull the lid down until the passive closing and active opening forces again match. By understanding these forces, it is possible to determine which element or elements of the lid system that are affected by a local, systemic, or neurologic disorder.

ANATOMY OF THE EYELIDS

The eyelids contain three main muscles innervated by three different neural networks. The oculomotor nerve (see Chapter 18) provides innervation to the levator palpebrae superioris muscle that keeps the eyelids open, a function assisted somewhat by Müller's muscle, which is innervated by the sympathetic nervous system. Eyelid closure is achieved by contraction of the orbicularis oculi muscle, innervated by the facial nerve (see later).

ANATOMY OF THE MUSCLES OF EYELID OPENING

The principal muscle involved in opening the upper eyelid and in maintaining normal lid posture is the levator palpebrae superioris. Two accessory muscles of lid opening, Müller's muscle and the frontalis muscle, play only minor roles.

Levator Palpebrae Superioris

The levator palpebrae superioris muscle originates at the annulus of Zinn and courses anteriorly along the superior aspect of the orbit, passing through a suspensory structure, Whitnall's ligament (also called the superior transverse ligament), to which it is attached by bands of connective tissue (Fig. 22.1). The levator does not extend all the way from its origin to the superior tarsus. Instead, it begins to gradually transition from muscle to tendon just posterior to Whitnall's ligament, such that anterior to Whitnall's ligament, it exists only as a tendinous aponeurosis. It is this aponeurosis that fuses with the orbital septum and attaches to the superior tarsus. The levator palpebrae superioris is innervated by branches of the superior division of the oculomotor nerve.

Müller's Muscle

Müller's muscle is a thin band of smooth muscle about 10 mm in width that inserts on the superior border of

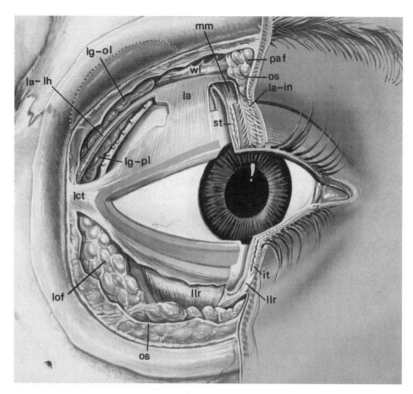

Figure 22.1. Anatomy of Müller's muscle. Anterior view of transected and partially dissected upper and lower eyelids. The lateral portion of the orbital septum and the levator have been excised to demonstrate adjacent relationships. Note that Müller's muscle (mm) is located just underneath the levator aponeurosis (la) and inserts directly into the upper aspect of the superior tarsus (st), whereas the levator aponeurosis inserts into the anterior aspect of the tarsus (la-in). it, inferior tarsus; la-lh, lateral horn of levator aponeurosis; lct, lateral canthal tendon; lg-ol, orbital lobe of lacrimal gland; lg-pl, palpebral lobe of lacrimal gland; llr, lower lid retractors; lof, lateral orbital fat; os, orbital septum (cut edge); paf, preaponeurotic fat; wl, Whitnall's ligament. (Reprinted from: Rootman J, Stewart B, Goldberg RA. *Orbital Surgery: A Conceptual Approach.* Philadelphia: Lippincott-Raven; 1995, with permission.)

the upper tarsus (Figs. 22.2). The muscle originates 10 to 12 mm above the tarsus from tendons inserted near the origin of the levator aponeurosis. Muller's muscle is innervated by fibers of the oculosympathetic pathway.

Although Müller's muscle is located in the upper eyelid, there is a similar, much smaller, sympathetically innervated muscle located in the lower eyelid. Hypofunction of this muscle (such as occurs in Horner syndrome results in slight elevation of the lower eyelid (upside-down ptosis).

Frontalis and Associated Muscles

The muscles controlling the eyebrow contribute to the eyelid appearance and, to a lesser extent, its elevation. Control of the eyebrow involves three sets of muscles: frontalis, procerus, and corrugator superciliaris (Fig. 22.3). The frontalis has cutaneous insertions at the level of the eyebrow, and frontalis fibers also intermingle with peripheral orbicularis oculi muscle fibers. Contraction of the frontalis raises the entire eyebrow and the upper eyelid through its cutaneous and

orbicularis oculi connections. The procerus muscle originates from the medial portion of the lower region of the frontalis muscle and inserts on the nasal bone. Contraction of this muscle pulls the medial portion of the eyebrow downward. The corrugator superciliaris originates from the frontal bone and llies beneath the frontalis and orbicularis oculi. It extends 2 to 3 cm laterally, where it blends with the frontalis and orbicularis oculi fibers. Contraction of the corrugator superciliaris pulls the eyebrow medially and downward.

ANATOMY OF THE MUSCLES OF EYELID CLOSURE

The primary muscle responsible for eyelid closure, the **orbicularis oculi,** is a typical striated muscle. It completely covers the orbital opening, forming concentric rings around the palpebral fissure and surrounding bone (Fig. 22.3). It is responsible not only for active eyelid closure but also for much of the facial expression around the eyes. It can be divided into three parts: orbital, preseptal, and pretarsal.

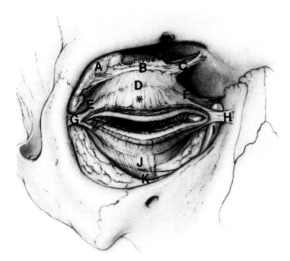

Figure 22.2. Anatomy of the levator palpebrae superioris muscle and its aponeurosis. This view shows relationship of the levator aponeurosis **(D)** to the superior tarsus (*) and to Whitnall's ligament **(B)**. **A:** lacrimal gland; **C:** superior oblique tendon sheath; **E:** lateral horn of the levator aponeurosis; **F:** medial horn of the levator aponeurosis; **G:** lateral canthal tendon; **H:** medial canthal tendon; **I:** lacrimal sac; **J:** lower eyelid retractors; **K:** inferior oblique muscle.

ABNORMALITIES OF EYELID OPENING

Abnormalities of eyelid opening include **ptosis**—insufficient opening of the eyelid—which can be caused by a variety of congenital and acquired disorders, many of which are of neuro-ophthalmologic importance, **apraxia of eyelid** opening caused by supranuclear inhibition of levator function, and eyelid **retraction,** a the

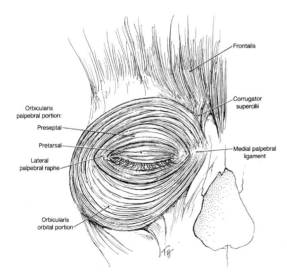

Figure 22.3. Anatomy of the orbicularis oculi, frontalis, procerus, and corrugator muscles.

only pathognomonic sign of thyroid eye disease and an important sign of other neuropathic, neuromuscular, myopathic, and mechanical disorders.

PTOSIS

A deficiency of levator tonus produces the clinical sign called blepharoptosis or ptosis. Ptosis may be produced by damage to the motor system controlling eyelid elevation and position at any point along the pathway, from the cerebral cortex to the levator muscle itself. Topical diagnosis of ptosis depends on the character of the deficiency and on evidence of neuropathic, neuromuscular, aponeurotic, developmental, mechanical, or myopathic disease.

The degree of ptosis can be quantified clinically by measuring the vertical length of the palpebral fissure—about 9 mm in normal subjects—assuming the lower eyelid is normally positioned. A more useful measure is the distance between the upper lid margin and the midcorneal reflex when the globe is in primary position. This is called the uMRD. Ptosis can be defined as an uMRD less than 2 mm or an asymmetry of more than 2 mm between eyes. Using this definition, most patients with ptosis exhibit a contraction of the superior visual field to 30 degrees or less.

Neurogenic Ptosis

Neurogenic ptosis may be caused by supranuclear, nuclear, or infranuclear dysfunction. In some cases, associated symptoms and signs make the distinctions among these causes obvious; in other cases, however, neither the location nor the nature of the lesion is clear.

Supranuclear Ptosis Unilateral ptosis is a rare manifestation of hemisphere dysfunction. This manifestation, called **cortical ptosis,** usually, although not invariably, is contralateral to the lesion. Unilateral ptosis has been described contralateral to lesions of the angular gyrus, to seizure foci in the temporal lobe, to hemispheric stroke, and to frontal lobe arteriovenous malformations (AVMs). It also has been described ipsilateral to ischemic hemispheric strokes (Fig. 22.4).

Bilateral cortical ptosis can also occur. It is associated most frequently with extensive nondominant hemisphere lesions. In most instances, the ptosis is accompanied by midline shift, gaze deviation to the right, and other signs of right hemisphere dysfunction, including left hemiparesis. The ptosis is often asymmetric. In the setting of cerebral infarction, the ptosis is transient, lasting from several days to 5 months or more.

Ptosis may develop in certain eccentric positions of gaze from congenital supranuclear inhibition of the levator; i.e., **supranuclear oculopalpebral synkinesia.** In such cases, lid position in primary gaze may be normal, or the lid may be slightly ptotic. When the patient adducts (or occasionally abducts) the eye on the

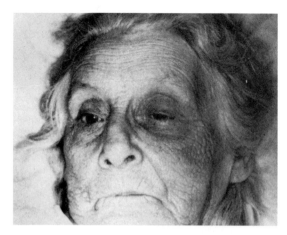

Figure 22.4. Unilateral supranuclear (cortical) ptosis. The patient developed a left ptosis associated with a left hemiparesis from a right hemisphere stroke. The patient also has a pre-existing right ptosis from dehiscence of the levator tendon. (Reprinted from: Caplan LR. Cerebral ptosis. *J Neurol Neurosurg Psychiatry.* 1974;37:1–7, with permission.)

affected side, however, the eyelid drops abruptly because of a loss of levator muscle tone. When the eye returns toward center, or toward the opposite side, the levator contracts and the eyelid returns to a normal position. The synkinesia may be unilateral (Fig. 22.5) or bilateral (Fig. 22.6). It may occur as an isolated phe-

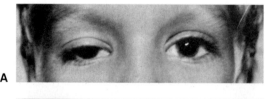

A

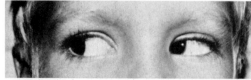

B

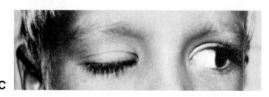

C

Figure 22.5. Congenital unilateral supranuclear oculopalpebral synkinesis. **A:** This young child has moderate right ptosis when looking straight ahead. **B:** When the patient looks to the right, the position of both upper eyelids is normal. **C:** On left gaze, there is almost complete right ptosis from inhibition of the levator muscle. Note that the left upper eyelid remains in a normal position in all positions of gaze. (Courtesy of Dr. C. Hedges.)

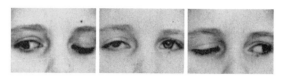

Figure 22.6. Congenital bilateral supranuclear oculopalpebral synkinesia. In primary position, the patient has a moderate right ptosis **(center)**. On right gaze **(right)**, the patient develops a marked left ptosis, whereas on left gaze **(left)**, the patient develops a marked right ptosis. (Courtesy of Dr. H. Rose.)

nomenon or in association with other congenital syndromes, such as the Duane retraction syndrome. The causes of supranuclear paradoxical levator inhibition are unclear. They may involve a variety of mechanisms, including ephaptic transmission or disturbances in the supranuclear pathways responsible for levator tonus, excitation, and inhibition.

Ptosis associated with mouth opening—**the inverse Marcus Gunn phenomenon**—is a rare condition in which the ipsilateral eyelid closes when the external pterygoid muscle moves the jaw to the opposite side (Fig. 22.7). Patients with this condition have mild ptosis of the affected eyelid when the eyes are in primary position and the mouth is closed. The associated ptosis is consequent to levator inhibition without contraction of the orbicularis oculi. This syndrome is an inverse of the Marcus Gunn jaw-winking phenomenon (see the subsequent text) and probably represents a supranuclear synkinesis affecting the oculomotor and trigeminal nerves.

Ptosis from Lesions of the Oculomotor Nucleus, Fascicle, or Nerve By far, the most common causes of acquired neurogenic ptosis are related to dysfunction of the oculomotor nucleus, fascicle, or nerve. Because the central caudal subnucleus of the oculomotor nucleus supplies bilateral equal innervation to the

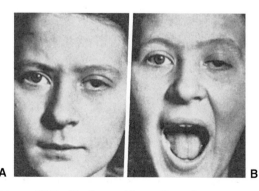

A   B

Figure 22.7. The Inverse Marcus Gunn phenomenon. **A:** When the patient looks straight ahead, she has a mild left ptosis. **B:** When the patient opens her mouth, the ptosis increases from inhibition of the left levator muscle.

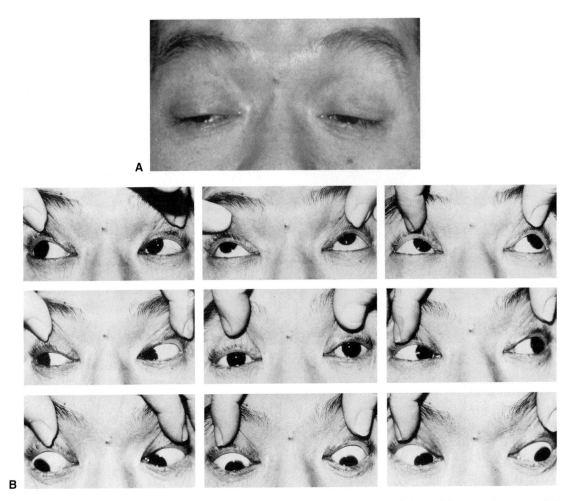

Figure 22.8. Midbrain ptosis. Isolated, bilateral ptosis in a patient with brainstem encephalitis and discrete inflammatory foci in the caudal mesencephalon. Ocular motility was completely normal. (Reprinted from: Conway VH, Rozdilsky B, Schneider RJ, et al. Isolated bilateral complete ptosis. *Can J Ophthalmol.* 1983;18:37–40, with permission.)

levator muscles, ptosis resulting from a nuclear midbrain lesion is always bilateral and symmetric as well as usually complete or at least very severe (Fig. 22.8). This **midbrain ptosis** is commonly associated with other signs of mesencephalic dysfunction. However, in some cases, only the central caudal subnucleus of the oculomotor nuclear complex is affected or is much more severely affected than the other oculomotor subnuclei, and bilateral, severe, symmetric ptosis is the predominant or only manifestation of the nuclear lesion.

Midbrain ptosis may be congenital, occurring as a consequence of dysplasia or aplasia of the oculomotor nucleus, or acquired. Acquired causes include ischemia, inflammation, infiltration, compression, and metabolic and toxic processes.

Lesions of the **fascicle of the oculomotor nerve** produce unilateral oculomotor nerve dysfunction that

may be mild or severe. The dysfunction may be isolated or associated with a contralateral hemiplegia, cerebellar ataxia, or rubral tremor, depending on whether adjacent structures in the midbrain (e.g., cerebral peduncle, red nucleus) are also affected by the lesion (see Chapter 18). For example, in some cases, the associated signs of midbrain dysfunction are minimal and consist of nothing more than an oculomotor nerve palsy and an abnormal masseter reflex. When ptosis occurs in patients with a lesion of the oculomotor fascicle, it is always unilateral, of variable severity, and, in our experience, associated with weakness of one or more of the extraocular muscles innervated by the oculomotor nerve (Fig. 22.9). Pupillary involvement is commonly but not invariably present.

The ptosis that accompanies a lesion of the **peripheral oculomotor nerve** is, like that caused by a fascicular lesion, unilateral and usually accompanied

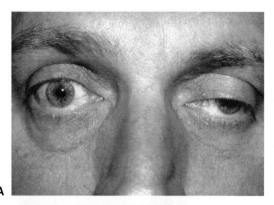

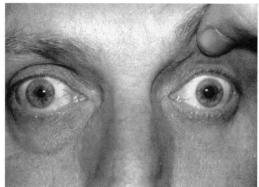

A

B

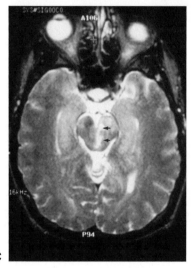

C

Figure 22.9. Unilateral ptosis associated with other evidence of a left third nerve paresis caused by damage to the fascicle of the third nerve from a left-sided midbrain infarct. **A and B:** Appearance of patient; **C:** MRI showing an extensive area of infarction along the path of the fascicle (*arrowheads*).

by ophthalmoparesis, pupillary involvement, or both (Fig. 22.10). Rarely, however, ptosis precedes the other signs of oculomotor nerve dysfunction by days, weeks, or even months, depending on the location and nature of the lesion. Isolated ptosis caused by peripheral oculomotor nerve dysfunction has been reported in patients with aneurysms, pituitary adenomas, meningiomas, and meningitis. Some of these cases are examples of truly isolated ptosis. In others, there are other symptoms, for example, headache, or subtle signs of oculomotor dysfunction, a mildly dilated but reactive pupil, an incomitant phoria, or asymptomatic underaction of the superior rectus that is only evident on extreme upgaze. Recurrent, isolated ptosis lasting 6 to 8 weeks has been described with ophthalmoplegic migraine. Isolated, complete, neurogenic ptosis can also occur from orbital trauma that generates forceful anterior displacement of the upper eyelid with denervation of the levator muscle. This form of ptosis usually resolves spontaneously within weeks.

Ptosis from Lesions of the Oculosympathetic Pathways Lesions of the oculosympathetic pathway produce **Horner syndrome,** a condition that is characterized in part by a partial, unilateral ptosis from hypofunction of Müller's muscle. The ptosis of Horner syndrome usually can be differentiated from the ptosis associated with oculomotor nerve dysfunction by their differing appearance and associated findings. The ptosis in Horner syndrome is often mild, variable, and always associated with ipsilateral miosis (Fig. 22.11). Involvement of a sympathetically innervated smooth muscle in the lower eyelid similar to Müller's muscle in the upper eyelid (see the previous text) results in elevation ("upside-down" ptosis) of the lower eyelid. The combination of ptosis of the upper eyelid and elevation of the lower eyelid produces the appearance of enophthalmos, although exophthalmometry invariably shows no asymmetry of the two eyes. Other signs of Horner syndrome include ipsilateral facial anhidrosis in patients with first-order or second-order neuron lesions, mildly reduced intraocular pressure in the

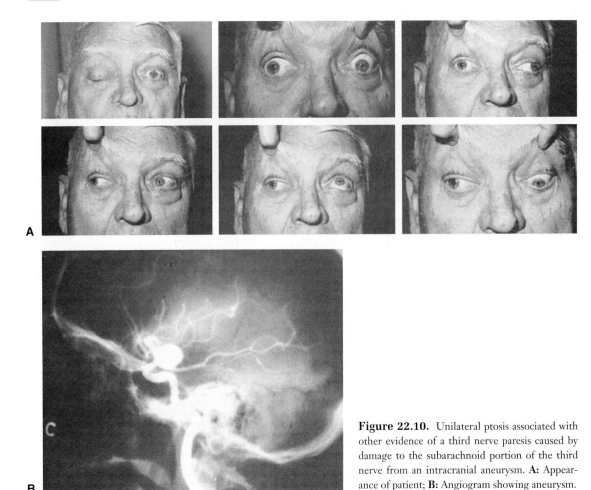

Figure 22.10. Unilateral ptosis associated with other evidence of a third nerve paresis caused by damage to the subarachnoid portion of the third nerve from an intracranial aneurysm. **A:** Appearance of patient; **B:** Angiogram showing aneurysm.

affected eye, heterochromia in congenital and very long-standing cases, and an increased accommodation amplitude. Horner syndrome is discussed in detail in Chapter 15 of this text.

The ptosis occasionally observed after conjunctival instillation of timolol maleate, a β-adrenergic blocking agent, may be caused by Müller's muscle blockade. Similarly, thymoxamine, an α-adrenergic blocking agent, may cause ptosis when given topically or parenterally.

Ptosis from Disinsertion, Dehiscence, or Thinning of the Levator Aponeurosis

The most common cause of acquired ptosis in adults is a dehiscence, disinsertion, or thinning of the levator aponeurosis (Fig. 22.12). Ptosis caused by such defects of the levator tendon may be bilateral or unilateral and can vary in its severity. In the early stages,

Figure 22.11. Horner syndrome. Note mild unilateral ptosis, anisocoria with smaller pupil on side of ptosis, and apparent enophthalmos caused by ptosis of affected upper lid and "upside-down" ptosis (i.e., elevation) of affected lower lid.

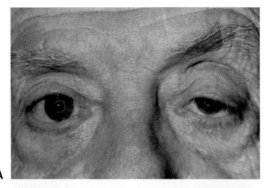

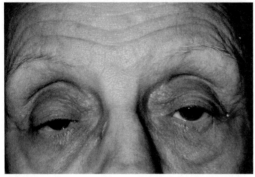

Figure 22.12. Ptosis from levator dehiscence. **A:** Unilateral ptosis. Note the difference in location of the superior lid folds, with the left being much higher than the right. Also note the deepened superior sulcus on the left side. **B:** Bilateral ptosis from levator dehiscence. Both eyelids show high superior lid folds and deep superior sulci. (Courtesy of Dr. Nicholas T. Iliff.)

the ptosis may be barely evident in primary position, but because it typically worsens in downgaze, the eyelid may obstruct the visual axis when the patient attempts to read. The presence of anisocoria (i.e., physiologic anisocoria that occurs in about 20% of normal individuals [see Chapter 15]) or a mild and asymptomatic heterophoria, or the frequent worsening of symptoms at the end of the day, may lead to the erroneous diagnosis of oculomotor nerve palsy or myasthenia gravis in such patients. However, the findings of normal levator excursion, an elevated or absent superior lid crease, a deep superior eyelid sulcus, worsening of ptosis in downgaze, and thinning of the skin above the tarsal plate should distinguish an aponeurotic ptosis from developmental, neurogenic, and myogenic causes.

Levator aponeurotic defects commonly occur in the elderly from involutional or degenerative changes that result in disinsertion, dehiscence, or thinning of the aponeurosis. Among patients between ages 15 and 50, aponeurotic ptosis is most commonly associated with a

long history of wearing rigid contact lenses. In such patients, repeated manipulation and traction of the upper eyelid while inserting or removing contact lenses causes disinsertion or thinning of the tendon.

Damage to the levator aponeurosis other than that associated with contact lens wear can occur from trauma, including that associated with ocular and orbital surgery. Thus, ptosis not infrequently occurs after cataract extraction, glaucoma surgery, radial keratotomy, orbital surgery, conjunctival procedures, enucleations, strabismus surgery, and blepharoplasty. Ptosis following orbital surgery or blepharoplasty in which there is deep orbital fat dissection or supratarsal fixation, is likely a result of direct injury to the levator aponeurosis. The aponeurosis also may be stretched or damaged from postoperative swelling, injection of an anesthetic into the upper eyelid, the use of a rigid lid speculum, ocular compression and massage, or attempts by the patient to open the eyelid against a tight patch. The myotoxic effects of anesthetic injections and trauma to the levator itself from bridle sutures or retrobulbar injections may also play a role in some cases.

In addition to the mechanisms described previously, ptosis from damage to or dysfunction of the levator aponeurosis may be associated with blepharochalasis, thyroid orbitopathy, pregnancy, and chronic use of topical steroids. Aponeurotic defects may also occur after episodes of eyelid edema caused by allergic reactions.

Myopathic Ptosis

Ptosis that occurs from damage to the levator palpebrae superioris muscle itself (as opposed to its tendon) may be either congenital (i.e., developmental) or acquired.

Congenital Myopathic Ptosis (Developmental Ptosis)
Although congenital ptosis occasionally is neurogenic (e.g., oculomotor nerve palsy, Marcus Gunn jaw-winking phenomenon, Horner syndrome) or traumatic (e.g., from a forceps delivery) in origin, the most common form is caused by a developmental myopathy of the levator palpebrae superioris muscle. Developmental ptosis is characterized by a deficiency in levator excursion (as opposed to ptosis caused by defects in the levator aponeurosis), an elevated or absent superior lid crease, and, most importantly, lid-lag on downgaze (Fig. 22.13). The majority of cases are unilateral, but about 20% are bilateral. Patients with severe developmental ptosis, particularly bilateral ptosis, may exhibit a compensatory chin elevation or frontalis contraction.

Developmental ptosis may exist in isolation, or it may be associated with other ocular findings, including strabismic or occlusion (deprivation) amblyopia, astigmatism, and anisometropia. Because the levator derives embryologically from the same anlage as the superior rectus, it is not surprising that underaction of

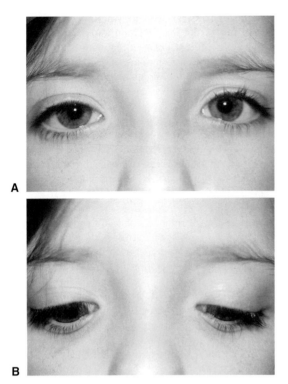

A

B

Figure 22.13. Congenital (developmental) ptosis. **A:** When the patient looks straight ahead, she has a very mild right ptosis. **B:** When the patient looks down, there is mild lid lag on the right but not on the left.

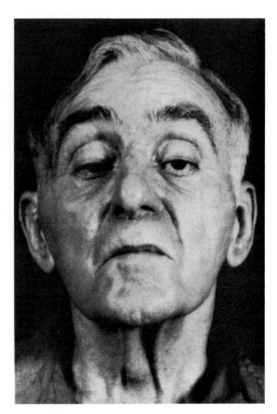

Figure 22.14. Ptosis in a patient with CPEO. Note also flat, expressionless facial features associated with continuous wrinkling of the frontalis muscles and a posterior head tilt in order to compensate for bilateral ptosis. (Courtesy of Dr. I. Lewis and the Canadian Medical Association Journal.)

the superior rectus frequently accompanies developmental ptosis.

Developmental ptosis may be associated with a variety of congenital ocular or systemic malformations. In some cases, the association is distinctive enough to constitute a well-defined syndrome, such as the blepharophimosis-epicanthus-ptosis syndrome, the congenital fibrosis syndrome, and Goldenhar syndrome. In other cases, developmental ptosis occurs in association with less clearly defined entities, including anomalies of the brain, heart, urogenital, skeletal, or auditory systems.

Acquired Myopathic Ptosis Acquired myopathic ptosis occurs in a number of the mitochondrial cytopathies characterized by chronic progressive external ophthalmoplegia (CPEO) (see Chapter 20). In some patients, the ptosis is the presenting sign and may persist in isolation for months to years before the development of ophthalmoplegia. Ptosis of this type usually is bilateral, relatively symmetric, and very slowly progressive. The superior palpebral lid fold may be completely absent. Excessive wrinkling of the brow and

backward head tilting are commonly employed to facilitate vision beneath the drooping lids (Fig. 22.14). Orbicularis oculi function, tested by forced lid closure, is frequently weak, and this combination of weakness of both eyelid opening and eyelid closure serves to distinguish the condition from other causes of ptosis except myasthenia gravis and myotonic dystrophy.

Because the manifestations of the disease are so slowly progressive and in part because they tend to be symmetric, patients with ptosis associated with CPEO are remarkably tolerant of their symptoms, and thus generally present relatively late in their course.

Bilateral partial ptosis contributes to the characteristic appearance of patients with myotonic dystrophy.

The levator palpebrae superioris muscle may be damaged by a variety of inflammatory, ischemic, or infiltrative processes affecting the orbit. Occasionally, ptosis is the most prominent manifestation. For example, lymphoid infiltration, sarcoidosis, amyloidosis, and idiopathic inflammatory disease of the orbit can sometimes selectively affect the levator and spare the

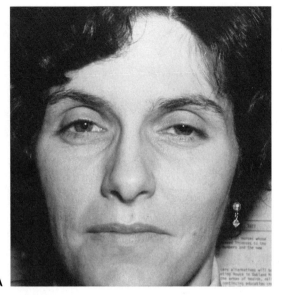
A

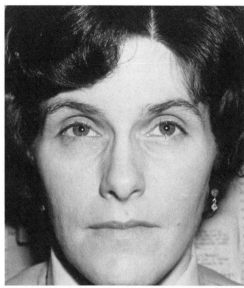
B

Figure 22.15. Ptosis in a patient with myasthenia gravis. **A:** Before injection of edrophonium, the patient has bilateral ptosis. **B:** One minute following an intravenous injection of 2 mg of edrophonium, the ptosis has disappeared.

extraocular muscles. Patients with diabetes mellitus also may develop unilateral or bilateral ptosis in association with other evidence of microangiopathic changes elsewhere in the body. Although most of these patients probably have a localized infarction in the midbrain, which affects either the oculomotor nerve nucleus or fascicle, or in the peripheral oculomotor nerve, chronic hypoxia of the levator muscle is responsible for this form of ptosis in some diabetic patients.

Neuromuscular Ptosis

Recognition of neuromuscular ptosis depends in part on the absence of clinical signs of an oculomotor or sympathetic lesion and the presence of clinical signs of neuromuscular disease. Ptosis in myasthenia gravis may occur in isolation, but it is more often associated with diplopia, varying degrees of ophthalmoparesis, weakness of the orbicularis oculi, and normal pupillary function by clinical testing (see Chapter 19). Ultimately, ptosis occurs in the majority of patients with myasthenia gravis. Regardless of when it develops, the ptosis of myasthenia gravis may be unilateral or bilateral, and when it is bilateral, it may also be symmetric or asymmetric (Fig. 22.15).

The hallmark of myasthenic ptosis is its fatigability and tendency to fluctuate in severity (Fig. 19), although this feature is by no means pathognomonic. A similar tendency to fatigue (although not to the same degree) occurs in patients with aponeurotic defects and oculomotor nerve palsies. Patients with ptosis from myasthe-

nia gravis, myasthenic syndromes, botulism, or drugs affecting neuromuscular transmission usually have sufficient signs and symptoms to allow the correct diagnosis to be made, such as the Cogan lid-twitch sign (Fig. 22.16), enhancement of ptosis with manual elevation of the contralateral eyelid (Fig. 22.17), and the orbicularis "peek" sign (Fig. 22.18). In addition, unless it is complete, myasthenic ptosis often improves when ice is held to the affected eyelid for 2 minutes (Fig. 22.19; see Chapter 19).

Ptosis may be produced by neuromuscular disorders other than myasthenia gravis, including botulism and certain envenomations. In such cases, the history as well as accompanying signs or symptoms—particularly pupillary involvement—allow the correct diagnosis. Neuromuscular disorders of neuro-ophthalmologic importance are described in detail in Chapter 19 of this text.

Mechanical Ptosis

Any process that increases the weight of the eyelid or mechanically interferes with the normal excursion of the eyelid can result in ptosis. The most common causes are neoplastic or inflammatory infiltration or mass effect on the eyelid (e.g., neurofibroma, capillary hemangioma, metastatic lesions, basal cell carcinoma, lymphoid lesions, and amyloidosis) and edema (e.g., after trauma or from blepharochalasis, inflammatory disease of the lid and orbit, acute thyroid eye disease, or giant papillary conjunctivitis). In contrast to conditions

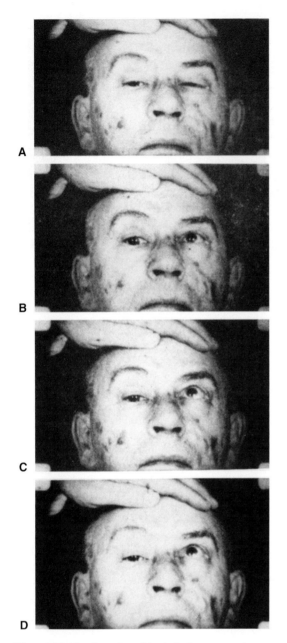

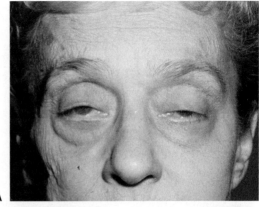

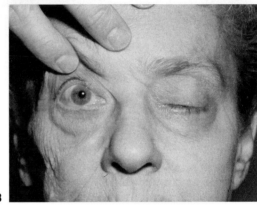

Figure 22.17. Enhancement of ptosis in a 78-year-old woman with myasthenia gravis. **A:** The patient has bilateral ptosis. **B:** When the right eyelid is elevated, the patient develops increased (enhanced) ptosis on the opposite side.

that increase the mass of the eyelid and cause ptosis in both primary and downward gaze, malignant and inflammatory infiltration of the superior orbital tissues may produce ptosis in primary gaze with "hang-up" (i.e., pseudoretraction) of the upper lid on downgaze. This can occur with minimal evidence of orbital disease

Figure 22.16. Cogan's eyelid twitch phenomenon in a patient with myasthenia gravis. The photograph is made from successive frames of a movie. As the patient looks upward, the left eyelid elevates fully while the right eyelid elevates only partially. The right eyelid then immediately becomes successively more ptotic. The entire process takes only a few seconds. In motion, this transient eyelid elevation gives the appearance of a twitch. (Reprinted from: Cogan DG. Myasthenia gravis: A review of the disease and a description of lid twitch as a characteristic sign. *Arch Ophthalmol.* 1965;74:217–221, with permission.)

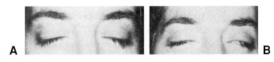

Figure 22.18. The orbicularis "peek" sign of myasthenia gravis. The patient is able to close the eyes tightly **(A)**, but the orbicularis then fatigues, and the inferior sclera becomes visible **(B)**. (From Osher RH, Griggs RC. Orbicularis fatigue: The "peek" sign of myasthenia gravis. *Arch Ophthalmol.* 1979;97:677–679.)

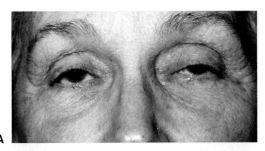

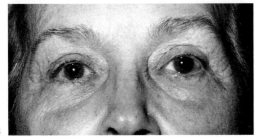

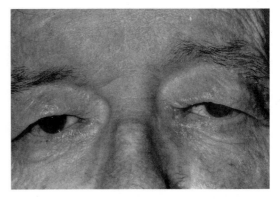

Figure 22.20. Pseudoptosis from dermatochalasis in an elderly man. Note folds of skin from the superior eyelids that obscure the upper half of both corneas. (Courtesy of Dr. Nicholas T. Iliff.)

Figure 22.19. The ice test for myasthenia gravis. **A:** Before placement of ice, patient has severe bilateral ptosis. **B:** After placement of ice for 2 minutes, the ptosis has resolved.

and can be an important sign of orbital malignancy or inflammation in patients with adult-onset ptosis.

Cicatricial changes from trauma and diseases such as trachoma, erythema multiforme, and pemphigoid may also result in an adhesive or restrictive type of ptosis. Entrapment of (e.g., from orbital roof fracture) or encroachment on (e.g., from bony fragments, intraorbital foreign bodies, subperiosteal and intraorbital hematomas, mass lesions) the levator can interfere mechanically with the movement and position of the eyelid. In such cases, the history and associated findings usually are sufficient to make the correct diagnosis.

Pseudoptosis

Pseudoptosis is an apparent ptosis unrelated to defects in the neural, neuromuscular, or myogenic components of eyelid elevation. Pseudoptosis may be present because the eye on the same side is abnormal in size, shape, or position; e.g., in patients with anophthalmos, phthisis bulbi, microphthalmos, or enophthalmos. Conversely, patients who present with isolated unilateral lid retraction and proptosis from thyroid orbitopathy are sometimes mistakenly thought to have ptosis of the other eye. In some persons, excessively loose skin (dermatochalasis) or prolapsed orbital fat (blepharochalasis) causes the skin of the upper eyelid to overhang the lid margin, simulating ptosis (Fig. 22.20).

Pseudoptosis often occurs in patients with a hypotropia who fixate with the higher eye. The position of the upper eyelid on the side of the hypotropia is

appropriate to the position of that eye, but because the patient is fixing with the higher eye, the eyelid on the side of the hypotropic eye appears ptotic. When the hypertropic eye is covered and the patient is forced to fixate with the previously hypotropic eye, the "ptosis" disappears (Fig. 22.21).

Pseudoptosis may occur in patients with downgaze paralysis. When such patients attempt to look downward, their eyes remain in the primary position, but their eyelids lower normally.

Narrowing of the lid fissure from hemifacial contracture, hemifacial spasm, blepharospasm, or previous facial nerve palsy may mimic ptosis. In such patients, the presence of other evidence of abnormal facial movement usually suggests the correct diagnosis.

Apparent ptosis can be caused by voluntary stimulation of one or both orbicularis oculi muscles. Patients with nonorganic overactivity of the orbicularis oculi usually show mild or pronounced wrinkling of the eyelids proportional to the amount of narrowing of the fissure and depression of the brow (although occasionally the brow is elevated). Indicative of levator tone, the upper eyelid crease is present in primary gaze and may deepen in upgaze. In addition, one can often see—and always feel—fine tremors of the affected eyelid as the patient attempts to maintain the "ptotic" lid position. Patients with organic ptosis do not show a delay in returning to their baseline lid position after manual elevation of the eyelid. In contrast, patients with nonorganic ptosis may sometimes exhibit a slight lag before the orbicularis oculi is factitiously reactivated. Nonorganic ptosis may occur in isolation or in association with other somatic complaints.

Treatment of Ptosis

A variety of surgical procedures can be used to treat ptosis. The treatment for any individual patient

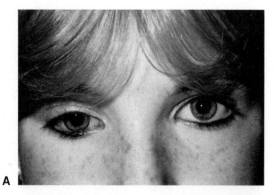

A

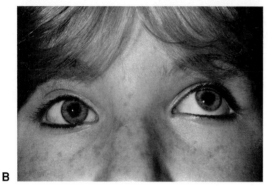

B

Figure 22.21. Pseudoptosis caused by with ipsilateral hypotropia and limitation of upward gaze in a patient who is fixing with the contralateral (hypertropic) eye. **A:** When the patient looks straight ahead and fixes with the left eye, she has a right hypotropia and appears to have a moderate right ptosis. **B:** When the patient fixes with the hypotropic right eye, however, the apparent ptosis disappears. (Courtesy of Dr. Nicholas T. Iliff.)

depends on the etiology of the ptosis, the amount of levator function, and the preference of the surgeon.

APRAXIA OF EYELID OPENING

A more common supranuclear insufficiency of eyelid opening than cortical ptosis is **apraxia of eyelid opening** (AEO). The main clinical features of AEO are as follows: (a) a transient inability to initiate lid opening; (b) the absence of any significant evidence of orbicularis oculi contraction, such as lowering of the brow beneath the orbital rim (Charcot sign); (c) frontalis contraction during attempts to open the eyelids; and (d) the absence of any other signs of neural or myopathic dysfunction. Most patients with AEO show a paucity of blinking interrupted by gentle closure of both eyelids that may last up to 30 seconds or longer. AEO occurs most commonly in patients with progressive supranuclear palsy, Parkinson disease, and atypical Parkinsonism including that induced by methyl-phenyl-tetrahydropyridine (MPTP). Other associations are listed in Table 22.2.

Table 22.2. *Disorders Associated with Apraxia of Eyelid Opening*

Progressive supranuclear palsy
Parkinson disease
Parkinsonism (including parksinsonism-dementia complex)
Shy-Drager syndrome
Adult-onset Hallervorden-Spatz disease
Huntington's chorea
Frontotemporal gunshot injury
Right hemisphere stroke
Wilson disease
Amyotrophic lateral sclerosis
Idiopathic

Treatment of involuntary eyelid closure caused by supranuclear inhibition of levator activity is not particularly successful. Individual case reports suggest that several drugs may be useful, including desipramine and L-dopa. Injection of the orbicularis oculi and frontalis muscles with botulinum toxin produces variable results, depending on the degree of orbicularis contraction that often accompanies the levator inhibition, and we believe this treatment is worth trying in patients with AEO, even though the results are less than satisfactory.

EYELID RETRACTION

Inappropriate and excessive elevation of the eye lids—eyelid retraction—makes a patient appear to be staring and also produces an illusion of exophthalmos. Mild degrees of lid retraction are frequently difficult to evaluate. The resting position of the upper lid is influenced by many factors, including age, alertness, and direction of gaze. Normal variations in resting lid position, or upper lid posture, are exemplified by the striking difference between infants and adults. The infant's eyelid, which barely touches the upper corneal limbus, may appear normal, whereas a similar lid position in an adult is abnormal and represents excessive lid elevation. In general, upper lid position is abnormal if it exposes sclera between the lid margin and the upper corneal limbus when the patient's head is straight and both of the patient's eyes are directed straight ahead.

Eyelid retraction may be unilateral or bilateral. The levator muscle is unique in being subjected to the influence of **two** yoke muscles—the contralateral levator and the ipsilateral superior rectus. Thus, eyelid retraction can result from inappropriate excitation or hyperactivity of ipsilateral levator neurons directly or indirectly via its yoke muscles, from oculosympathetic excitation or inappropriate hyperactivity, and from contracture or shortening of the levator muscle

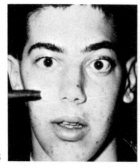
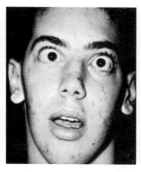
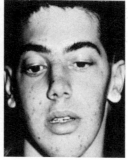

A,B   **C**

Figure 22.22. Bilateral eyelid retraction in a patient with a dorsal mesencephalic syndrome (Collier sign). **A:** The patient has moderate bilateral eyelid retraction when looking straight ahead. **B:** On attempted upward gaze, the eyes do not elevate, but the eyelids elevate normally, producing marked eyelid retraction and stare. **C:** On attempted downward gaze, the eyelids move normally with the eyes, and the eyelid retraction and stare disappear.

or its tendon, Müller's muscle, or the superior rectus muscle. Causes of eyelid retraction may be classified as neuropathic, neuromuscular, myopathic, and mechanical.

Neuropathic Eyelid Retraction

Neuropathic eyelid retraction may be caused by supranuclear, nuclear, or infranuclear mechanisms. In some cases, the pathophysiology is clear; in others, it is either unknown or multifactorial.

Supranuclear Eyelid Retraction   Although true retraction of the eyelids does not usually occur from lesions in the cerebral hemisphere, intermittent or prolonged inappropriate eyelid opening sometimes develops in patients with unilateral nondominant or bilateral cerebral hemisphere disease. Such patients may be unable to close their eyelids on command (i.e., compulsive eye opening), or they may close their eyes only briefly before opening them again (i.e., motor impersistence). These patients have a supranuclear disturbance of orbicularis control and have normal levator relaxation.

Supranuclear bilateral eyelid retraction—**Collier sign**—most commonly occurs with lesions of the dorsal mesencephalon. This type of lid retraction is almost invariably associated with other evidence of dorsal mesencephalic dysfunction, most often a deficiency of upward gaze but also convergence-retraction nystagmus and pupillary light-near dissociation. The dorsal mesencephalic syndrome, also called Parinaud syndrome, is discussed in Chapter 17 of this text. It suffices here to emphasize that the eyelid retraction that occurs with lesions of the dorsal mesencephalon is usually symmetric and sustained as long as the patient directs the eyes straight ahead or slightly upward, increases as the patient looks up, and follows the eyes in a normal fashion when the patient looks down (Fig. 22.22). These features distinguish eyelid retraction from lesions of the dorsal mesencephalon from the more

common form of lid retraction seen in thyroid orbitopathy, in which lid lag is invariably present.

The nucleus of the posterior commissure (nPC) appears to be the premotor structure responsible for mesencephalic lid retraction. As noted previously, lesions that damage this structure in the dorsal mesencephalon generally produce bilateral lid retraction; however, in addition, they may damage the oculomotor nerve fascicle on one side, producing a ptosis on the side of the fascicular damage. This results in a condition characterized by ptosis on one side and primary eyelid retraction (i.e., not secondary to the contralateral ptosis) on the other. This condition is called the "plus-minus syndrome" (Fig. 22.23). Imaging studies in patients with this syndrome show unilateral paramedian lesions, usually infarctions, dorsal and rostral to the red nucleus in the area of the nPC, extending ventrocaudally to the fascicle of the oculomotor nerve on the ptotic side. Thus, damage to the nPC apparently causes bilateral supranuclear lid retraction that may be masked on one side by an associated fascicular oculomotor nerve palsy.

Sustained eyelid retraction may be observed with any of the disorders known to produce a dorsal mesencephalic syndrome. Some common causes include hydrocephalus, stroke, MS, shunt malfunction, and both intrinsic and extrinsic tumors (Fig. 22.24).

Neurodegenerative conditions that cause supranuclear disturbances in upgaze may cause lid retraction. For example, lid retraction is common among patients with progressive supranuclear palsy, Parkinson disease, and Machado-Joseph disease (spinocerebellar ataxia, type 3), and some patients with severe Guillain-Barré syndrome (GBS) demonstrate marked bilateral limitation of upper lid descent during the acute phase of their illness.

Lid retraction and slight downward gaze of both eyes in response to a sudden decrease in ambient light is a physiologic reflex seen in infants between 1 and 5 months of age. Sometimes called the "eye-popping

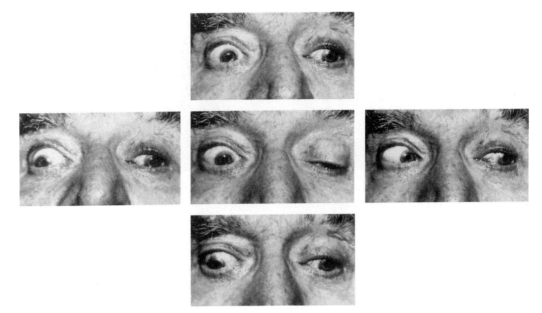

Figure 22.23. Unilateral ptosis associated with contralateral upper eyelid retraction from a lesion of the dorsal mesencephalon that also damages the fascicle of the oculomotor nerve on one side (plus-minus syndrome). The patient has marked eyelid retraction on the right and marked ptosis on the left. There is a paresis of upward gaze, a left third nerve palsy, and lid-lag on downgaze. Computed tomographic scanning showed a paramedian midbrain infarct located ventrally and laterally to the aqueduct, extending from the midline to the area of the red nucleus laterally. (Reprinted from: Gaymard B, Lafitte C, Gelot A, et al. Plus-minus syndrome. *J Neurol Neurosurg Psychiatry.* 1992;55:846–848, with permission.)

reflex" or "nonpathologic lid retraction," it is a useful way of assessing levator function in infants. Transient, clonic, bilateral lid retraction with spastic downward gaze deviation that resolves after several weeks also occurs in otherwise healthy neonates. This may be a variant of the benign, transient, supranuclear disturbances of ocular motility that frequently occur in such infants.

Coma and stupor are commonly associated with eyelid closure caused by an absence of levator tonus. Occasionally, however, levator tonus persists and produces the incongruous picture of intermittently open lids in an unresponsive patient (coma vigil). This sign usually indicates disease of the ventral mesencephalon and pons, but it may occur with diffuse hemisphere disease (persistent vegetative state). Comatose patients with Cheyne-Stokes respiration sometimes open their eyes during the rapid-breathing phase and close them during the slow-breathing phase.

Some patients with extrapyramidal syndromes (e.g., postencephalitic Parkinsonism, progressive supranuclear palsy) have defective inhibition of their eyelids during downward gaze. Such patients have normal lid position when they look straight ahead; however, the lids lag behind briefly as the eyes follow an object downward. Patients with a unilateral midbrain lesion dorsal to the red nucleus may also exhibit lid lag without lid retraction. The lesion in these patients is postulated to disrupt the pathways between the rostral interstitial nucleus of the medial longitudinal fasciculus (MLF) and the central caudal subnucleus of the oculomotor nuclear complex while sparing the nPC.

Synkinetic Eyelid Retraction Elevation of the ipsilateral eyelid may be observed in normal subjects during abduction and, less commonly, on adduction. Lid retraction on attempted abduction in patients with Duane retraction syndrome and in patients with acquired abducens nerve palsies may represent an exaggerated expression of this physiologic synkinesis (Fig. 22.25).

The **Marcus Gunn jaw-winking phenomenon** is a paradoxical elevation of one eyelid that occurs with certain movements of the jaw. It is caused by a synkinesis between the pterygoid muscles and the levator. The associated movements of lid and jaw are termed a "trigemino-oculomotor" synkinesis and are subdivided into an external pterygoid-levator synkinesis and an internal pterygoid-levator synkinesis. Stimuli other than movement of the pterygoids can also produce the same kind of eyelid retraction in some of the patients with this condition.

Simultaneous contraction of the levator with the external pterygoid muscle is the most common form of the Marcus Gunn jaw-winking phenomenon. The

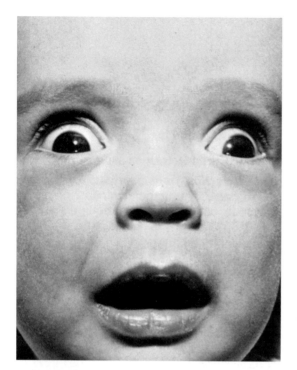

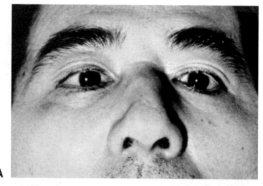

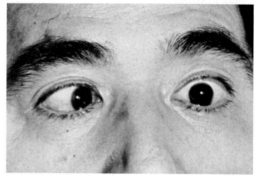

Figure 22.24. Bilateral eyelid retraction in a baby with communicating hydrocephalus. On attempted upgaze, there is no upward movement of the eyes (in fact, the eyes are resting slightly below the horizontal midline), but the eyelids elevate normally. This appearance is often called (the "setting sun" sign).

Figure 22.25. Eyelid retraction associated with left abduction paralysis. **A:** Primary position, the patient's upper eyelids are in normal and equal position. **B:** On attempted gaze left, the left eye abducts only to the midline, and there is elevation of the left upper lid and eyebrow.

affected eyelid is usually ptotic when the jaw muscles are at rest; however, when the jaw muscles contract, the eyelid elevates to a normal position or may even retract and will remain in this position as long as the jaw muscles are active. Elevation of the upper lid may occur (a) when the mandible is moved to the opposite side (contraction of the ipsilateral external pterygoid muscle); (b) when the mandible is projected forward or the tongue is protruded (bilateral contraction of the external pterygoid muscles); or (c) on wide opening of the mouth (i.e., strong depression of the mandible) (Fig. 22.26). In all of these settings, the abnormal levator contraction is most evident when the patient is looking downward.

In most instances, external pterygoid-levator synkinesis is congenital and is first recognized during the act of sucking soon after birth. The condition improves with age in some patients but not in others.

Patients with the Marcus Gunn phenomenon commonly have associated ocular abnormalities, including strabismus, amblyopia, anisometropia, and congenital nystagmus. The most common ocular motor disturbances are double elevator palsy, unilateral superior rectus palsy, Duane retraction syndrome, and adduction palsy with synergistic divergence.

The cause of the synkinesis between the pterygoid muscles and the levator muscle in the Marcus Gunn jaw-winking phenomenon is unknown.

Treatment of patients with the Marcus Gunn jaw-winking phenomenon depends on their ophthalmologic and cosmetic status. Amblyopia should always be treated aggressively, and vertical strabismus should be corrected before attempting surgical repair of ptosis. Eyelid surgery should only be contemplated after the patient (when age permits), parents, and surgeon agree that the jaw-winking, ptosis, or both, are objectionable. Surgery usually consists of weakening the levator aponeurotic complex combined with a lid elevation procedure.

Eyelid Retraction Caused by Oculomotor Nerve Dysfunction   The most common cause of this type of retraction is congenital or acquired **aberrant regeneration of the oculomotor nerve.** In this setting, the retraction is not present at all times and, in fact, ptosis may be present when the patient is looking straight

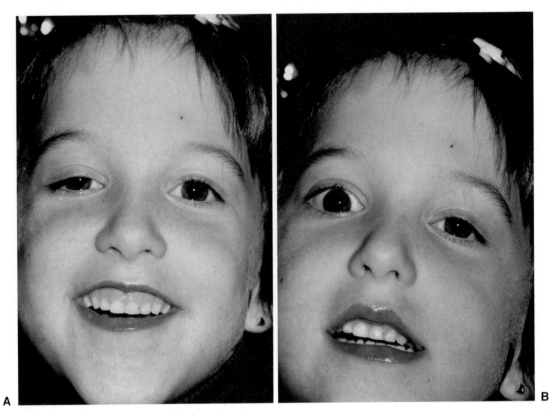

Figure 22.26.   The Marcus Gunn jaw-winking phenomenon. **A:** The child has a congenital right ptosis. **B:** When the child moves her jaw to the left, the right eyelid elevates, and the ptosis disappears. (Courtesy of Dr. Nicholas T. Iliff.)

ahead; however, the lid retracts or at least "hangs up" during attempted infraduction, adduction, or both.

Lid retraction due to aberrant regeneration of the oculomotor nerve usually develops several months after an acute, non-ischemic oculomotor nerve palsy, in which case the condition is known as **secondary aberrant regeneration of the oculomotor nerve.** However, when a slowly progressive compressive process (such as an aneurysm, meningioma, or schwannoma that is usually, but not always, located within the cavernous sinus; see Chapter 18) damages the nerve so slowly that the nerve has time to regenerate, the condition is called **primary aberrant regeneration of the oculomotor nerve.**

Other conditions involving the oculomotor nerve that may cause periodic eyelid retraction are oculomotor palsy with cyclic spasms, a condition that usually is congenital, and ocular neuromyotonia, an acquired condition that usually occurs after radiation therapy for a basal skull mass (see Chapter 18). In both conditions, the eyelid retraction usually is unilateral and associated with pupillary constriction and spasms of one or more of the extraocular muscles innervated by the oculomotor nerve.

Unilateral Eyelid Retraction Associated with Contralateral Ptosis   Patients with unilateral ptosis who, for any of a number of reasons (e.g., congenital or acquired strabismus, amblyopia, cataract), fixate with the eye on the side of the ptosis, may develop retraction of the eyelid on the opposite side (Fig. 22.27). This phenomenon can most easily be diagnosed by prolonged (>5 minutes) occlusion of the eye on the side of the ptosis, which will result in the retracted eyelid assuming a more normal position. Conversely, brief occlusion of the eye on the side of the ptosis probably is the least sensitive method, because the contralateral retracted eyelid may not reposition immediately.

The explanation for the phenomenon of unilateral eyelid retraction associated with contralateral ptosis is based on Hering's law. Intended to explain the conjugate movement of both eyes, Hering's law states that yoked extraocular muscles receive equal degrees of innervation. This law also applies to the levator muscles. Thus, in an attempt to maintain the normal position of a ptotic eyelid, the innervational drive to both lids increases, causing the ptotic lid to assume a more normal position, and the unaffected lid to retract. Secondary retraction of the eyelid in patients with contralateral

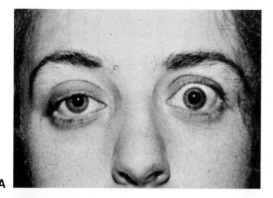

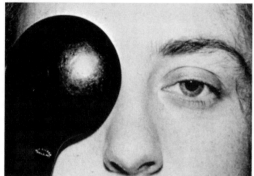

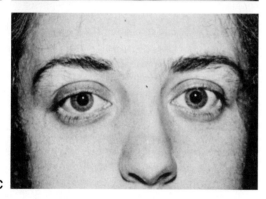

Figure 22.27. Unilateral eyelid retraction secondary to contralateral ptosis (secondary eyelid retraction) in a patient with myasthenia gravis. **A:** The patient has moderate right ptosis and marked left upper eyelid retraction. **B:** When the right eye is covered with an occluder, the left eyelid retraction disappears as levator tonus is reduced bilaterally. **C:** After an intravenous injection of edrophonium chloride (Tensilon®), the right eyelid elevates, and the left eyelid retraction disappears. Eyelid retraction occurs in this setting because Hering's law of equal innervation to agonist muscles applies to the levator muscles as well as to the extraocular muscles.

ptosis is most likely to occur when the ptosis is severe, acquired, and ipsilateral to the dominant eye. The failure to recognize this phenomenon may lead to the erroneous diagnosis of thyroid orbitopathy.

Eyelid Retraction from Sympathetic Hyperfunction
Patients with neck trauma may develop a syndrome of recurrent throbbing headaches and oculosympathetic hyperactivity characterized by ipsilateral lid retraction, hyperhydrosis, and mydriasis—the **Claude-Bernard syndrome**. During the headache-free interval, some of these patients have a Horner syndrome. The syndrome is thought to be caused by sympathetic irritation or hyperactivity.

Sympathetic hyperactivity is thought to be responsible for some cases of lid retraction observed in patients with thyroid orbitopathy (see later). Indeed, dilute solutions of both direct and indirect adrenergic stimulants (e.g., cocaine, hydroxyamphetamine, phenylephrine, apraclonidine, naphazoline) will widen the palpebral fissure in such patients.

Neuromuscular Eyelid Retraction

Transient, spontaneous eyelid retraction may occur in patients with **myasthenia gravis** without evidence of thyroid dysfunction. This phenomenon, which usually occurs on return of the eyes from upward gaze to primary position, appears to be caused by post-tetanic facilitation of the levator muscle. Like the lid retraction of midbrain disease (i.e., Collier sign), neuromuscular lid retraction may be bilateral and symmetric, bilateral but asymmetric, or completely unilateral. Unlike the eyelid retraction of the dorsal mesencephalic syndrome, however, in patients with neuromuscular eyelid retraction, the levator usually fails to "relax" smoothly and completely, and the lid fold fails to smooth out as the eyes move downward. Momentary lid retraction also may be seen in patients with myasthenia after the patient makes an upward saccade from downgaze to primary position (Cogan lid-twitch) (Fig. 22.16). Finally, patients with myasthenia may develop retraction of the eyelid secondary to ptosis of the contralateral eyelid (Fig. 22.27).

Eyelid retraction may result from topical or systemic administration of drugs that affect the neuromuscular junction. The anticholinesterase agents edrophonium chloride (Tensilon®) and neostigmine methylsulfate (Prostigmin®) produce eyelid retraction in some patients with myasthenia gravis. In addition, subparalytic doses of succinylcholine can produce shortening of the levator muscle fibers associated with the depolarization effect of the drug, resulting in lid retraction.

Myopathic Eyelid Retraction

Congenital myopathic eyelid retraction can be unilateral or bilateral and may be associated with nonspecific

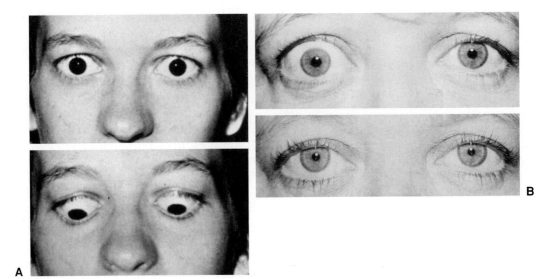

Figure 22.28. Eyelid retraction in patients with dysthyroid orbitopathy. **A:** Bilateral **(top)** associated with lid lag on downward gaze **(bottom)**; **B:** Unilateral before **(top)** and after **(bottom)** eyelid surgery.

strabismus, underaction of the superior rectus on the side of the retraction, or lower lid retraction. The condition also may be associated with other developmental anomalies, including optic disc hypoplasia, craniosynostosis, and Down syndrome. In such cases, levator excursion is normal and there often is lagophthalmos on downgaze, indicating either failure of appropriate inhibition of levator tonus or decreased elasticity of the levator or its suspensory ligaments.

Dysthyroid orbitopathy is the most common cause of acquired unilateral and bilateral sustained lid retraction in both children and adults. The retraction results from pathologic shortening of the levator muscle, resulting in inability of the muscle fibers to lengthen normally. Thus, patients with dysthyroid disease may show retraction of one or both upper eyelids associated with infrequent or incomplete blinking (Stellwag sign), abnormal widening of the palpebral fissure (Dalrymple sign), lid lag on attempted downward gaze (Graefe sign), or a combination of these signs. The retraction itself may be unilateral or bilateral and transient or persistent (Fig. 22.28). It can occur in isolation but is more often associated with other signs of dysthyroid orbitopathy, including proptosis, chemosis, and strabismus. The treatment of eyelid retraction in patients with dysthyroid orbitopathy is primarily surgical and consists of various levator-lengthening procedures.

Eyelid retraction occurs with increased frequency in patients with severe liver disease (Summerskill sign). The appearance is similar to that seen in patients with thyroid orbitopathy.

Myotonic eyelid retraction, lid lag, or both may be observed in patients with familial periodic paralysis (Fig. 22.29). A similar myotonic lid lag may occur in patients with myotonic dystrophy and in patients with congenital myotonia (see Chapter 20).

Mechanical Lid Retraction

Various local processes can damage the eyelid and produce mechanical lid retraction. For example, cutaneous cicatricial changes of the upper eyelid can produce eyelid retraction. The most common causes are burns and deep lacerations. Less commonly, cicatricial eyelid

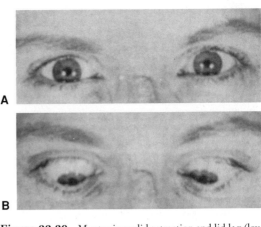

Figure 22.29. Myotonic eyelid retraction and lid lag (levator myotonia) in a patient with hyperkalemic periodic paralysis. **A:** When the patient looks straight ahead, the eyelids are slightly retracted. **B:** On downward gaze, there is marked eyelid lag. (Reprinted from: Layzer RB, Lovelace RE, Rowland LP. Hyperkalemic periodic paralysis. *Arch Neurol.* 1967;16:455–471, with permission.)

retraction occurs from damage to the eyelid from orbital cellulitis with necrosis (particularly from staphylococci and group A streptococci), herpes zoster, scleroderma, or atopic dermatitis.

Eyelid retraction can occasionally be caused by contact lens wear. It resolves when the contact lens is removed. In other cases, a contact lens becomes displaced superiorly but is thought by the patient to have been lost. The retained lens causes an inflammatory reaction in the superior fornix and eventually becomes embedded in an inflammatory cyst, the nature of which may not be appreciated until the cyst is opened surgically and the contact lens is found within it.

Postsurgical lid retraction is most often seen as an overcorrection after surgery for ptosis, although a variety of other orbital and ocular procedures can also result in lid retraction. Mechanisms causing postsurgical lid retraction include damage to the superior rectus muscle, fibrosis of the inferior rectus muscle, and cicatricial adhesions.

Blowout fractures of the orbit may cause lid retraction by entrapment of the surrounding connective tissue. Lid retraction can also occur during an effort to elevate or fixate with a hypotropic or restricted eye.

ABNORMALITIES OF EYELID CLOSURE

As with eyelid opening, abnormalities of eyelid closure may occur from disorders involving any part of the pathway for contracture of the orbicularis oculi, from the cerebral cortex to the muscle itself. Such disorders may be congenital or acquired and may be caused by either hypofunction or hyperfunction of the orbicularis muscle and, to a lesser extent, by the muscles that assist the orbicularis in eyelid closure (i.e., the frontalis, procerus, and corrugator superciliaris).

INSUFFICIENCY OF EYELID CLOSURE

As with eyelid opening, insufficient eyelid closure can be neuropathic, neuromuscular, or myopathic in origin. Arriving at the correct diagnosis thus requires a careful history and complete examination, sometimes followed by appropriate ancillary studies.

Neuropathic Insufficiency of Eyelid Closure

Neuropathic causes of insufficient eyelid closure may be supranuclear, nuclear, or infranuclear. In some cases, the cause is clearly neuropathic but the precise mechanism is unknown or multifactorial.

Supranuclear Insufficiency of Eyelid Closure Voluntary eyelid closure is mediated by the pyramidal system. Patients with localized subcortical capsular lesions usually can close both eyes, although the force of closure is diminished, and the ability to wink

may be lost on the contralateral paretic side (Revilliod sign). In some cases, paresis is profound and yet spontaneous involuntary or emotional movements of the facial and orbicularis muscles remain undisturbed (automatic-voluntary dissociation) (Fig. 22.30).

Bilateral inability to voluntarily close the eyelids may result from a unilateral lesion, usually in the nondominant frontal lobe, but it more commonly develops with bilateral frontal lobe lesions. This phenomenon is called **supranuclear paralysis of voluntary lid closure** or compulsive eye opening. Patients with this syndrome are unable to initiate voluntary closure of either eyelid, even though they retain their ability to comprehend the task and have intact reflex eyelid closure (Fig. 22.31). Supranuclear paralysis of eyelid closure can occur in patients with unilateral or bilateral infarcts or tumors in the frontal lobe, Creutzfeldt-Jakob disease, progressive supranuclear palsy, and motor neuron disease.

Motor **impersistence** of eyelid closure also occurs in patients with bilateral or unilateral hemispheric lesions. When such patients are instructed to close the eyelids and keep them closed, they are unable to obey. The eyelids close, often develop a fine tremor, and then almost immediately reopen. This phenomenon most frequently is seen in patients with a nondominant hemisphere stroke and is most evident during the first week after the stroke. Occasionally, the condition is unilateral.

Nuclear and Fascicular Insufficiency of Eyelid Closure Unilateral weakness of eyelid closure and facial movement may result from unilateral damage to the facial nerve nucleus or fascicle. In such instances, other evidence of brainstem disease is almost always present, including reduction in corneal sensation, ipsilateral abducens nerve paresis or horizontal gaze paralysis, and ipsilateral cerebellar ataxia.

Bilateral weakness of eyelid closure occurs as part of the facial diplegia that is caused by lesions of the pontine tegmentum. Such lesions may be congenital or acquired. Acquired processes include ischemia, inflammation, infiltration, and compression.

When insufficiency of eyelid closure results from damage to the facial nerve fascicle within the brainstem, there usually is complete facial paralysis associated with other signs of brainstem dysfunction, such as ipsilateral horizontal gaze palsy from damage to the ipsilateral abducens nucleus or paramedian pontine reticular formation, ipsilateral abduction weakness from damage to the ipsilateral abducens nerve fascicle, and contralateral hemiparesis from damage to the ipsilateral pyramidal tract (Fig. 22.32). The combination of ipsilateral facial nerve palsy, ipsilateral abduction weakness, and contralateral hemiparesis is called the Millard-Gubler syndrome (see Chapter 18).

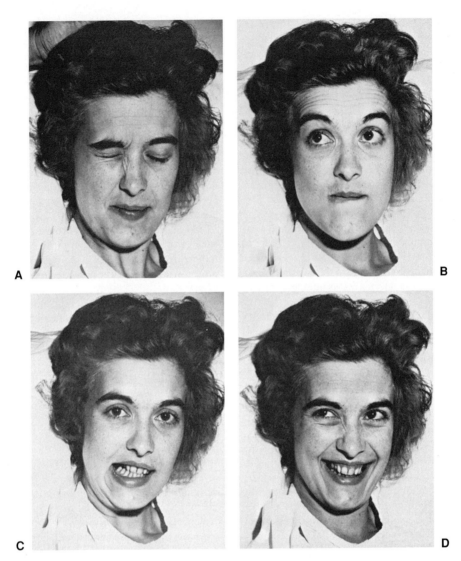

Figure 22.30. Central volitional (supranuclear) paralysis of the orbicularis oculi after a subcortical hematoma that caused a left hemiplegia and a left facial nerve paresis. **A:** When the patient is told to close her eyes tightly, the left orbicularis oculi, left corrugator muscle, and the other muscles of the left lower side of the face fail to respond. **B:** Volitional control of the forehead is normal. **C:** Left lower facial weakness is evident when the patient attempts to show her teeth. **D:** A spontaneous smile (emotional-extrapyramidal-facial innervation) evokes symmetric contraction of all facial muscles, including the orbicularis oculi, indicating that nuclear and infranuclear pathways are intact.

Insufficiency of Eyelid Closure from Peripheral Facial Nerve Palsy Insufficiency or weakness of eyelid closure associated with lesions of the facial nerve is usually combined with weakness of other facial muscles supplied by that nerve. Topographic diagnosis of facial nerve paresis may be facilitated by the relationship of the facial nerve to surrounding structures and by the fact that along its course, the nerve gives off various branches that subserve specific functions. The facial nerve, in addition to innervating the facial musculature, is also responsible for reflex tearing (via the greater superficial petrosal nerve), hearing (via the nerve to the stapedius muscle), taste on the anterior two thirds of the tongue (via the chorda tympani), and salivation (via nerve branches to the sublingual and submandibular glands) (Fig. 22.33). Thus, by testing reflex tearing, hearing, taste, and ability of an individual with peripheral facial weakness to produce saliva, one often can determine the location of the responsible lesion. In addition, various electrodiagnostic tests, including nerve excitability, electromyography, blink reflex, and electroneurography help determine

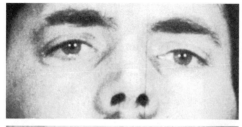

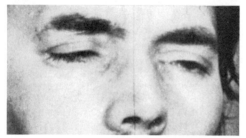

Figure 22.31. Supranuclear paralysis of voluntary eyelid closure (compulsive eyelid opening) in a patient with Creutzfeldt-Jakob disease. **A:** The patient has no movement of the eyelids when told to close his eyes, even though he understands what he is being told to do and is attempting to do it. **B:** The patient shows some ability to blink to a visual threat. (Reprinted from: Russell RW. Supranuclear palsy of eyelid closure. *Brain.* 1980;103:71–82, with permission.)

the extent of dysfunction and prognosis for facial nerve recovery.

Lesions in the cerebellopontine angle (CPA) that produce unilateral facial nerve paresis usually also produce signs and symptoms related to dysfunction of the vestibulocochlear and trigeminal nerves. Common manifestations thus include unilateral sensorineural hearing loss, tinnitus, vertigo, facial pain and numbness, corneal hypesthesia, and unsteadiness of gait. All of the components of the facial nerve may be affected. Less common manifestations include hemifacial spasm, nystagmus, evidence of cerebellar dysfunction (e.g., ataxia and tremor), and hydrocephalus. Nevertheless, although most patients with lesions in the CPA present with multiple neurologic findings, facial nerve paralysis may be the only manifestation, particularly in children.

Lesions of the CPA that may cause a facial nerve paresis include vestibular and trigeminal schwannomas, meningiomas, epidermoids, lipomas, arachnoid cysts, aneurysms, metastatic lesions, and glomus jugulare tumors (Fig. 22.34). Granulomas associated with tuberculosis, sarcoid, syphilis, or certain fungal infections can also damage the facial nerve in the CPA.

A facial nerve lesion located within the facial canal between the internal auditory meatus and the geniculate ganglion produces many of the same signs as those encountered with lesions in the CPA, except that

brainstem signs are absent, and there is no evidence of dysfunction of the trigeminal nerve. Lesions between the geniculate ganglion and the branch to the stapedius muscle produce similar manifestations except that reflex lacrimation is preserved because the lesion is distal to the superficial petrosal nerve. Damage to the facial nerve between the branch to the stapedius muscle and the chorda tympani produces facial paralysis, loss of taste on the anterior two thirds of the tongue, and diminution of salivary secretion.

Lesions of the facial nerve distal to the takeoff of the chorda tympani produce only facial motor paralysis. Facial neuropathies that localize to the intratemporal portion of the facial nerve may be caused by fractures of the temporal bone, herpes zoster (Ramsey Hunt syndrome), otitis media, and neoplasms. The condition called "Bell's palsy" belongs in this category. Lesions distal to the stylomastoid foramen may affect one or more peripheral branches of the facial nerve and are usually caused by facial trauma, facial surgery, or disease of the parotid gland.

Most isolated facial nerve palsies are idiopathic and are called Bell's palsy. The diagnosis of Bell's palsy is based on a constellation of findings and the exclusion of other known causes. The condition usually is unilateral. About 60% of patients with Bell's palsy have a history of a viral prodrome. The onset of facial motor weakness is acute and frequently accompanied by pain or numbness of the face, neck, or tongue. The pain is characteristically located in the retroauricular area. Hypesthesia or dysesthesia in the distribution of the trigeminal or glossopharyngeal nerve occurs in 25% to 35% of patients. Sensory findings may precede the onset of facial paresis and usually do not persist beyond 7 to 10 days. Dysgeusia and dysacusis are fairly common accompaniments. Both subjective and objective signs of dry eye may be present, and epiphora from exposure or paralytic ectropion is common. Mounting evidence implicates a viral etiology in the pathogenesis of Bell's palsy, most likely herpes simplex. Nevertheless, some authors maintain that the crucial factor is swelling of the facial nerve (from inflammation, ischemia, or both) within the facial canal.

Overall, about 85% of patients with Bell's palsy eventually recover completely or are left with only slight residual deficits. The remaining 15% have permanent deficits consisting of residual weakness, tonic contracture, synkinesis, spasms, or gustatory lacrimation (crocodile tears). Clinical factors that adversely affect recovery include advanced age (over 60), diabetes mellitus, complete paralysis, decreased tearing, hyperacusis, and delay in the onset of recovery.

The efficacy of systemic corticosteroids in the treatment of Bell's palsy is somewhat controversial. Patients treated with prednisone appear to have less denervation and greater improvement in functional grade at

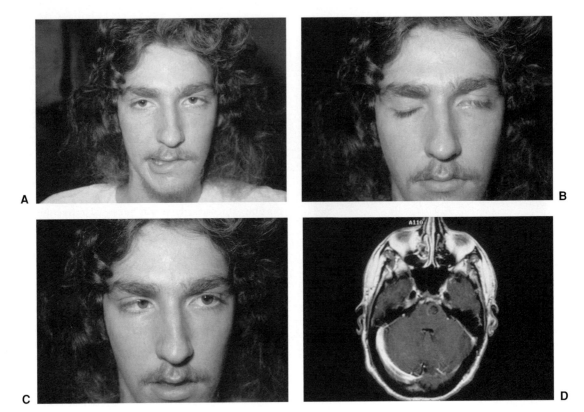

Figure 22.32. Insufficiency of eyelid closure in a patient with a left-sided fascicular seventh nerve paresis caused by an intrapontine hemorrhage from a cavernous angioma. **A:** The patient has left-sided facial weakness; **B:** The patient cannot close the left eyelid completely; **C:** The patient has an ipsilateral abducens nerve paresis. **D:** MRI shows a large lesion on the left side of the ventral pons consistent with a cavernous angioma.

recovery than patients who are not treated in some studies but not in others. Although steroids may not entirely prevent partial denervation or contracture, their use may speed recovery and may also reduce the risk of gustatory lacrimation from autonomic synkinesis and of progression from incomplete to complete paralysis. Thus, most physicians treat patients with prednisone in a dose of 1 mg/kg/day for 10 to 14 days followed by a rapid taper.

Because herpes simplex virus has been implicated in the pathogenesis of Bell's palsy, many physicians treat patients with the condition with acyclovir along with systemic corticosteroids. However, there is no difference in the outcome of patients treated with steroids alone compared with patients treated with both steroids and acyclovir.

An isolated facial nerve palsy that may mimic Bell's palsy can occur in a number of systemic disorders. These include infections and inflammations (herpes zoster oticus, acquired immune deficiency syndrome, otitis media, mastoiditis, Lyme disease, syphilis, sarcoidosis, tetanus), ischemia (diabetes mellitus, hy-

pertension), and immunemediated inflammatory diseases (periarteritis, GBS, postvaccination demyelination, MS). Neoplastic causes of isolated peripheral facial palsy include vestibular and facial nerve schwannomas, meningiomas, glomus jugulare tumors, lipomas, dermoids, epidermoids, parotid tumors, carcinomatous meningitis, cholesteatomas, metastatic tumors, and lymphoid lesions. Miscellaneous causes include toxic agents (thalidomide, ethylene glycol, organophosphate poisoning), trauma (temporal bone fractures, facial injuries, barotrauma from scuba diving), iatrogenic injuries (from local anesthetic blocks and facial surgery), amyloidosis, Paget disease, and benign intracranial hypertension.

Because so many conditions can cause an acute, initially isolated, facial nerve paresis, progression of a facial palsy for longer than 3 weeks, lack of recovery after 3 to 6 months, development of hemifacial spasm, prolonged otalgia or facial pain, or recurrence of paralysis after recovery should prompt closer investigation of a "Bell's palsy" to rule out an underlying systemic inflammatory or infectious etiology or a neoplasm.

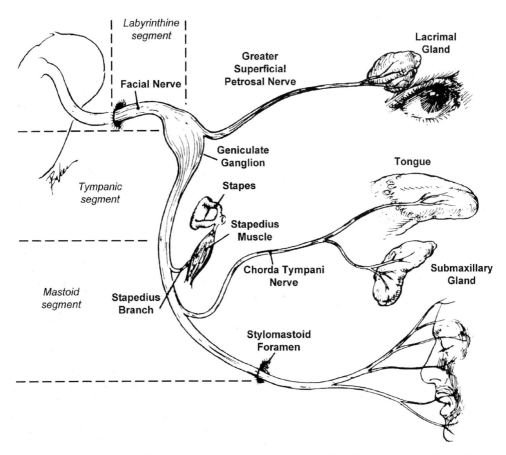

Figure 22.33. Schematic drawing of the branches of the facial nerve showing the different functions of those branches. The branches and their functions include the greater superficial petrosal nerve (reflex tearing), the nerve to the stapedius muscle (stapedius reflex), the chorda tympani nerve (taste on the anterior two thirds of the tongue and submaxillary gland secretion), and peripheral motor branches to the facial muscles. (Reprinted from: Alford BR, Jerger JF, Coats AC, et al. Neurophysiology of facial nerve testing. *Arch Otolaryngol.* 1973;97:214–219, with permission.)

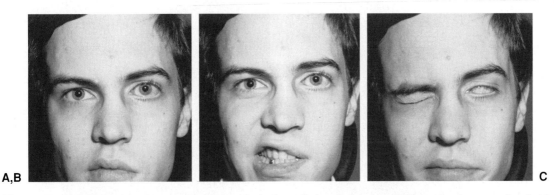

Figure 22.34. Peripheral facial nerve palsy after removal of a vestibular schwannoma. **A:** The patient has a complete facial nerve palsy. Note the widened left lid fissure and sag of the left lower eyelid. **B:** When the patient attempts to show his teeth, lower facial weakness is evident. This weakness did not improve when extrapyramidal facial innervation was stimulated. **C:** On attempted eyelid closure, there is almost complete paralysis of the left orbicularis oculi muscle. Note intact Bell's phenomenon.

In patients with congenital or developmental facial nerve paresis, there may be other evidence of incomplete development (i.e., hypoplasia) or agenesis of the facial nerve. Such patients may have Möbius syndrome, congenital unilateral lower lip paralysis (CULLP), hemifacial microsomia, or other associated developmental defects, such as aural atresia and microtia. Acquired prenatal causes include birth trauma and exposure to thalidomide or rubella virus.

Less than 1% of all facial nerve palsies are bilateral and simultaneous. Such cases usually are idiopathic (i.e., Bell's palsy) or caused by Lyme disease, sarcoidosis, GBS, Fisher syndrome, brainstem encephalitis, or neoplasia (e.g., carcinomatous meningitis, glioma). Less common causes include meningitis (e.g., from syphilis, tuberculosis, cryptococcus), diabetes mellitus, head trauma, pontine hemorrhage, systemic lupus erythematosus, ethylene glycol ingestion, benign intracranial hypertension, and Wernicke-Korsakoff syndrome.

The rehabilitation and supportive management of patients with a facial nerve palsy depend on the stage and severity of facial weakness. During the acute phase, treatment should be directed at preventing the complications of corneal exposure by using topical lubricants and, in some cases, cellophane wrap occlusive dressings or self-adhesive occlusive bubbles. If supportive therapy fails, a temporary or permanent tarsorrhaphy should be performed. When the facial nerve has been severed or severely damaged, and recovery is not likely to occur, procedures that juxtapose the upper and lower eyelids and improve eyelid (and other facial muscle) function should be considered, including permanent tarsorrhaphy, lateral canthoplasty to treat the effects of paralytic ectropion, and insertion of a gold weight or palpebral spring (cerclage) to reanimate the upper eyelid. Facial reanimation can sometimes be accomplished using a variety of techniques, including direct facial nerve repair, autogenous nerve grafts, cross facial nerve grafting, and nerve crossovers using the hypoglossal nerve. In addition, temporalis muscle transfers, free-muscle grafts, and facial suspension with fascia lata, tendon, or alloplastic materials can be used.

Abnormal Eyelid Closure Associated with Aberrant Regeneration of the Facial Nerve Aberrant regeneration of the facial nerve (AFR) may occur after damage to the facial nerve, particularly after compression, trauma, or Bell's palsy. The previously paralyzed side of the face is invariably weak and may appear contracted (Fig. 22.35). Typically, each closure of the eye occurs simultaneously with a twitch at the corner of the mouth that also may be accompanied by dimpling of the chin and contraction of the platysma. During forced lid closure, there is an exaggerated contraction of all facial muscles on the side of the previously paretic facial nerve. Conversely, both voluntary and involuntary movements of the lips or the corner of the mouth precipitate co-contraction of the orbicularis oculi on

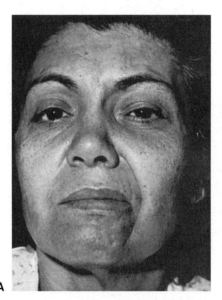
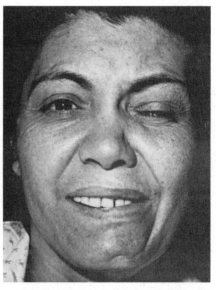

A   **B**

Figure 22.35. Aberrant regeneration of the left facial nerve after an acute peripheral facial nerve paresis (Bell's palsy) producing facial contracture and partial closure of the left eyelid associated with certain movements of the mouth. **A:** The patient has a narrowed left interpalpebral fissure and a deepened left nasolabial groove. **B:** Any spontaneous or voluntary movement of the lower face, such as trying to smile, produces co-movements of all muscles on the left side of the face, resulting in eyelid closure.

the affected side that may superficially resemble hemifacial spasm or the inverse Marcus Gunn jaw-winking phenomenon (see the previous text); however, unlike hemifacial spasm, which occurs spontaneously (see the subsequent text), the eyelid and facial spasms that occur in patients with aberrant regeneration of the facial nerve are induced by voluntary or involuntary movements of the eyelid or mouth. Similarly, unlike the inverse Marcus Gunn phenomenon, in which the eyelid closure is caused by levator inhibition, narrowing of the lid fissure in aberrant regeneration of the facial nerve is caused by inappropriate contraction of the orbicularis oculi muscle.

Neuromuscular Insufficiency of Eyelid Closure

The orbicularis oculi often is weak in diseases that affect the neuromuscular junction. **Myasthenia gravis** characteristically produces weakness of eyelid closure, usually combined with ptosis. This weakness of orbicularis function is responsible for the "peek phenomenon," in which a patient with myasthenia gravis initially is able to close the eyelids, but as closure is maintained, the orbicularis fatigues and the eyelids separate, exposing the globe. Weakness of the orbicularis oculi in patients with neuromuscular disease also may be characterized by retraction of the lower eyelid. Botulism also can cause weakness of the facial muscles, including the eyelids, as can certain envenomations (e.g., snake and spider bites) that affect the neuromuscular junction. The diagnosis of neuromuscular disease, particularly myasthenia gravis, should be considered in any patient with weakness of eyelid closure associated with ptosis, ophthalmoparesis, or both.

Myopathic Insufficiency of Eyelid Closure

The orbicularis oculi muscle is almost always weakened by any disease that weakens the facial musculature. Weakness of the orbicularis muscle may be characterized not only by weakness of spontaneous or forced eyelid closure but also by lack of upper facial expression, wasting of eyelid tissue, and fatigue of the eyelids during attempted sustained closure. In addition, there may be retraction of the lower eyelid or paralytic ectropion (Figs. 22.34 and 22.36). Myogenic weakness of the orbicularis oculi is usually bilateral. Weakness in the pretarsal segment impairs blinking but must be significant before blinking is overtly impaired. Because lacrimal drainage depends in part on normal muscle action in the lower eyelid, weakness of contraction may result in epiphora. The most common causes of myopathic insufficiency of eyelid closure are congenital muscular dystrophy, myotonic dystrophy, and the mitochondrial cytopathies associated with CPEO (Fig. 22.37).

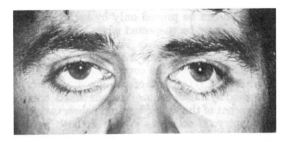

Figure 22.36. Bilateral, symmetric lower eyelid retraction in a patient with myotonic dystrophy and generalized facial weakness. (Reprinted from: Cohen MM, Lessell S. Retraction of the lower eyelid. *Neurology.* 1979;29:386–389, with permission.)

EXCESSIVE OR ANOMALOUS EYELID CLOSURE

Unlike insufficient eyelid closure, which can be caused by neurologic, neuromuscular, or myopathic causes, excessive or inappropriate eyelid closure usually is neurologic in origin.

Essential Blepharospasm and the Blepharospasm-Oromandibular Dystonia Syndrome (Meige Syndrome; Brueghel Syndrome)

Blepharospasm is an involuntary closure of the eyelids evoked by contraction of the orbicularis oculi. When blepharospasm occurs in isolation without other

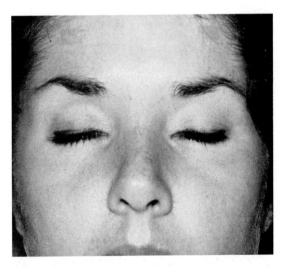

Figure 22.37. Bilateral orbicularis oculi weakness in a patient with the Kearns-Sayre syndrome variant of CPEO. The patient is attempting to close her eyelids as tightly as possible. Note lack of folds in the upper eyelids and inability to bury the lashes.

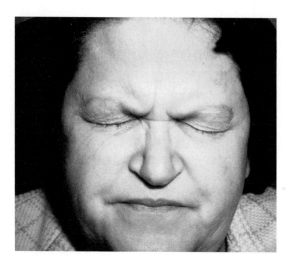

Figure 22.38. Essential blepharospasm. The patient first noted intermittent spasms of lid closure several years earlier. By the time she was examined, she was experiencing almost continuous, bilateral symmetric spasms of the orbicularis oculi muscles.

evidence of neurologic or ocular disease, the condition is called essential blepharospasm (Fig. 22.38). When these focal dystonic eyelid movements spread to other cranial muscles, the syndrome is called blepharospasm-oromandibular dystonia or Meige syndrome. The disorder occurs most frequently in women over 50 years of age. Initially, there is an increased frequency of blinking, particularly in response to sunlight, wind, noise, movement, or stress. This blinking progresses to involuntary spasms, initially on one side, but inevitably on both. Certain maneuvers like touching the eyelid, coughing, vocalizing, or chewing gum may alleviate the spasms, which increase in frequency and severity as the disease progresses.

Patients with Meige syndrome may experience involuntary chewing movements, lip pursing, trismus, wide opening of the mouth, spasmodic deviations of the jaw, abnormal tongue movements (protrusion, retraction, and writhing), spasmodic dysphonia, and, rarely, difficulty swallowing. In addition to orofacial spasms, such patients may have oculogyric crises, platysmal contractions, torticollis, retrocollis, or other forms of focal dystonia. Generalized dystonia is rare, however.

Many patients with essential blepharospasm and Meige syndrome stop reading, watching television, and driving; some become depressed, occupationally disabled and, in some cases, functionally blind. The disorder may plateau at any point along its progression. Remissions are rare but occur in about 11% of patients, almost always within 5 years of the onset of symptoms.

Most cases of essential blepharospasm and Meige syndrome are sporadic, although there are familial occurrences. In addition, patients with essential blepharospasm and Meige syndrome often have a family history of other movement disorders, or they may give a past history of tics or excessive blinking, sometimes dating back to childhood. Thus, familial blepharospasm and craniocervical dystonia may be phenotypically heterogeneous and autosomal-dominantly inherited with incomplete penetrance.

Many patients with blepharospasm, whether of the essential variety or part of Meige syndrome, complain of dryness, grittiness, irritation, or photophobia. Some of these patients have evidence of dry eyes or ocular surface disease by slit-lamp biomicroscopy or Schirmer testing, whereas in others, there is no apparent reason for their complaints.

The cause of essential blepharospasm and Meige syndrome is unknown, but there is abundant clinical and neurophysiologic evidence that essential blepharospasm and Meige syndrome are **focal dystonias** caused by dysfunction of the basal ganglia or brainstem

Botulinum toxin type A is the primary form of therapy for patients with blepharospasm. Its effect generally lasts 2 to 4 months. Other drugs, such as clonazepam, trihexyphenidyl, and tetrabenazine, can also be used to treat essential blepharospasm and Meige syndrome, but they are less efficacious. Essential blepharospasm also can be treated surgically by removing all or part of the orbicularis oculi muscle; however, complications, variable effectiveness, and frequent recurrence are major limitations of this approach. We believe that surgery should be reserved for patients with disabling blepharospasm that does not respond to botulinum toxin, oral medications, or a combination of these treatments, or for patients who cannot tolerate these treatments.

Patients with essential blepharospasm often have associated dermatochalasis, ptosis, or both. These can be treated with blepharoplasty and ptosis surgery, both of which often reduce the severity of the blepharospasm to some extent. However, these procedures are merely adjuncts to the treatment of blepharospasm and should not be considered as primary treatments for the condition.

Blepharospasm Associated with Lesions of the Brainstem and Basal Ganglia

Blepharospasm may be caused by a variety of lesions and disorders of the basal ganglia and mesodiencephalic region. These include strokes, MS, progressive supranuclear palsy, Parkinson disease, Huntington disease, Wilson disease, Lytico-Bodig syndrome, Hallervorden-Spatz syndrome, olivopontocerebellar atrophy, communicating hydrocephalus, and encephalitis lethargica.

Blepharoclonus

Typical blepharospasm is characterized by repetitive episodes of tonic contractions of the orbicularis oculi, and EMG studies show that the orbicularis contractions in many such patients consist of rhythmic phasic bursts at a rate of 3 to 6 Hz. When such contractions result in visible repetitive upward jerks of the eyelids, the term **blepharoclonus** is used. Blepharoclonus occurs in patients with brainstem syndromes caused by stroke or trauma, hydrocephalus from aqueductal stenosis in the setting of Parkinsonism, and MS.

Ocular Blepharospasm

Blepharospasm occasionally is caused by irritative or painful ocular disease. Photophobia and lacrimation are also present in patients with this form of blepharospasm, often called **ocular blepharospasm.** The most common causes of ocular blepharospasm are disturbances of the eyelids (e.g., blepharitis, trichiasis, entropion), disturbances of the corneal epithelium, severe dry eyes, iritis, scleritis, and angle-closure glaucoma. Although less common, patients with ocular albinism, congenital achromatopsia, aniridia, or posterior subcapsular cataracts may experience blepharospasm and photophobia in response to bright light. Chemotherapeutic agents such as cyclophosphamide, doxorubicin, fluorouracil, tegafur (furanyl-5-fluorouracil), and mitomycin-C may produce ocular irritation and severe blepharospasm, as may a variety of topical medications.

Rarely, patients with strabismus develop what appears to be a unilateral tonic blepharospasm to avoid diplopia. This is particularly common in patients with acquired paralytic strabismus and in patients with intermittent exotropia. It is most obvious in bright light.

In our experience, true ocular blepharospasm is rare. Nevertheless, ocular causes of blepharospasm should always be excluded before a search for a neurologic cause of blepharospasm is undertaken or a diagnosis of essential blepharospasm is made.

Blepharospasm Associated with Drug-Induced Tardive Dyskinesia

Patients with tardive dyskinesia have blepharospasm and facial tics similar to those seen in patients with Meige syndrome (see the previous text); however, patients with tardive dyskinesia have choreic movements of the extremities as opposed to the more sustained, dystonic movements observed in patients with Meige syndrome. The most important distinguishing feature of tardive dyskinesia, however, is that it is always drug-induced, usually developing 1 to 2 years after starting the medication. In most instances, the responsible agents are antipsychotic or neuroleptic drugs, such as dopamine-blocking or dopamine-stimulating agents.

Drug-induced dyskinesia can also occur after the use of antiemetics, anorectics, or nasal decongestants that contain sympathomimetic agents and antihistamines.

The blepharospasm and facial tics of tardive dyskinesia may improve if the drug responsible is identified and discontinued. If the symptoms persist, or if the drug cannot be stopped for medical reasons, botulinum toxin can be used to control the spasms.

Facial Tics and Tourette Syndrome

In contrast to the sustained, dystonic movements typical of blepharospasm, facial tics are usually brief, clonic, and jerk-like. They tend to be stereotyped and repetitive. They can vary in frequency, increasing when the patient is bored, tired, or anxious. Eye-winking tics are most commonly observed in childhood, tend to be unilateral, and affect boys more often than girls. They resolve spontaneously after months or years.

When facial tics begin between 2 and 15 years of age, last more than 1 year, fluctuate in severity, and are associated with tics in multiple other bodily locations, vocalizations (e.g., grunting, sniffing, barking, throat-clearing, utterance of obscenities), obscene gestures, and other aberrancies of behavior, Tourette syndrome (also called Gilles de la Tourette syndrome) is the likely diagnosis. Ocular manifestations are common in this condition and include increased blinking, blepharospasm, forced staring, and involuntary gaze deviation.

Nonorganic Blepharospasm

Nonorganic blepharospasm generally has a sudden onset and usually is preceded by an emotionally traumatic event. Although quite rare, it is more common among children and young adults with serious psychologic problems. The blepharospasm is frequently bilateral and may last for hours, weeks, or even months, at which point it may resolve spontaneously. The eyelids are sometimes gently, sometimes forcibly, closed. In some patients, psychotherapy, behavior therapy, hypnosis, or biofeedback are of benefit. In others, a single injection of botulinum toxin is sufficient to eliminate the spasms permanently.

Focal Seizures

Several eyelid phenomena are associated with seizures. An adversive (jacksonian) seizure from an irritative focus in the frontal eye fields can evoke contralateral spasmodic eyelid closure, twitching of the face, and "spastic" lateral gaze. Blinking or fluttering of the eyelids also may be observed in psychomotor or absence seizures. Blinking is usually bilateral and symmetric, although unilateral blinking ipsilateral to the seizure focus has been described.

Lid-Triggered Synkinesias

Eyelid closure occasionally triggers movements of muscles that are not innervated by the facial nerve, presumably from a central or supranuclear disturbance. In some patients with such eyelid-triggered dyskinesias, firm external stimulation of the cornea elicits a brisk anterolateral jaw movement to the side opposite the stimulus associated with eyelid closure: the **corneomandibular reflex**. In other patients, an acquired **palpebromandibular synkinesia** is present that is similar to the corneomandibular reflex except that the jaw movements that regularly accompany spontaneous eye blinks can occur without an external corneal stimulus. The palpebromandibular reflex usually is associated with bihemispheric or upper brainstem pathology.

Facial Myokymia (with and without Spastic Paretic Facial Contracture)

The term *facial myokymia* refers to involuntary, fine, continuous, undulating contractions that spread across facial muscles. The contractions are usually unilateral. Electrophysiologically, affected muscles show brief tetanic bursts of motor-unit potentials that recur in a rhythmic or semirhythmic fashion several times a second as singlets, doublets, or groups. These bursts recur at a rate of 3 to 8 Hz.

The most common type of facial myokymia occurs in otherwise normal persons and affects only the orbicularis oculi of the lower (or, occasionally, the upper) eyelid on one side. This **eyelid myokymia** often begins at times of excessive fatigue or stress. It usually lasts for several days, but it may persist for a few weeks and even for several months. During this time, it is usually intermittent, lasting for several hours at a time. Patients with this condition may become alarmed, particularly because they can feel the eyelid fasciculations. They often believe that their eye is "jumping," and some patients actually experience oscillopsia from the effects of the myokymic eyelid against the globe; however, this type of transient eyelid myokymia is almost always benign.

Eyelid myokymia that persists continuously for several months or even years is usually an isolated phenomenon of no systemic or neurologic significance; however, it also may be the first sign of MS or an intrinsic lesion near the facial nerve nucleus in the dorsal pons. Thus, we believe that patients in whom isolated eyelid myokymia persists for more than 3 months should undergo MR imaging, as should patients with eyelid myokymia who have or develop other neurologic manifestations.

Many disorders characterized by involuntary movements of the facial muscles can begin with eyelid myokymia, including essential blepharospasm, Meige syndrome, hemifacial spasm, and **spastic-paretic facial contracture**. This last disorder is characterized by myokymia that first begins in the orbicularis oculi muscle and gradually spreads to most of the muscles on one side of the face. At the same time, associated tonic contracture of the affected muscles becomes evident. Over a period of weeks or months, the nasolabial groove slowly deepens, the corner of the mouth is drawn laterally, the palpebral fissure narrows, and all the facial muscles become weak. As the contracture becomes more pronounced, voluntary facial movements on the affected side diminish (Fig. 22.39). Spastic-paretic facial contracture is a sign of pontine dysfunction in the region of the facial nerve nucleus. Disorders that may produce it include MS, intrinsic brainstem neoplasms (particularly gliomas but also metastatic tumors), extra-axial neoplasms compressing the brainstem (e.g., chordomas), syringobulbia, brainstem vascular lesions, GBS, obstructive hydrocephalus, subarachnoid hemorrhage, basilar invagination, Machado-Joseph disease, brainstem tuberculoma, cysticercosis, and autosomal-dominant striatonigral degeneration. In most instances, the phenomenon and the pathology that causes it are unilateral, but bilateral facial myokymia from bilateral pontine disease may occur in patients with GBS, following cardiopulmonary arrest, during the course of a lymphocytic meningoradiculitis, and following exposure to a variety of toxins.

The pathophysiology of transient facial myokymia is unknown; however, MR imaging in patients with MS who have continuous facial myokymia often shows changes consistent with demyelination in the postgenu portion of the fascicle of the facial nerve in the dorsolateral pontine tegmentum. In all autopsy cases in which a brainstem tumor is responsible for the condition, the tumor infiltrates the pontine tegmentum, basis pontis, or both, sparing the facial nerve nucleus and its neurons. It has therefore been suggested that the lack of direct damage to the ipsilateral facial nerve nucleus in the presence of more rostrally placed lesions produces a functional deafferentation, possibly of local circuit neurons. This, in turn, results in hyperexcitability of facial nerve neurons, thus causing myokymia or spastic-paretic facial contracture. When the facial nerve nucleus itself is damaged by the pathologic process, the facial spasm resolves, leaving only facial paralysis and contracture.

Hemifacial Spasm

Hemifacial spasm (HFS) is characterized by involuntary paroxysmal bursts of painless, unilateral, tonic or clonic contractions of muscles innervated by the facial nerve (Fig. 22.40). It occurs most commonly in middle-aged adults, but it may develop at any age. The condition is almost always sporadic, but there are

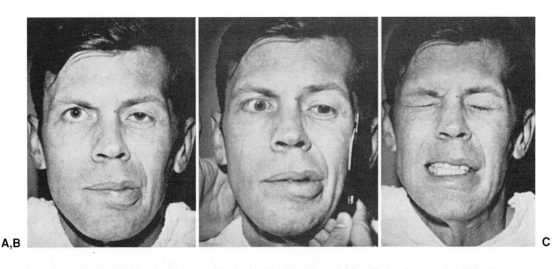

A,B
C

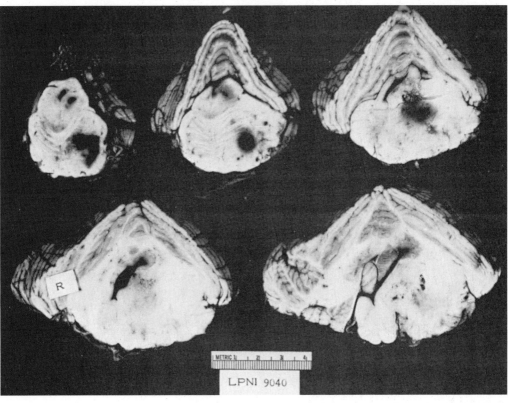

D

Figure 22.39. Spastic paretic facial contracture associated with a pontine astrocystoma. **A:** The patient's face is at rest. Note deepened nasolabial groove and narrowed palpebral fissure on the left. **B:** On attempted left gaze, the patient shows a horizontal gaze palsy. **C:** Voluntary forced eyelid closure exposes the paresis of the left orbicularis oculi and the left side of the face. The patient subsequently died and an autopsy was performed. **D:** Serial sections through the brainstem of the patient show a left-sided astrocytoma. (Reprinted from: Sogg RL, Hoyt WF, Boldrey E. Spastic paretic facial contracture: A rare sign of brain stem tumor. *Neurology.* 1963;13:607–612, with permission.)

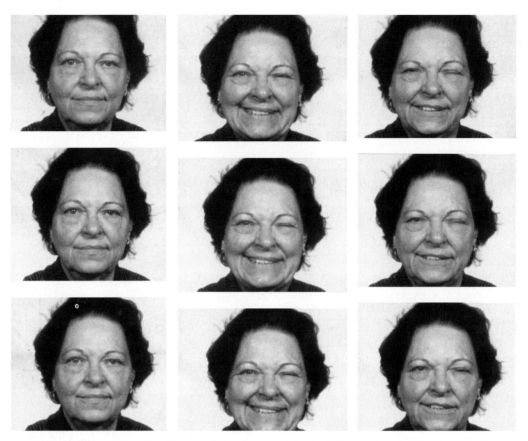

Figure 22.40. Left hemifacial spasm. Photograph is a composite of multiple frames of a video that shows the development of the hemifacial spasm. Note that between spasms, the patient's face appears normal; however, when the spasms occur, the left side of the mouth draws up, the midfacial muscles contract, and the left eyelid closes. (Reprinted from: Garibaldi DC, Miller NR. Tortuous basilar artery as etiology of hemifacial spasm. *Arch Neurol.* 2003;60:626–627, with permission.)

familial cases. Bilateral cases occur but are exceptionally rare, and most reported cases probably are examples of essential blepharospasm or Meige syndrome.

HFS usually first appears as spasms of the orbicularis oculi and then spreads slowly to the lower facial muscles over months to years. The spasms may occur spontaneously or be triggered by voluntary facial movements or changes in position, and they may worsen with fatigue, stress, or anxiety. Long-standing HFS almost always is associated with ipsilateral lower facial weakness, although this may be hard to detect, either because it usually is fairly mild or because of the constant spasms. In addition, many patients with HFS have clinical evidence, EMG evidence, or both, of synkinesis between the orbicularis oculi and orbicularis oris muscles.

Most cases of HFS are thought to be caused by pulsatile compression of the proximal region of the facial nerve at the root entry zone (the transitional zone between central and peripheral myelin) by normal vessels in an aberrant location or by dolichoectatic vessels. The blood vessels most commonly responsible for the compression are the anterior inferior cerebellar artery, the posterior inferior cerebellar artery, and the vertebral artery. Less commonly, one or more veins accompanying these vessels appear to be responsible. A variety of imaging techniques, including CT scanning, MR imaging, MR angiography, and CT angiography may show ipsilateral displacement, tortuosity, or enlargement of the basilar or vertebral arteries in patients with HFS (Fig. 22.41).

Although HFS appears to be caused by vascular compression from otherwise normal arteries or veins in over 99% of cases, a variety of other structures also can compress the facial nerve at the root entry zone, producing HFS. These lesions include aneurysms, AVMs, infratemporal hemangiomas, and arterial dissections as well as extra-axial tumors located in the CPA such as epidermoids, vestibular schwannomas (acoustic neuromas), meningiomas, cholesteatomas, and lipomas. Occasionally, HSF is produced by intraparenchymal brainstem lesions, including tumors and granulomas.

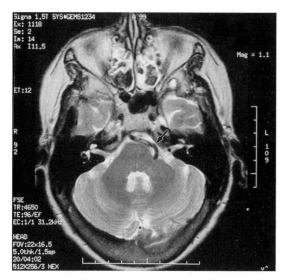

Figure 22.41. Neuroimaging showing vascular compression of the left facial nerve in a the patient with ipsilateral hemifacial spasm shown in Figure 22.40. Proton-density magnetic resonance image, axial view, shows compression of the left facial nerve (*) by a tortuous basilar artery (*arrow*). The patient was treated successfully with botulinum toxin A. (Reprinted from: Garibaldi DC, Miller NR. Tortuous basilar artery as etiology of hemifacial spasm. *Arch Neurol.* 2003;60:626–627, with permission.)

Other rare causes include arachnoid cysts, MS, pontine infarction, hemosiderosis, arachnoiditis, and lesions or structural abnormalities of the bone of the skull base. In some cases, HFS is associated with evidence of hyperactivity of other cranial nerves. The most common association is with trigeminal neuralgia.

The only way to cure most cases of HFS is to decompress the facial nerve at the root entry zone by moving the offending vessel or vessels. Although this procedure has potential mortality and a well-defined morbidity, including permanent ipsilateral hearing loss, facial weakness, or both, the results are generally excellent. When performed by an experienced surgeon, the overall cure rate is about 90% or greater. In most patients who are cured, the HFS disappears within 3 to 10 days after surgery, although in a smaller group, resolution can take weeks to months. Among patients whose HFS persists or recurs after apparently successful surgery (i.e., the vessel compressing the nerve is identified and moved), the majority are cured after a second operation.

The results of medical therapy for HFS are generally disappointing. The most commonly used drugs are carbamazepine (Tegretol), diphenylhydantoin (Dilantin), and dimethylaminoethanol (Deanol). Gabapentin (Neurontin) has also been reported to be of value in selected patients.

Intramuscular injections of botulinum toxin can be used to control, but not cure, HFS. In our opinion, this mode of therapy is the best alternative for patients who are unwilling or unable to undergo posterior fossa microvascular decompression of the facial nerve. Other injectable drugs are under investigation.

Excessive Eyelid Closure of Neuromuscular Origin

Neuromuscular hyperexcitability of the orbicularis oculi usually is part of a generalized disorder. The excitability may be latent, spasmodic, or constant. In hypoparathyroidism or during hyperventilation, a tap over the lateral orbital margin produces contraction of the ipsilateral orbicularis muscles and the surrounding facial muscles (latent hyperexcitability). Strychnine poisoning causes spasmodic hyperexcitability and tetanus causes a constant or sustained neuromuscular hyperexcitability manifested in the facial muscles as **risus sardonicus** (Fig. 22.42).

Excessive Eyelid Closure of Myopathic Origin

Myotonia of the orbicularis oculi may occur in association with a number of disorders. For example, patients can develop eyelid myotonia in association with

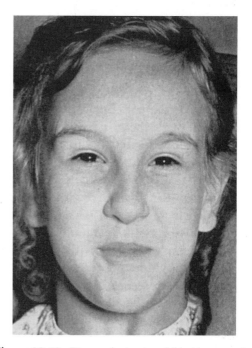

Figure 22.42. Risus sardonicus in a child with tetanus. Increased tone of all facial muscles is evident. Note that the child appears to be smiling. Her apparent bilateral ptosis is caused by myotonia of the orbicularis oculi muscles. (Reprinted from: Ford FR. *Diseases of the Nervous System in Infancy, Childhood and Adolescence.* 5th ed. Springfield, IL: CC Thomas; 1966:621, with permission.)

primary hypothyroidism. The myotonia typically disappears after such patients are treated with replacement thyroid medication.

Patients with both the congenital and adult forms of myotonic dystrophy may show myotonia of the orbicularis oculi. In adults with myotonic dystrophy, EMG studies demonstrate evidence of prolonged contraction in the orbicularis oculi following a blink (see Chapter 20).

Myotonia of the orbicularis oculi may occur in patients with hyperkalemic familial periodic paralysis.

Slowness of eyelid opening or temporary narrowing of the palpebral fissure may occur following sustained eyelid closure, application of ice to the lids, or administration of potassium salts. Eyelid myotonia can also occur in patients with chondrodystrophic myotonia (Schwartz-Jampel syndrome) (see Chapter 20).

FOR FURTHER INFORMATION

See *Walsh & Hoyt's Clinical Neuro-Ophthalmology*, 6th edition, Volume 1, Chapter 24.

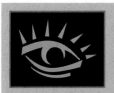

P atients who have physical signs and symptoms for which no adequate organic cause can be found may receive any one of a large range of diagnostic labels, including functional illness, functional overlay, hysteria, hysterical overlay, conversion reaction, psychophysiological reaction, somatization reaction, hypochondriasis, invalid reaction, neurasthenia, psychogenic reaction, psychosomatic illness, malingering, and Münchhausen syndrome. This plethora of labels highlights the confusion that occurs when one tries to fit patients with nonorganic disease into a formal classification.

GENERAL CONSIDERATIONS

The **nature of the symptom** and the manner of its communication are crucial in the understanding of a nonorganic disorder. The patient may be stoic and restrained, or histrionic and dramatizing. The symptom may take the form of a physical dysfunction (e.g., strabismus) that is displayed with a minimum of verbal description, or the symptom may be described verbally during the examination. Thus, one must also determine the **nature of the physical dysfunction** and the

degree of disability. It is important to determine why the symptoms have focused in a particular area (e.g., the visual system).

Another consideration is the amount of time a patient spends thinking about his or her symptoms and the precise nature of the thoughts in phenomenological terms. This concept is called **ideation.** For example, is the patient phobic or deluded?

A patient's **affect** may tell the physician much about the patient's complaints. Some patients clearly are depressed, whereas others are truly indifferent, and still others are anxious. Of particular interest is a patient's **attitude toward those involved in the diagnosis and treatment of his or her condition.** These are persons with whom one would expect the patient to cooperate in an attempt to get well. Is the patient hostile, suspicious, fearful, flirtatious, pleading, aloof, or excessively cooperative and agreeable?

Understanding a patient's **motivation** or incentive for achieving the "sick role" and the degree to which he or she is conscious of it may be the most difficult part of the diagnostic process, but it may be the most crucial. The nature of motivation may range from an unconscious seeking of the dependency-gratifying and guilt-allaying aspects of the "sick role" to the overtly conscious attempt to obtain attention, sympathy, material gain, or a combination of these.

---

*Adapted from Chapter 27 by Neil R. Miller, Neuro-Ophthalmologic Manifestations of Nonorganic Disease.

TERMINOLOGY

Most nonorganic disturbances are categorized by three types: (a) malingering; (b) Münchhausen syndrome; and (c) psychogenic.

MALINGERING

Patients whose symptoms are consciously and voluntarily produced are said to be **malingering.** Malingering can be divided into several different categories, including simulation of nonexistent disease, elaboration of preexisting disease, and attribution of a disability to a different cause. The most common settings in which malingering occurs are potential compensation after a real or feigned injury, avoidance of a particular task, such as military service or a simple school examination for which the patient is unprepared, or an attempt to seek special attention from family or friends.

MÜNCHHAUSEN SYNDROME

Malingering must be differentiated from **factitious disorder with physical symptoms,** also called the **Münchhausen syndrome.** Patients with this condition intentionally produce physical symptoms and signs, some of which may be ocular. Manifestations might include swelling and redness of the conjunctiva simulating an orbital cellulitis, scarring of the eyelids and conjunctiva, and even chorioretinal scarring, all of which are then presented to members of the medical profession. Patients with Münchhausen syndrome are thought to harbor a psychological internal need to adopt the role of a sick person.

PSYCHOGENIC DISTURBANCE

Patients whose symptoms seem truly independent of volition are said to have a somatoform disorder or **psychogenic disturbance.** Examples of psychogenic disturbances include body dysmorphic disorder, conversion disorder (hysteria, conversion reaction), hypochondriasis, and somatization disorder.

A **body dysmorphic disorder** is characterized by a patient's perception of a single physical defect, most often in the facial region, including the eye. The patient is preoccupied with this sign even though it is minimal (e.g., a mild ptosis or anisocoria) or is not present at all.

A **conversion disorder** is diagnosed if alterations or a loss of physical functioning are present that seem to express a psychological conflict or need rather than indicating organic illness. This disorder comprises the clinical syndromes that were previously classified as "hysteria" or "conversion neurosis." Patients in whom such disorders occur may subconsciously obtain both primary gain (e.g., protection from trauma or reduction of stress) and secondary gain (e.g., increased attention).

Hypochondriasis is the fear of, or strong belief in, specific serious physical conditions accompanied by ex-cessive self-observation and the reporting of numerous physical signs and symptoms. It differs from body dysmorphic disorder in that it includes both symptoms and signs from multiple organ systems throughout the body.

A **somatization disorder** features recurrent and multiple somatic complaints. As in hypochondriasis, multiple organ systems may be mentioned, but the patient's descriptions are vague, and anxiety or depression usually is present.

Unfortunately, there remains a large group of patients in whom a clear distinction between malingering, Münchhausen syndrome, and psychogenic or somatoform disturbances simply cannot be made. In such cases, the physician must recognize that there is no organic basis for the patient's symptoms and signs and manage the patient accordingly.

SPECIFIC NONORGANIC NEURO-OPHTHALMOLOGIC DISORDERS

From a neuro-ophthalmologic standpoint, there are five areas that may be affected by nonorganic disease:

1. Vision, including visual acuity and visual field
2. Ocular motility and alignment
3. Pupillary size and reactivity
4. Eyelid position and function; and
5. Corneal and facial sensation.

The physician faced with a patient complaining of decreased vision or some other disturbance related to the **afferent** or **efferent** visual systems for which there is no apparent biologic explanation has two responsibilities. First, the physician must ascertain that an organic disorder is not present. Second, the physician must determine if the patient can see or do something that would not be possible if the condition were organic in nature. To best achieve these goals, the physician must adopt an **empathetic** attitude toward the patient regardless of the patient's history, attitude of the patient toward the physician or the disease, or the clinical findings. If the physician has or is perceived to have a cynical, disbelieving, or confrontational attitude, the patient may not cooperate fully during the examination and the results will be unsatisfactory.

NONORGANIC DISEASE AFFECTING THE AFFERENT VISUAL PATHWAY

Nonorganic disease that affects the **afferent** visual system is extremely common. It may occur as monocular or binocular decreased visual acuity, abnormal visual fields, or both. Color vision often is abnormal in such patients (depending on the manner in which it is tested), but abnormal color vision is rarely a primary complaint.

Decreased Visual Acuity

Decreased visual acuity is probably the most common nonorganic disturbance in ophthalmology. It occurs most often in children and young adults, but it may be observed in patients 60 years of age and older. It may be psychogenic or caused by malingering. Nonorganic visual loss that is psychogenic seems to be more common in children, with females being affected much more often than males. Malingerers are most often adult males, perhaps because men are more often involved in motor vehicle and work-related accidents than are women.

Patients with nonorganic loss of visual acuity complain of a variable loss of vision in one or both eyes that is not accompanied by a refractive error, a disturbance of the ocular media, or other evidence of retinal or optic nerve dysfunction. Abnormal color perception, an abnormal visual field, or both, may accompany the visual loss.

In many cases, the physician may suspect that the patient's visual loss is nonorganic during the medical history interview which, as noted previously, is perhaps the most crucial aspect of the evaluation. In addition, the way the patient acts during the history taking may be helpful. Patients who are truly blind in both eyes tend to look directly at the person with whom they are speaking, whereas patients with nonorganic blindness, particularly patients who are malingering, often look in some other direction. Similarly, patients claiming complete or nearly complete blindness often wear sunglasses, even though they do not have photophobia, and the external appearance of the eyes is perfectly normal. In any event, the physician who suspects a nonorganic visual process may be able to orient

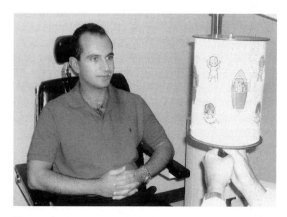

Figure 23.1. Use of the optokinetic drum to detect nonorganic bilateral blindness. The patient is asked to look straight ahead with both eyes open while the drum is rotated, first in one direction, then in the other.

the examination in a way to bring out the nonorganic nature of the visual disturbance.

If a patient claims no perception of light, light perception only, or perception of hand motions by one or both eyes, one can use a rotating optokinetic drum or horizontally moving tape to produce a horizontal jerk nystagmus that indicates intact vision of at least 20/400 (Fig. 23.1). It is important in this regard that the images on the tape or drum be sufficiently large so that the patient is not able to look around them. When testing a patient who claims complete loss of vision in one eye only, the test is begun by rotating the drum or moving the tape in front of the patient, who has **both** eyes open. Once good optokinetic nystagmus is elicited, the unaffected eye is suddenly covered with the palm of the examiner's hand or a handheld occluder (Fig. 23.2). Patients with nonorganic loss of vision in one eye will continue to show a jerk nystagmus.

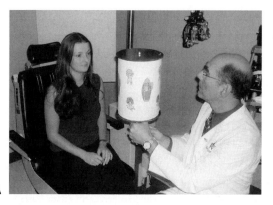 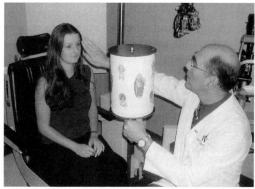

A **B**

Figure 23.2. Use of an optokinetic drum to detect nonorganic unilateral blindness. **A:** In a patient claiming unilateral blindness, the drum is first rotated while the patient is instructed to look straight ahead with both eyes open. **B:** Once nystagmus is elicited, the examiner continues to rotate the drum and suddenly covers the "normal" eye with the palm of the hand and observes the "blind" eye for continued nystagmus.

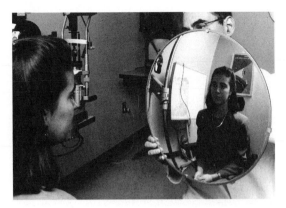

Figure 23.3. Use of a mirror to detect nonorganic blindness. The affected eye is occluded if the patient claims blindness in only one eye; otherwise, both eyes are left open. The patient is instructed to look straight ahead into the mirror, and the mirror is then rotated and turned from side to side. The development of nystagmus or a nystagmoid movement of the eyes indicates that the patient can see moving images in the mirror and thus is not blind.

A second test that is helpful in detecting visual function in an eye or eyes that are said to have either no perception of light or light perception only is the "mirror test." A large mirror is held in front of the patient's face, and the patient is asked to look directly ahead (Fig. 23.3). The mirror is then rotated and twisted back and forth, causing the images in the mirror to move. Patients with vision better than light perception will show a nystagmoid movement of the eyes, since they cannot avoid following the moving reflection in the mirror.

An excellent way to detect nonorganic visual loss in a patient who claims to be unable to see shapes or objects in one or both eyes is to ask the patient to touch the tips of the first fingers of both hands together. If the patient claims loss of vision in one eye only, the opposite eye is patched before the test is performed. As every physician knows, the ability to touch the tips of the fingers of two hands together is based not on vision but on proprioception. Thus, patients with organic blindness can easily bring the tips of the first fingers of both hands together, whereas patients with nonorganic blindness, particularly those who are malingering, will be unable to do so (Fig. 23.4). Similarly, a patient with organic blindness can easily sign his or her name without difficulty, whereas patients with blindness caused by malingering may produce an extremely bizarre signature.

A variety of tests may be performed in patients who claim vision in the range of 20/40 to hand motions in one or both eyes. None of these tests is invariably reliable, but one or more usually is sufficient to provide convincing evidence that visual acuity loss either

is nonexistent or not as severe as the patient claims. Visual acuity may be tested not by starting from the largest letters or numbers and moving progressively to smaller ones, but by beginning with the **smallest** line. Assuming that the patient cannot see this first line after being allowed to concentrate for several minutes, the physician tells the patient that the size of the print is now going to be "doubled" in size, and the patient is shown the next larger line and given several minutes to read it. This process is continued until the patient is able to read the line. This method of testing often produces visual acuity better than that initially claimed by the patient. In addition, some projector slides have several 20/20 lines, and these lines may be shown to the patient in succession as the examiner tells the patient the size of the letters is increasing.

Testing of near vision is also important in patients claiming decreased acuity. A discrepancy in the distance and near-visual acuity that is not attributable to a refractive error or a disturbance of the media, such as an oil drop cataract, usually is evidence of a nonorganic disturbance.

Patients claiming decreased vision in one eye only may undergo a "refraction" in which the normal eye is fogged with a high plus lens (e.g., a +5.00 or higher sphere), and a lens with minimal power (e.g., a ±0.50 sphere or cylinder) is placed before the worse eye. The patient is then told to read the chart with "both eyes." A variation of this test is the use of paired cylinders. A plus cylinder and a minus cylinder of the same power (usually 2–6 diopters) are placed at parallel axes in front of the "normal" eye in a trial frame. The patient's normal correction is placed in front of the affected eye. The patient is asked to read, with both eyes open, a line that previously had been read with the normal eye but not with the affected eye. As the patient begins to read, the axis of one of the cylinders is rotated about 10 to 15 degrees. The axes of the two cylinders thus will no longer be parallel, blurring vision in the normal eye. If the patient continues to read the line, or can read it again when asked to do so, he or she must be using the affected eye.

Red-green glasses used with a red and green duochrome slide superimposed on the normal vision chart can be used to induce a patient to read with an eye that supposedly cannot see (or cannot see well) by making the patient think that he or she is using both eyes. In this test, the eye behind the red lens will see the letters on both sides of the chart, whereas the eye behind the green lens will see only those letters on the green side of the chart. The lenses are arranged so that the red lens is over the eye with decreased vision, and the patient is then asked to read the chart with both eyes open. If the patient reads the entire line, it is obvious that the abnormal eye must be functioning better than the patient claims.

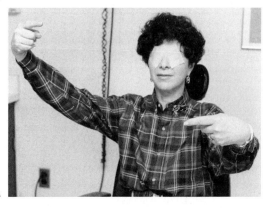
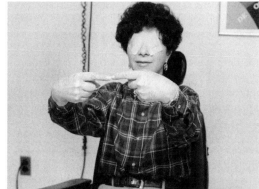
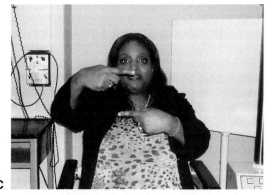
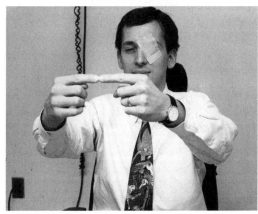
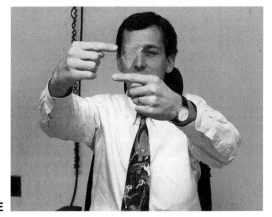

Figure 23.4. Testing nonorganic visual loss by asking a patient who claims monocular or binocular blindness to touch the tips of the first fingers of each hand together. **A and B:** A person who is truly blind can easily touch the tips of the fingers together, using proprioception, as the person in these photographs is doing despite having both eyes occluded. **C:** A woman with nonorganic loss of vision in both eyes is unable to touch the tips of the fingers together, even though she should be able to do so. A person with monocular nonorganic visual loss may touch the tips of the fingers together when viewing with the "normal" eye **(D)**, but may claim to be unable to do so when viewing with the "blind" eye **(E)**.

A variant of the red-green glasses/duochrome chart test that employs the red-green glasses and Ishihara color plates can be performed in patients with presumed nonorganic monocular visual loss that is worse than 20/400. The patient should first be tested for "congenital" color vision as described later. Once it has been established that color vision is normal, the patient is asked to view the Ishihara color plates while wearing red-green glasses with the red lens over the affected eye. With the exception of plates 1 and 36, the numbers and lines on the Ishihara plates cannot be seen by the eye over which the green filter is placed. Even with visual acuity of 20/400, however, all of the color plates can be seen through a red filter. Thus, a patient who has normal color vision in at least the unaffected eye, who then views the plates through red-green spectacles with the red lens in front of the affected eye, and who correctly identifies the figures on the plates, must have visual acuity of 20/400 or better in the affected eye.

Polarizing lenses can be used in several ways to detect nonorganic visual loss in a patient with decreased vision in one eye only. In the American Optical Polarizing Test, the patient wears polarizing glasses, and the test object, a Project-O-Chart slide, projects letters alternately so that one letter is seen by both eyes, the next by the right eye, the next by the left eye, etc. Another test uses a polarizing lens placed before a projector. The patient is asked to read the chart while wearing polarizing lenses, with one eye or the other being allowed to see the whole projected image at a time.

A prism that is 4 diopters in strength can be used to detect vision in an eye said to have reduced or no vision. The patient is asked to look with both eyes at the vision chart. A 4-prism diopter loose prism is then placed, base-out, over the "affected eye." A patient with normal binocular vision will show a movement of both eyes toward the direction of the apex of the prism followed by a shift of the fellow eye back toward the center. A patient with true decreased or absent vision in the eye over which the prism is placed will show no conjugate movement at all. Similarly, when the prism is placed over the "better eye" of a patient whose other eye truly is blind or has extremely reduced sight, only the first conjugate binocular shift will occur. There will be no compensatory movement of the fellow eye back toward the center.

Several **prism dissociation tests** can be used to detect mild degrees of nonorganic monocular visual loss. In this test, the patient is first asked if he or she has experienced double vision in addition to loss of vision in the affected eye. If the answer is negative, the patient is told that the examiner will test the alignment of both eyes and that the test should produce vertical double vision. A 4-prism diopter loose prism is then placed base down in front of the unaffected eye at the same time that a 1/2-prism diopter prism is simultaneously placed with the base in any direction over the eye with decreased vision. In this way, the patient does not become suspicious that the examiner is paying specific attention to one eye or the other. A 20/20 or larger size Snellen letter is then projected in the distance, and the patient is asked if he or she has double vision. When the patient admits to diplopia, he or she is then asked whether the two letters are of equal quality or sharpness, and an assessment of visual acuity can then be made.

Patients in whom visual acuity is reduced and there is no evidence of a refractive error, disturbance of the ocular media, or a macular abnormality by ophthalmoscopic examination are often assumed to have an underlying optic neuropathy even if the optic disc appears normal. Patients with a true optic neuropathy, however, almost invariably have a disturbance of color vision that can be detected using various types of color plates, such as the Hardy-Rand-Rittler Pseudoisochromatic Plates or the Ishihara Color Plates. It is useful to "prepare" the patient suspected of having nonorganic visual loss for the test by asking if he or she was ever diagnosed as having "congenital color blindness." Assuming the patient gives a negative answer, he or she is told that the color vision test the physician is going to perform is a test of congenital color blindness and that the patient should therefore be able to see the figures or numbers.

Testing of stereopsis may be valuable in detecting nonorganic visual loss. There is a definite correlation between binocular visual acuity and stereopsis (Table 23.1). For instance, a patient with 20/20 vision in one eye and organic visual loss producing visual acuity of 20/200 in the fellow eye has stereoacuity of only about 180 seconds of arc, whereas a patient with 20/20 visual acuity OU has stereoacuity of 40 seconds of arc. A variety of stereoacuity tests are available, all of which have advantages and disadvantages.

Examination of pupillary responses can be helpful in diagnosing nonorganic visual loss. Patients who report complete blindness in both eyes should have pupils that do not react to light stimulation unless the process affects the postgeniculate visual pathways. Thus, the pupils of a patient who cannot perceive light with either eye because of bilateral retinal, optic nerve, or optic tract lesions, or because of damage to the optic chiasm, do not react to light stimulation, whereas the pupils of a patient who is blind from bilateral lesions of the optic radiations or striate cortex will react relatively normally to light. Pupils that react to light stimulation in a patient who claims complete loss of vision in both eyes indicate either that the patient is cerebrally blind (usually from damage to the striate cortex—cortical blindness) or that the patient has nonorganic loss of vision.

Patients with unilateral or asymmetric optic neuropathy invariably have a relative afferent pupillary

Table 23.1. *Relationship of Visual Acuity and Stereopsis*

Visual Acuity	Average Stereopsis[a]
20/20	40
20/25	43
20/30	52
20/40	61
20/50	78
20/70	94
20/100	124
20/200	160

[a]Measured in seconds of image disparity.
(Modified from: Levy NS, Glick EB. Stereoscopic perception and Snellen visual acuity. *Am J Ophthalmol.* 1974;78:722–724.)

defect (RAPD) that can easily be detected by performing a swinging flashlight test (see Chapters 14 and 15). The absence of an RAPD in a patient with monocular visual loss indicates either that the patient does not have a unilateral optic neuropathy (and thus may support a diagnosis of nonorganic visual loss) or that the patient has a **bilateral** optic neuropathy that is asymmetric. It must be emphasized that patients with electrophysiologic evidence of bilateral optic neuropathy may nevertheless have very asymmetric visual acuity in the two eyes unassociated with an RAPD. Thus, if there is no indication of nonorganic disease in a patient with unexplained, unilateral visual loss without an obvious relative afferent pupillary defect, such a patient should undergo electrophysiologic testing, particularly full-field and multifocal electroretinography and pattern-reversal and flash-evoked visual evoked potentials.

The management of patients who have nonorganic loss of visual acuity is problematic and often depends on whether the patient is a child or an adult and whether the condition is thought to be psychogenic or caused by malingering. Nonorganic visual loss in children usually occurs as a situational phenomenon caused by a wide range of academic, social, or familial difficulties. Once it is certain that the condition is nonorganic, one can first attempt to "cure" the visual loss by informing the child that the only problem is a slight refractive error. A minimal correction is then placed into a trial frame or phoropter, and the patient is told that they "should see normally" with this set of glasses. If this is successful, the patient is told not to worry about the visual process and that the refractive error is sufficiently minimal that it probably is not necessary for glasses to be worn. If this maneuver is unsuccessful, the parents can be privately informed of the findings so that they will not continue to be concerned about an organic process. The child is then informed that, fortunately, there is **no irreversible damage to the eyes** and that vision should improve spontaneously with time. No particular time frame is indicated during which this will occur, and the child is encouraged to "do as well as you can" in school, at home, etc., until vision improves. This approach usually is sufficient to solve the problem in the vast majority of cases. Nevertheless, dealing with children whose visual loss is associated with complex interpersonal relationships within the family, such as sexual abuse or other social difficulties, is much more difficult and may require the services of a psychotherapist, child psychiatrist, or other specialist.

The treatment of adults with nonorganic loss of visual acuity is more complicated than the treatment of children, particularly when there is evidence of malingering, and the outcome usually is much less satisfactory. As long as there is a motivation for material secondary gain, it may be impossible to "treat" such a patient for his or her visual loss. In many cases, the physician must be content that the loss of vision is nonorganic and to record this fact in the patient's chart. There is no purpose in confronting the patient with our belief that the visual loss is nonorganic unless one can convince the patient that ultimately it is not in his or her best interest to continue the charade because there is objective evidence that the visual loss is nonorganic and that such evidence will eventually cost the patient time, money, or even freedom.

Visual Field Defects

Nonorganic visual field defects can be of several types. The most common nonorganic visual field defect is a nonspecifically constricted visual field. When the field is tested kinetically, using either a Goldmann perimeter or a tangent (Bjerrum) screen, the field may have a spiraling nature, becoming smaller and smaller as the test object is moved around the field (Fig. 23.5). Alternatively, the visual field may remain the same size or nearly the same size regardless of the size or brightness of the test stimulus, or it may be inconsistent when tested repeatedly in one or more meridians. Other nonorganic visual field defects, however, include unilateral or bilateral central scotomas, unilateral hemianopia, bitemporal hemianopia, binasal hemianopia, and even homonymous hemianopia.

A nonorganically constricted visual field may be diagnosed in a variety of ways. In some cases, the patient can be cajoled into enlarging the field. After completion of perimetry, the patient is told that he or she did fine but that it was clear to the examiner that the patient was responding only when he or she was "absolutely certain" that he or she saw the test object. The examiner then explains that the test is to be repeated and encourages the patient to respond at an earlier stage when he or she just barely detects the stimulus.

Nonorganic visual field constriction can also be detected by testing the field using a tangent screen with the patient at two different distances from the screen (usually 1 and 2 meters). The size of the test object is varied so that the ratio of the size of the test object and the distance of the patient from the screen remain constant; i.e., a 9-mm-diameter white test object is used when the patient is 1 m from the screen, and an 18-mm-diameter white test object is used when the patient is 2 m from the screen. Patients with an organically constricted visual field (e.g., patients with retinitis pigmentosa) will show an increase in the absolute size of the visual field under these conditions when they are moved from 1 m to 2 m away from the screen, whereas patients with nonorganic visual field constriction will maintain the same absolute size of the field

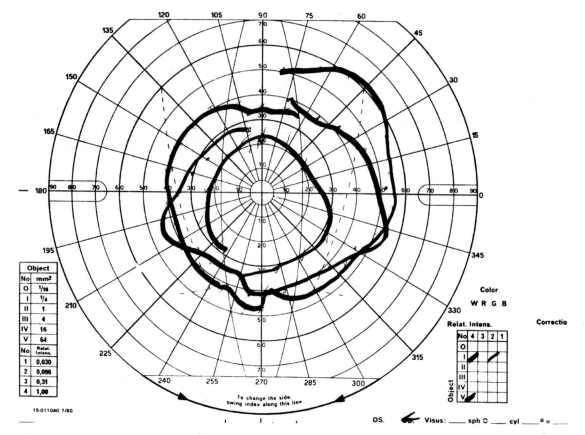

Figure 23.5. In a patient claiming visual difficulties in the right eye, there is a nonorganic spiral field when the eye is tested kinetically using a Goldmann perimeter.

constriction. Automated kinetic perimetry can give similar results.

Nonorganic monocular hemianopias and scotomas as well as both binasal and bitemporal hemianopic defects usually can be diagnosed by first performing visual field testing monocularly and then binocularly (Fig. 23.6). If the field defect is present in only one eye when the eyes are tested separately, but is still present when binocular simultaneous field testing is performed, the defect can be assumed to be nonorganic. This method cannot distinguish between organic and nonorganic homonymous hemianopic defects or bilateral central scotomas.

A quick and easy method of detecting nonorganic visual field loss of all types is to test saccadic eye movements into the supposedly absent portion of the field. The patient assumes that the eye movements and not the visual fields are being tested. This assumption is strengthened by first asking the patient if it hurts to move the eyes. Regardless of the patient's answer (which, interestingly, is often affirmative), the patient is told that the examiner is going to test the eye movements, and the patient is asked to pursue an object in

various directions. The patient is then asked to look from the straight ahead position to an eccentric location where the examiner holds an object. The object is subsequently moved from one location to another with the patient being asked each time to look from the center to the object. If the patient complains that he or she "cannot see" that far in the periphery, the examiner explains that he or she understands and that is why the patient should look **directly** at the object rather than to try to see it in the peripheral vision.

It should be noted that patients can create reproducible nonorganic visual field defects not only when tested with kinetic perimetry but also when tested using automated static perimetry (Fig. 23.7). Such patients do not necessarily show an increased number of fixation losses or false-positive or false-negative errors.

The management of patients with nonorganic visual field constriction is similar to that of patients with nonorganic visual loss. Children and adults who do not seem to be malingering are told that they eventually will improve, and this usually is the case.

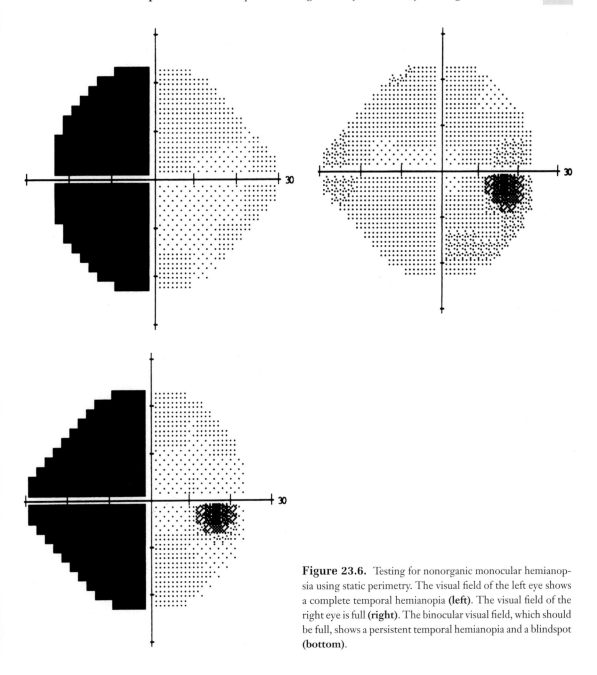

Figure 23.6. Testing for nonorganic monocular hemianopsia using static perimetry. The visual field of the left eye shows a complete temporal hemianopia **(left)**. The visual field of the right eye is full **(right)**. The binocular visual field, which should be full, shows a persistent temporal hemianopia and a blindspot **(bottom)**.

Interestingly, most patients with nonorganic visual field loss deny that their visual field disturbance significantly limits their daily activities or state that despite their visual difficulties they are able to maintain their normal lifestyle. Such patients thus rarely require psychiatric or psychological counseling for these patients. It is generally inadvisable to confront adults whose visual field defects are caused by malingering unless it seems likely that one can end the charade with a few well-chosen words.

Monocular Diplopia

Most patients who complain of double vision are suffering from misalignment of the visual axes. In such cases, the diplopia immediately resolves as soon as one eye is covered. Patients in whom diplopia remains despite occlusion of one eye are said to have **monocular diplopia.** This condition is caused most often by a refractive error, particularly by uncorrected or improperly corrected astigmatism; by incorrectly fitted glasses; or by some irregularity of the cornea or

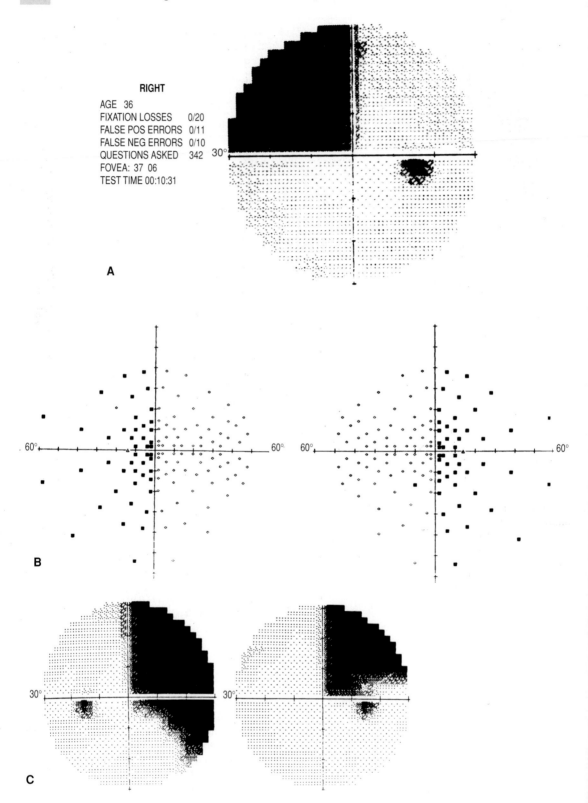

RIGHT
AGE 36
FIXATION LOSSES 0/20
FALSE POS ERRORS 0/11
FALSE NEG ERRORS 0/10
QUESTIONS ASKED 342
FOVEA: 37 06
TEST TIME 00:10:31

Figure 23.7. Fabricated visual field defects. **A:** Artificially produced quadrantanopsia with the Humphrey field analyzer, using a 24-2 program. Note the excellent reliability. **B:** Fabricated bitemporal hemianopia, using the Humphrey Full Field 120-point screening test **(left and right)**. **C:** Fabricated incongruous right homonymous hemianopia, using Humphrey Central 30-2 threshold test.

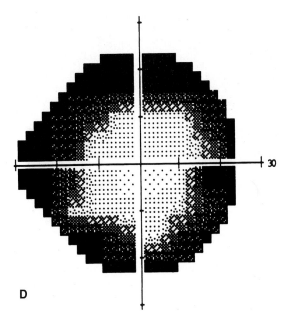

D

Figure 23.7. (*Continued*) **D:** Fabricated constricted visual field in a patient with no clinical or electrophysiologic evidence of retinopathy or optic neuropathy. Note the "squaring" of the field defect, a phenomenon common to nonorganic visual field constriction recorded by automated perimetry. (**A:** Reprinted from: Glovinsky Y, Quigley HA, Bissett RA, et al. *Am J Ophthalmol.* 1990;110:90–91, with permission. **B and C:** Reprinted from: MacLeod JDA, Manners RM, Heaven CJ, et al. Visual field defects. *Neuroophthalmology.* 1994;14:185–188, with permission.)

lens. Most patients with this type of organic monocular diplopia will recognize a difference in the intensity of the two images that they see. One image will be fairly clear, but the second image will be perceived as "fuzzy" and may be described as a "ghost image" that overlaps the clear image. The "diplopia" in such cases usually resolves with a pinhole, a better refraction or fitting of spectacles, or a contact lens.

True monocular diplopia (i.e., two separate and equal images of an object seen with one eye only) is almost never caused by organic disease. It is seen most often in children who have found themselves in stressful academic, social, or family situations. Once both the child and the parents are reassured as to the benign nature of the condition, it usually resolves within a short period of time.

NONORGANIC DISEASE AFFECTING FIXATION, OCULAR MOTILITY, AND ALIGNMENT

Nonorganic disturbances of ocular motor function include disturbances of fixation, ocular motility, and alignment.

Disturbances of Fixation: Voluntary Nystagmus and Voluntary Saccadic Oscillations

Saccadic oscillations in most patients are involuntary eye movements caused by a neurological disease affecting the brainstem, cerebellum, or both. Nevertheless, some persons can produce saccadic oscillations that resemble nystagmus, ocular flutter, or opsoclonus.

Voluntary nystagmus is characterized by a rapid to-and-fro movement of the eyes that is willfully initiated. It can be produced by 5% to 8% of the population and may occur as a familial trait. Voluntary nystagmus consists of rapidly alternating saccades with frequencies that range from 3 to 42 Hz and amplitudes that range from 0.5 to 35 and that can be sustained for only a few seconds. Voluntary nystagmus usually is horizontal; however, it can be vertical or torsional, and it can be produced in the light or dark and with the eyelids open or closed. It is almost always binocular but has been reported as a monocular phenomenon.

Patients with voluntary nystagmus typically complain of oscillopsia and reduced vision. Such patients have fluttering of the eyelids and a strained facial expression during the episodes of nystagmus. In addition, the eyes tend to converge during the nystagmus.

Voluntary nystagmus has no pathologic significance. It may, however, be mistaken for certain pathologic conditions that affect fixation, including acquired nystagmus and saccadic intrusions (see Chapter 19).

Rare patients appear to be able to produce large-amplitude, to-and-fro rapid eye movements. These **voluntary saccadic oscillations** are actually bursts of conjugate saccades in opposing directions, with no intersaccadic interval. Unlike the saccades of voluntary nystagmus, they are multidirectional (horizontal, vertical, or oblique), have amplitudes up to 40, and sometimes have curvilinear trajectories. These characteristics are similar to those of ocular flutter and opsoclonus; however, patients with true ocular flutter or opsoclonus generally have other neurologic manifestations. Thus, when saccadic oscillations that appear to be ocular flutter or opsoclonus are found in patients who do not have other neurologic signs or symptoms, the possibility of a nonorganic cause should be considered.

Disorders of Ocular Motility and Alignment

Several nonorganic disorders of ocular motility and alignment may be observed in patients both with and without visual complaints. These disorders include insufficiency or paralysis of convergence, spasm of the near reflex, supranuclear horizontal and vertical gaze paresis, and forced downward deviation of the eyes.

Convergence Insufficiency or Paralysis Convergence insufficiency or paralysis may be nonorganic in

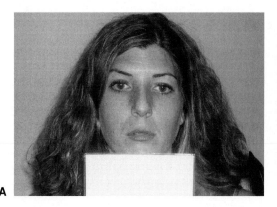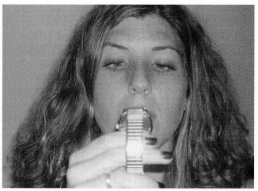

A **B**

Figure 23.8. Nonorganic convergence insufficiency. **A:** Inability to converge upon a near target despite encouragement. **B:** Normal near-reflex elicited by asking patient to tell the time by looking at a wristwatch.

nature. We have seen several cases, usually in adolescents, but also in adults. Such patients often have associated insufficiency or paralysis of accommodation, although either disturbance may exist independently. Patients with apparent weakness of convergence may nevertheless show normal convergence when asked to read a paragraph at length during which the eyes are alternately covered. Asking the patient to perform other near tasks such as telling time by looking at his or her wristwatch, may also be associated with normal convergence (Fig. 23.8).

Spasm of the Near Reflex The most common nonorganic disturbance of ocular motility and alignment is **spasm of the near reflex** (Fig. 23.9). The syndrome is characterized by episodes of intermittent convergence, increased accommodation, and miosis. The degree of convergence is variable. Some patients exhibit marked convergence of both eyes, resulting in a marked esotropia. Others show a lesser degree of convergence such that one eye remains relatively straight while the other converges. In all cases, however, the patient seems to have unilateral or, more often, bilateral limitation of abduction during testing of versions although not necessarily during testing of ductions. The degree of accommodation spasm also is variable. Some patients produce only a few diopters of myopia, whereas others produce 8 to 10 diopters of myopia. Miosis is invariably significant in patients who exhibit spasm of the near reflex regardless of the degree of accommodation and convergence spasm.

Spasm of the near reflex may be mistaken for unilateral or bilateral abducens nerve paresis, divergence insufficiency, horizontal gaze paresis, or even myasthenia gravis. However, the lack of other neurological deficits, the variability of the eye movements, and the constant occurrence of miosis associated with the adductive eye movements generally permit the correct

diagnosis to be made. In addition, despite apparent unilateral or bilateral abduction weakness during testing of versions (with both eyes open), when ductions are tested directly with one eye occluded or indirectly using oculocephalic testing, both eyes invariably have full abduction and the miosis seen when the eyes are in the esotropic position immediately resolves. Covering one eye during a typical spasm also may cause dramatic reversal of the miosis. Finally, refraction with and without cycloplegia during a period of spasm establishes the presence of pseudomyopia.

Several organic conditions, in addition to abducens nerve paresis and horizontal gaze paresis, may mimic spasm of the near reflex. Pretectal esotropia, also called pseudo-abducens paresis or pseudo-6th nerve palsy, is a general disordered co-contraction of extraocular muscles and is not related to the near reflex. Convergence nystagmus jerks are not accompanied by miosis in this condition. Convergence substitution sometimes occurs when patients with supranuclear horizontal gaze paresis use convergence to move the adducting eye into the limited field of gaze. The resulting eye movement may suggest spasm of the near reflex.

True convergence spasm may occasionally be caused by organic lesions, such as intrinsic lesions of the mesencephalon or extrinsic lesions compressing the dorsal mesencephalon. Thus, the examiner who is unsure whether or not spasm of the near reflex is organic must be prepared to give the patient the benefit of the doubt and perform appropriate neuroimaging studies.

Management of persons with nonorganic spasm of the near reflex may consist only of reassurance. Psychiatric counseling may be appropriate in other cases. In some patients, symptomatic relief may be produced using a cycloplegic drug combined with bifocal spectacles or reading glasses, or even glasses with an opaque inner third of the lens such that they occlude vision when the eyes are esotropic. Spasm of the near reflex

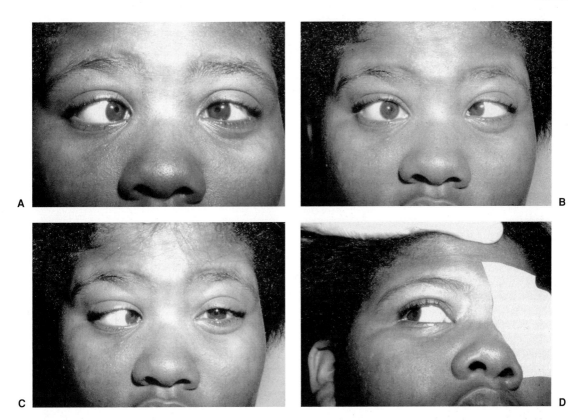

Figure 23.9. Spasm of the near reflex. The patient is a healthy 15-year-old girl. **A:** In primary position, the eyes are esotropic, and the pupils are constricted. **B:** On attempted right gaze, the right eye does not abduct, even to the midline, and the pupils become more constricted. **C:** On attempted left gaze, the left eye does not abduct beyond the midline, and the pupils become more constricted. **D:** When the left eye is patched and the patient is asked to pursue a target to the right or is asked to fixate a stationary target while the head is rotated to the left, the right eye abducts fully and the pupil becomes less constricted.

should never be treated with strabismus surgery as it will not eliminate the esotropia that is present during the spasms and will produce an exotropia between spasms.

Paralysis of Horizontal and Vertical Gaze   Patients with nonorganic **paralysis of horizontal and vertical eye movements** will not make voluntary horizontal or vertical saccades or pursuit movements and will not fixate on a distant object to allow oculocephalic testing; however, when such patients are observed through a one-way mirror, they can be seen to make absolutely normal pursuit and saccadic eye movements. In addition, measurements of eye movements during chair rotation in light and darkness indicate normal pursuit and saccadic systems.

Forced Downward Deviation of the Eyes in Nonorganic Coma and Seizures

The typical response of a patient with organic coma is either no movement of the eyes, such as occurs in pa-

tients with brainstem disease or drug-induced coma, or a smooth movement of the eyes in the direction **opposite** of a head turn (the normal "doll's eyes" response, see Chapter 16). The eyes of a patient feigning a comatose state, however, are often deviated tonically toward the floor as if to avoid looking at the observer. On moving the head to the opposite side, the eyes will either saccade directly to the side facing the floor (i.e., in the **same** direction as the head turn) or they occasionally will dart from side to side before coming to rest. Although a true seizure focus may certainly produce a deviation of the eyes to one side, turning the head from side to side in such a setting will not affect this deviation.

NONORGANIC DISORDERS OF PUPILLARY SIZE AND REACTIVITY

A variety of pupillary phenomena has been described in patients with various types of psychiatric and psychogenic diseases. For example, anxious patients occasionally have widely dilated and poorly reacting pupils

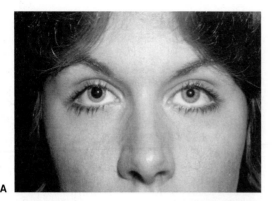

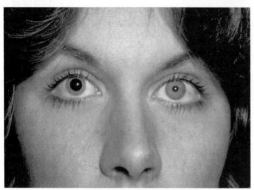

Figure 23.10. Diagnosis of unilateral pupillary dilation caused by voluntary use of a topical parasympatholytic drug using 1% pilocarpine. **A:** Before instillation of pilocarpine, the right pupil is markedly dilated (much more so than in a third nerve palsy). The size of the left pupil is normal. The right pupil was nonreactive to both direct and consensual light stimulation. **B:** 45 minutes after instillation of 1% pilocarpine in both lower cul-de-sacs, the right pupil is still markedly dilated but the left pupil is markedly constricted.

that fail to dilate further to a psychosensory stimulus as they are already maximally dilated. The pupils of schizophrenic patients are sometimes dilated and unreactive, and some patients develop widely dilated pupils during acute attacks of panic and that are associated with generalized autonomic disturbances consistent with sympathetic hyperfunction, including profuse sweating, trembling, tachycardia, and tachypnea. The pupils of such patients appear normal between attacks.

Perhaps the most common induced pupillary disturbance seen in ophthalmologic practice is a unilateral (and occasionally bilateral) fixed, dilated pupil caused by purposeful topical administration of a mydriatic agent (Fig. 23.10A). Pharmacologically dilated pupils are extremely large—larger than the dilated pupils associated with an oculomotor nerve palsy—and usually completely nonreactive to light or near stimulation.

They are unassociated with ptosis, diplopia, or strabismus unless there is a preexisting disturbance of eyelid function or ocular motility. The diagnosis of a pharmacologically dilated pupil is made by placing 1 to 2 drops of 1% pilocarpine in each lower cul-de-sac. A neurologically dilated pupil (i.e., oculomotor nerve paresis, tonic pupil) will constrict maximally within 30 minutes; however, a pharmacologically dilated pupil either is not affected and remains widely dilated (Fig. 23.10B) or constricts minimally. Unresponsiveness or even partial responsiveness of a dilated, fixed pupil to a solution of pilocarpine that is of sufficient strength to constrict the opposite, normally reacting pupil is absolute evidence of pharmacologic blockade, regardless of the patient's protestations to the contrary.

NONORGANIC DISTURBANCES OF ACCOMMODATION

The role of accommodation spasm in the condition called spasm of the near-reflex is discussed previously. In addition, however, nonorganic **weakness or paralysis of accommodation** may occur, primarily in children and young adults. Such patients are unable to read unless provided with an appropriate plus lens, and even then may claim an inability to read clearly. Indeed, it is the failure of a patient with normal distance vision and an inability to read despite an appropriate reading aid

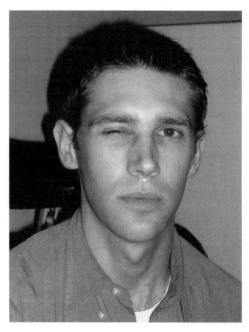

Figure 23.11. Nonorganic (voluntary) unilateral ptosis. Note elevation of the right **lower** eyelid and slight ptosis of the right eyebrow.

that should alert the physician to the possibility that the condition is nonorganic.

NONORGANIC DISTURBANCES OF EYELID FUNCTION

Nonorganic **ptosis** (pseudoptosis) is rare. In most cases, one can see or feel a fine spasm of the supposedly ptotic eyelid. There also tends to be elevation of the lower eyelid and variable relaxation of the elevators of the ipsilateral eyebrow, producing a mild brow ptosis (Fig. 23.11).

Blepharospasm may rarely be psychogenic in nature. Most cases of psychogenic blepharospasm occur in children and young adults and seem to be triggered by a particular emotionally traumatic event.

Patients who are anxious or upset often have variable bilateral eyelid **retraction.** This condition can usually be distinguished from the eyelid retraction of dysthyroid orbitopathy by its intermittent, variable nature and the lack of any other evidence—clinical or by imaging—of an orbitopathy.

NONORGANIC DISTURBANCES OF OCULAR AND FACIAL SENSATION

Anesthesia of the skin of the eyelids and of one or both corneas may be nonorganic, as may hypersensitivity, with the latter being associated with lacrimation, blepharospasm, photophobia, or a combination of these. Sensitive spots along the upper or lower margins of the orbits are common in patients with such complaints.

NONORGANIC DISTURBANCES OF LACRIMATION

Excessive secretion of tears may be nonorganic and may be associated with nonorganic blepharospasm. **Bloody tears** may be produced by depositing blood from self-induced nosebleeds into the conjunctival sacs.

FOR FURTHER INFORMATION

See *Walsh & Hoyt's Clinical Neuro-Ophthalmology*, 6th edition, Volume 1, Chapter 27.

Note: Page numbers followed by *f* and *t* indicate figures and tables.